"In a time when children have been largely silenced during this global pandemic, Drs. Ginger Calloway and Margaret Lee have given careful, thoughtful and compassionate voice to children involved in our legal systems. Featuring internationally known legal and mental health scholars with impeccable reputations in the legal community, this edited book provides a key resource for learning about the various legal systems that impact children, including juvenile justice, dependency, family law, immigration and criminal. Written by practitioners for practitioners, this book is both comprehensive and easy to read with several case studies to expand on concepts and to showcase the voices of children. This book is a must read for both mental health and legal professionals working with children in the legal system and for students interested in children and the law."

Michael Saini, PhD, MSW, RSW, *associate professor,*
Factor-Inwentash chair in Law and Social Work,
University of Toronto, Ontario, Canada

T0298413

Handbook of Children in the Legal System

This handbook brings together the relevant literature on children and their developmental characteristics, the legal venues in which they may appear, and the systemic issues practitioners must consider to provide a thorough guide to working with children in the legal system.

Featuring contributions from leading mental health and legal experts, chapters start with an overview and history of the juvenile justice system along with discussion of critical developmental areas imperative to consider for work with children, and idiosyncratic issues that arise. The book ends with a case presentation section that illustrates the varied roles and venues in which children appear in the legal system. An extended bibliography provides additional resources and literature to investigate specific topics in greater length.

This accessible and useable guide is designed to appeal to a broad range of people encountering children in the legal system, including social workers, psychologists, psychiatrists, attorneys, and judges. It will also benefit professions such as law enforcement as well as probation officers, child protective workers, school personnel, and medical personnel.

Ginger C. Calloway, PhD, is a clinically trained psychologist whose areas of forensic expertise include evaluation for Atkins' cases, evaluations of juveniles, evaluations for various legal competencies, and specific areas of consultation to attorneys.

S. Margaret Lee, PhD, is a psychologist whose work focus is providing services to divorcing families and family law attorneys. Dr. Lee is a frequent presenter at national and international conferences in different areas of psychology/family law.

Handbook of Children in the Legal System

Edited by Ginger C. Calloway and S. Margaret Lee

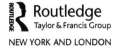

Routledge
Taylor & Francis Group

NEW YORK AND LONDON

First published 2022
by Routledge
605 Third Avenue, New York, NY 10158

and by Routledge
2 Park Square, Milton Park, Abingdon, Oxon, OX14 4RN

Routledge is an imprint of the Taylor & Francis Group, an informa business

Library of Congress Cataloging-in-Publication Data
Names: Calloway, Ginger, 1947- editor. | Lee, S. Margaret, editor.
Title: Handbook of children in the legal system / edited by Ginger C. Calloway
and S. Margaret Lee.
Identifiers: LCCN 2020052921 (print) | LCCN 2020052922 (ebook) | ISBN
9780367027773 (hardback) | ISBN 9780367027810 (paperback) | ISBN
9780429397806 (ebook)
Subjects: LCSH: Children's rights–United States. | Children–Legal status,
laws, etc.–United States. | Juvenile courts–United States. | Psychic
trauma in children–United States.
Classification: LCC HQ789.A5 H35 2021 (print) | LCC HQ789.A5 (ebook) |
DDC 346.01/3083–dc23
LC record available at https://lccn.loc.gov/2020052921
LC ebook record available at https://lccn.loc.gov/2020052922

ISBN: 978-0-367-02777-3 (hbk)
ISBN: 978-0-367-02781-0 (pbk)
ISBN: 978-0-429-39780-6 (ebk)

DOI: 10.4324/9780429397806

Typeset in Times New Roman
by KnowledgeWorks Global Ltd.

Contents

List of Contributors   ix
Foreword   xi
Acknowledgments   xiii

Introduction   1
GINGER C. CALLOWAY AND S. MARGARET LEE

PART ONE
Overview   7

Section I: Overview of Juvenile Justice System

  1 **The Push-Me-Pull-You of Juvenile Justice**   9
     MARY C. WILSON

  2 **A View from the Bench: Perspectives of a Former Juvenile Court Judge**   43
     MARCIA MOREY

Section II: Developmental Variables

  3 **Children's Memory for Forensically Relevant Experiences**   55
     LYNNE BAKER-WARD, PETER ORNSTEIN, AND TAYLOR E. THOMAS

  4 **Navigating Tricky Waters: Understanding and Supporting Children's Testimony**
     about Experiencing and Witnessing Violence   84
     DEBORAH GOLDFARB, HANA CHAE, AND LAURA SHAMBAUGH

PART TWO
Assessment   111

  5 **Assessment: Methods, Measures, Protocols, and Report Writing**   113
     S. MARGARET LEE

PART THREE
Case Studies

125

6   **Out of Home Care: Depending on the Kindness of Strangers**   127
    BARBARA L. MERCER

7   **Attachment Relationships for Attorneys: Using Expert Testimony to Guide the Court's Determination of Children's Best Interests in Family Court Cases**   152
    ALICIA JURNEY
    INTRODUCTION BY GINGER C. CALLOWAY

8   **Considerations when Working with Central American Immigrant Children in the Legal System**   164
    GISELLE A. HASS

9   **Adolescent Post-Traumatic Stress Disorder in the Civil Arena**   182
    AMY LEVY

10 **Interviewing Children about Sexual Abuse**   196
    JACQUELINE SINGER

11 **Interpersonal Violence and Children**   224
    NANCY W. OLESEN

12 **Giving Voice to Children in Non-Traditional Families**   235
    DEBORAH WALD AND S. MARGARET LEE

13 **Hague Convention Cases**   257
    S. MARGARET LEE AND BRENT D. SEYMOUR

14 **Resist Refuse Dynamics in Family Law with a Young Child**   277
    GINGER C. CALLOWAY AND S. MARGARET LEE

15 **A Case of Juvenile Homicide with Complex Issues of Mental Illness and Developmental Disorder**   295
    GINGER C. CALLOWAY

16 **The Role of Advocates for Children in Dependency Court**   311
    SALLY WILSON ERNY

Appendix A   316
Appendix B   339
Bibliography   360
Index   371

Contributors

Lynne Baker-Ward, PhD, Professor, Department of Psychology, North Carolina State University.

Ginger C. Calloway, PhD, clinically trained Psychologist whose areas of forensic expertise include evaluation for Atkins' cases, evaluations of juveniles, evaluations for various legal competencies, and specific areas of consultation to attorneys.

Hana Chae, MA, BS, MA, is a doctoral student in the legal psychology program at Florida International University. She earned her BS in Criminal Justice and Psychology from SUNY Oneonta and MA in Forensic Psychology from John Jay College of Criminal Justice in New York. Her research interests include children's memory, impacts of direct/indirect violence on children's memory, and children's participation in the legal system.

Sally Wilson Erny, Deputy CEO, National CASA/GAL Association for Children.

Deborah Goldfarb, PhD, is a legal psychology professor at Florida International University. She obtained her JD from the University of Michigan Law School and her PhD in Developmental Psychology from the University of California, Davis. Deborah also practiced for a number of years as an attorney, including as a law clerk in the federal courts. She studies a number of topics at the intersection of law and developmental psychology, including legal attitudes, developmental intuitive jurisprudence, and memory in victims and eyewitnesses.

Giselle A. Hass, PsyD, ABAP, Clinical and Forensic Psychologist.

Alicia Jurney, JD, Partner, Smith Debnam Law Firm, Raleigh, North Carolina.

S. Margaret Lee, PhD, Psychologist whose work focus is providing services to divorcing families and family law attorneys. Dr. Lee is a frequent presenter at national and international conferences in different areas of psychology/family law.

Amy Levy, PsyD, Clinical Psychologist in private practice in California and North Carolina, Civil Forensics and Assessment Practice, Psychoanalytic Psychotherapy Practice, Clinical Member, Psychoanalytic Center of the Carolinas.

Barbara L. Mercer, PhD, West Coast Children's Clinic, Oakland, California. Clinical Psychologist in Seattle, Washington.

Marcia Morey, JD, North Carolina House of Representatives, 30th District; Former Chief District Court Judge, 14th Judicial District, North Carolina; Member Governor James Hunt's Commission on Juvenile Crime and Justice.

Nancy W. Olesen, PhD, Clinical and Forensic Psychologist, San Rafael, California.

Peter Ornstein, PhD, F. Stuart Chapin Distinguished Professor, Emeritus, Department of Psychology and Neuroscience, University of North Carolina at Chapel Hill.

Michael Saini, Associate Professor, Factor-Inwentash Chair in Law and Social Work, University of Toronto, Ontario, Canada.

Brent D. Seymour, JD., Seymour Family Law, San Francisco, California.

Laura Shambaugh, MS, is a PhD student at Florida International University. Her primary area of interest in research is eyewitness memory. She has explored the effectiveness of an explicit "not sure" pre-lineup instruction, the ability of pre-identification confidence judgments to predict lineup decision accuracy, and jailhouse informant testimony as post-identification feedback.

Jacqueline Singer, PhD, Private Practice, Forensic Psychologist, Sonoma, California.

Taylor E. Thomas, PhD, Research Associate, Department of Psychology and Neuroscience, University of North Carolina at Chapel Hill.

Deborah Wald, JD, The Wald Law Group, San Francisco, California.

Mary C. Wilson, JD, Chief Juvenile Public Defender, Wake County, North Carolina.

Foreword

A book about children's voices and effective ways to assess and consider their views could not be more timely. While the past century has seen dramatic improvements in legislative and policy changes to better address children's views, rights and best interests, the current global pandemic has shifted the focus to primarily protecting children against the spread of the virus. Measures aimed at physical distancing from the deadly COVID-19 virus, have resulted in families sheltering-in-place, self-isolating, and distancing from friends and family not in their immediate bubble. As many courts closed their physical doors and went online for emergency only cases, children were also coping with school closures, canceling of their sports and extracurricular activities and the missed opportunity to be connected face-to-face with peers. These protection measures, although required to stop the spread of the virus, have tended to silence the voices of our most vulnerable, and especially our children.

The social science research about the impact of the pandemic on children is only now starting to emerge. Anecdotally, while children have been hidden away in their homes and on their phones, many are experiencing a sharp decline in their sense of safety, normalcy, and connection. Isolated from their peers, school friends, teammates, and community, it is being suggested that children are experiencing higher rates of stress, adjustment problems, and higher risk of maltreatment, neglect, and exploitation.

While Drs. Ginger Calloway and Margaret Lee did not plan to write this book during a pandemic, their project provides new hope for ways we can again listen to the voices of children.

Drs. Calloway and Lee have purposefully and thoughtfully assembled together several complementary chapters that showcase the importance of understanding the unique needs of each child, while also improving the types of services offered to children to better address their needs.

As an academic, I am impressed by the inclusion of the most relevant social science research that creates the foundation for many of the positions put forward in this book. As a practicing social worker in the legal system, I am keenly aware of the importance of the ecology of children's experiences and the various systems (e.g., parents, peers, teachers, therapists, the courts) that influence children's sense of belonging, development, and adjustment. Although not named as a guiding framework, the ecological transactional model seems evident throughout the book. At times, the book is concentrated on children's brains and memories, while other times, the book features the work of the professionals within the courts. Understanding the connections to the various systems interacting in law is critical to appreciate the application of law, especially as it relates to children.

I was delighted to learn about this project a couple of years ago. While both Drs. Calloway and Lee were already well established in their fields of practice and both had significant publication and presentation experiences at international conferences and were no stranger to the spotlight, this project marked their first adventure of writing a book together. I recall my enthusiasm about the potential for this book and my anticipation for having a key resource that would address the various ways that children interact with the legal system. I was also drawn to the range of topics, the diversity of approaches, and the remarkable scholars on their list of contributing authors.

While I was keen about the premise of the book, the actual content exceeded my expectations. The writing is sharp, relevant, and consistent throughout. The information is well-researched, detailed, and useful for both mental health and legal practitioners. This book clearly and effectively refocuses our attention to the needs of children and it provides us with critical considerations to best support, advocate, assess, listen, protect, and intervene with children in the legal system.

Drs. Calloway and Lee clearly considered the various forms of law that intersect with children, as witnesses (e.g., testifying), victims (e.g., out-of-home placements), and offenders (e.g., juvenile detention). As a result, the book provides both legal and mental health professionals with a single source edited volume that provides a compact and comprehensive reference for all areas of the law that intersect with children. By focusing on children as witnesses, victims, and offenders, the book is both far-reaching and provides clues to the complex pathways that lead to children taking on multiple roles with the various legal systems. The integration of the various legal systems fits well with the growing attention towards crossover cases and the impact on certain types of legal encounters (e.g., as a child victim of violence) on future encounters with other legal systems (e.g., as a youth offender).

The range of children and legal issues covered in the book are further enhanced by the esteemed list of chapter authors from across disciplines, including a Chief District Court Judge, a Juvenile Public Defender, Academics, Psychologists, Lawyers, Immigration Specialists, Hague Convention Specialists, Experts from Specialized Courts, including Juvenile, Dependency, Criminal and Family, Trauma Specialists, Children's Advocates, and Program Officers. The unique and varied backgrounds of the authors certainly contribute to the range of considerations, the varied viewpoints, and the richness of the case studies and chapter implications offered. The capable and experienced specialists in law provides a timely, thorough and attuned analysis of the historical considerations, the current tides, and the future implications for effective service for children involved in legal matters.

There are many opportunities within this book to learn about children and the various roles that professional take on to support children in the courts, including qualifying experts, custody evaluators, advocates, and attorneys who represent children in the courts.

Another significant strength of this book is the writing style. This book is written by practitioners for practitioners. The content, tone and pitch are delivered for easy consumption of concepts and so this book has general appeal to a wide variety of legal and mental health practitioners, such as judges, lawyers, psychologists, psychiatrists, social workers, and advocates working with or on behalf of children.

Each chapter provides explication of complex concepts, supporting literature from the social sciences, and practical consideration for working with children. The book is broken down into four parts, each with its own purpose and format. While the first part of the book is to provide an overview of the book, the second part provides an overview of children involved in legal matters. Drs. Calloway and Lee's expansive expertise in assessment and measurement is on full display in part three. In part four, case studies guide the discussion, making this a practical, useful and descriptive method for drawing out the applications and implications across the various forensic and legal contexts of practice with children.

There is an important focus on children's overall development as they interact with legal systems, and I find this refreshing as a focus in a book about children and the law. The chapters are replete with descriptions of the science regarding children's cognitive developments, language and vocabulary acquisitions, attachment formations, and the development of memories. The developmental milestones are then used to guide discussions about children's suggestibility, decision-making, and risk and resiliency as these pertain to children's involvement in the legal system. The depth and range of these topics covered provide the reader with an important balance to both consider the voices of children and to assess their capacity to provide independent, accurate, and credible views.

Drs. Calloway and Lee's provide a valuable contribution to the field and I am overjoyed to see just how well this has all come together for their first book on such an important area. The wisdom and expertise shared within the pages will have broad appeal for both mental health and legal practitioner who work with children in the legal system. This is one of those books that even after you read it, you will keep it on your desk for easy referencing to specific sections, while you look to effectively intervene with children involved in the legal system.

Michael Saini
PhD, MSW, RSW
Associate Professor
Factor-Inwentash Chair in Law and Social Work
University of Toronto, Ontario, Canada

Acknowledgments

We first want to thank all the authors who contributed to this volume. To all who contributed tremendous amounts of time to this effort and willingly accepted our comments for revisions, we are deeply grateful. It has been so gratifying and inspiring to work with all of you in this effort.

We appreciate the many colleagues, family and friends who have listened to us talk about this book across the time it has taken to complete. We could not have done this without your support and willing, open ears. Particularly, we thank our own children and grandchildren who have constantly rekindled our fascination with watching children grow, develop, and teach us on a daily basis. Our grandchildren have been incredibly wonderful to keep us focused in the present – so THANK YOU: Wilson, Coleman and Galileo!

We are especially thankful to Mark Worthen, PsyD, and David DeMatteo, JD, PhD, who responded quickly and comprehensively to our requests for their expert review of some chapters.

And as always, we are grateful to the many children whose lives we have entered over the years and who have taught us about humor, listening, and forthrightness.

And last, thank you to the editors at Routledge who have been incredibly flexible and who asked us to write this volume.

Introduction

Ginger C. Calloway and S. Margaret Lee

Little did we imagine when we agreed to co-edit this book that we would, in the process of completing it, encounter a worldwide pandemic that has, in many ways, decimated and upturned the U.S. economy and usual patterns of everyday life. Nor could we have anticipated that we would witness our society in the U.S. undergo an intense soul searching about racism, fairness, and justice in the aftermath of the George Floyd killing and others like his, previously and afterward. On a personal level, the pandemic has affected our deadlines, some of our contributing authors' health, and our ability to get together in real time and place, as we live on different coasts. Observing the impact of shelter in place policies has made us keenly aware of the ravages of ambiguity and uncertainty on the well-being and peace of mind of ordinary and not so ordinary people. The energy, enthusiasm, and extraordinary appeal to multiple, diverse groups of individuals within our society from the protests that emerged following George Floyd's death have been remarkable. And most certainly, all of the foregoing have affected our practices with children in myriad ways.

We started our work on this book as a team several decades ago when we met at the Society for Personality Assessment. As enthusiasts of the Rorschach Inkblot Measure, as child psychotherapists, as child custody evaluators, as single mothers raising boys, and with histories of knowing that we have learned and benefited so much from our own children and the children with whom we have had the privilege to work clinically and forensically, we immediately shared common perspectives, outlooks, and values. Dr. Lee introduced me to the Association of Family and Conciliation Courts. Thus began a collegial partnership that has spanned literally across the U.S. and in which we often presented together nationally and internationally, wrote articles together, and critiqued each other's written work over a couple of decades.

In all that we have learned and benefited from working with and truly "hearing" children's voices, it was an easy "yes" to the editors at Routledge to build on our written work, presentations, and collegiality to produce this book. At the outset, we need to clarify that we have defined "children" broadly as individuals spanning pre-school to adolescence, in order to provide practitioners with the range of individuals, venues, and circumstances with whom and in which we have worked. We have both worked as child and family practitioners in clinical settings and with children and adolescents in a variety of forensic settings as well. We are not academicians or researchers and so our handbook is not an exhaustive tome on the nuances of all variables inherent to and that characterize children uniquely, nor does it exhaustively treat and consider all variables inherent to working with children. We have relied on our contributing authors to provide the most up-to-date research findings in the specific areas for which they have written. This handbook is aimed at other practitioners, including attorneys, law enforcement, social workers, psychologists, other mental health workers, guardians, and the like, who may benefit from our experience and knowledge as well as the incredible knowledge and experience of our contributing authors.

DOI: 10.4324/9780429397806-1

Although our intention was not to produce a book with primarily female authors, that has been the outcome. We invited professionals we knew to be excellent in their work, most with long histories of writing articles and chapters, and authors whose focus has been on assisting children in the legal system. Although some male professionals approached declined to contribute, mostly due to time constraints, we also believe that the predominance of female authors also reflects the cultural tendency for women to work in areas serving children.

Working with children in any setting immediately places a practitioner in a system and thus requires systemic thinking. Those various systems range from narrowly defined, such as the family of origin and the child only, more broadly defined as a particular child in a specific school or school system, or extensively defined as a juvenile offender who offends in a school or other setting and subsequently encounters the juvenile justice system. A more extensively defined system might also include a child in foster care who must be considered in the context of guardians, guardian attorneys, dependency court, social service, and child protection workers and agencies, school system(s), out-of-home and in-home placement, multiple therapeutic and residential caregivers, and various psychotherapeutic interventions including multiple practitioners. The point is that working with children is a complex matter that involves attention to diverse parts of the system and individuals within that system or those systems that touch on the welfare of the child. What must not be lost above all is the child and his/her ability to consent and to understand consent to interventions, explanations, and evaluations, sensitivity to the privacy of the information children offer and balancing children's needs with those of the court. Adherence to ethical and professional standards is critical and requires practitioners to continually re-visit ethical issues in light of children's unique needs, diversity, contexts, special developmental differences, and culture.

This handbook is divided into three parts. Part One, Section I is an overview of the juvenile justice system and one judge's view from the bench. Part Two, Section II covers developmental variables to consider when working with children. Part Two is assessment methods, measures, protocol, and report writing specific to children and adolescents. Part Three presents case studies that illustrate the problems, issues, and concepts that are covered in earlier parts of the book.

By way of introduction, we first consider the roles and venues in which children can function and appear in the legal system. Included with roles and venues, we give the evidentiary standards needed for legal decision-making. Last, we note the critical variables to consider when working with children in the legal system.

With regard to roles and venues, children can show up as victims in the legal system, perhaps one of the most obvious being direct and indirect emotional, sexual and/or physical abuse and neglect, as a function of reports to or other contact with Child Protective Services and Department of Social Services. In many jurisdictions in the United States, witnessing domestic violence is also considered child abuse. According to the National Center for Biotechnology Information (www.ncbi.nlm.nih.gov), approximately 10% of children are exposed to domestic violence annually and 25% of children are exposed to at least one event of domestic violence during their childhood. These children routinely encounter multiple law enforcement officers, multiple social workers, guardians, and a plethora of mental health professionals. This book is written to assist various professionals to more completely understand and therefore more effectively assist the children they encounter. Children identified by child protective agencies are typically served in dependency court, where the weight of evidence is the least stringent of evidentiary standards, preponderance of evidence, for most issues. The burden of proof, therefore, occurs when the party with the burden convinces the trier of fact, a solitary judge in dependency court, that there is a greater than 50% that the claim is true. An exception to this burden of proof is when there is a question of terminating parental rights and putting a child up for adoption. In this situation, the burden of proof is clear and convincing evidence. Given the fact that there may be different standards in different states related to different proceedings having different burdens of proof, it is wise to learn the specifics in the state where you practice.

Children in family court matters are also victims, with regard to exposure to domestic violence, substance abuse, mental illness, and the pernicious effects of their parents' unrelenting quarrels and inability to compromise. While the percentage of children whose parents litigate their custodial time is small relative, under 5%, to the larger number, and percentage of families who resolve disputes without litigation, the families that do litigate are often dramatic and compelling in presentation and their children more often than not suffer in apparent ways. When families do litigate, the prevailing standard of proof is either "preponderance of evidence" or "clear and compelling" evidence, depending on the state and the issue being adjudicated. Clear and convincing is the typical standard of proof for most civil matters. The trier of fact, typically a sole judge, must be convinced by firm belief or conviction that the evidence is sufficient to show that a given proposition is more probable than not. The only state that uses jury trials in child custody matters is Texas, where a parent can make the request for a jury trial. Other civil matters where children might appear as victims occur in personal injury matters, one example of which is covered by Dr. Levy in Chapter 9 of this book.

Trauma for and various forms of abuse to children can result in referrals for children as victims to the criminal justice system. These cases are varied, with regard to type of trauma and variant of abuse. The Goldfarb and associates chapter in this book covers the relevant features of these kinds of cases for which it is necessary that professionals master an understanding. Of particular import in their chapter are the effects of trauma on children's ability to testify. Referral to the criminal justice system is a weighty matter for all concerned, requires nuanced understanding of roles and procedures for experts, and challenges sometimes fiercely held presumptions and potential biases on the part of mental health or other professionals.

> A criminal prosecution occurs when the government (federal or state) charges an individual with the commission of an act that is forbidden by statute and punishable by imprisonment or a fine. Conviction of and punishment for a criminal offense have traditionally been viewed as the most severe actions society can take against one of its members. Accordingly, the criminal process is the most highly formalized of any adjudicatory proceeding. The prosecution must prove each element of the crime "beyond a reasonable doubt" (a level of certainty that can be reasonable quantified at above 90%).

Children or adolescents may commit misdemeanors or felonies and hence present as offenders in the juvenile justice system, they may be deemed "delinquent" and disposed of by the court in various ways, they may be transferred to adult court and thereby be subject to the same standards as adult offenders, and they may be transferred back from adult court to juvenile court.

> There are other legal questions facing juvenile court justices regarding justice-involved youth, of course. Indeed, there are numerous points along the juvenile justice continuum where assessments conducted by different professionals, both informally and formally, affect how youths are subsequently treated. These points have been described

as follows: pre-arrest diversion, arrest procedures, filing of criminal charges, pretrial detention, transfer to and from adult court, competency to stand trial, adjudication, disposition, sentencing, rehabilitation intervention planning, and supervision planning.

Wilson's chapter (1) and Morey's chapter (2) cover a history of the juvenile justice system and specific experiences of sitting as a juvenile court judge.

In Chapter 1 our contributing author covers a history of the juvenile justice system, the influences it has experienced and incorporated or rejected, recent decisions by the Supreme Court of the United States (SCOTUS) that have dramatically influenced the course of decision-making in juvenile justice and the impact of adolescent brain science on these SCOTUS decisions. She discusses how children have variously been treated protectively, relative to adults, and yet on the other hand how children have been deprived of essential Constitutional rights by these various trends in the perception and treatment of children. She gives some thought to ways in which the "school to prison" pipeline has been reinforced and provides detail about certain, seminal cases in juvenile justice with citations provided for specific case law. The school-to-prison pipeline in part evolved when typical misbehavior in adolescence was criminalized instead of being dealt with by the schools, parents, or a community. She ends with a discussion of newly adopted "Raise the Age Legislation" and her thoughts about necessary directions for the juvenile justice system. The impact of societal trends on how disposition in juvenile court is handled are noteworthy and combined with reliance by SCOTUS on science from adolescent brain research make evident the need for greater nuance in understanding and handling juveniles who offend, with even greater input required from the scientific community to reform this system for more equitable resolutions. Informing the trier of fact about these multiple issues and about adolescent development is a critical role for forensic evaluators and mental health and other professionals who interact with the juvenile system on behalf of this age child.

Chapter 2 is one judge's view from the bench in juvenile court and the various challenges with which she was presented as a juvenile court judge. This contributing author's experiences provide a personal perspective and experiential depth to ideas, problems, trends, and issues outlined by our contributing author who covers a history of the juvenile justice system. The notion of "super predator," a fascinating yet disturbing phenomenon, is one covered by both authors with somewhat different perspectives. This former judge concludes with her thoughts about how to improve juvenile justice courts and dispositions of juveniles. Her impact as one individual in a complex, monolithic, and immovable system is illuminating. This stands as an example of the indispensable requirement for practitioners interacting with the juvenile justice system to be well prepared, transparent, and anchored in their approaches by reliance on the latest data available through research and study and on solemn consideration of ethical principles as they uniquely apply to younger children and adolescents.

In Section II of Part One, developmental variables are covered in two chapters. Chapter 3 covers "Children's Memory for Forensically Relevant Experiences." This chapter covers substantial, extant literature that has accumulated about children's memory and language skills, especially as these affect children's ability to testify. These authors from North Carolina State University and the University of North Carolina, Chapel Hill trace memory development, the operation of memory, age related changes in memory, with a particular focus on memory over time, central to an understanding of children's memory for forensically relevant experiences. Especially applicable for practitioners interacting with children in forensic settings are the variables this group considers that impact memory performance, including stress and repeated interviewing. Their recommendations for practices that help limit memory distortion and support children in their use of memory content aid practitioners in an ethical and scientifically informed practice with regard to children they encounter in the forensic arena.

Chapter 4 complements and adds to Chapter 3 by delving into specific issues of testimony in experiencing and witnessing violence. These authors, from Florida International University, review research on trauma and when children are directly or indirectly victimized. They review research on trauma and psychopathology, review how trauma impacts children's abilities to accurately recall and testify about events, and explore interventions to help child victims testify in legal proceedings. Their conclusions propose future research that can assist children to navigate legal proceedings. Throughout these two chapters on memory and effects on memory run the parallel fundamentals and interaction of language, suggestibility, and social pressure that are unique to children and adolescents and that also influence testimony and recall.

Part Two of this handbook covers assessment methods, measures, protocol, and report writing that are common for evaluators, specific for certain referral questions and psycholegal issues, and specific for particular ages. Part Three brings the first three parts together by way of case studies, illustrating the issues highlighted in Parts One and Two. We are grateful to all contributing authors for their hard work, their willingness to accept ongoing feedback, and their thoughtfulness with the cases they present. Every effort possible was made by our contributing authors who present case studies to disguise the particular situations and cases to protect confidentiality of all subjects.

Part Three reflects our goal to reach a wide range of professionals who work with children in the legal system and provide the reader with a broad understanding of how various facets of the legal system, various venues, and people involved in interrelationship with each other. To provide this breadth of information we asked authors from most possible legal venues serving children to contribute, while also requesting that they provide case examples involving children of different ages and stages of development. These chapters also cover a range of socio-economic levels. Chapters 6 and 9 involve cases primarily in dependency court, chapters 7, 11, 12, and 14 involve children primarily in family court, although the reader will note that these are cases where children find themselves in multiple court venues. Children also seen in the Federal Court system as exemplified in Chapter 8 with immigration issues and in Chapter 13 with international parental abduction involving the Hague Convention. Chapter 10 focuses on child sexual abuse in a range of venues. Chapter 15 is a criminal case involving an adolescent.

Despite these differences, certain themes and issues emerged across many chapters. The most striking issue that arose in the majority of chapters was that of the presence of trauma and secondarily a common issue was that of attachment; difficulties in attachment between parents and their children and or loss of attachment figures. Many chapters also address the issue of children's voices, how are they heard, how are their opinions are weighed, and how children can be assessed regarding the meaning and reliability of their words.

Chapter 6 by Barbara Mercer involves out-of-home placement and dependency court, with cases involving the issues of trauma and attachment, and complex loss. Chapter 7 by Alicia Jurney and Ginger Calloway also looks specifically at attachment in a young child whose adoption is being contested raising the issue of the role of biology in determining who should be a parent. The question of who is a parent and issues of biological and psychological factors in determining parentage is further developed in Chapter 12 written primarily by Deborah Wald, who looks at a wide range of non-traditional families and explores the impact of advances in medically assisted conception. Trauma or potential trauma is an element in all of the chapters with case examples, even in Chapter 15 by Ginger Calloway who describes the evaluation of an adolescent murderer but also incorporates a deep and complex understanding of how the crime occurs but also notes the trauma experienced by the youngster in response to the crime and its aftermath.

Several chapters have trauma as their main focus with Chapter 9 by Amy Levy presenting cases from civil cases involving personal injury suits, in Chapter 10 Jaqueline Singer explores the evaluation of several cases involving child sexual abuse. Nancy Olesen describes in Chapter 11 the impact of domestic violence on family systems as seen in family court custody cases. In both Chapter 11 and in Chapter 14 written by Ginger Calloway, describe typical cross-allegations in divorce that often lead to a need to determine whether a parent is allegedly abusive or whether there are "refuse/resist" dynamics in the family, i.e. was a child's fear of and refusal to have contact with a parent due to abuse or from a more complex dynamic., that can include alienating behaviors.

Both Chapter 13 by S. Margaret Lee and Brent Seymour and Chapter 8 by Giselle Hass present views of how children are dealt with in a more global sense. International decisions about children hold out the probability of loss, possible trauma, and in international cases the need to hear the children's voices are important elements.

Finally, it is expected that a portion of our readership will be mental health evaluators who either perform forensic evaluations with children or are interested in doing so. Chapter 5 by S. Margaret Lee provides an overview of issues to consider and points the reader to more in-depth resources. Several chapters have very in-depth evaluation information, primarily Chapter 9 by Dr. Levy who explores types of tests used and the controversies regarding their usefulness, Chapters 14 and 15 by Dr. Calloway provide detailed assessment information and are good examples of how findings from evaluations can be useful to the court for addressing the psych-legal questions in front of the court.

Part One

Overview

Section I

Overview of Juvenile Justice System

1 The Push-Me-Pull-You of Juvenile Justice

Mary C. Wilson

Part One: The Juvenile Delinquency Court Dichotomy

Early Treatment of Children

In early common law brought to the colonies from England, children who committed crimes were generally brought to the same courts as adults. Children under 7 years of age were presumed to be incompetent to stand trial so were not charged. Children between 7 and 13 where charged and, if it appeared to the court that the child could discern the difference between good and evil, the child could be found guilty. All children 14 and older were tried as adults. By law, children had no inherent rights. They were deemed to be chattel, owned by their father who had a possessory interest in the child's labor.

Judges in criminal courts understood that children sent to adult prisons would just become better criminals, so a system arose of placements for these delinquent youth to house them away from adults. In 1825, New York opened the first House of Refuge as a place to send children convicted of crimes. However, not all children were spared from adult prison. Only if the court found that the child was "reformable" would they be sent to one of these placements for rehabilitation and education. These "reform schools" spread and by the mid 1800s, many states had a House of Refuge, where courts sent children not only found guilty of crimes but also simply for being poor. While some states maintained separate facilities for youth convicted of crimes than those children simply found to be "vagrants" or "incorrigible," many states housed them all in the same reform schools. Courts saw themselves as protecting poor children from a life of idleness by placing them in alms houses where they were supposed to be fed, housed, given some education and eventually placed in jobs.

In 1839, Pennsylvania had the first known case to invoke the doctrine of *parens patriae* in a court matter. In *Ex parte Crouse* (1839), the child had been brought to court originally for being beyond her mother's control, not for any criminal offense, and was sent to Philadelphia's House of Refuge. When the father filed a writ of habeas corpus to try to bring the child home again, the courts denied the release, using the power of *parens patriae*, Latin for "the State as Parent," to hold that the state had the inherent power to maintain custody of someone who is incapable of taking care of themselves. The Court stated that "the House of Refuge is not a prison, but a school" and "the object of charity is reformation, by training its inmates to industry" (*Ex parte Crouse*, 1839, p. 11). This doctrine of *parens patriae* became the primary focus for the treatment of any juvenile brought to court, whether they were accused of criminal behavior or just misbehavior. The notion was that the court would protect the child from poverty and thus a life of crime or "delinquency."

DOI: 10.4324/9780429397806-2

The Rise of Juvenile Courts

The Illinois Juvenile Court Act of 1899 has been credited as forming the first "Juvenile Court" as distinct from adult criminal court. Using the doctrine of *parens patriae*, this new court sought to provide guidance to wayward youth, as opposed to criminally punish them. However, during the drafting of the law, little attention was given to the actual procedural process. The law simply acknowledged that children should not be sent to adult criminal court, so a judge or a magistrate talked to the child, "adjudicated" him, and ordered services. Believing that these judges were removing the child from regular adult criminal court and that the judge would act as a parent looking after the child, they saw no need to create criminal procedural safeguards. Thus, the modern juvenile court system was built on the idea of protection of society from wayward children by placing these youth in "reform schools" but also built on protection of the child by removing them from adult criminal courts and jails.

By 1925, most states had laws creating a specific "Juvenile Court" of some sort that removed youth from the adult system. These new juvenile courts varied greatly, as the process was generally left up to the presiding judge. Judge Ben Lindsey was an outspoken leader in the early movement with the creation of Denver Juvenile Court in 1900, which he ran as an informal court of equity. He believed children did not need criminal procedural protections, such as the Fifth Amendment privilege against self-incrimination, stating that children ought to be encouraged to admit their wrong-doing because the court's goal was to provide treatment. Because of the belief that the courts were attempting to rehabilitate and educate children rather than punish them, there was little perceived need to provide legislative protections for procedural due process in these juvenile court statutes. Defense attorneys, if indeed there were any, played little part in the disposition of the case.

Whether this new juvenile court system actually functioned to rehabilitate children rested solely on the personal beliefs regarding benevolence of the judge overseeing the system and the services a community could provide. Model programs, like the Juvenile Court of Allegheny County in Pennsylvania operating from 1933 to 1968 under its own charter, developed elaborate procedures to handle both delinquent and "incorrigible" youth by training probation officers and social workers to present the "facts" and provide the court with recommendations for necessary treatment to reform the child. This medical model persisted throughout the early part of the 20th century. However, public criticism arose because of the wide disparities, seen from one county to the next even within the same state, that resulted from the lack of formal procedures and the complete discretion of the individual juvenile court judges.

The Constitution Applies to Youth

In the 1960s, legal scholars began to publish articles critical of the *parens patriae* model because juvenile courts were functioning more like adult criminal courts, seeking punishment and locking children in "reform schools," that were often just juvenile prisons, for petty crimes and simple poverty. Case law changes move slowly because each individual case that a court decides can deal only with the issues of that specific case. Occasionally the Supreme Court will decide a case that brings about sweeping changes in a field of law. That is exactly what happened with two famous cases in the mid 1960s in juvenile delinquency law with *Kent v. United States* (1966) and *In re: Gault* (1967) (see Part Three, this chapter).

This shift towards granting Constitutional rights to children within the informal setting of juvenile court was a dramatic change from the *parens patriae* culture. As juvenile courts became more like adult court in the punitive aspect, the culture shifted to the protection of children from the law and shifted away from protection of society from children. The inherent conflict in the duties of a paternalistic juvenile judge began to grow more apparent as more stories began to creep out from the secret world of these confidential courts indicating that some were more punitive than rehabilitative. This cultural shift led many states and the federal government to conduct studies and pass legislation addressing juvenile law in attempts to standardize the ways that children were being dealt with in courts across the nation.

Federal Legislation to Protect Children

As law review articles and Supreme Court cases began to shift towards the view that the Constitution does indeed apply to children, federal legislation to protect youth began to take form. In 1967, the President's Commission of Law Enforcement and Justice devoted a full chapter to many various problems with how juvenile courts were being conducted throughout the country. In 1968, Congress passed the Juvenile Delinquency and Prevention Control Act to encourage removing children who had not committed a crime, called "status offenders," from locked facilities. When little changed, the Federal Juvenile Justice and Delinquency Prevention Act of 1974 (JJDP) was passed in attempt to mandate change in states' juvenile laws. This landmark legislation was the first federal attempt to support a nationwide comprehensive approach to the problems in juvenile justice. The Office of Juvenile Justice and Delinquency Prevention (OJJDP) was formed to provide training and assistance to develop community-based treatment services and oversee and disburse federal grants to model programs. Receipt of the federal grant monies for juvenile services was based on whether states complied with the two core principles of deinstitutionalization of status offenders (DSO) and separation of juvenile delinquents from adult offenders, called "sight and sound separation." The deinstitutionalization principle aimed to protect children by not allowing status offenders to be locked up for non-criminal misbehavior, like running away or skipping school. The "sight and sound separation" principle stated that delinquents should not be housed in a facility where they could see or hear any adult offender, thus striking a balance between protecting society by locking up the delinquent child and protecting the child from the damage of incarceration with adults.

The JJDP Act was re-authorized and amended in 1980 to establish jail removal requirement as a third core principle, stating that juveniles should not be placed in adult jails at all. However, because some large cities were continuing to struggle with too many "out-of-control" youth who misbehaved, ran away, or skipped school but did not get charged with breaking a law, it also included the "Valid Court Order" exception, creating a loophole to allow judges to incarcerate status offenders if they had violated an order from a juvenile court judge to abide by certain conditions. This loophole returned some control to juvenile judges to protect society from misbehaving children. In an attempt to improve and standardize procedures in juvenile courts nationwide, the JJDP Act has been amended many times to address growing or new concerns within juvenile justice. Currently it has 28 requirements; however, the Federal grant funding is only decreased for non-compliance in any of the four "core requirements:" 1) deinstitutionalization of status offenders (DSO); 2) separation of juveniles from adult inmates (sight and sound separation): 3) removal of juveniles from adult jails and lockups (jail removal); and 4) addressing disproportionate minority contact (DMC). This brought the pendulum swinging back to protection of the child. However, media reports of youth committing violent crime did not allow it to swing this way for long.

The "Super Predator" and "Youth Gangs"

As the twentieth century was winding down, the pendulum swung back towards protection of society from dangerous children. The last three decades are frequently referred to as the "get tough" era of juvenile justice. In the mid 1970s, states began toughening laws regarding juveniles by easing transfer processes to allow more youth and more offenses to be brought back into adult court. The National Advisory Committee of Juvenile Justice began to criticize the requirements of the JJDP Act regarding deinstitutionalization. Courts across the nation began to focus on delinquency deterrence by heavy punishment. In 1995, criminologist John Dilulio coined the phrase "super-predator" to describe youth he claimed had "no respect for human life" and "no concept of future" based on studies of youth involved in criminal gangs. Crime statistics were blaming youth and "youth gangs" for the increase in violent crime. While there was a brief spike in juvenile crime from the mid 1980s to early 1990s, review of Federal Bureau of Investigation (FBI) statistics over time belie the myth that teens were becoming more violent. In fact, the FBI reports of crime statistics found that 70% of the recent increase in violent crime had been committed by adults. However, this perception that youth crime was spiraling upward spurred states to strengthen laws against juveniles in effort to deter youth violence.

As fear of the "super-predator" spread through media attention, social culture began to call for a shift from looking at the individual offender (protecting the child) to concentrating on the offense (protecting society from the child). By the end of the 1990s, all 50 states had laws making transfer to adult court easier for more types of crimes and for even younger children, thus putting more youth back into adult criminal courts, facing long incarcerations. Many states allowed prosecutors to "direct file" criminal charges in adult court, thus completely bypassing the juvenile system meant as a gatekeeper to use individualized court transfer hearings to send only the most violent or "non-amenable" youth to adult court. Because of the notoriety of a few violent incidents involving youth, many of these legislative changes also opened juvenile courts to the public and made it harder to seal the confidential juvenile records, thus making it even harder to protect the children from their poor decisions.

The notorious "Central Park jogger" case is an example of how a rush to send children to adult court in a highly publicized and emotional case can go horribly wrong. There is ample evidence that a large group of older teens were "wilding" in the park on the night of April 19, 1989 and there were several victims of various assaults and robberies. However, the five younger teens who were convicted of the jogger's terrible beating and rape had nothing to do with it. All were tried in adult court on scant evidence other than what later proved to be false confessions that were made after days of police interrogation without their parents present. In 2002, all five were fully exonerated when DNA and his confession proved Matias Reyes had committed the attack alone. While the public does need protection from horrendous acts, these five innocent children deserved protection from a system fraught with problems. The public was not protected by this travesty of justice because the real culprit, never charged with the jogger's attack, went on to commit several more rapes and a murder before he was caught. The five innocent children certainly deserved the protections that more Constitutional procedural safeguards would have offered their cases.

In response to this social perception of out-of-control youth and the reaction from law enforcement efforts to combat youth crime, the Office of Juvenile Justice and Delinquency Prevention started the National Youth Gang Center (NYGC) in 1995 to gather and compile national statistics on these so-called "youth gangs." Their definition of youth gangs included children as young as 10 years old up to age 22. They excluded motorcycle gangs, hate groups, and prison gangs, thus claiming that these "youth gangs" sprang up in and of themselves. In effort to study and combat the perceived problems of youth violence, the NYGC conducted regular nationwide surveys of law enforcement agencies in large and small cities and rural counties. What they later determined (in 2009) was that these youth were actually being recruited by adult gang members.

In the early 1980s the "broken windows" policing theory began gaining traction in large cities throughout the nation. This theory, stemming from a study by Stanford psychologist Philip Zimbardo in 1969, held that where conditions deteriorated, crime followed; therefore, the police should crack down on vagrancy, drunks, and teens hanging out on neighborhood streets in order to make them safer. The belief was that if one broken window in a building was left unattended, the rest would be broken soon. This led to pushing police out of their cars to walk beats through poverty-ridden neighborhoods to arrest petty criminals for acts of vandalism and vagrancy. By the mid 1990s, "broken windows" policing policies evolved into zero-tolerance policies and more and more youth were arrested for petty crimes or just "hanging out" with their friends (loitering). This drove the theory that violent juvenile crime was on the rise, while it was actually just that juvenile arrest was rising, mostly for petty crimes, because of these zero-tolerance policies. Rather than taking little Johnny home to pay for the neighbor's broken window, officers were arresting and charging him. This criminalization of normal teenaged behavior drove up the arrest numbers.

Another reason for the perception of a "spiraling" crime rate that triggered the "get tough era" was the proliferation of police officers placed in schools. While the first known program for School Resource Officers (SRO) started in the 1950s in Flint, Michigan, it did not receive national recognition until 1973 when the National Advisory Commission on Criminal Justice Standards and Goals recommended large law enforcement agencies, those over 400 employees, to provide an officer to every junior high and high school. As the concept spread across the country during the turbulent 1960s, the focus of these programs was to improve relationships between youth and law enforcement. Individual SROs were expected to minimize their law enforcement roles and work on improving the young people's image of cops. In 1991, the National Association of School Resource Officers incorporated and began spreading training models and funding resources across the nation. The original purpose of these officers in the schools was to build relationships with children, not to arrest them for petty offenses. However, the combination of law enforcement officers in schools and zero-tolerance policies led to what has become known as the "School to Prison Pipeline," as more youth were not just suspended for minor misconduct but also charged and brought to juvenile court.

By the early 1990s, the SRO had morphed from a plain-clothes officer placed in the school to teach classes, such as the D.A.R.E. program, and build relationships with children to a uniformed officer there to enforce zero-tolerance policies by charging and arresting children. At the close of the 20th century, in April 1999, the school shooting in Columbine High School in Colorado solidified the role of the SRO as the law enforcement protector of the school, not the teacher and relationship-builder. While a full discussion of the school-to-prison-pipeline is beyond the scope of this chapter, it is to be hoped that recent trends in criminal justice reform will include removing officers from schools or, at the very least, returning them to the original purpose of relationship-building teachers/ mentors rather than arresting officers.

Studies of juvenile justice in the 1990s were showing that the majority of youth lacked attorney representation, including most of youth who were placed out-of-home. Some studies suggested serious concerns about the quality of representation for those who did have lawyers. The few lawyers that were involved in juvenile courts typically acted more like Guardian Ad Litem attorneys, representing the best interest of the child, from the perspective of "the system," as opposed to the criminal defense attorney's ethical duty to represent their client's expressed interest, i.e., what the individual client actually wants the attorney to do with their case. The juveniles' attorneys were often just in court to help the probation officer move the case through the court system, plead the child guilty and "get them help." So, while the emphasis of juvenile justice was becoming "get tough" on youth to protect society, the protections of individual children charged with crimes were not living up to the Constitutional mandates of due process being expressed in many United States Supreme Court decisions. During the "get tough" era, the pendulum swung far out toward protection of society from the child in a perfect storm of misperception: kids now have lawyers, so are protected, but youth arrest rates are rising as a result of zero-tolerance and broken windows policies.

Twenty-First Century Juvenile Law

The pendulum is now swinging back toward protection of children as advances in the science of adolescent brain development push legislatures in many states to revamp their juvenile court systems to provide more treatment and to raise the age of criminal responsibility. More scientific studies are being published that utilize new MRI technology to show the slow development of the brain from a person's mid adolescence until mid or even late 1920s. As this science becomes more widely known, public opinion has begun to shift to the belief that teens are less culpable than adults who commit crimes, so they should be protected by returning them to juvenile court, with its emphasis on treatment and rehabilitation.

In 2009, the National Youth Gang Center merged with the National Gang Center as experts began to recognize that street gang activity encompassed all ages, and thus a comprehensive effort to combat gangs was needed. The belief that these "youth gangs" were organized and run by the mythical "super-predator" and were somehow different from ordinary adult street gangs gave way to the reality that adult gang members actually recruited juveniles, partly because of the belief that the juvenile system wouldn't punish them harshly for these very adult crimes. OJJDP's comprehensive gang model now emphasizes efforts to prevent youth from joining gangs. Also in 2009, Congress enacted the federal Gang Prevention, Intervention and Suppression Act which recognized the brain science now showing the lesser culpability of teens and so included attempts to combat this recruitment of younger members by enhancing the sentence of those adults who used juveniles for crimes believed to have been committed to promote gang culture. Many states followed suit, enacting their own gang suppression laws that included more protection of minors in efforts to discourage adult criminals from recruiting youth.

In 2018, the Juvenile Justice and Delinquency Prevention Act was amended again, adding more protections for juveniles. Specific changes were made to strengthen the Core Requirement to address disproportionate minority contact (DMC), modifying the name of this requirement to Racial and Ethnic Disparities (RED) to more accurately reflect the issues. Numerous studies reviewing the data show that a disproportionate number of youths of color come into the juvenile system at each point of contact. The 2018 amendment added a requirement to not just study data to identify disparities but also to implement actual policy and procedural changes to reduce racial and ethnic disparities within the juvenile justice system. The history of racism that exists in the United States affects the rates of charges, adjudications, and incarceration as well as the policies in place throughout the justice system. While a full discussion of racial disparities is beyond the scope of this chapter, it should be recognized that these issues must be addressed. This new amendment may help pave the way to actual change.

Modern juvenile courts act very like the adult criminal courts; however, they have developed a different language for the various processes. Typically, a child is charged on a petition, as opposed to a citation, warrant, or indictment in adult court. Children don't plead guilty or have a trial: they admit responsibility or have an adjudicatory hearing. Guilty adults are sentenced; whereas, if a juvenile is found responsible and adjudicated to be a delinquent youth, he has a disposition hearing and the conditions of probation are imposed by disposition order meant to impose treatment services that are in the best interest of the juvenile. Not only is the language different, there are many procedures in juvenile court that have no equal in adult criminal court. Because early juvenile court arose having "court counselors," euphemism for juvenile probation officers, to assist the judge with decisions about what to do with the child, a system developed that children can only be petitioned to court by these court counselors. Law enforcement officers decide to charge an adult, but these same officers must go to juvenile court counselors/probation officers to seek petitions to charge a juvenile. The court counselor conducts an intake evaluation process to determine whether to file the petition in court to formally charge a child or to divert the case. In diversion, they can simply dismiss the petition or put the child on a behavior contract for some short period and mandate counseling, community service, or other sanctions and treatment services. Because this process has government officials talking with the child about the crime before they are ever brought to court, the child's Fifth Amendment right against self-incrimination can potentially be violated. Adults do not meet with their future probation officer until after they are convicted of a crime. Court counselors who work with kids at intake and make decisions about whether to bring the case to court are the same people who become their probation officers when they are adjudicated delinquent. These very processes that are meant to protect children from adult criminal court consequences show why procedural safeguards to protect the juvenile's rights are necessary. This dual role that the juvenile court counselor/probation officer must navigate in processing juveniles into and through the system creates an inherent conflict of interest that mandates the Court's need to provide procedural safeguards for youth to prevent the railroading of children seen so often in the *parens patriae* model of early juvenile court systems.

In the dichotomy of purpose, juvenile court judges still have a difficult balance in each case before them. The U.S. Constitution, and most states' Juvenile Codes, mandate that the judges grant procedural safeguards to youth that protect their rights throughout the court process. But most states also have "purpose of juvenile court" clauses that mandate the judges to consider protection of society in any given decision in juvenile court. The current culture of many juvenile court systems seems to have pushed the pendulum back towards protection of the children based on scientific evidence of adolescent brain development.

Part Two: Scientific Studies of Brain Development

Any parent can tell you that they know their teenagers are not fully equipped to function in the adult world, but now doctors can pinpoint why. As medical technology has advanced since the turn of the century, so has the scientific understanding of how the human brain functions and develops. Advances in functional magnetic resonance imaging (fMRI) technology allow for studies that show the actual parts of the brain that are at work as test subjects conduct various tasks. This has led to advances in the understanding of brain development from childhood through adolescence and into full adult maturation. Some scientists now state that the brain is not fully developed until the mid to late 20s, long past legal adulthood. This understanding has led to changes in how society views adolescents, resulting in changes in both policy and law regarding how to treat youth who violate the law.

"What were you thinking?" is so often heard from parents and juvenile court judges when discussing with children their criminal behavior, or merely the poor decision-making behind their misbehavior. But to understand why kids do thoughtless things, we must realize that it is not so much *what* they were thinking, but *how*. Adults often believe that teens act out because they are rebelling against authority or needing to establish themselves as separate from parental authority. While these *psychological* reasons may sometimes play a part in poor choices, brain science indicates that teens' frustrating behaviors are more often a *physiological* response. Their behavior stems from the fact that their brain is still not fully developed.

Adolescent Brain Development

Our brains are made up of several distinct parts that develop at different times, but all of these parts must work together to allow a person to function as a healthy adult. The cerebrum consists of the outer layer or cerebral cortex, often called the "gray matter," and the inner layer or cerebral medulla, often called the "white matter." The cerebellum is a structure near the back of the brain that coordinates movement and speech. The amygdala and hippocampus control emotion and memory. The brain stem connects the brain to the spinal cord, telling the rest of our body how to function by regulating such things as breathing, heart rate, and blood pressure. The cerebral cortex, what lay people think of as The Brain, is divided into four lobes: the frontal, the parietal, the temporal, and the occipital lobe, each housing different functions and needing to connect effectively to communicate with each other.

These various parts of the brain don't grow much bigger in size past age ten; however, the brain develops in connectivity to increase its functioning as these brain parts communicate better with each other. This connectivity process, called myelination, starts in the back of the brain, with the frontal lobe not reaching full maturation till the mid-to-late 20s. The frontal lobe is what controls executive functioning or "higher reasoning," such as the cognitive abilities to organize information and make decisions by weighing risks. It is what causes a person to stop and think about short- and long-term consequences before acting or reacting. Because teen frontal lobes are not fully functioning, adolescents often *re*act from emotions rather than *pro*act from the cognitive deliberations of thinking fully about their situation and responding with a "good," measured decision. The amygdala, located in the temporal lobe, is part of the limbic system and it primarily controls emotions. Thus, kids are said to act from their amygdala, or emotions, rather than their frontal lobe, or reasoning.

Synaptic pruning, the process by which the unused connections are eliminated, happens mostly during early adolescence. This is why teens appear to be developing cognitive skills and can exhibit adult-like intellect with the ability to make decisions. However, their brain is not actually developed enough to use the frontal lobe executive functioning that allows critical thinking and weighing of risks. Instead, they are processing information with their amygdala, the emotion center. Studies of youth show that young teens "think with their feelings." In studies that use magnet resonance imaging (MRI) to watch what parts of the brain are being used during certain tasks, a teen brain shows the most activity in the amygdala, thus showing the subject reacting out of emotion (Scott, *et al.*, 2018; Steinberg, 2012). An adult brain functions more from the frontal lobe, thus showing the ability to stop and think about what is presented before deciding upon a correct choice of action. As a teen grows, their gray matter becomes less dense and the white matter increases.

This myelination process allows for more complex thinking skills to emerge. As the frontal lobe develops, these cognitive skills and processing speeds improve, allowing the person to make better decisions faster.

This slow development of the frontal lobe is also why teens appear so self-centered. Because myelination occurs well into adulthood, even late-teen brains often don't have the capacity to regulate their emotions necessary to exercise self-control. Juvenile court judges frequently ask a teen who has committed a crime what their victim may have felt. However, this is not something the child has even considered because, frequently, their brain is not yet capable of weighing the consequences to their actions or viewing their behavior from outside of themselves. The amygdala develops more quickly and is being affected by the rushing hormones of adolescence, so the young brain doesn't effectively send signals to the frontal cortex fast enough to regulate their emotion and think through consequences before reacting. This is also why their behavior can be so impulsive and risk-taking. The limbic system, responsible for reward/sensation seeking, is stimulated by social pressures, thus making the teen susceptible to the peer pressure that can seem to control their every decision, from the colors that they dye their hair and the fashion of their clothes to their acting out in thoughtless ways.

These effects of peer pressure peak in mid adolescence, from age 15 to 17. While teens are intellectually capable of making good choices when calmly discussing behavior, e.g. in a classroom or with parents, their frontal cortex does not get the signal to stop and think when they are confronted with the rush of immediate decisions in everyday life, especially with their friends watching. The increased susceptibility to peer pressure even shows in studies where the test subjects were told peers were watching from another room, without the actual presence of their friends. Some studies utilizing MRIs to track what part of the brain is most active show that this hypersensitivity to peer pressure which increases risk-taking behavior, is still present even when the test subjects are specifically told about its effects prior to the study (Scott *et al.*, 2018). This indicates that the teens were reacting out of emotion, as seen by activity in the amygdala, without stopping to consider what they understood cognitively, as seen by the lack of frontal lobe activity. In other words, when asked by an adult in a neutral, non-excited setting, such as a classroom, teenaged Johnny has the cognitive skills to reason through a hypothetical situation and state that robbery is wrong. However, when "chilling" with his friends on a Saturday at the local park and someone suggests they all go take a kid's brand-new bicycle across the street, Johnny does not have the brain capacity to stop to consider the consequences. His sensitivity to the emotions aroused in the amygdala, his tendency to seek risky stimulation, and his brain-driven susceptibility to peer pressure all work to override any executive functioning that would stop him or give him an ability speak up to say that's wrong and to go home.

Simulated driving experiments that show teens taking more risk, such as speeding or running stop lights, when peers are in the car watching them has led to changes in driver's licensing laws (Scott *et al.*, 2018). This heightened sensitivity to peer pressure can influence teens for good as well as antisocial acts. Participation on sports teams, academic competitions, and peer-counseling programs can give youth the pro-social impetus to succeed. Indeed, positive peer culture models have been utilized successfully in numerous adolescent residential treatment centers across the nation. Now brain science shows that to be a best-practice model.

The processes by which the brain parts communicate with each other involve chemical and electrical reactions through neurotransmitters. Norepinephrine is involved in arousal, alertness, memory, and attention. It stimulates the "fight or flight" response. Dopamine is an inhibitory transmitter that blocks neurons from firing and is associated with the reward system of the brain, often called the "feel good" chemical. Serotonin, also an inhibitor, regulates emotions, mood, anxiety and impulse control. Low serotonin is associated with depression, panic attacks, and suicide. Changes in hormones in adolescents cause an increase in the number of dopamine receptors in the brain. Thus, the reward system of the teen's brain has a heightened sensitivity to this "feel good" chemical, causing the teen to seek excitement. Brain imaging studies show a much stronger response in the reward-processing areas of the brain in teens than either children or adults (Scott *et al.*, 2018). This process drives much of the "thrill-seeking," risk-taking behavior that is seen to peak in mid adolescence. Some studies specifically show that teens learn more from "rewarding" experiences than from "costly" ones, thus the evidence shows they don't learn well from their mistakes (Steinberg, 2012). These studies indicate why the "scared straight" programs from the 1990s have shown to be ineffective with teens; their brains enjoy the thrill rather than process the cognitive reasons to avoid bad consequences.

Effect on the Developing Brain of Drugs, Trauma, and Mental Health Issues

The teen brain is very excitable because the brain chemistry of adolescents is wired to be responsive to every little thing in their environment in order to form new connections within the brain. This connection growth of young brains makes learning easier. Known as plasticity, this process means the teen brain changes and adapts to the environment much more quickly than an adult brain. The old phrase "you can't teach an old dog new tricks" is based in brain science. But this high responsivity also leads to over-stimulation when youth are in stressful environments. This is why trauma negatively affects young brains more profoundly and why teens can become addicted to drugs more quickly than adults. Studies in addiction show that brains of teens who smoke marijuana are affected for much longer periods than adults (Weir, 2015). Teens will still perform poorly on cognitive tests days later, while the adult brains have returned to baseline functioning scores by the next day. Because the teen brain is still "learning" how to connect as it develops neural pathways, any adolescent substance use is "teaching" the teen brain to rely on these introduced chemicals. While debate continues over the use of marijuana in America, there is definite scientific evidence that its chronic use in teens interferes with normal brain development.

Trauma also is shown to have heightened and negative effects on the developing brain (Denno, 2019). Much research has been done on the long-term effects of poverty and trauma on children showing that it affects not only their physical and mental health, it can also contribute to medical diseases later in life. The effects of stress lead the brain to create more cortisol, the "fight or flight" chemical, which in turn inhibits normal development of the brain. This early over-activation of cortisol leads the children to be more sensitive to trauma as their brain has adapted to the problem.

The tendency to seek risky stimulation is what drives teens to engage in the very conduct that leads to more stress in their lives and thus more interference with their brain development and, ultimately, to their legal trouble. Experimentation with alcohol and drugs, "acting out," fighting, bullying-victimization, and "caving in" to peer pressure are just a few of the behaviors that lead a teen into involvement with the criminal system. As every parent knows, if teens are not protected from themselves during this critical time, their impulsivity and drive to take risks couple together to lead them into trouble. Brain science is now providing evidence to show why societal policies should lean towards protecting the adolescent from himself (Steinberg, 2012; Scott, *et al.*, 2018).

Brain Development and Legal Policy

This social policy effort to include brain science can be seen in many areas. However, since science cannot state to a medical certainty when a specific individual's brain has fully matured, it is difficult for the law to set a bright-line rule for when a person becomes an adult. While the brain is showing cognitive intelligence abilities as young as 15, the brain does not reach full mature reasoning ability until as late as 26. This difficulty is seen in the varying ages at which legal rights are determined across settings. A person cannot legally enter a contract until age 18 whereas some states allow a person as young as 14 to make medical decisions about abortion without parental notice. Adolescents can die for their country at 18 but cannot buy a beer to celebrate until 21. Teens can legally drive at 16, whereas the insurance rates are exceedingly high until the mid 20s.

The timing of brain development shows why some of these different ages may make sense. Because Susie can make a well-reasoned decision when given time to reflect, away from peer pressure, it is reasonable to allow her to make a medical decision about her body in young teenage. But because she may drive recklessly with her friends in the car, it is also reasonable to enforce graduated license rules from 16 to 18 to protect her, as well as those driving in the next lane. Because alcohol and other drugs have shown to put teens at higher risk for addiction, it is reasonable to enforce alcohol restrictions till later in life. Brain science provides for sound reasoning behind these apparent legal discrepancies. This science is also beginning to affect other areas of societal policy regarding teens. Schools across the nation are adopting later start times to account for studies showing that teens' natural sleep cycles keep them awake late, so they need to rise later in the morning.

In recent years, the use of brain science to justify a reduction in criminal culpability of teens has impacted legal reasoning and social policy and led to the adoption of policies that protect the child, rather than protect society from the child. Belief, now based in this science, that teens have lower actual ability to control their behavior and higher impulse to seek risky behaviors leads society to lean towards protecting the teens from themselves and their thoughtless conduct. All of these studies justify more treatment for adolescents and a trend away from harsh punishment in adult courts. For the past 50 years in opinions that effect adolescents, the Supreme Court of the United States has been saying what all parents know: that kids are different, more impulsive, immature, and in need of guidance. In the past, the Supreme Court based these opinions on the slowly shifting law, not on hard scientific facts. As studies advanced our understanding of adolescent brain development, the Court began to take notice and cite these scientific studies to swing the law towards more protection of children.

Part Three: The Constitution Applies to Kids Too!

Juvenile Court was born and grew up under the theory of *parens patriae* with the idea that the state, through the all-powerful juvenile judge, was to protect youth and provide for their proper education and maturation. However, as legal scholars published more reviews of what was actually happening in the privacy of juvenile courts across the country, some even comparing them to Star Chambers and kangaroo courts, the Supreme Court had to take notice and question the lack of procedural due process in what were clearly courts of punishment and deprivation of liberty, not courts of treatment or guidance.

In 1963, the lawyer Abe Fortas argued and won the landmark *Gideon v. Wainwright* case before the U.S. Supreme Court, granting the right to counsel in adult criminal cases. Just a few years later, and then on the Supreme Court of the United States, Justice Fortas wrote the opinion for *Kent v. United States* (1966) that legally addressed only the statutory law in the District of Columbia, but that hinted heavily at the Constitutional implications for adolescents. Thus, began a line of jurisprudence that reassured juvenile justice warriors that the Constitution does indeed apply to kids. In *Kent*, the Court based its opinion on statutory law, holding that the judge's waiver, or legal transfer, of Kent to adult court for trial was invalid because the judge had not followed the statute's mandate to base the waiver on a "full investigation" (*Kent v. United States*, 1966).

Morris Kent was a 14-year-old when first put on juvenile probation in 1959. Two years later he was arrested on burglary and rape charges and incarcerated in the District of Columbia Receiving Home for Children. His mother hired an attorney who, upon conferring with juvenile officials learned that the prosecutor planned to try Morris as an adult. His attorney immediately filed motions opposing the transfer to adult court, requesting access to the court counselor's thick file on young Morris from his years on probation and, additionally, requesting a formal hearing. Without ruling on any of these motions, the juvenile court judge declined to grant any hearing and ordered the matter transferred to adult court with no findings of fact. Kent was eventually convicted of some offenses in adult court and sentenced to 30 years in prison.

In *Kent v. U.S.*, Justice Fortas based his opinion on the D.C. statute under which Kent was charged. However, the opinion included several Constitutional arguments, hinting broadly that juvenile courts nationwide should allow for basic due process protections within their juvenile statutes. He expressed "concern that the child receives the worst of both worlds: that he gets neither the protections accorded to adults nor the solicitous care and regenerative treatment postulated for children" under the *parens patriae* model (*Kent v. United States*, 1966, p. 556). Indeed, reading the footnotes in the opinion is like reading a scathing rebuke of juvenile courts for not living up to their intended purpose as protectors of children, from criticizing the police procedures with juveniles to noting the "impossibility of the burden" on juvenile court judges and even calling into "question whether the *parens patriae* plan of procedure is desirable" (*Kent v. United States*, 1966, p. 554).

The *Kent* decision held that for a waiver to adult court to be valid there must be: 1) a hearing, even if informal, 2) entitlement to counsel for the juvenile, and 3) attorney access to the juvenile's confidential records, for assistance of counsel to be meaningful. Was Fortas bringing his beliefs from *Gideon* into juvenile court? While the holding of the *Kent* opinion did not actually extend the right of counsel to all juveniles, Fortas did state in non-binding dicta that the "right to representation is not a formality ... it is the essence of justice" (*Kent v. United States*, 1966, p. 561). Neither did this opinion clearly state that the juvenile defender's duty is that of express interest, as opposed to best interest. However, Fortas again hinted that the juvenile's counsel was to act as a **defense** attorney, not simply a guardian ad litem, by stating that the attorney's role was not to simply state facts about the child that would help the judge decide on what rehabilitation to impose, but to actually challenge the evidence put forward by the judge's staff, social workers, and probation officers. *Kent* set the stage for the case that is considered by juvenile defenders to be the birth of Constitutional rights for children and thus, highly significant and consequential for juvenile justice.

Case law moves very slowly because the Court can only address the issue(s) presented in the case at bar. However, *In re: Gault* (1967) was a giant leap for juvenile delinquency court. Again, Fortas wrote the opinion for the Court and, while he had to limit the holding to the issues raised in the trial court, the dicta suggested other rights that needed to extend to children. In reviewing the history of the doctrine of *parens patriae* in juvenile court, Fortas gave a nod to the good intentions but cited many studies to explain that the reality of how courts were working did not meet those lofty goals. The intent was to provide treatment, but he noted the high recidivism rates. The intent was to maintain confidentiality of records to protect children's future, but he cited the reality that many records were released and hurt young adults' ability to join society as productive members with jobs. While the informal nature of juvenile court was intended to benefit children, the reality was that many of the courts' stern, disciplinarian punishing procedures and sentences had the opposite effect, causing delinquent youth to turn further into lives of crime.

Gerald "Jerry" Gault was accused of joining a friend in making a lewd phone call to a neighbor lady. Without any notice of the specific charges, without a trial, without any evidence presented and without any discussion of the facts of the case, the judge sentenced 15-year-old Jerry to commitment in the State Industrial School until he was 21. Six years of incarceration for a prank phone call! An adult convicted in a trial for the same offense could have received no more than two months in jail. The *Gault* opinion discussed what should have happened to young Jerry if the juvenile system worked as intended, instead of the "kangaroo court" that had occurred (*In re: Gault*, 1967, p. 28). Fortas opined that if the judge had taken the time to talk to Jerry he would have learned that he had two working parents that could have provided proper discipline and a big brother who could be a good influence and so Gault could have stayed in the home and grown up to be a productive member of society.

The actual holding in *Gault* granted four specific rights to children: 1) to notice of charges, 2) to counsel, 3) to confrontation of accuser with cross-examination, and 4) to the privilege against self-incrimination. The opinion discussed at length how the informal nature of juvenile proceedings had degenerated into a farce and why Constitutional limits must be applied when children were being incarcerated like adults. In discussing the right to counsel, the opinion stated the obvious fact that probation officers cannot act as counsel for the child because they are typically the person filing the charges and telling the judge why the juvenile should be found to be a delinquent. In explaining the necessity of procedural limits on the adjudication hearings, the Court stated that, without counsel expressly guarding the child's rights, the right to a hearing with sworn testimony and cross-examination is meaningless. Citing the now-famous *Miranda v. Arizona* (1966) case which had come down the year before, Fortas expressed concern regarding the unreliability of juvenile "confessions" and stated that the juvenile judge must exercise care when discussing confessions in court. The majority opinion discussed the need for more formality in the adjudication process to assure that confessions were trustworthy, through a defense attorney holding the court to the safeguards of the privilege against self-incrimination and the cross-examination of sworn testimony. While Gault's appellate attorney had requested other rights, the Court did not reach them in this matter.

The original idea of a benevolent judge talking with a child who "confessed" his wrong-doing as a component of rehabilitation is not what most juvenile courts had become. Fortas cited cases from various state courts that were beginning to grant Constitutional rights to children because of just such egregious stories of long incarcerations instead of beneficial treatment. The *Gault* case attempted to address these travesties of justice by imposing procedural restraints on how juvenile judges reached adjudication without taking away the benefits of a paternalistic judge at the disposition phase. Stating "[t]here is no reason why the application of due process requirements should interfere with" the juvenile receiving treatment, the Supreme Court tried not to throw out the baby with the bath water (*In re: Gault*, 1967, p. 24).

While *Gault* granted many rights to juveniles, the right to an attorney is paramount. Without an attorney protecting those rights, the procedural safeguards would not actually be implemented in hearings. Indeed, what began to happen in courts after the Supreme Court mandated the right to an attorney was that probation officers or judges simply downplayed the right and convinced parents and children to waive the right to representation so the courts could continue to function just as they had. This has continued into the 21st century and has allowed such abuses as the Pennsylvania "Kids for Cash" scandal where two juvenile court judges were imprisoned after being convicted in 2011 of taking money in return for sentencing children in their courtrooms to long incarceration in private, for-profit juvenile detention centers.

The Supreme Court continued to expand Constitutional rights to children when, just three years later, they decided *In re: Winship* (1970). This case held that the state must prove the allegations in court beyond a reasonable doubt. Winship was a 12-year-old boy accused of stealing $112 dollars who was imprisoned in a "reform school" for 18 months, with a possibility that incarceration could extend till he turned 18. Again, the Court specified that providing procedural safeguards at the adjudication phase would not interfere with the overall purpose of juvenile court, i.e., rehabilitation of the child. The New York Court of Appeals had upheld the sentence, stating that an adjudication is not a criminal conviction. In striking down the New York statute allowing preponderance of the evidence to suffice as the standard of proof in juvenile courts, the Supreme Court cited its lengthy discussion in *Gault* regarding the failure of the juvenile justice system to fulfill its intended beneficial purposes. Writing for the *Winship* majority, Justice Brennan stated that "civil labels and good intentions do not themselves obviate the need for criminal due process safeguards in juvenile courts" (*In re: Winship*, 1970, p. 366). However, he went on to state that, because these safeguards were being applied to the adjudication phase, the trial judges could continue to be informal at the dispositional phase and exercise wide discretion in providing individual treatment for the children brought before them.

The *Winship* decision gets to the very heart of the on-going dichotomy of purposes of juvenile delinquency court, protection of the child versus protection of society from the child. No matter what a state may call it, the adjudication stage of juvenile court is a criminal-like proceeding whose function is to determine if a child broke the law, thus protecting society from "criminal" children. Because a child can be incarcerated in prison-like "reform schools," procedural safeguards must be mandated so that these trial courts can maintain the confidence of their communities that they are indeed dispensing justice, not acting as the kangaroo courts that the *Gault* Court had called them. As Justice Harlan discussed in his concurrence, the "fundamental value determination of our society that it is far worse to convict an innocent man than to let a guilty man go free" should apply to children as well (*In re: Winship*, 1970, p. 372). Because children are known to falsely "confess" and the evidence may not be sufficient to find them "guilty," as required in adult criminal court, these procedural safeguards must rigorously test the facts to get to the truth of the matter before proceeding to disposition (sentence). Therefore, the guilt-innocence phase of adjudication should function as an adult criminal trial court, with a lawyer helping the child in a contested hearing with Constitutional Due Process rights to determine actual guilt, while the dispositional phase should continue to informally seek treatment that is in a child's best interest, thus protecting the child.

The next year, however, in *McKeiver v. Pennsylvania*, the Supreme Court stated that, while *Gault* and *Winship* said that some of the Constitution applies to children, not all of it must. The Court held that the Sixth Amendment Constitutional right to trial by jury did not extend to juvenile adjudication hearings. The Court specifically acknowledged the dichotomy of purpose in juvenile court, pointing out the different goals of the adjudication stage, which it compared to adult trial stage, and the disposition/sentencing stage, which should be non-punitive. The Court discussed its "appreciation" of the benevolent juvenile judge who should protect the child with a disposition aimed at guiding the child with rehabilitation, rather than punishment. However, the Court expressed "disturbed concern" over judges who were "untrained" in the ideal of the juvenile court's "understanding approach" and who thus gave punitive, long sentences of incarceration (*McKeiver v. Pennsylvania*, 1971, p. 534). The opinion acknowledged that the actual process of modern juvenile court had not lived up to the original ideal. However, the Court did not want to turn juvenile court away from the beneficial rehabilitation efforts into a "fully adversarial process" that would "put an effective end to what has been the idealistic prospect of an intimate, informal protective proceeding" (*McKeiver v. Pennsylvania*, 1971, p. 545). While holding that the Constitution did not mandate the protection of a jury trial for juveniles, the Court specifically stated that the states are free to statutorily extend this right, as many states have legislatively done.

In 1975, the Court extended an additional Constitutional right to juveniles. In a unanimous decision in *Breed v. Jones* (1975), the Court held that the Fifth Amendment bar against Double Jeopardy applied to juveniles. Following a hearing and adjudication of armed robbery in juvenile court, 19-year-old Jones was ordered transferred to adult court for trial because the juvenile judge decided at the disposition (juvenile sentencing) phase that Jones was not amenable to treatment and therefore was unfit for juvenile court. He was subsequently found guilty in a new trial in adult criminal court. In a relatively brief opinion, the Court concluded that a juvenile adjudication was the same as an adult court criminal trial and that Jones was therefore put at risk of jeopardy (tried) twice for the same crime.

In its analysis, the Court laid out the basic dilemma every juvenile defender faces in the juvenile court dichotomy of protecting the child versus protecting society. If the defender allows the child client to participate in pre-adjudication evaluations and reports by the probation officer in order to stay in juvenile court and/or receive favorable adjudication and disposition, the child may be risking the information being used against him if the case is transferred to adult court. If the attorney does his duty to protect his client's Fifth Amendment right to remain silent by non-cooperation, he risks the probation officer or prosecutor recommending transfer *because* the juvenile's "non-cooperation" renders the child not amenable to treatment. While many state's statutes mandate that this information is not admissible against the child, in footnote 23 the Court cited the juvenile judge as admitting that "nobody is going to eradicate from the minds of the district attorney or other people the information they obtained" from an evaluation of the juvenile during the intake process (*Breed v. Jones*, 1975, p. 541). While the Court left the exact procedures of transfer to the states to legislate, they required that the decision on **whether** to transfer a child to adult court must be made before any adjudication hearing.

Early Constitutional cases focused on procedural rights while the next major U.S. Supreme Court case addressing juvenile law turned to protection of juveniles from harsh adult sentences. In *Eddings v. Oklahoma* (1982), the Court vacated a death penalty sentence for a 16-year-old boy who killed the highway patrolman who had pulled him over. The Supreme Court remanded the case back to the Oklahoma trial court for a re-sentencing hearing that would take into account not just his age, but also the other mitigating evidence his lawyer presented regarding his mental and emotional development and the child abuse he had suffered at the hands of his policeman father. In its reasoning, the Court cited a 1967 Juvenile Delinquency Task Force Report that extensively described children as different from adults, more impulsive, less culpable, and therefore deserving of less punishment. The Court acknowledged that because they could base their decision to reverse the lower court on case law, they would not reach the Constitutional issue of whether the Eighth Amendment ban on cruel and unusual punishment prohibits execution of juveniles. However, their analysis foreshadowed the decision to reach that conclusion two decades later in *Roper v. Simmons* (2005).

Just two years after *Eddings*, the Court started citing studies regarding the rise in teen crime rates from the "get tough" era of juvenile justice in their decision in *Schall v. Martin* (1984). *Schall* was a class action habeas corpus case involving 34 children held in "preventative detention" prior to trial. The federal district court struck down the New York statute allowing for pre-trial detention of juveniles because it lacked due process procedures. The federal appellate court agreed to strike down the statute for a different reason; stating that, because most juveniles were held for only a short period of time and released to probation upon the adjudication of their case, pre-trial detention was punishment without a finding of guilt. The U.S. Supreme Court reversed the lower courts, holding that New York's pre-trial detention statute was indeed Constitutional because it served a legitimate state interest, e.g. protection of society and the child, and that it did provide sufficient procedural safeguards. While the ruling was based on complicated legal analysis behind methods of Constitutional scrutiny, the dicta in the case showed the Supreme Court followed the "get tough" era by minimizing the punishment aspect: 1) finding that pre-trial detention is usually brief and only temporary and 2) "juveniles, unlike adults, are always in some form of custody," i.e., parents have custody of their children (*Schall v. Martin*, 1984, p. 265). The Court went on to state that "the juvenile's liberty interest may, in appropriate circumstances, be subordinated to the state's *parens patriae* interest in preserving and promoting the welfare of the child" (p. 265). This return to the paternalistic theory of juvenile justice marked a setback in the movement towards protection of the child.

A few years later, Justice Stevens cited psychological theories about adolescent immaturity suggesting lessened culpability in his ruling in *Thompson v. Oklahoma* (1988), when the Court, once again, overturned a death penalty sentence for a child from Oklahoma. Thompson was only 15 when he participated with three adults in the murder of his brother-in-law, a man who had abused Thompson's sister. Because the legal question specifically centered on the Constitutionality of the death penalty as applied to a 15-year-old, the Court made the sweeping holding that the Eighth Amendment ban on cruel and unusual punishment prohibited the death penalty for children under the age of 16. In its reasoning, the Court looked at legislation regarding death sentences for youth across the country. The Court considered how juries applied the death sentence in trials of young people to arrive at the "unambiguous conclusion that the imposition of the death penalty on a fifteen-year-old offender [was] generally abhorrent to the conscience of the community" (*Thompson v. Oklahoma*, 1988, p. 832). The Court also cited child psychologists Erik Erickson's and Lawrence Kohlberg's theories of stages of childhood development (p. 835 fn. 43) to show that children are different and less culpable than adults: "Inexperience, less education and less intelligence make the teenager less able to evaluate the consequences of his or her conduct while at the same time he or she is much more apt to be motivated by mere emotion or peer pressure than is an adult" (p. 835). However, basing court decisions on the medical studies of the adolescent brain would have to wait 17 more years for the actual hard science to catch up with findings in the field of adolescent brain development.

Finally, in 2005, the Supreme Court heard Christopher Simmons' case and extended the Eighth Amendment prohibition on death penalty to all juveniles under the age of 18 in *Roper v. Simmons* (2005). Seventeen-year-old Chris was the uncontested instigator of a planned and heinous murder of a woman he had chosen as his victim because of his involvement with her in a prior car accident. At his trial, in 1994, both the prosecutor and the defense argued that his age should be a factor in sentencing. The prosecutor appealed to the "get tough" era's rising fear of the juvenile as "super-predator" to argue that his age should count against him. By the time his case got to the Supreme Court in 2005, the Court had begun to recognize that medical studies in adolescent brain development provided scientific confirmation regarding what psychologists had opined about the immaturity of teens. The Court based its holding on the prior reasoning of *Thompson* that looked to current social morals as reflected by contemporary decisions of state legislatures and juries, i.e., more states banning capital punishment for juveniles and fewer states executing them. However, the Court added citations of the scientific studies of adolescent brain development to bolster their discussion of why juveniles are different from adults, comparing the reasoning to its 2002 holding in *Atkins v. Virginia* regarding mentally handicapped adults' lesser culpability.

Background on this culpability issue shows that, in 1989, the Court had released two opinions declining to find a categorical ban on capital punishment: for juveniles in *Stanford v. Kentucky* (1989) and for mentally handicapped adults in *Penry v. Lynaugh* (1989). In 2002, though, the Court reconsidered the issue regarding handicapped adults and overruled *Penry* in *Atkins v. Virginia* (2002), citing "the lesser culpability of the mentally retarded offender" among other factors regarding cognitive capabilities (*Atkins v. Virginia*, 2002, p. 319). Although young Simmons had exhausted his appeals, his attorney re-filed for post-conviction relief following the 2002 holding in *Atkins*, contending that the same brain science issues that led to the prohibition on execution of mentally handicapped adults should apply to children as well. Just as the *Atkins* Court had revisited and overruled *Penry*, the Court used *Roper* to overrule their decision in *Stanford*.

Much of the *Roper v. Simmons* (2005) opinion examined changing societal beliefs about use of the ultimate punishment on those with lesser culpability. However, the Court cited scientific studies to discuss three main differences between children and adults resulting from their still-developing brains: 1) adolescents' lack of maturity and underdeveloped sense of responsibility; 2) their vulnerability to negative influences and peer pressure; and 3) the juvenile's transitory, less fixed personality traits that allow for rehabilitation. These three points about adolescents were subsequently relied upon and elaborated in the *Miller v. Alabama* decision that will be discussed later in this chapter.

The Court based some of its reasoning on the fact that two of the main reasons behind capital punishment, retribution and deterrence, are undermined for juveniles by these advances in brain science. They stated that "[r]etribution is not proportional if the law's most severe penalty is imposed on one whose culpability or blameworthiness is diminished … by reason of youth and immaturity" (*Roper v. Simmons*, 2005, p. 571). The Court added that these characteristics "suggest as well that juveniles will be less susceptible to deterrence" (p. 571). The Court solidly based this Constitutional protection of juveniles on the growing scientific evidence, stating "[t]he differences between juvenile and adult offenders are too marked and too well understood to risk allowing a youthful person to receive the death penalty despite insufficient culpability" (p. 572). In non-binding dicta, the Court foreshadowed its willingness to also protect youth from the next highest punishment, stating that "it is worth noting that the punishment of life without the possibility of parole is itself a severe sanction, in particular for a young person" (p. 571). Because the Court must wait for legal issues to come to them, rather than mandating new law, they had to wait five years for this issue to arise.

In 2010, in *Graham v. Florida*, the Supreme Court utilized the same reasoning in *Roper v. Simmons* (2005) to extend the Eighth Amendment Constitutional ban on cruel and unusual punishment to sentences of life without the opportunity for parole (LWOP) for juveniles in non-homicide crimes. In this case, Terrence Graham was originally given probation for a burglary charge, committed when he was just 16, but was sentenced to LWOP when he admitted violating the terms of that probation. Citing *Roper*, the Court treated it as a given that "because juveniles have lessened culpability they are less deserving of the most severe punishments" (*Graham v. Florida*, 2010, p. 68). In deciding to extend this right as a categorical rule for all juveniles under age 18, the Court specifically discussed and rejected the idea of allowing trial court judges to discern the individual culpabilities of the teen offender because "it does not follow that courts taking a case-by-case proportionality approach could with sufficient accuracy distinguish the few incorrigible juvenile offenders from the many that have the capacity for change" (*Roper v. Simmons*, 2005, p. 77). Thus, the advances in brain science encouraged the protection of **all** teens from the thoughtlessness of their actions.

Historically, Eighth Amendment jurisprudence looks at whether a particular punishment is "cruel and unusual" through an exhaustive statistical look at how the punishment is being imposed, e.g., how many state legislatures allow it, how often it is actually imposed, and whether these numbers are trending up or down. However, in *Graham*, as the dissent pointed out, the evidence before the Court showed that 37 states allow LWOP for juveniles and it appeared to be frequently imposed. Therefore, the Court's majority opinion based its reasoning primarily on considering the proportionality of the sentence, i.e., whether the "sentence fits the crime" when applied to a juvenile. Therefore, the accumulated scientific findings about adolescent brain development drove the Court to ban LWOP for juveniles convicted of non-homicide offenses.

As part of their rationale to apply this bright-line rule to all persons under 18, the *Graham* Court made an interesting observation that the "features that distinguish juveniles from adults" may also "impair the quality of the juvenile defendant's representation" (*Graham v. Florida*, 2010, p. 78). Since the *Gault* Court originally mandated the right to an attorney for juvenile proceedings in 1967, there has been much debate about the quality of their actual representation, particularly in law review articles. National legal organizations have been created to train lawyers in how to provide zealous advocacy for youth. States have developed standards to mandate express interest advocacy and raise the bar in the effectiveness of juvenile defense. With the *Graham* decision, this appeared to be the first time that the Supreme Court acknowledged that the very reasons that kids are different from adults may make it harder for juvenile defenders to do their job. That is, teens' characteristic mistrust of adults, impulsivity, and difficulty in thinking long-term to make reasoned decisions impairs their ability to assist the attorney in their defense. This finding becomes critically important in evaluating juveniles' capacity to proceed.

Just two years later, the Court extended *Graham* by mandating that the Eighth Amendment ban on cruel and unusual punishment also prohibited life without parole for adolescents through the mechanism of **mandatory** sentencing schemes, even in circumstances where the individual adolescent committed a homicide. Two such homicide cases were combined for the ruling in *Miller v. Alabama* (2012). One defendant, Evan Miller, was a 14-year-old boy convicted in adult court in Alabama of murder in the course of arson. Miller and his friend Colby Smith were smoking marijuana and playing drinking games with an adult neighbor, Cole Cannon (who had just sold drugs to Miller's mother before bringing the teens to his own house). The boys stole $300 from Cannon's wallet, beat him with a baseball bat and, later that night, set fire to the trailer in attempt to cover up their crimes. Smith was allowed to plead guilty to lesser crimes in exchange for the testimony that convicted Miller under the felony murder rule (death resulting during commission of a felony – in this case, the arson).

The second defendant was Kuntrell Jackson, a 14-year-old boy also tried as an adult, in Arkansas. Jackson was minimally involved in an armed robbery of a video store in which the clerk was killed. Jackson did not know of the existence of the gun until they were driving to the store and he saw it in a companion's coat sleeve; moreover, he stayed in the car at first and was not the shooter. When he was convicted of felony murder and aggravated robbery, Arkansas law mandated life without parole. Both of these states' statutory sentencing schemes mandated the sentence of LWOP without allowing either of the boys' attorneys to present any of the abundant mitigating factors about their respective clients' lack of culpability, evidence of juvenile characteristics regarding capacity for change, or other relevant sentencing information.

In writing for the majority in the *Miller* decision, Justice Kagan started with the premise that *Roper* and *Graham* both "establish that children are constitutionally different from adults for purposes of sentencing, [b]ecause juveniles have diminished culpability and greater prospects for reform" (*Miller v. Alabama*, 2012, p. 471). She went on to cite the reasoning provided by research in brain development from *Roper* and even, in footnote 5, stated that "neuroscience continues to confirm and strengthen the Court's conclusions" (p. 472). While the Court acknowledged that *Graham* applied to non-homicide offenses, not to murder, they justified extending *Graham* to homicide crimes because "none of what is said about children – about their distinctive (and transitory) mental traits and environmental vulnerabilities – is crime-specific" (*Miller v. Alabama*, 2012, p. 473). However, this holding did not state that juveniles can not be given LWOP. It simply stated that **mandatory** sentencing to LWOP was unconstitutional, limiting the holding to a mandate that trial courts must consider the individual characteristics of the juvenile before imposing a sentence of life without parole. This opinion also foreshadowed a possible extension of Constitutional protections to the procedures for transferring a juvenile to adult court. Stating "[t]he key moment for exercise of discretion is the transfer," the majority hinted that they might ban the various mandatory transfer schemes extant in many states that allow prosecutors the discretion to try juveniles in adult court without judicial review, if this specific issue is brought before the Court (p. 488). (See Part Five, this chapter)

While many of the recent Supreme Court cases focused on reduced punishment for juveniles based on reduced culpability, the Court recently expanded Constitutional protections to apply to legal procedures used in dealing with juveniles. These procedural protections rely on the same brain science showing "that children cannot be viewed simply as miniature adults" (*J.D.B. v. North Carolina*, 2011). In *J.D.B.*, a 13-year-old boy in the seventh grade was brought into a conference room in his middle school by the uniformed school resource officer for local law enforcement officers to question him regarding suspected involvement in neighborhood break-ins. J.D.B. was questioned by two officers, accompanied by two school officials, in a closed room for 30 to 45 minutes without any notice to a parent or any Miranda warnings.

Most Americans, even children, are familiar with *Miranda v. Arizona* (1966), from the many television shows that quote the rights: "You have the right to remain silent. Anything you say can and will be used against you. You have the right to an attorney." Because this is heard coming from every cop in any show as they arrest a person, most Americans falsely believe that these rights are what a cop has to say when arresting someone. Miranda warnings, as they are frequently called in the legal field, are only mandated to be administered to any person before being questioned by an officer if the suspect is being held "in custody," whether he has been formally arrested or not. Indeed, if the officer does not plan to question the person, the officer does not have to "read them their rights" to arrest them. These guarantees are meant to protect persons "in custody" from bowing to the pressures of custodial interrogation and confessing in violation of their Constitutional Fifth Amendment right against self-incrimination. Most states have some sort of legislation now mandating how these rights are to be administered and including an additional right for juveniles that they can have their parent or guardian present at the questioning. It is the government's responsibility to ensure that any confession taken from a suspect was done legally and within Constitutional bounds. Therefore, the legal issue in most confession cases when the person was not mirandized becomes: Was the person "in custody" at the time of the interrogation? Since *Miranda* was decided, much case law has developed to help officers decide where the line is that determines when a person is "in custody." This line falls somewhere *after* the officer first encounters a suspect on the street and stops them to ask a question and *before* the formal "booking" at the police station. For any confession to be admissible in court, the state must show the defendant was read his rights prior to answering questions if he was in custody. The law mandates that the test to determine whether a suspect is in custody is an objective one that considers all the circumstances surrounding the interrogation process and asks whether a reasonable person in the defendant's position would believe that he is free to leave without answering. In J.D.B.'s case, the trial attorney moved to suppress his statements to the officers, arguing that he was "in custody" in the school office and was not read his Miranda rights prior to the questioning.

J.D.B. was a middle-schooler pulled out of class and questioned by cops in a closed room with school officials standing by. The state trial court denied J.D.B.'s motion to suppress his statement, ruling that he was not in custody because he was at school (not a police station) and was allowed to get on the bus at the end of the day and go home without ever being arrested. Under the current test, one could believe that a reasonable adult would know he could leave the school without answering a cop's questions, but all kids know they will get in trouble if they leave school, especially if they've been called to the principal's office! The majority opinion pointed out the "absurdity" of applying the "reasonable person" adult standard to consider how a child would perceive his ability to get up and walk out of school during the middle of the school day (*J.D.B. v. North Carolina*, 2011, p. 276). They mandated that a suspect's age, when it is known or obviously apparent to the officer, must be considered among the custodial interrogation factors. Ultimately the Court held that "to ignore the very real differences between children and adults would be to deny children the full scope of the procedural safeguards that *Miranda* guarantees to adults" (p. 281).

In summary, the trend in Constitutional law indicates that the Supreme Court is using modern brain science to change laws to protect children from their poor decisions. While many of the juvenile law cases examined sentencing laws and mandated that juveniles be protected from the harsher punishments reserved for hardened adult criminals, other cases transferred this knowledge of children's cognitive deficits to provide more procedural rules that mandate treating children differently throughout the criminal process. In response to this trend in case law, some states are also amending their Juvenile Codes away from the harsh laws enacted during the "get tough" era to provide more protection to youth.

Part Four: Modern "Raise the Age" Legislation

At the start of the 21st century, the pendulum began swinging back toward protection of the child. Advances in understanding of adolescent brain development are becoming accepted as peer-reviewed, hard science, not simply psychological theories of child development, and more states are reconsidering how their justice systems treat youngsters who break the law. While the "get tough" era of the 1980s and 1990s saw most states enacting laws to put more youth into adult criminal prosecution by easing transfer processes, the trend is now towards bringing more back into juvenile courts. Called "Raise the Age" laws, these legislative efforts have seen all but three states raise the age of juvenile jurisdiction to 18.

There were widely different practices among the states regarding the age at which youth were included in juvenile jurisdiction. Research in adolescent brain development made its way into the court systems through professional publications and citations in case law. As societal attitudes began to recognize that adolescents' underdeveloped brains meant that teens were less able to control their impulsivity and make reasoned decisions, juvenile justice policies began to shift toward finding adolescents less culpable than adults who break laws. And thus, the trend moved to keeping youth in juvenile courts in order to provide more treatment services, rather than transferring to adult court. In 2005, the Campaign for Youth Justice began a nationwide initiative to push all states to raise the age of criminal responsibility to 18. This non-profit organization works in Washington D.C. to provide assistance to individual states to push "raise the age" legislation as well as other laws and policies that benefit youthful offenders.

Connecticut was the first of the three most punitive holdout states to raise the age of criminal responsibility for juveniles from 16 to 18. Youth advocates in Connecticut cited U.S. Supreme Court decisions and studies in adolescent brain development to push their legislators to create the Juvenile Jurisdiction Implementation Team in 2003. By 2006 they had passed reform legislation: 1) to raise the age from 16 to 18 on July 1, 2009, 2) to initiate more court diversion and community-based treatment services, and 3) to improve pre-trial detention practices for youth. To push the bill through the legislature over law enforcement resistance, advocates cited numerous studies that show that handling youth in juvenile justice systems actually improved public safety and lowered criminal justice costs over the long term because youth were provided treatment and rehabilitation rather than incarcerated with adults. Current data indicate that these efforts are paying off in both improved public safety and cost savings. Spending is less for juvenile justice, despite the added population. The juvenile arrest rate has dropped dramatically since 2009, and the state has closed a detention facility. Connecticut is a state to watch for best practices in juvenile justice.

As of August of 2020, only three states have yet to raise the age from 17 to 18: Wisconsin, Georgia, and Texas. Each of these states currently has pending reform bills and they appear to be following the national trend and research from the brain scientists. Critics of the "raise the age" movement have primarily been 1) law enforcement organizations who believe that older teen offenders understand what they are doing when they commit crimes despite the brain science to the contrary and 2) fiscally-conservative legislators who believe that treatment of more youth in juvenile court will simply cost too much. However, the science regarding brain development is becoming more generally acceptable for recommending less punitive ways to deal with youthful offenders. And all evidence from the states that have raised the age is that the overall cost to society goes down. Handling youth in juvenile courts has had the positive effects of 1) better outcomes for youth by providing treatment services as opposed to adult incarceration, and 2) better protection of society, e.g., safer communities by lower arrest and recidivism rates and long-term cost savings. These documented positive effects of raising the age have led some states to push further. For example, Vermont passed a bill in 2018 to raise the age to 19 by 2022, citing the brain science showing **all** teens are still developing and able to be rehabilitated. Connecticut, Illinois, Massachusetts, and Mississippi are each considering this option as well.

Statistics show that raising the age has led to a drop in the number of youths transferred to adult court. Judicially waived cases have dramatically dropped since its peak in 1994 of 13,000 youth. Numbers have been steadily declining since 2006, ranging from 7,200 youth in 2006 to 4,200 in 2013 and 2014 (Juvenile Justice Geography, Policy, Practice & Statistics. 2017). All states continue to support various legal processes to transfer cases to adult court if the offense warrants adult punishment. Some data suggests that the actual number of African American youth transferred is the highest it has been in 30 years (Campaign for Youth Justice. 2017. p. 9). Current statistics show that youth in adult incarceration are 36 times more likely to commit suicide (National Juvenile Justice Network. 2020). A look at some states that raised the age over ten years ago shows that removing the youthful offenders from adult prosecution and providing treatment services within the juvenile system has been so successful at reducing recidivism that these states are considering raising the age further, to 21 or higher, to keep "emerging adults" out of the adult criminal justice system as well.

As the scientific research continues to show that brains do not fully develop until the mid to late 20s, criminal justice reform advocates will continue to push for better ways to protect children, and now emerging adults, from their impulsivity and poor decision-making. The data from these early states continues to show that treating youth with services and keeping them out of the criminal justice system, be it the adult or the juvenile system, does in fact protect society from the child as well as the child from himself. Known as the "raise the age effect," this phenomenon shows that rehabilitative services work to lower juvenile crime rates and, in turn, lower long-term expenses for the criminal justice system and, not inconsequentially, make communities safer.

Thus, the push-me-pull-you dichotomy of whether criminal justice systems should protect the child or protect society from the child can be resolved by expanding the juvenile system to serve older youth as well as expanding the services to keep them out of **any** criminal court system. The raise the age trend appears to be moving forward. Now it is time to increase the number and types of services available in juvenile court to keep children, teens and young adults from entering "the system" at all through diversion programs, restorative justice policies, and other innovative programs that protect the young brain from itself.

Part Five: Where Does This Lead Us?

In the dichotomy of pitting the *parens patriae* model of juvenile court against Constitutional Due Process safeguards for juvenile offenders, the juvenile justice system does not have to sacrifice one to achieve the other. All evidence from studies conducted in those states that are implementing creative new laws, programs and treatment services to keep kids out of court and provide more rehabilitative treatment is showing that this protection of children actually also protects society from them because recidivism rates decline after implementation of the new policies. Trends in juvenile justice appear to be turning away from the "get tough" era and back to the original purpose of providing a separate court system for juveniles: to protect them from their poor decisions and to raise "good kids." While science has not advanced to the point of being accurate enough to apply individually from one child to another by use of a particular medical test that can show Johnny's brain is X percentage immature because of Y results on an MRI, overall science supports the trend in Constitutional law to increasingly provide more procedural protections for children.

The changes to each state's juvenile court system must come from its own legislators changing laws and the local juvenile justice stakeholders changing policies. While the courts can mandate certain rules be implemented by overturning cases and laws as they are appealed, the court's job is to interpret the laws, not to make new laws. Courts can only address specific issues that are presented by each individual case. As an example, the Supreme Court cannot prospectively issue rules that states must follow. However, occasionally the Court uses dicta to foreshadow how they **might** rule on an issue that is not squarely before them. This happened in *Kent v. United States* (1966), when the Supreme Court based its ruling narrowly on statutory law but hinted widely at the Constitutional implications, ultimately changing the landscape of juvenile justice. Therefore, juvenile justice advocates need to continue to put pressure on their state legislators and their local communities to push for better systems to assist more youth. Findings about juvenile brain development and data-analysis of new programs as they are implemented in juvenile systems across the nation can be used to advocate for the adoption of more creative new policies everywhere. This section suggests just some of the systemic legal and procedural changes that would better assist wayward youth while still assuring protection of society.

Reforms Needed in Juvenile Court

Continue to Raise the Age for Juvenile Court Jurisdiction

The trend to raise the age of criminal responsibility to 18 needs to push the final three states (Georgia, Texas, and Wisconsin) to come into parity with the nation. Juvenile courts should, at the very least, include all teens under 18. This is the logical cut off based on society's general view that 18 constitutes formal adulthood. Indeed, Justice Kennedy pointed out in his opinion in *Roper v. Simmons* (2005) that expert psychologists and psychiatrists are not allowed to diagnose a patient under 18 as having antisocial personality disorder because the Diagnostic and Statistical Manual of Mental Disorders V (DSM V) does **not allow** such a diagnosis for someone so young (p. 648). Indeed, the DSM V discourages the diagnosis of **any** personality disorders for youth under 18 precisely because their personality is still developing. In the discussion of the diagnosis of personality disorders, the DSM warns doctors that it "should be noted that the traits of a personality disorder that appear in childhood will often not persist unchanged into adulthood" (p. 647). Because medical science recognizes age 18 as a logical bright-line rule to allow certain diagnoses based on brain development, the courts should set a legal bright-line rule of 18 for prosecution to be in juvenile courts. While some laws, such as alcohol possession, put adult responsibility at older ages, most Americans view an 18-year-old as an adult. Science showing that reasoned decision-making abilities within the brain are not fully developed until 25 or later does suggest that the trend to raise the age to 20 or even 21 is a logical next step.

Raise the Minimum Age for Juvenile Court Jurisdiction

Another trend towards protecting youth that needs to continue is that of raising the minimum age of criminal responsibility to 12. The same medical advances in understanding brain development that indicate the teen has not fully developed his executive functioning also show that these cognitive functions are even less developed in pre-teen children. Children under 12 are predominantly still concrete thinkers, indicating their underdevelopment in the abstract thinking skills necessary to truly appreciate the concepts of criminal responsibility. Younger children's criminal misbehavior can and should be handled within the family, school, and community by providing treatment services and youth programs rather than criminal punishment and incarceration. As of January 2020, 22 states set a minimum age for criminal prosecution. Massachusetts and California set it at 12 and Nebraska sets it at 11. Fourteen states will prosecute youth at age ten: Arkansas, Arizona, Colorado, Kansas, Louisiana, Minnesota, Mississippi, Nevada, North Dakota, Pennsylvania, South Dakota, Texas, Vermont, and Wisconsin. While Washington sets the minimum age at 8 and Connecticut and New York set that age at 7. North Carolina, the last to raise the age from 15, has the youngest minimum age of six years old. While this leaves the majority of states not having any minimum age, meaning theoretically they can prosecute a 4 or 5-year-old child for any offense, most juvenile justice stakeholders would admit that a child that young would probably not pass a test for capacity to stand trial.

It is a Constitutional and statutory mandate that the government cannot prosecute any individual that lacks the capacity to stand trial. It is the ethical duty of juvenile defenders to seek specialized evaluations when they suspect their client does not understand the process or cannot assist them in defending the case. Brain science supports the notion that many, if not most, young children lack such capacity. If the minimum age was raised to 12, the number of defenders having to seek these expensive evaluations by adolescent psychology experts for capacity to stand trial would greatly reduce the costs of "the system," while the children, often called a "child in need of assistance" instead of a juvenile delinquent, could be served in the social welfare system. A return to the days when little Johnny can apologize to the neighbor for breaking a window and be told to work off the costs by doing some chores is in order. He does not need to be charged with a crime and brought to a formal courtroom.

The critics that speak out against raising the minimum age cite the need for services for these delinquent children as one of their main concerns. However, those states that do have higher minimum age of criminal responsibility still find systems, such as social service systems, to provide needed prevention services for wayward children and the accountability for their parents. The same systems that now provide services without court intervention to teen status offenders can be utilized to assist young children who criminally misbehave without ever involving the criminal justice system.

Eliminate Transfer to Adult Court without a Judicial Amenability Hearing

A court-structure change that is supported by brain science and by Constitutional Due Process case law is that of eliminating all **mandatory** transfer procedures and statutes. Every state has laws that allow juveniles to be transferred to adult criminal court for prosecution. These transfer laws vary widely. Some states allow transfer for certain minimum ages and only for certain high felonies. Other states have no minimum age, such that a 5-year-old child could theoretically be prosecuted in adult criminal court. The legal procedures required to waive jurisdiction from juvenile to adult courts also vary widely, with three primary methods for prosecuting youth in adult court. 1) Judicial waiver laws allow the juvenile court judge to hear the prosecutor's motion to transfer a child on a case-by-case basis. Often called "fitness" or "amenability" hearings, these procedures allow the defense to put on evidence of the client's lowered culpability and amenability to treatment and be heard as to reasons why the child's case should be retained in juvenile court. All transfers should require an "amenability" hearing and judicial review of the transfer. 2) Prosecutorial discretion laws, often called "direct file," that are allowed in some states give the prosecutor discretion to decide to skip juvenile court altogether and file the charges directly in adult criminal court without judicial oversight. The problem with this mechanism is that it looks only at the crime, not the individual juvenile. Even a very progressive prosecutor who might consider retaining in juvenile court a child who has mitigating factors would not know about those factors until a scheduled hearing allows opportunity for the defense to present them. 3) Statutory exclusion and automatic transfer laws mandate that certain high crimes originate in or go straight to adult court without the child ever seeing a juvenile court judge for an amenability hearing. These last two processes that **mandate** certain ages or certain crimes to transfer should be abolished. Brain science would suggest that any **mandatory** transfer, which does not allow juvenile judges to weigh an individual child's culpability and fitness for treatment, is unconstitutional. Justice Kegan foreshadowed this very idea in footnote three in her opinion in the *Miller* case (*Miller v. Alabama*, 2012, p. 469).

While the *Miller* holding could only address the issue of mandatory sentencing schemes that was presented, footnote three in the majority opinion stressed the importance of the transfer hearing (*Miller v. Alabama*, 2012, p. 469). Miller's attorney had requested funds from the trial court to hire a "mental expert" for the transfer hearing. The trial court judge denied his request and the Alabama Court of Criminal Appeals affirmed this denial because state case law precedent held that formal due process procedures were not required at this preliminary stage. At least one appellate judge urged the Alabama Supreme Court to address the issue, stressing the importance of transfer hearings, and stating that allowing this mental evaluation once the child is already in adult court was "in effect, too little, too late" (p. 469). This specific issue must reach the Supreme Court before the Justices can mandate judicial review of transfer decisions and give juvenile judges a chance to weigh each child's individual culpability and amenability. However, state legislatures could 1) abolish direct file, statutory exclusion, and automatic/mandatory transfer procedures by passing laws mandating that all ages under 18 and all crimes start in juvenile court and 2) mandate that an amenability hearing must be held for a judge to weigh evidence and be the one to decide whether to transfer any case to adult court.

All youth who are eligible for transfer should have their cases heard before a juvenile court so individual characteristics can be weighed by an impartial judicial official trained in handling juvenile cases prior to any transfer. Additionally, younger teens and children should not be transferred to adult court. Brain science and Constitutional trends support setting the minimum age of 15 for any child to be prosecuted as an adult. In footnote five of the *Miller* opinion, the Court points out that "the science ... supporting *Roper*'s and *Graham*'s conclusions ha(s) become even stronger," and "neuroscience continues to confirm and strengthen the Court's conclusions" (*Miller v. Alabama*, 2012, p. 472). While the Court may be reluctant to set bright-line rules regarding age, the science supports the notion that treating children in juvenile court is a better protection of society than sending them to adult prisons.

Prohibit the Felony Murder Rule for All Juveniles

Justice Breyer's concurring opinion in *Miller v. Alabama* (2012) supports states passing legislation that prohibits the application of the felony murder rule to juveniles. The felony murder rule allows for the conviction of all persons involved in any felony that goes awry and ends in a killing, even unplanned, to be found guilty of murder. This law is frequently misunderstood even by adults. Many an adult offender has asked his attorney "How can I be found guilty of a murder that I didn't commit, and didn't even know might happen, because I didn't know my accomplice had a gun, and I wasn't even there when it went down, because I was simply sitting in the back of the car during a robbery gone bad?" A teenage brain cannot be expected to foresee and understand this legal concept of transferred intent, difficult enough for an adult offender to grasp. Justice Breyer clearly understood that conundrum when he foreshadowed in his concurring opinion and gave the non-binding advice to the trial court that "this type of 'transferred intent' is not sufficient to satisfy the intent to murder that could subject a juvenile to a sentence of life without parole" (*Miller v. Alabama*, 2012, p. 491). Following the medical science, Breyer's concurrence provides advocacy for the categorical protection of any juvenile from a felony murder conviction. This is because brain science shows "the ability to consider the full consequences of a course of action and to adjust one's conduct accordingly is precisely what we know juveniles lack capacity to do effectively" (*Miller*, p. 492). Applying the brain science to legal rules should lead states to change their laws to prohibit the use of the felony murder rule on juveniles.

Eliminate Coercive Interrogation Techniques on All Juveniles

Another practice that adherence to adolescent brain science would eradicate from juvenile courts is the use of coercive methods in police interrogation of juveniles. These techniques, widely taught and utilized by law enforcement agencies throughout the nation, are guilt-presumptive methods that employ coercive and psychologically manipulative practices to get a suspect to admit what the police think he did. The purpose of using coercive techniques is to elicit a confession, not to seek the truth of what happened. Certain instructors of interrogation teach that coercive techniques are supposed to be used only when there is reasonable belief that the suspect is guilty, i.e., following a more open-question interview to detect deception in attempt to determine if the suspect is lying. Thus, it should never be used as an investigative tool, while police are still trying to ascertain what actually took place. Some training directions caution against using coercive interrogation on juveniles and persons with intellectual disabilities. However, a review of cases across the nation shows that coercive interrogation is still routinely used on youth by many law enforcement agencies and is frequently the basis of overturned convictions based on invalid confessions.

The "Central Park Five" case cited in Part One gave widespread publicity to the problem of police coercion and youthful false confessions. Data regarding false confessions from both youth and adults continues to grow as more convictions are being vacated by DNA evidence proving the convicted person did not commit the crime to which he confessed. Studies indicate that up to 33% of these exonerations involved youth under 18 making false confessions, while 49% were under 21 (Innocence Project, 2020).

Two primary issues may contribute to the high number of innocent youth who falsely confess: 1) Innocent youth may be more likely to be subjected to coercive interrogation than innocent adults because the very behavioral indicators that police are taught to see as indicating deception (avoids eye contact, squirms in chair, slouches, repeated denials, and other fidgety behaviors) are behaviors common to simple adolescence. These behaviors lead police to believe the child is lying, presume that he's guilty and trigger the coercive interrogation tactic. 2) Youth are known to be at higher risk than adults of admitting to something they did not actually do under these coercive interrogations with psychologically manipulative questioning. Adolescent brain development can help explain why youth may falsely confess at higher rates than adults.

Juveniles are particularly susceptible to giving false confessions for several reasons based on their limited life experience, high suggestibility, and limited executive functioning abilities. 1) Not only are they susceptible to outside influences from peers as well as adult authority figures like teachers and police, they have been taught to trust adults and frequently want to appear to comply or give the correct answer. 2) Because youth lack the executive functioning for proper decision-making, they are unable to see the long-term effects of confessing. Thus, they tend to simply tell the officer what he wants to hear so they can go home, taking the most expedient, short-term way out of the stressful situation of custodial interrogation. 3) The very nature of the coercive interrogation techniques used by police that is designed to psychologically overwhelm adults produces even more stress on the youthful suspect. As discussed in Part Two, this stress and trauma lead to more difficulty with the teen brain attempting to utilize frontal lobe executive functioning, thus overcoming any cognitive ability to reason through the process and withstand the psychological pressure to confess, even to something the suspect did not do. The teen's amygdala pushes him to say whatever is needed to get out of the interrogation room.

This fear of forced or false confessions was part of the Supreme Court's reasoning behind the 2011 holding in *J.D.B.* that age must be considered in determining whether a suspect is "in custody" in juvenile matters. Writing for the majority, Justice Sotomayor discussed the problem of false confessions and stated that "the risk is all the more troubling –and recent studies suggest, all the more acute—when the subject of custodial interrogation is a juvenile" (*J.D.B. v. North Carolina*, 2011, p. 269). The Court recognized 50 years ago that judges understood that juveniles frequently gave false confessions. For example, part of Justice Fortas' reasoning in 1967 in *Gault* that children needed attorneys was his discussion of the unreliability of juvenile confessions. He stated that "the greatest care must be taken to assure that the admission ... was not coerced or suggested ... and not the product of ... adolescent fantasy, fright or despair" (*In re: Gault*, 1967, p. 55). With brain science showing the reasons why youth are more susceptible to suggestion, their desire to please the interrogator with the "right" answers and their inability to see the long-term consequences of a false admission, the need for laws banning these coercive interrogation techniques on juveniles is apparent.

Expand Alternatives to Detention

Court policies need to utilize the studies being done across the nation that indicate that incarceration of teens, even in juvenile detention facilities and away from adults, actually has negative results. The practice does not protect society because the youth that are sent to Youth Development Centers, euphemism for youth prisons, tend to re-offend more and commit higher level crimes than similar youth who were given community-based services rather than incarceration. Detention of juveniles has been shown to raise school drop-out rates, increase recidivism, exacerbate, and even cause mental health problems, and negatively affect future employment prospects. In addition, detention is much more expensive than providing community-based treatment services. With the overwhelming evidence that this punishment model and other "scared straight" programs simply do not work, it is troubling that court counselors, prosecutors, and judges still rely so heavily on incarceration in juvenile courts. To effectively protect society from the criminal misconduct of children, the juvenile court system must provide treatments and services within the community that meet the child's specific needs, rather than just "lock them up." It follows that all stakeholders in the system, including the judges, should have specialized training in dealing with children and teens, from education on adolescent brain science to effective ways to better communicate with young people. While some juvenile systems are creating programs for more community-based services and instituting local policies against incarceration, this trend toward science driving more and better treatment should be mandated by law and spread throughout the nation.

Mandate Juvenile-Specific Pattern Jury Instructions

Because there are some youth that commit horrendous crimes, it is inevitable that some will be transferred and tried as adults. While general standards for juvenile defense dictate that the criminal defense attorneys who handle juvenile cases become knowledgeable about how adolescent brain development affects the culpability and amenability issues of their clients and zealously advocate for each client, Superior Court judges and juries do not have this specialized knowledge. Therefore, all states should develop juvenile-specific pattern jury instructions. These are the instructions that the judge gives to the jury before they begin their deliberations as to the prevailing law regarding this specific crime in this specific case. When a juvenile is being tried, juries should be instructed as to how relevant brain science changes certain legal concepts. For example, in the preliminary instruction the judge gives regarding the function of the jury, a pattern instruction should add language reminding the jury that the defendant in this trial is a juvenile and that the jury must take into account the information they heard from the witness stand regarding specific characteristics about adolescent brain development regarding this juvenile.

Mandate More Diversion from Any Court System

These suggested changes may come about slowly, only after the Supreme Court is able to mandate legal procedures by addressing each individual issue as children's cases wend their way through the appellate system. Another alternative is for state legislators to initiate these changes by re-writing Juvenile Codes based on learning from youth advocates and adhering to findings from studies regarding brain development. However, while waiting for appellate mandates to come from the Supreme Court or for reform advocates to gather enough support to lobby for legislative change, the stakeholders within each local juvenile court system could begin making beneficial improvements by changing their policies and procedures.

Scientific studies show that most juveniles "age out" of delinquency as executive functioning skills develop within their frontal lobe, giving them the ability to make better decisions. Longitudinal studies also show that the deeper a child is pushed into "the system," the worse the outcomes for both the child and society. More incarceration in either the juvenile or adult system leads to more recidivism and higher level offenses. This knowledge implicates the need to develop better policies, procedures, and programs to divert youth away from ever entering the criminal justice system.

Judge Steven Teske, from Clayton County, Georgia, has been a preeminent leader in the juvenile justice field for 20 years, traveling the nation teaching about many of the best practices his local court has instituted that have not only helped juvenile offenders but also increased community safety. He points to an obvious notion, yet one completely overlooked by most juvenile justice stakeholders, that distinguishes those "kids that scare us" from those "kids that make us mad." He talks about providing more discipline without court intervention for those "kids that make us mad" and preserving court intervention and system resources for those "kids that scare us." This common sense approach is behind the national trend to implement School-Justice Partnerships that keep the "kids that make us mad" with their bad behavior from ever entering the courtroom (https://www.school-justicepartnership.org/).

A School-Justice Partnership (SJP) is a model that brings together personnel from local schools, juvenile courts, law enforcement, and the community juvenile service providers to form an agreement to provide referrals to services rather than criminal charges against youth who commit minor crimes within the schools. North Carolina's new Juvenile Justice Reinvestment Act, raise the age law, includes a provision that 1) mandates the N.C. Administrative Office of Courts to develop a toolkit and model SJP agreement and 2) encourages each community statewide to implement these proven best practices. Former Judge and now representative Marcia Morey, who contributed a chapter to this book, was intently involved in North Carolina's efforts toward "Raise the Age" legislation. Judge Jay Corpening, the Chief District Court Judge in New Hanover County, North Carolina, is a leader in science-driven juvenile justice reform. In training stakeholders throughout N.C. about the positive results of New Hanover County's School-Justice Partnership, he states "the **only** road out of poverty is through the schoolhouse," not the courthouse, nor the jail house. In promoting SJPs, he advocates "changing our toolbox" by using more community-based treatment and less use of detention, emphasizing the need to "use a flashlight, not a hammer." This analogy of light leading the way to teach wayward youth rather than punishment to correct or deter them is a natural outgrowth of using adolescent brain development to inform effective policy. Implementing SJPs nationwide could virtually eliminate the School-to-Prison-Pipeline mentioned in Part One.

The national Office of Juvenile Justice and Delinquency Prevention (OJJDP) has numerous programs and models to improve juvenile court systems. Its mission statement begins

"OJJDP provides national leadership, coordination, and resources to **prevent** and respond to juvenile delinquency" (emphasis added). However, the very idea of "delinquency prevention" needs to undergo a fundamental attitude shift toward viewing its mandate as preventing the **criminalization** of normal teen behavior, including minor misbehavior that breaks a law, rather than preventing juvenile crime. That is not to say that preventing crime by using evidence-based programs that get teens involved in pro-social programs is not a necessary component of good delinquency prevention. What is needed is a mental shift away from the idea that all juvenile "crime" needs to be prosecuted because evidence has shown that keeping kids out of "the system" does increase public safety. Diverting more wayward youth from courtrooms and into positive, skill-building programs helps them mature into productive members of society rather than angry adults who feel disenfranchised.

Not all bad behavior needs to be prosecuted as a criminal offense. For example, many juvenile defenders, and even juvenile court judges, lament the charge of Disorderly Conduct ever being brought to court. A typical petition alleging disorderly conduct can be "little Johnny ran down the hall shouting obscenities and banging the lockers, disrupting classroom teaching." While this behavior is not to be condoned and certainly infuriates school personnel, it should not be a crime. Thus, Judge Teske is a true leader in differentiating between "kids that make us mad" and "kids that scare us." His successes in Clayton County, Georgia, show that delinquency prevention should focus on the decriminalization of normal teen behaviors that make adults mad.

Other evidence-based programs use mediation and restorative justice practices in lieu of prosecution. These programs bring the victim and the offender together with trained professionals to discuss the juvenile offender's behavior and allow the offender to hear the victim's experience from the victim's perspective in an effort to hold the offender accountable in a way that fosters healing for all involved. The idea behind restorative justice is simply that crime causes harm and both the offender and the victim will heal better, or recover from the trauma of the crime, if they decide together how to redress the harm. The juveniles learn empathy by hearing how the victims were hurt and offenders are able to take responsibility by making amends. The victims recover more successfully when they have an opportunity to be heard about how they have been harmed by the offense and have a voice as to the appropriate redress. This model returns juvenile discipline to its root, discipulus, Latin for pupil, in that research shows teaching kids the right way to act works better and lasts longer than simply punishing their bad behavior. The use of restorative justice practices has spread as its effectiveness with youth has become more widely publicized. In 2019, the Office of Juvenile Justice and Delinquency Prevention convened a Restorative Justice Working Group, consisting of experts in the field from across the nation, to develop a resource guide to assist communities to implement these proven practices more consistently.

There are many new and varied programs being implemented across the nation that divert youth from court. A complete list of these innovative programs is beyond the scope of this chapter. However, the following sources of information provide details about some of them. There are many nationwide organizations funding research in best practices in treatment of youthful offenders. Founded in 1948, the Annie E. Casey Foundation is one that has been funding programs and research that benefit disadvantaged children in more fields than just juvenile justice (www.aecf.org). Its Juvenile Detention Alternatives Initiative led numerous communities to institute programs to find better ways to address delinquency than locking kids up (https://www.aecf.org/work/juvenile-justice/jdai/jdaiconnect/). Its Models for Change: Juvenile Diversion Guidebook is an excellent resource that juvenile justice stakeholders should access to begin to effect change within their local systems (www.modelsforchange.net). The OJJDP website has a Model Programs Guide that is an excellent avenue to find programs that have been proven effective as well as guides to assist in implementation (https://www.ojjdp.gov/mpg). The National Juvenile Justice Network assists reformers on a statewide level to bring about necessary changes within their own systems for better treatment of all juvenile offenders (https://www.njjn.org/). The 21st century has brought the winds of change to juvenile justice that should blow away the "get tough" era's harsh punishment models and lead to real advances in protecting juveniles while also protecting our communities from their thoughtless delinquent behavior.

A Novel, Bifurcated Juvenile Court Structure

In balancing the dichotomy of rights in juvenile court, a possible structure that would divorce the adjudication stage from the disposition stage could provide the most protection to both the child and the community. As Justice Blackmon stated in 1971 in his opinion in *McKeiver*, "adjudication of the factual issues on the one hand and disposition of the case on the other are very different matters with very different purposes" (*McKeiver v. Pennsylvania*, 1971, p. 528). Adjudication is just like a criminal trial in adult court where the purpose is to challenge and filter the evidence against the accused to determine if a crime was actually committed by this individual. Disposition in juvenile court is to provide the best possible rehabilitation and treatment alternatives after an individualized evaluation of this particular child. The *McKeiver* opinion discussed the ideals of the original purpose of juvenile court and many of its failures to achieve these lofty goals. Comparing juvenile justice to a great experiment, the Court stated "[w]e are reluctant to disallow the States to experiment further and to seek in new and different ways the elusive answers to the problems of the young" (p. 547). Continuing that experimental idea, some innovative juvenile judge should consider the possibility of implementing a bifurcated procedure in juvenile court: one judge to conduct the adjudication hearing, thereby granting the juvenile all the rights and safeguards afforded to adults in criminal trials, and another judge to hold the disposition hearing, such judge who has training in both adolescent brain development and the specific needs and treatment issues of children.

This totally new, split court would divert lower level crimes into community programs, bringing only the most serious offenses to court. Only after the juvenile is adjudicated delinquent, i.e., found guilty, would the court counselors/probation officers become involved in conducting the individualized assessments for mental health and substance abuse in order to craft recommendations for the judge to impose a truly rehabilitative disposition order. This would make the juvenile process more like the adult process in that the accused's Constitutional rights would be protected from any government interference such as probation officers' questions and service plans until after a judicial finding of guilt/responsibility. This model would not necessitate different judges. Separating the adjudication hearing from the disposition hearing would allow the juvenile judge to change hats from the legal mind-set during trial, that of seeking truth and protecting children's rights, to the paternalistic mind-set at disposition that the original juvenile courts envisioned would provide benevolent guidance to wayward youth. One week of court could be dedicated to adjudication hearings, wherein the judge's perspective is that of the legal factfinder. The next week, for disposition hearings, would allow for *Gault*'s image of the "fatherly judge touch[ing] the heart and conscience of the erring youth by talking over his problems" and providing "benevolent and wise" discipline in his disposition order (*In re: Gault*, 1967, p. 26). The time in between hearings would allow for the court counselors to conduct their individualized evaluations only after a youth has been found responsible for a criminal offense. This bifurcated system would change the juvenile court from the "the worst of both worlds" (*Kent v. United States*, 1966, p. 556) with no procedures and considerable punishment into the best of both worlds with 1) strong safeguards to reach appropriate verdicts and 2) benevolent judges, well versed in adolescent brain science, who craft wise orders based on individualized evaluations for treatment. It would protect the juvenile's right to remain silent as court counselor evaluations would only be conducted after a finding of guilt, thus saving children from having to talk about their alleged offenses with state officials before a finding of responsibility. It would save time and money, as only those found guilty would need these lengthy personalized evaluations.

Conclusion

Many innovative local programs are being implemented across the nation that divert youth from court, and many states are passing laws to grant Constitutional procedural safeguards to juveniles. However, the confidentiality of the juvenile system that protects juveniles' records also has allowed these "secret" courts to become so widely different in practice that a veteran juvenile justice stakeholder with 20 years of experience in one state could move to another and suddenly find themselves a stranger in a strange land trying to understand the new state's system. Granted, it would be impossible to standardize juvenile courts to all look alike; criminal laws vary across the nation, and even adult criminal courts differ widely in their procedures. However, every juvenile justice system in the nation should strive to adapt their processes to implement common sense reforms based on the evolving brain science that shows how treating kids instead of punishing them helps everyone. With these reforms, the push-me-pull-you of juvenile court can be reconciled into a functional animal moving in one direction. This is because protecting the juvenile's rights, by providing treatment rather than punishment and criminal records, does protect society from the child, by lowering recidivism and preventing the creation of a true "super-predator" as a teen grows up in an adult prison.

Bibliography

American Psychiatric Association. (2013). *Diagnostic and Statistical Manual of Mental Disorders* (5th ed.). Washington, D.C.

Annie E. Casey Foundation. (8–9–2018). Retrieved from: https://www.aecf.org/blog/get-involved-advocates-for-change-in-juvenile-justice/

Arain, M., Haque, M., Johal, L., Mathur, P., Nel, W., Rais, A., Sandhu, R. Sharma, S. (2013). Maturation of the Adolescent Brain. *Neuropsychiatric Disease and Treatment*, Vol. 9, pages 449–461.

Blackstone's Commentaries on the Laws of England. (1765–69). Retrieved from: https://avalon.law.yale.edu/subject_menus/blackstone.asp.

Brown, Sarah Alice. (June 2012). *Trends in Juvenile Justice State Legislation: 2001–2011*. National Conference of State Legislatures. Retrieved from: https://www.ncjrs.gov/App/Publications/abstract.aspx?ID=261423

Campaign for Youth Justice. (3–26–2019). *OJJDP Data Supports the "Raise the Age Effect."* Retrieved from: http://cfyj.org/2019/item/ojjdp-data-supports-the-raise-the-age-effect

Casey, B J., Bonnie, Richard J., Davis, Andre, Faigman, David L., Hoffman, Morris B., Jones, Owen D., Montague, Read, Morse, Stephen J., Raichle, Marcus E., Richeson, Jennifer A., Scott, Elizabeth S., Steinberg, Laurence, Taylor-Thompson, Kim A., Wagner, Anthony D. (2017). "How Should Justice Policy Treat Young Offenders?" *MacArthur Foundation Research Network on Law & Neuroscience*. Nashville, Tenn.

Clayton County Georgia Juvenile Court (2020) *Annual Report FY20*. Clayton County Youth Development & Justice Center. Retrieved from: https://www.claytoncountyga.gov/home/showdocument?id=154

Connecticut Juvenile Jurisdiction Planning and Implementation Committee. (2–12–2007). Final Report. Retrieved from: www.raisetheagect.org/resources/JJPIC-report.pdf

Cook, Lauren. (2019). Central Park Five: What To Know about the Jogger Rape Case. *AM New York*. Retrieved from: https://www.amny.com/news/central-park-five-1-19884350/

Dennis, Andrea L. (2017). Decriminalizing Childhood. *Fordham Urban Law Journal*, Vol. 45, pages 1–44.

Denno, Deborah. (2019). How Courts in Criminal Cases Respond to Childhood Trauma. *Marquette Law Review*, Vol. 103, pages 301–363.

Drum, Kevin. (2016). A Very Brief History of Super-Predators. *Mother Jones*. Retrieved from: https://www.motherjones.com/kevin-drum/2016/03/very-brief-history-super-predators.

Egley, Arlen Jr., and Ritz, Christina, E. (2006). *Highlights of the 2004 National Youth Gang Survey*. (Report No. OJJDP Fact Sheet 01; FS-200601). Retrieved from: https://www.hsdl.org/?view&did=476637.

Evans, Brian. (2019). *2019 State Legislation Review: Fewer Children in Adult System*. Campaign for Youth Justice. Retrieved from: www.campaignforyouthjustice.org/2019/item/2019-state-legislation-review-fewer-children-in-the-adult-system

Feld, Barry C. (2017). My Life in Crime: An Intellectual History of the Juvenile Court. *Nevada Law Journal*, Vol. 17, pages 299–329.

Geraghty, Diane. (2016). Bending the Curve: Reflections on a Decade of Illinois Juvenile Justice Reform, *Child Legal Rights Journal*, Vol. 36:2, pages 71–89.

Griffin, Patrick, Addie, Sean, Adams, Benjamin, Firestone, Kathy. (2011). *Trying Juvenile as Adults: An Analysis of State Transfer Laws and Reporting*. National Report Series Bulletin. Office of Juvenile Justice & Delinquency Prevention. Retrieved from: https://ojjdp.ojp.gov/library/publications/trying-juveniles-adults-analysis-state-transfer-laws-and-reporting

Guckenburg, S., Stern, A., Sutherland, H., Lopez, G., Petrosino, A. (2019). *Juvenile Detention Alternatives Initiative Scale-Up: Study of Four States*. San Francisco, CA: WestEd.

Guggenheim, Martin. (2017). Barry Feld: An Intellectual History of a Juvenile Court Reformer. *Nevada Law Journal*, Vol. 17, pages 371–392.

Hartley, C. A. and Somerville, L. H. (2015). The Neuroscience of Adolescent Decision-making. *Current Opinion in Behavioral Sciences*, Vol. 5, pages 108–115.

Harvard Health Blog. (2011). *The Adolescent Brain: Beyond Raging Hormones*. Retrieved from: https://www.health.harvard.edu/mind-and-mood/the-adolescent-brain-beyond-raging-hormones

Howell, K. Babe. (2016). The Costs of "Broken Windows" Policing: Twenty Years and Counting. *Cardozo Law Review*, Vol. 37, pages 1059–1073.

Innocence Project. (2019). *DNA Exonerations in the United States*. Retrieved from: https://www.innocenceproject.org/dna-exonerations-in-the-united-states/

Innocence Project. (2019). *Exoneration Statistics and Databases*. Retrieved from: https://www.innocenceproject.org/exoneration-statistics-and-databases/

Joyner, Alfred. (6–14–2019). *Who is Matias Reyes? Serial Rapist and Murderer in Central Park Five Series "When They See Us."* Retrieved from: https://www.newsweek.com/who-matias-reyes-serial-rapist-murderer-central-park-five-series-when-they-see-us-1442045

Justice Policy Institute. (3–7–2017). *Raise the Age: Shifting to a safer and more effective juvenile justice system*. Retrieved from: www.justicepolicy.org/research/11239

Juvenile Justice Geography, Policy, Practice & Statistics. (7–14–2017). *Transfer Reported Data Trends Updated*. Retrieved from www.jjgps.org/news/article/73/transfer-reported-data-trends-updated

Juvenile Justice Initiative. (2017) *Dialogue, Education & Advocacy*. Retrieved from: https://jjustice.org/wp-content/uploads/Newsletter-Fall.pdf

Juvenile Justice Initiative (2009) Fact Sheet. Retrieved from: https://jjustice.org/wp-content/uploads/Public-Act-1.pdf

Juvenile Justice Initiative. (2012). *HB 2404 Raising the Age*. Retrieved from: https://jjustice.org/wp-content/uploads/RTA-HB2404-Fact-Sheet.pdf

Kassin, Saul M. (2014) False Confessions: Causes, Consequences, and Implications for Reform. *Policy Insights from the Behavioral and Brain Sciences*, Vol. 1:1, pages 112–121.

Kelling, George, and Wilson, James. (1982). Broken Windows: The Police and Neighborhood Safety. *The Atlantic Monthly*, March 1982.

Luna, Marco. (2018). Juvenile False Confessions: Juvenile Psychology, Police Interrogation Tactics, and Prosecutorial Discretion. *Nevada Law Journal*, Vol. 18, pages 291–316.

MacArthur Foundation Research Network on Adolescent Development and Juvenile Justice. (9–1–2006). *Less Guilty by Reason of Adolescence*. (Issue Brief 3) Retrieved from: https://www.issuelab.org/resource/less-guilty-by-reason-of-adolescence.html#

MacArthur Foundation Research on Adolescent Development and Juvenile Justice. (2015) *Juvenile Justice in a Developmental Framework* (2015 Status Report). Retrieved from: https://www.macfound.org/media/files/MacArthur_Foundation_2015_Status_Report.pdf

Models for Change. (3–1–2011). *Juvenile Diversion Guidebook*. Baltimore, MD: MacArthur Foundation, Model for Change. Retrieved from www.modelsforchange.net/publications/301

Mumola, Samantha A. (2018). The Concrete Jungle: Where Dreams Are Made of … and Now Where Children Are Protected. *Pace Law Review*, Vol 39:1, pages 539–567.

National Gang Center (2020). History of the National Gang Center. Retrieved from: https://www.nationalgangcenter.gov/#about

National Juvenile Defense Center. (August 2019). *A Right to Liberty: Resources for Challenging the Detention of Children*. Retrieved from: https://njdc.info/wp-content/uploads/2019/A-Right-to-Liberty-Resources-for-Challenging-the-Detention-of-Children-1.pdf

National Juvenile Defense Center. (January 2014). *Juvenile Justice Purpose Clauses* (Multi-Jurisdiction Survey). Retrieved from: https://njdc.info/practice-policy-resources/state-profiles/multi-jurisdiction-data/

National Juvenile Defense Center. (2019). *Minimum Age for Delinquency Adjudication* (Multi-Jurisdiction Survey). Retrieved from: https://njdc.info/practice-policy-resources/state-profiles/multi-jurisdiction-data/minimum-age-for-delinquency-adjudication-multi-jurisdiction-survey/

National Juvenile Defense Center. (2019) *State Profiles*. Retrieved from: https://njdc.info/practice-policy-resources/state-profiles/

National Juvenile Justice Network. (2020). *Keep Youth out of Adult Courts, Jails and Prisons*. Retrieved from: https://www.njjn.org/about-us/keep-youth-out-of-adult-prisons

National Juvenile Justice Network. (November 2012). *Competency to Stand Trial in Juvenile Court: Recommendations for Policymakers*. (Policy Update). Retrieved from www.njjn.org/uploads/digital-library/NJJN_MfC_Juvenile-Competency-to-Stand-Trial_FINAL-Nov2012.pdf

Office of Juvenile Justice and delinquency Prevention (July/August 2019). *Administrator Harper Convenes Restorative Justice Working Group*. OJJDP News @ a Glance. Retrieved from: https://ojjdp.ojp.gov/sites/g/files/xyckuh176/files/newsletter/252941/topstory.html

Office of Juvenile Justice and Delinquency Prevention (June 2019). *Key Amendments to the Juvenile Justice and Delinquency Prevention Act Made by the Juvenile Justice Reform Act of 2018*. Retrieved from: https://ojjdp.ojp.gov/sites/g/files/xyckuh176/files/pubs/252961.pdf

Office of Juvenile Justice and Delinquency Prevention. (2019). *Model Program Guide*. Retrieved from: https://www.ojjdp.gov/mpg

Office of Juvenile Justice and Delinquency Prevention. (July 1999). *National Gang Survey of 1996*. Retrieved from: https://www.ncjrs.gov/pdffiles1/173964.pdf. Washington D.C. U.S.Department of Justice.

Peng, An. (2019). *The Unforeseen Directions of Raising Juvenile Court Ages in Massachusetts*. Boston University Statehouse Program. Retrieved from: https://www.telegram.com/news/20190403/unforseen-directions-of-raising-juvenile-court-ages-in-massachusetts

Reader, Hon. W. Don. (1996). The Laws of Unintended Results. *Akron Law Review*, Vol. 29, pages 477–489.

Schuppe, Jon. (8–12–2015). *Pennsylvania Seeks to Close the Books on "Kids for Cash" Scandal*. NBC News article. Retrieved from: https://www.nbcnews.com/news/us-news/pennsylvania-seeks-close-books-kids-cash-scandal-n408666

Scott, Elizabeth, Duell, Natasha, and Steinberg, Laurence. (2018). Brain Development, Social Context, and Justice Policy, *Washington University Journal of Law & Policy*, Vol. 57, pages 13–74.

Scott, Elizabeth S, and Grisso, Thomas. (1997). The Evolution of Adolescence: A Developmental Perspective on Juvenile Justice Reform, *Journal of Criminal Law & Criminology*. Vol. 88, pages 137–189.

Spergel, Irving. (October 1991). *Youth Gangs: Problem and Response.* (National Criminal Justice Reference Service Report). Retrieved from: https://www.ncjrs.gov/txtfiles/d00027.txt.

Spierer, Ariel. (2017). The Right to Remain a Child: The Impermissibility of the REID Technique in Juvenile Interrogations. *New York University Law Review*, Vol. 92:5, pages 1719–1750.

Steinberg, Laurence. (2012). Should the Science of Adolescent Brain Development Inform Public Policy? *Issues in Science and Technology*, Vol. 28, pages 70–76.

Tamilia, Hon. Patrick R. (1996) In Search of Juvenile Justice: From Star Chamber to Criminal Court. *Akron Law Review*, Vol. 29, pages 509–529.

Thomas, J.M. (2017). *Raising the Bar: State Trends in Keeping Youth Out of Adult Courts (2015–2017).* Washington, DC: Campaign for Youth Justice.

U.S. Department of Justice. (1994). Juvenile Crime Facts. Retrieved from: https://www.justice.gov/jm/criminal-resource-manual-102-juvenile-crime-facts

U.S. Department of Justice. (2011). *Trying Juveniles as Adults: An Analysis of State Transfer Laws and Reporting.* (National Reporting Series). Retrieved from: https://www.ncjrs.gov/pdffiles1/ojjdp/232434.pdf

Weir, Kirsten. (2015). Marijuana and the Developing Brain. *Monitor on Psychology.* American Psychological Society. Vol. 46:10, page 48. https://www.apa.org/monitor/2015/11/marijuana-brain

Table of Cases

Ex parte Crouse, 4 Whart. 9 (1839)

Gideon v. Wainwright, 372 U.S. 335 (1963)

Kent v. United States, 383 U.S. 541 (1966)

Miranda v. Arizona, 384 U.S. 436 (1966)

In re: Gault, 387 U.S. 1 (1967)

In re: Winship, 397 U.S. 358 (1970)

McKeiver v. Pennsylvania, 403 U.S. 528 (1971)

Breed v. Jones, 421 U.S. 519 (1975)

Eddings v. Oklahoma, 455 U.S. 104 (1982)

Schall v. Martin, 467 U.S. 253 (1984)

Thompson v. Oklahoma, 487 U.S. 816 (1988)

Stanford v. Kentucky, 492 U.S. 361 (1989)

Penry v. Lynaugh, 492 U.S. 302 (1989)

Atkins v. Virginia, 536 U.S. 304 (2002)

Roper v. Simmons, 543 U.S. 551 (2005)

Graham v. Florida, 560 U.S. 48 (2010)

JDB v. North Carolina, 564 U.S. 261 (2011)

Miller v. Alabama, 567 U.S. 460 (2012)

2 A View from the Bench

Perspectives of a Former Juvenile Court Judge

Marcia Morey

1989: My Time as Prosecutor

I came to juvenile court after two years of doing enforcement work with NCAA. I was charged with investigating colleges and universities suspected of violating provisions of the Association. Traveling the country, I was struck by how frequently the NCAA held the student-athletes accountable for various acts of wrongdoing but so rarely could truly make a dent in the often problematic cultures of big-time of athletics programs. A 17-year-old kid who was treated to dinner by a scout was a much easier target than an athletic director or even a head coach.

Little did I know that this theme – the individualization and punishment of wrongdoing rather than addressing structural problems of a system – would recur throughout my time in the juvenile court.

In 1989, the Durham County District Attorney hired me to work as an assistant district attorney. Here's my memory of the interview. Interested in my Olympic swimming[i] and NCAA experience, he asked: "You got any trial experience?" Me: "None." Durham DA: "Ever worked with kids?" Me: "No." Durham DA. "Do you have any kids?" Me: "No." Durham DA: "You like kids?" Me: "They're ok." I was hired and assigned to juvenile court.

An Undervalued Institution

While this assignment may seem surprising given my singular lack of experience; in fact, there is a long tradition of sending the most inexperienced prosecutors and defense attorneys to juvenile court. I was told "kiddie court" was where I was being sent to learn the ropes. Once I got some experience, they assured me, I would move on to prosecute adults in criminal cases in "real" court. In other words, juvenile court was the lowest rung on the ladder for new lawyers –a dumping ground (Sanborn, J.B. Jr. (2000), 1 Barry L. Rev. 7, 40) at worst, and, if one was reasonably competent, a launching pad toward something more visible and more prestigious.

Why is juvenile court so devalued? Partly it has to do with its history. Child advocates, social workers mostly, created the juvenile court in late 19th century Chicago (Fedders, B., 2010 in 14 Lewis & Clark L. Rev. 771; Tanenhaus, D.S., 2004) They were troubled that children were tried and jailed with adults. These advocates envisioned a separate, and different, system for juveniles that would be informal and flexible, with all parties focused on the child's best interest and rehabilitation. Recent historical scholarship (Feld, B.C., 1999; Ward, G., 2012; Butler, C.N., 2013) complicates the narrative of juvenile court architects as "child savers." This work notes that law-and-order impulses were also predominant: law enforcement was tired of being unable to get convictions against young people in adult court because of perceptions that judges were lenient. Anti-immigrant fears meant that

DOI: 10.4324/9780429397806-3

elected officials wanted an institution that could get immigrant youths off the street. Once created, juvenile court was not equally accessible to all youths – a separate and inferior system existed for Black youth through the Jim Crow era. In all events, the court was as much meant to function as a social-welfare institution as it was to adjudicate crime.

The vocabulary of the juvenile court that evolved from these various perspectives reflected this distinctive mission. Instead of "complaints" or "indictments," charging documents were phrased "in the welfare of the child." Rather than verdicts of "guilty," youths would be found "delinquent." Instead of "sentences," youths received "dispositions." As one commentator put it, "[t]he reformers' aim was to protect children from the law, not to bring more law to bear on them (Sutton, J.R., 1988). In short, the juvenile court was ideally to act as would a "kind and just parent" (Ayers, W., 1997).

The Supreme Court's decision in *in re Gault* (387 U.S. 1 (1967)) instituted due process protections the right to notice of the charges, the right to counsel, the right to confrontation and cross-examination, and the privilege against self-incrimination. Subsequent cases established that the Double Jeopardy Clause would apply in delinquency prosecutions (*In re* Winship (397 U.S. 358 (1970)) and that cases needed to be proved against juveniles beyond a reasonable doubt (Breed v Jones (421 U.S. 519 (1975)). But the juvenile court has never lost its "best interests" overlay; nor has it shed its rehabilitative aspirations. Indeed, the Court in Gault made explicit that due process could co-exist with the unique, putatively benevolent aspirations of the juvenile court. It held that

> [w]hile due process requirements will, in some instances, introduce a degree of order and regularity to Juvenile Court proceedings to determine delinquency, and in contested cases will introduce some elements of the adversary system, nothing will require that the conception of the kindly juvenile judge be replaced by its opposite, nor do we here rule upon the question whether ordinary due process requirements must be observed with respect to hearings to determine the disposition of the delinquent child.
>
> (In re Gault, 387 U.S. 1, 16)

For many lawyers, the perceived social work nature of juvenile court is a turnoff. Legal education tends to stress certain skills – incisive cross-examination, erudite oral advocacy, sophisticated legal argumentation in briefs – over the so-called "soft skills" of interviewing, counseling, negotiation, collaboration, and using developmentally appropriate language and techniques that are necessary in juvenile court (Fedders, B., 2010). In reality, these perceived differences are somewhat overstated: in both juvenile *and* criminal court, plea bargaining dominates proceedings (Yoffe, E., 2017) and in both forums, astute counseling is important and sometimes constitutionally required (Reimer, N.L., 2012). Still, the pre-*Gault* understanding that juvenile court is paternalistic and thus requires less a lawyer than a social worker or parent figure long has deterred lawyers from embracing juvenile court practice.

The social-work label of juvenile court sticks in part because of the portion of the docket devoted to what we call in North Carolina "undisciplined" cases – known elsewhere as CHINS (Child in Need of Services) or PINS (Person in Need of Services). These are status offenses – misbehavior that makes a person subject to court jurisdiction only because of the age of the person who allegedly commits them. So, for example, if a child is missing curfew consistently, or skipping school, or just "beyond the control of the parent," (N.C.G.S. §7B-1501 (2019)) a school official or parent can initiate proceedings in juvenile court (Id). If a court finds that a child has done any of these things, the court can place the child on what is known as "protective supervision" for a defined period and order a series of restrictions on the child's liberty. Such restrictions might include things like remaining on good behavior, attending school regularly, getting passing grades, keeping to a curfew, and reporting to a court counselor (N.C.G.S. §7B-2504 (2012)).

At first blush, these requirements might not seem like a big deal, and might even seem to be good for a child. But that seemingly intuitive response ignores three things: first, much of what constitutes a status offense is developmentally typical misbehavior out of which a child is mostly likely to eventually grow; second, more severe risk-taking and misbehavior may be a symptom of a deeper problem – a learning disability or trauma history, for example – that is better addressed through the education, mental health, or child welfare systems and third and finally, court intervention for minor misbehavior may sometimes make problems worse through making youth feel stigmatized. Indeed, one meta-analysis found that youth whose technically illegal but still minor misconduct fared no better with juvenile court intervention than without (Gatti, U., 2008.) As with delinquency cases, racial and ethnic disparities exist in undisciplined proceedings; it seems that even the most well-intentioned juvenile court reforms cannot ameliorate the bias that pervades the juvenile court.

Nonetheless, in undisciplined cases, just as in delinquency cases, throughout my time in the prosecutor's office and in fact nationwide until recently, I found that most system actors believed that juvenile court intervention was at worst an appropriate consequence for antisocial behavior and, at best, a response consisting of services and supports that a child was actually fortunate to receive. Like my colleagues, I truly believed that the juvenile court was a place to reform wayward youth – hearkening back to our pre-*Gault*, "kind and just parent" forbears – and expose them to help to which they would otherwise not be entitled. In other words, we all thought we were helping. So, even for young people who found themselves in court for extremely minor misbehavior – shoplifting, say, or pushing someone on the playground – we could justify a prosecution on the grounds that the consequences, like the children, were minor.

The Age of the "Superpredator"

As soon as I got into the prosecutor's office, I realized that, contrary to what I'd been told, juvenile court *was* real court. And I had real power. Discretion is one of the most important parts of a prosecutor's toolbox, and I was determined to use mine wisely (Marowitz, P.L., 2017). With minimal statutory and constitutional constraints, I was empowered to decide whether to dismiss charges, recommend pre-hearing detention, and suggest terms of disposition. In one area, however, I was not free to use my discretion. I was discouraged from engaging in plea bargaining. Thus, any law-breaking behavior that *could* constitute a felony, in my office, was in fact be charged and prosecuted as such. A kid who took his mother's credit card and made unauthorized charges at a video game store, for example, would be charged with felonious larceny. Similarly, kids were not to be given the "break" of having multiple counts consolidated into one. If the allegation was that 25 mailboxes were vandalized, 25 separate petitions would be taken out, one for each count of injury to personal property. I was told by my superiors and colleagues that young people would draw problematic lessons from being allowed to plead their cases down from a felony to a misdemeanor.

The reason for this tough-on-crime approach to charging and resolution of cases? Despite the rehabilitative trappings of the juvenile court, this time period was the beginning of the era of the "superpredator" (Equal Justice Initiative, 2014). In 1995, Princeton political scientist John Dilulio Jr. coined this racially coded term, warning of a coming wave of "feral youths devoid of impulse control or remorse" who are "fatherless, Godless, and jobless" (Birckhead, T., 2017). He predicted that the number of juveniles in custody would increase threefold in the coming years and that, by 2010, there would be "an estimated 270,000 more young predators on the streets than in 1990" (Equal Justice Initiative, 2014). Criminologist James Fox joined in the rhetoric, saying publicly, "Unless we act today, we're going to have a bloodbath when these kids grow up" (Scott, E. and L. Steinberg, 2003). These predictions set off a flurry of legislative activity designed to make the prosecution of young people more punishing. Between 1992 and 1999, dozens of states passed laws that made it easier for prosecutors to try children as adults (Birckhead, 2017, at 409). Media outlets piled on; crime coverage grew increasingly racialized and biased, publicizing images of Black youth in shackles to exploit fears and sell newspapers.

In Durham, a turning point occurred in 1993. That year, a 13-year-old boy named Gregory used an ax to murder his 90-year-old neighbor. He had raked leaves for this woman and noticed her car parked in the garage one evening. He broke the front door windowpane, entered the house, and then demanded the woman's car keys. When she refused, he killed her; he drove her car for three days around Durham. The case landed on my docket. At the time, North Carolina law did not allow for transfer of juveniles under the age of 14 to the adult system. The public was outraged and picked up the "adult time for adult crime" mantra that was sweeping the country (Levick, M., 2017).

The next year, the General Assembly moved swiftly, creating legislation that anyone charged with a homicide crime as young as 13 would mandatorily be prosecuted in adult court and considered as an adult for any subsequent felony offenses (N.C.G.S, §7B-2200) At the same time, children as young as 13 could, after a hearing initiated by the DA's office, be transferred to adult court for any felony (N.C.G.S., §7B-2200).

The predicted crime wave never materialized. There *was* a spike in the lethality of violence in the mid-1990s, but that was attributable as much to the easy availability of firearms as any other factor (N.C.G.S., §7B-2200 at 408). As an assistant prosecutor, I recall that in just one week I once transferred five juveniles to adult court on armed robbery and attempted murder. Perhaps predictably, treating kids as adults didn't work as proponents of the transfer law had hoped. For example, I recall one 14 year-old who was transferred to adult court on a murder charge. Likely because of his comparatively small stature, and immaturity, the Superior Court judge approved a deal in which he plead guilty to involuntary manslaughter and received probation. Judges accustomed to dealing with grown men and women, often with lengthy records, treated young people less punitively but, problematically in my view, as an afterthought. The 14-year-old who pled to manslaughter didn't get any of the services or treatment he would have received had he been sent to one of our state's training schools which, while certainly imperfect, were better than getting nothing on probation. Tragically, this young man killed someone else just two years after his first transfer.

The Punitive Tide Begins to Turn

It gradually became clear to me that the hammer of juvenile transfer laws and no-plea-bargaining positions made too many issues seem like nails. In other words, it just couldn't be that all wrongdoing by kids required a tough and punitive approach. Something new was required. In 1994, I worked with local stakeholders to form the Durham County Teen Court. (Durham County Teen Court & Restitution Program, http://durhamteencourt. org/). Teen court is an alternative system of justice for middle and high school students who are first-time alleged offenders. It was the first such diversionary program in the state (and second in the nation) for first-time youthful offenders charged with misdemeanors.

The idea was to hold young people accountable for what they did, yet at the same time to provide them with a process outside the traditional juvenile court delinquency proceeding that might spare them the stigma and collateral consequences of a delinquency adjudication. A jury of their adolescent and teen peers hands out consequences like community service. The process exposes youth – both the jurors and the participants – to other volunteer judges and lawyers in a courthouse setting that is nonthreatening. The idea is to let kids know that they can be the authors of their fate rather than just having things happen to them. I am proud that the program is still running, and that it has in fact spread to other counties. At the national level, things were beginning to soften a bit as well. The lethality of the crime spike of the 1990s levelled off. Arrest rates began to go down. The crack cocaine epidemic subsided. Between 2003 and 2013 (the most recent data available), the rate of youth committed to juvenile facilities after an adjudication of delinquency fell by 47%. Every state witnessed a drop in its commitment rate, including 19 states where the commitment rates fell by more than half. It took longer for the laws and policies generated from this overheated rhetoric to change – but that eventually began to happen, too.

In 1997, perhaps the apex of punitive rhetoric and policies, North Carolina governor James B. Hunt created a Commission on Juvenile Crime and Justice. This move occurred fresh on the heels of the case that spurred the changing of the law that made juvenile transfer to adult court mandatory in first-degree murder cases and discretionary in other felonies for youths as young as 13. The Crime Commission had made unsettling projections about what was likely to happen in North Carolina, which mirrored those of Dilulio and other academics and prognosticators. One prediction was that violent juvenile crime was going to increase more than 146% in the coming decade. Governor Hunt, a Democrat, was one of many elected officials for whom being, and seeming, tough on crime was a political boon. This phenomenon has long been bipartisan; there's long been little downside politically to being tough on crime (Beckett, K. and T. Sasson, 2004). In fact, part of his campaign platform had been a pledge to "stop the punks and thugs" (Weaver, C., 2016).

I agreed to serve on the Commission, but did so on the condition that the governor come to juvenile court himself so that he could see the reality beneath the rhetoric. I wanted him to see the faces of the kids. To hear their stories. Looking at those kids, listening to accounts of their lives, I myself had begun to learn things that no prior work or life experience had taught me – about generational poverty, trauma, and learning disabilities that went undiagnosed or poorly managed.

Within one hour of sitting in a juvenile courtroom, the governor saw enough to change his mind about the system being populated by punks and thugs. During that time, three kids were sent to what were then known colloquially as "training schools," the end of the line for the juvenile delinquency system – essentially prison for young people. In 1997, we had 1,500 commitments. Under the existing juvenile delinquency code, a court could send kids to training school no matter the offense of which they were proven delinquent or undisciplined. Kids went to training school for running away, smoking marijuana, skipping school. This near-lawlessness was facilitated not only by the politics of the time but also by more mundane facts about juvenile court. For one, courtrooms were not open to the public. The idea was that closing courts meant more confidentiality for kids, but the reality was that this lack of transparency enabled the worst and most punitive excesses of prosecutors and judges.

The Juvenile Code at the time gave enormous discretion to judges in terms of dispositions. Third, the defense bar largely subscribed to the notion shared by all other actors, namely, that they should act not according to what the child wanted, or even to achieve the least restrictive alternative, but instead to further children's best interests, however amorphously defined and susceptible to race and class bias this standard turned out to be (Fedders, B., 2010). "Best interest" thinking has long had a hold on defense attorneys, for a variety of reasons, not least of which was the lack of authoritative guidance from courts about exactly whose interests an attorney should serve (Fedders, B., 2010). Today, despite the fact that the academic and professional consensus is that the "expressed interests" of the child are what a juvenile defense attorney ought to pursue (Fedders, B., 2010), defense attorneys continue to act according to what they, the court counselor, or a child's parents deem best.

The governor had his mind changed that day about what needed to happen in juvenile court, why, and by whom. The next year, I joined the Commission. We revamped the entire code. We created a sentencing grid to hem in judicial discretion about which children were eligible for the most restrictive dispositions. We proposed – and got – legislative changes that required parental attendance in court and involvement in their children's dispositions. We also added language making clear that the juvenile court had as part of its mission not only public safety but also the provision of uniform procedures to assure fairness and equity. We wanted to decrease the number of kids pulled out of their homes and sent to institutions, improve public safety, and stop spending inordinate amounts of taxpayer money on a system that seemed unmoored from best practices. In short, we sought to make the promises of the pre-*Gault* juvenile court a reality: to be a separate, gentler institution for youthful wrongdoing that could more successfully rehabilitate children than the criminal system. We wanted, as well, to implement reforms that would ensure the due process protections that *Gault* mandated would be observed. Having both goals in mind was important. During my time on the Crime Commission, juvenile crime rates were reduced by approximately 40%. There are multiple reasons for explanations social scientists give to the rise and fall of crime rates.

Ascent to the Bench

In 1999, Governor Hunt appointed me to the district court bench in Durham. Juvenile court had not risen in the esteem of most system actors since my time as an assistant district attorney. As a result, it was not difficult to quickly win a rotation into the juvenile court. For me, it quickly felt like the work I had been born to do.

My vantage point as a judge gave me new insight into the myriad ways that bureaucracies – and bureaucrats – fail children. Perhaps I should be clearer. Bureaucracies and those who staff them repeatedly fail *poor* children – which is who overwhelmingly populates our juvenile courts (Birckhead, T., 2012). Whereas as a prosecutor I tended to think of alleged criminal wrongdoing as the result of individual bad thoughts and actions, I began to see how crime converged with a host of other structural factors.

My sense as a prosecutor that juvenile court was a dumping ground for inexperienced lawyers took on new meaning as I got my feet under me as a judge. I gradually came to see how other systems used juvenile court as a dumping ground for their tough-to-handle kids. In public schools, for example, overworked teachers might push administrators or school police to file petitions against misbehaving students (Fedders, B., 2016). While it might be the case that those students had in fact broken the law – they pushed someone on the playground (assault) or took a classmate's ear buds (larceny) or had a loud meltdown in the hallway (disorderly conduct) – the decision to file delinquency charges rather than to handle it in the school felt to me like a result of insufficient resources in the school (Fedders, B., 2016).

Sometimes, unfortunately, it seemed that the schools were sending kids to court because they had given up on them. Indeed, it was around this time that the idea that there was a school-to-prison pipeline for Black and brown kids, along with low-income kids, started to gain traction (Advancement Project, 2016). The language of the War on Drugs was imported into schools, as administrations began to impose "zero tolerance" disciplinary consequences for myriad infractions (Advancement Project, 2016). Once suspended from school, a child faced a host of adverse consequences. High suspension rates correlate with low academic achievement and an increased likelihood of dropping out, which in turn is linked to a higher chance of involvement in the criminal system (Advancement Project, 2016).

Along with schools, the child welfare system often didn't seem to step up to show investment in the kids in their care, preferring instead to shunt "difficult" kids into juvenile court. The North Carolina Juvenile Code provides that, when a judge is taking a child into custody pending resolution of her case, she has as a placement option a foster home or other facility operated by DSS (N.C.G.S. 7B_1905). Despite this provision, DSS would often appear in court to oppose "having" to take a child into care. At the same time, DSS caseworkers for kids who were already in their care would with some frequency appear at court dates and argue for very restrictive dispositions, always on the ground that the child "needed" it but often, it seemed to me, to make their jobs easier. They reasoned, sometimes correctly, that a child who failed at probation would be committed to a detention or commitment facility, thus greatly lessening the amount of work they needed to put into their cases.

Perhaps the biggest system problem I saw as a juvenile court judge was the privatization of mental health that occurred in North Carolina in 2001. That year, the General Assembly passed a law requiring local jurisdictions to bifurcate management of mental health services from the service delivery. Before the law's passage, regional and county agencies delivered mental health services through the direct employment of care providers. The 2001 law required local management entities (LMEs) to contract with private providers (North Carolina Mental Health System, 2012). Austerity cost-control measures also meant that it seemed that the right treatment was never available for long enough. Kids would be ordered to therapy but have to wait weeks and sometimes months for the referral to go through. Or they would be cut off after three months. Or the therapist would leave, frustrated by the low pay that resulted from the various law changes to mental health.

Initially, it seemed that I had limited ability to affect these systemic issues. Many judges speak of themselves as just "calling balls and strikes"; in other words, as refereeing and adjudicating disputes, but not really having any power to change the game. To some extent, they are right – separation of powers doctrines and institutional expertise mean that there are limits on how involved a judge can get in matters unrelated to the specific case before her.

As time went on, however, I grew to appreciate how I could hold individuals to account *other* than just kids. Instead of just, for example, finding a kid in violation of probation for failing all of her classes, I could subpoena in someone from the school to find out why no one had ever suggested that she be evaluated pursuant to the provisions of the Individuals with Disabilities Education Act. Instead of just adjudicating a kid delinquent for the offense of resisting arrest, I could on my own ask the testifying officer why he had approached her in the first place. Rather than simply acquiesce to multiple continuance requests from the state for more time while a child languished in detention awaiting trial, I could demand that they proceed or dismiss the case. Juvenile court can feel like being stuck in peanut butter underwater – it has a culture of its own, things can drag on, kids may come back multiple times, court counselors keep doing the same things over and over. Sometimes the only person who could shake things up was a judge, and I did so more and more as I got more experience. The importance of not just agreeing to more time for the state was brought home to me in one case that I remember vividly still today. A child charged as a juvenile sex offender was awaiting a placement in a treatment facility. The Department of Juvenile Delinquency and Prevention had already asked for two continuances because they said they had been unable to find an appropriate placement. After the second request, I learned from the child's defense attorney that he had tried to commit suicide. Weeks had gone by and no placement had been found. I brought in everyone involved for a contempt of court hearing, at which I demanded to know how the lapse in communication had happened, and why the child was continuing to be held at all.

I also came to understand more and more the unique convening power that judges have to help make systems change for the betterment of children (Teske, S.C., et al., 2012). As people who have and, importantly, are *seen as having* community-wide legitimacy, juvenile court judges can get people to the table to discuss what they should all have in common – how to improve outcomes for kids. We can invite school officials, people from mental health, representative from child welfare, law enforcement officers, community-based program representatives, and parents to come in and talk with each other to try to develop jointly arrived at solutions that all stakeholders will feel invested in. That's the best way to get buy-in from everybody involved.

Here's one example. North Carolina was the last state in the nation to raise the maximum age of juvenile court jurisdiction (Powell, L., 2017). The reader can access additional information about the "raise the age" legislation in the chapter by Mary Wilson, J.D., that appears in this book. Despite the fact that *Roper vs. Simmons* and its progeny had declared what all of us who work with kids know – that they are more impulsive, more susceptible to peer pressure, and have less well-developed characters than adults – the North Carolina legislature had steadfastly refused to treat kids as kids. Sitting in adult district court, the ridiculousness of this policy was made clear time and time again. Once, I had to oversee the prosecution of a 16-year-old girl who was cited for littering. She didn't come to court because, like many teenagers, she was maybe slightly disorganized and lost the citation. Or she read it and didn't understand its significance. The prosecutor asked for and had gotten a $500 bond. The sheriff picked her up on a warrant and brought her to court in handcuffs. When I asked her if she knew why she was there, she was utterly befuddled. When I explained it, she exclaimed, "this is stupid!"

Because I did not and could not disagree with her, I decided in 2013 to stop waiting for the legislature to do the right thing in terms of 16 and 17 year-olds. I convened the sheriff, chief of police, District Attorney, chief public defender, and a host of community-based organizations to create the Misdemeanor Diversion Program (MDP). The idea behind MDP was similar to the juvenile teen court, which I had helped create nearly 20 years earlier. Prior to any charges being filed, an officer would start a referral to a coordinator stationed at the court. With the consent of the parent, a 16- or 17-year-old who would otherwise have been prosecuted for a series of misdemeanors would instead come to court for a mock trial. The teen would then be "sentenced" to some work that would help his community and, once he completed it, the case would be over. He would thereby escape having any record of his wrongdoing anywhere whatsoever.

Race

Durham is the site of a long and proud history of Black activism and civil rights advocacy, often leading the way in desegregation efforts and other progressive reforms (*New York Times*, 1971). After initially resisting the order of *Brown vs. Board of Education* that schools were to desegregate "with all deliberate speed," public school districts in the South eventually became, in the wake of a series of Supreme Court opinions in the late 1960s and early 1970s, home to the nation's most desegregated public schools (Wilson, E., 2016). In 1969, Black students occupied Duke University to demand a series of reforms, including the creation of an African American Studies department. In 1971, the visionary Ann Atwater, chronicled in the film *The Best of Enemies*, was able to see beyond the virulently racist beliefs and past of a Ku Klux Klan member and make an alliance with him in order to further school desegregation efforts begun by *Brown*. Today, Durham boasts one of the most progressive city governments in the country in terms of affordable housing development and criminal justice reform (Gullapalli, V., 2019).

Notwithstanding this tradition of civil rights activism, dramatic racial and ethnic disparities exist in the juvenile court population in Durham – as they do nearly everywhere. These disparities begin at arrest or citation and intensify throughout the process. Cases that arise out of misbehavior in school comprise nearly half of most delinquency dockets. Youth of color remain far more likely to be committed than white youth. Between 2003 and 2013, for example, the racial gap between Black and white youth in secure commitment increased by 15%.

In thinking about racial disparity, the old adage about fish comes to mind.

> There are these two young fish swimming along and they happen to meet an older fish swimming the other way, who nods at them and says "Morning, boys. How's the water?" And the two young fish swim on for a bit, and then eventually one of them looks over at the other and goes "What the hell is water?"

In other words, it can be darned hard to even recognize where racial disparity begins, much less what accounts for it or how to end it. Inequity is the literal water in which juvenile court system actors swim. Racial disparities persist even amidst otherwise encouraging trends. Despite the fact that detention, prosecutions, and commitments have decreased, the racial disparities seemingly endemic to the juvenile justice system have not improved. While we have gotten more comfortable talking about racial bias and racism, we are much less good at committing to fix it. Here too, though, I learned over time to ask tough questions of the state and its witnesses to try to push back against the disproportionate prosecution of Black and brown kids. Even though we know that smoking marijuana is terrible for the developing teen brain – and I did what I could in fashioning dispositions to get kids to stop smoking it – I was frequently frustrated by the fact that so many Black kids were in court for possession of marijuana. How did they get found out in the first place? Hard to avoid the conclusion that racial profiling had something to do with it. And why couldn't school officials or even police officers do something *besides* initiate a court case to deal with it? I knew of friends and colleagues with kids in private school who told me about kids caught *selling* their parents' anti-anxiety drugs, or their own ADHD drugs, in school to classmates. While those kids might face school discipline, they would *never* be in court. The difference? Schools, police, child welfare, prosecutors, us judges – all of us have been guilty at one time or another of thinking that while *some* kids get to make mistakes, learn from them, get slapped on the wrist, but still be entitled to the bright future that seems their birthright, *other* kids need to be taught a lesson through a court case. And, sadly, even in 2019, which kid gets a break is still all too often based on the color of his skin.

Epilogue

My time on the juvenile court bench was instructive, enraging, and humbling. I saw first-hand the enormity of structural challenges that young alleged delinquents face. I was frustrated by how shredded our social safety net has become. The meager resources we could offer were never enough. Even though I could see they had their own challenges, parents sometimes hurt more than they helped, throwing up their hands and trying to turn their kids over to the system. Sometimes, thinking they were doing the right thing, they urged their kids to confess to crimes – even ones they didn't commit. Some days, it felt like I couldn't get through to anybody.

But there were other days when the work was worthwhile – it was enormously gratifying to see kids actually grow out of their misbehavior, to start to succeed in school, to come up to the bench and shake my hand after completing probation. Sometimes, we made a difference.

But, with the passage of time, I've come to think that juvenile court should be reserved for only the most serious of crimes – if not abolished altogether. Most of what we hold kids accountable for is either the direct result of poverty, racism, and system failure, or selectively prosecuted based on race or socioeconomic status. Much of what prosecutors and judges do is based not on evidence but on hunches. There's still too much misguided do-gooderism, a sense that if we can only get a kid put on probation then we can "fix" him. But what kids need is not, for the most part, to be found in any delinquency court, no matter how well intentioned and how well run. It's in their homes, their schools, and their communities. We need to invest in *that*.

Because I came to feel that I had done what I could on the bench, I moved in 2017 to the North Carolina General Assembly, in the House of Representatives. I was honored to co-sponsor the "Raise the Age" bill that finally passed. I wanted to work to do what I could to shift financial resources toward those who needed it. To stop the funneling of poor, Black and brown kids into oppressive systems through the creation of evidence-based policies and laws.

It's been, to say the least, another learning experience. The fractiousness that characterizes American politics is so disheartening. Sometimes it feels like an uphill battle that will never end.

But when I think about the challenges facing the kids who I saw on a daily basis as a juvenile court judge, slugging it out with politicians feels like child's play.

Note

i After winning several national and international individual swimming titles, I co-captain ed the 1976 Olympic swimming team. The entire American team performed second to the East Germans, who infamously later were revealed to have been involuntarily doped. The experience was documented in the 2016 movie, "The Last Gold." https://www.swimmingworldmagazine.com/meet/the-last-gold-documentary-world-premiere.

References

Advancement Project. (2016) The Origins of the School to Prison Pipeline. https://americadivided-series.com/wp-content/uploads/2016/08/Divided-One-Pager-PDF.pdf

Ayers, W. (1997) A Kind and Just Parent: The Children of Juvenile Court.

Beckett, K. & Sasson, T. (2nd ed. 2004) The Politics of Injustice: Crime and Punishment in America.

Birckhead, T. (2012) Delinquent by Reason of Poverty, 38 *Wash. U. J.L. & Pol'y* 53, 58–60.

Birckhead, T. (2017) The Racialization of Juvenile Justice and the Role of the Defense Attorney, 58 *B.C. L. Rev.* 379, 409 (2017).

Blakely, S.S. (2014, April 7) Law Firms Shouldn't Overlook the Value of Soft Skills, *ABA Journal*.

Equal Justice Initiative (n.d.) The Superpredator Myth, 20 Years Later. https://eji.org/news/superpredator-myth-20-years-later

Fedders, Barbara (2010) Losing Hold of the Guiding Hand: Ineffective Assistance of Counsel in Juvenile Delinquency Representation, 14 *Lewis & Clark L. Rev.* 771.

Fedders, Barbara (2016) The Anti-Pipeline Collaborative, 51 *Wake Forest L. Rev.* 565.

Feld, Barry C. (1999) Bad Kids: Race and the Transformation of the Juvenile Court.

Gatti, U., (2008) Iatrogenic Effect of Juvenile Justice, 50 *Journal of Child Psychology & Psychiatry* 991

Gullapalli, Vaidya. (2019) Spotlight: A City Says no to More Police, The Appeal (6/10/19) (detailing how Durham City Council refused to greenlight funding for hiring of more police officers in favor of increasing minimum wage for part-time city workers).

In the Public Interest. (2012) "North Carolina Mental Health System". Archived from the original on March 20, 2012.

Levick, M. (2017) Through Rose-Colored Glasses: The Twenty-First Century Juvenile Court, 42 *Hum. Rts.* 23

Markowitz, Peter L. (2017) Prosecutorial Discretion Power at its Zenith, 97 *Boston University Law Review* 489.

Powell, LaToya B. (2017) "Raise the Age" is Now the Law in North Carolina, School of Government (8/31/17).

Reimer, N.L. (2012) Much Ado About What we do and what Prosecutors and Judges Should not Do, The Champion.

Sanborn, Joseph B., Jr., (2000) Striking Out on the First Pitch in Criminal Court, 1 Barry L. Review

Scott, Elizabeth S. & Steinberg, Laurence (2003) Blaming Youth, 81 *Tex. L. Rev.* 799.

Sutton, J.R. (1988) Stubborn Children: Controlling Delinquency in the United States.

Teske, Steven C., Huff, B. & Graves, C. (2012) Collaborative Role of Courts in Promoting Outcomes for Students: The Relationship Between Arrests, Graduation Rates, and School Safety 134 in Keeping Kids in School and out of Courts. https://www.sog.unc.edu/sites/www.sog.unc.edu/files/articles/05-2-Teske_Collaborative%20Role%20of%20Courts_1.pdf

Ward, Geoff (2012) *The Black Child Savers*: Racial Democracy and Juvenile Justice

Weaver, C. (2016) Program Report: Judge Marcia Morey, Rotary Club of Durham (6/18/16) http://durhamrotaryclub.org/2016/06/program-report-judge-marcia-morey

Wilson, E. (2016) The New School Segregation, 102 *Cornell L. Rev.* 139, 151

Yoffe, E. (2017, September) Innocence is Irrelevant, The Atlantic.

Section II
Developmental Variables

3 Children's Memory for Forensically Relevant Experiences

Lynne Baker-Ward, Peter Ornstein, and Taylor E. Thomas

Dora Villanueva returned home from work on March 17, 2012, after receiving three telephone calls from her increasingly distressed boyfriend, Ever Mendez. When she entered the apartment where Mendez was caring for her children, she found her 4-year-old daughter, K. V., staring "zombie like" at the television. Her 2-year-old son, I. V., was cold and did not respond to her attempts to revive him. EMTs transported I. V. to a hospital where he was declared deceased on arrival. Photographs of his body documented multiple injuries.

Later that same day, a Child Advocacy Center interviewer talked with K. V. In response to questions about Mendez' actions, she told him that she saw Mendez kick I. V.'s torso and then she saw I. V die. In his police interview, Mendez admitted striking I. V. but denied using force sufficient to cause his death.

Mendez' trial took place five years later, when K. V. was 9 years old. She testified that she saw Mendez punch I. V. in the stomach after the boy soiled himself and that I. V. did not move or get up. Two pathologists testified that I. V.'s death occurred when his liver split due to blunt force trauma but disagreed about the time of death. The jury convicted Mendez of capital murder of a person under 6 years of age, and he received a mandatory life sentence. Mendez appealed the verdict in 2019. Although a number of technical legal issues were involved, the question of K. V.'s competence to give testimony was central to the challenge of the conviction. Can very young children remember and report events occurring before age 5, or, as argued by an expert witness, do they have very poor memories? Did the initial interviewer's questions, which implied that Mendez attacked I. V., lead K. V. to form false memories? Did some contradictions in K. V.'s testimony call into question her credibility?

This case, *Mendez v. State*, No. 08–17–00076-CR, 2019 Tex. App. LEXIS 3093 (Tex. Ct. App. April 17, 2019) (unpublished), illustrates the centrality of memory development for an understanding of children's legal testimony. A number of factors are clearly involved in children's capabilities in reporting important events they have observed or experienced. It has long been understood, however, that at a fundamental level, children cannot report what they cannot remember (Brainerd & Ornstein, 1991; Ornstein, Gordon, & Baker-Ward, 1992). In this chapter, we examine children's memory within the context of legal proceedings. Our objective is to provide forensic and mental health practitioners with an understanding of basic memory development as well as the contextual and individual difference variables that influence memory performance. Given the relevance to practice, we emphasize the maintenance and change of children's memories over time.

DOI: 10.4324/9780429397806-4

Children's Memory in Legal Proceedings

Witnesses in legal proceedings rely on *episodic memory*, or memory for an event that occurred at a specific time and place. Our episodic memories include such everyday events as car inspections or committee meetings, as well as significant personal experiences that define our identities and constitute our life stories, described as *autobiographical memory* (see Fivush, 2011). Episodic memory contrasts with *semantic memory*, the store of knowledge that an individual possesses, including facts and definitions encoded without the inclusion of contextual information. However, semantic memory is important in forming and maintaining episodic representations. Semantic memory influences the likelihood that specific aspects of an experience are encoded and also impact the nature of the resulting representation in memory, which, in turn, affects the likelihood of the maintenance or distortion of stored information over time (see Baker-Ward, Ornstein, & Principe, 1997). Further, autobiographical memory operates in such a way that information necessary to understand an experience – including knowledge about the self as well as knowledge of events germane to this self-knowledge (see Marsh & Roediger, 2013) – is incorporated automatically. Hence, understanding memory within the context of legal proceedings requires attention to both episodic and semantic representations, as discussed below. Further, both episodic and semantic memory undergo profound developmental change, necessitating an understanding of age-related changes in memory.

The long spans of time often involved in legal proceeding amplify the importance of an understanding of memory for professionals who work with child witnesses. In *Mendez vs. State*, five years transpired between the death of I. V. and the trial of the accused. In other cases, an additional, extensive period may transpire between the alleged occurrence of a crime and a child's disclosure of the experience (e.g., see Alaggia, Collin-Vezina, & Lateef, 2017). Such delays may involve conversations and other naturally occurring interactions that can convey potentially inaccurate information about the events in question. As such, these delays provide not only the likelihood of some forgetting but also increased opportunities for memory distortion and suggestibility. Given the increasing rates of prosecution of cases of child abuse alleged to have occurred years and even decades in the past (i.e., historical child abuse; Connolly, Coburn & Chong, 2017), retention intervals are likely to increase. In an analysis of all felony child abuse cases adjudicated over a four-year period in Los Angeles County, Stolzenberg and Lyon (2014) reported that the average length of time between filing charges and the beginning of a trial was 245 days, and this long "delay interval" most likely will rise. Because clinical assessments and therapy as well as multiple interviews are often involved, questions about memory interference and forgetting are particularly salient when there is an extended delay before going to trial.

It also seems certain that children's capabilities in regulating their own behavior become increasingly important as the retention period increases. Testimony begins with *incidental memory*, with the witness observing or experiencing an event and spontaneously forming a memory for the experience. The child's understanding of the event as it transpires drives this unintentional memory. When the child subsequently responds to questions about the experience, *deliberate memory processes* take over. Children's capabilities in guiding their own memory search and retrieval processes, influenced by their understanding of the purpose of the proceedings and their willingness to cooperate, are increasingly significant factors in their provision of information. Individual differences in intellectual performance, coping, and other variables are relevant at each stage of information processing, but may be particularly significant as the delay interval increases and retrieving material from memory becomes more difficult. The role of the interviewer in applying practices that may compensate in part for a child witness' limitations can thus help to determine the outcome of questioning.

In this chapter, we examine the implications of an understanding of memory and its development for obtaining and evaluating children's testimony. We begin with an overview of the operation of the memory system, followed by a discussion of typical age-related changes in the storage and retrieval of information. Our particular focus is on the status of memory over time, including an examination of distortions that can occur from both naturally occurring processes and deliberate exposure to misinformation. We then explore the impact of the typical characteristics of forensically relevant events, including stress and repeated interviews, on memory performance. Our final section introduces some of the individual differences that are likely to influence children's testimony. Our goal is to provide practitioners with information that can assist them in identifying multiple influences on children's memory from the occurrence of an event to the last formal report of what they witnessed or experienced. Further, we offer recommendations for practices that should help limit memory distortion and support children's provision of useful information.

The Basic Operation of the Memory System

Psychologists agree that remembering reflects the operation of a series of cognitive processes that start with the entry of information in memory and conclude with a report of the remembered experience. The individual's direction of attention and understanding is crucial at the outset, as some but not all information enters memory. What is encoded results in the establishment of memory traces or representations that may vary as a function of many factors, including age. These representations may be affected by a number of experiences that occur while information is in storage, including conversation, rumination, and exposure to inconsistent information. Remembering depends on being able to retrieve information from these memory representations later and then in being able to use culturally determined narrative skills to report the initial experience.

It may be helpful to think of these processes involved in remembering as representing the flow of information through an imperfect and dynamic memory system. In this regard, consider five basic principles that comprise a general characterization of the literature on memory and its development (Gordon, Baker-Ward, & Ornstein, 2001; Ornstein, Larus, & Clubb, 1991):

1 *Not everything gets into memory.* Not every aspect of an event experienced by the individual is encoded into memory. Attention and knowledge-based expectations determine the information that is represented in memory, and aspects of an experience that do not receive attention will not be entered into memory (e.g., Mack & Rock, 1998).

2 *The representation of information in memory varies in strength.* Information about an encoded experience is said to "reside" in storage in a representation or trace. However, the strength of the trace (or the coherence of the representation) typically increases with development (see Baker-Ward et al., 1997).

3 *The status of information in memory varies over time.* Memory representations are not static, but rather are subject to change as a function of time and subsequent experiences. With the passage of time, memory representations may decay and become more difficult to retrieve subsequently. In addition, what happens as time passes is of critical importance for the survival – or the modification – of a memory representation. Naturally occurring conversations with others, misleading questioning, and exposure to similar events can alter the memory representation (e.g., Principe, Turnbull, Gardner, Van Horn, & Dean, 2017; Brubacher, Glisic, Roberts, & Power, 2011).

4 *Not everything in memory is retrieved.* According to this consensus view of the operation of memory, remembering involves searching through the memory system. However, not everything that has been encoded and placed in memory storage can be "found"

at any one point in time, and thus retrieval is often quite imperfect. In general, the search strategies used by older children and adults, in comparison to those of young individuals, are more effective, with corresponding benefits for the retrieval process.

5 *Not everything that is retrieved is reported.* Successfully searching memory is, of course, necessary for the final step of reporting on one's experiences. However, not everything that is recovered during the search process is reported, as both children and adults can make decisions concerning whether or not to "go public" with what they have remembered. This may be particularly relevant in some abuse situations in which young witnesses do not disclose what they have retrieved because of embarrassment, fear, or other reasons.

Following an overview of the typical course of memory development, we examine each of these general principles in detail and explore their implications for understanding memory performance among child witnesses.

Age-Related Changes in Children's Memory

The emergence of children's abilities to remember past events occurs in early childhood. Innovative research involving nonverbal measures of memory highlights the remarkable abilities of infants to encode, store, and retrieve information about their previous experiences over increasingly long periods of time (Rovee-Collier, 1997; Bauer, 1996). For example, under some conditions, newborns can recognize voices and passages that they heard while in utero (DeCasper & Spence, 1986). Infants, moreover, are able to reproduce a series of actions (e.g., assembling a gong) that an experimenter previously modeled (Bauer, 1996). Successful reproduction of these action sequences among 13-month-olds occurs even after delays of eight months (Bauer, Hertsgaard, & Dow, 1994). However, because of the nonverbal nature of the information "reported" during these elicited recall tasks, this early memory capability has limited forensic relevance.

The capacity to remember and report verbally information about personal experiences emerges in the early preschool years. Children's delayed reports of events that transpired before they could talk are "sparse and/or riddled with errors" (Brubacher, Peterson, La Rooy, Dickinson, & Poole, 2019, p. 74). However, as soon as they can talk, children verbally encode and subsequently report their experiences. Decades of research by Robyn Fivush and her colleagues (e.g., see Fivush, 2011) have established that even 2-year-old children can provide accurate information in response to specific questions about recent, everyday experiences. Nonetheless, substantial development occurs across the preschool and early elementary school years (see Gordon et al., 2001). By age three, children can typically respond to general, open-ended prompts ("Tell me what happened at Will's house"), as well as probes for specific event components and yes/no questions. However, in contrast to the recall of even 5-year-old children, the amount of information that preschoolers provide in response to general questions is quite limited. Across the elementary school years, children generate increasingly extensive reports that include descriptive details and elaboration of the actions reported. Moreover, after middle childhood, event memory development corresponds largely to the acquisition of narrative skill. Early adolescents can provide coherent narratives describing their experiences, in that they convey information about the context in which the event occurred, report the order in which actions transpired, and include their thoughts and feelings about the events (Reese, Haden, Baker-Ward, Bauer, Fivush, & Ornstein, 2011).

An early investigation in our laboratory (Baker-Ward, Gordon, Ornstein, Larus, & Clubb, 1993) documented changes in children's event memory across the preschool through early elementary school years and serves to illustrate a method used to investigate children's event memory. This age span was of interest in part because of questions regarding young children's abilities to testify in legal proceedings and the importance of their reports in proceedings involving questions of abuse. In this investigation, we chose to examine children's memory for the components of a routine pediatric examination. Studies of children's recall of medically-related experiences provide a unique platform for characterizing children's memory, as the events under consideration (i.e., medical visits involving an adult touching of a child's body) are similar in some regards to events about which children are asked to testify (i.e., sexual abuse). The verifiable knowledge of what occurs during each physical examination also permitted us to assess directly children's retention of event-related information over time, as well as the accuracy of their reports.

At each age level, the children were interviewed twice, first immediately after their check-ups and then again after a delay of one, three, or six weeks. The interviews made use of a structured protocol designed to assess memory for the various component features of the physical examination. Beginning with open-ended probes (e.g., "Tell me what happened during your check-up."), the examiner continued with more specific questions (e.g., "Did the doctor check any parts of your face?"), and then moved on to yes/no questions about features that had not yet been volunteered (e.g., "Did she [he] check your eyes?"). The children also responded to potentially misleading yes/no questions about activities not included in the check-ups. Overall, the findings indicated that young children's reports of a salient event can be quite impressive, with recall averaging approximately 83% of the component features of the physical examination. Nonetheless, there were striking age-related changes in various aspects of memory performance. In contrast to the older children, the 3-year-olds showed lower levels of overall recall, greater dependency on yes-no types of questions, more forgetting, and a reduced ability to differentiate between activities that had and had not been included in their medical check-ups. The performance of the 5-year-olds was midway between that of the 3- and 7-year-olds.

Based on research documenting preschoolers' memory capabilities, most psychologists would not question 4-year-old K. V.'s capability in providing information about her brother's death earlier in the day, as described in the case summary that opened this chapter. But would such a young child retain even the most important component of this memory over a period of five years, the interval between the death and the trial in *Mendez*? Psychoanalytically-oriented psychologists once believed that adults and even older children would be unlikely to recall events that took place before they were 2 to 4 years of age or even older (see Pillemer, 1998, for review). This phenomenon was referred to as *childhood amnesia* or *infantile amnesia*. Researchers subsequently established that memories for some very early experiences persist into adulthood, although there is a relative paucity of memories from early childhood among adults' recollections (Peterson, 2002), especially memories of events that transpired before age 2 (Aktar, Justice, Morrison, & Conway, 2018). Moreover, longitudinal research examining children's long-term retention of highly salient events clearly establishes the persistence of children's memories. Notably, Peterson (2015) examined 39 adolescents' recall of a salient injury that occurred more than a decade earlier, when most of the participants were between 3 and 5 years old. On average, the participants recalled 70% of the components of the injury, as identified shortly after it occurred, and additionally provided 45 unique details. Although accuracy decreased somewhat over time, the adolescents correctly reported about 85% of the components and unique details.

Additional prospective analyses have identified characteristics of early memories that can predict whether these memories would survive over time. In one investigation (Morris, Baker-Ward, & Bauer, 2010), 4-, 6-, and 8-year-old children reported personal experiences (e.g., family outings) initially and after a delay of one year. Breadth of content in the initial report, based on the children's responses to directed probes (e.g., who was there? where was the event?) did not predict the survivability of the memory over the year. However, the thematic coherence of the initial report added to the prediction of survivability of the memory, over and above the contribution of the child's age. Using a similar approach, Peterson and colleagues (Peterson, Morris, Baker-Ward, & Flynn, 2014) examined the survivability of children's earliest memories over a two-year interval. The inclusion of emotion terms in the initial memory report and each of three measures of narrative coherence added to the prediction of the survival of the memory after age was in the model. However, the presence of reminders (e.g. photos) of the event, the category (e.g., outing, injury) and the uniqueness of the experience and the word count of the report did not contribute to the prediction. Narratives that are more coherent are likely to have a stronger representation in memory (see Baker-Ward et al., 1997). As examined below, emotion contributes to the distinctiveness of an experience and hence its memorability.

The depiction of children's changing abilities to remember presented in this section draws primarily on research conducted in supportive contexts. However, as discussed below, the setting, the characteristics of the events under discussion, and the interviewers' behavior strongly affect the depiction of children's competence that can emerge.

Context Specificity

As summarized above, empirical work on the development of children's memory highlights rapid changes across early childhood in children's abilities to remember and report events from the personal past. That said, it is nonetheless important to emphasize that estimates of children's memory skills must be viewed as "context specific" such that our assessments of these abilities can vary markedly as a function of both the nature of the event being remembered and the conditions prevailing at the time of assessment (e.g., Ornstein, Baker-Ward, & Naus, 1988; Ornstein & Myers, 1996). Concerning the nature of the event, it is necessary to consider, among other things, both the knowledge (and hence understanding) that the child brings to the experience as well as the arousal and/or stress that may be elicited. In this regard, consider differences in children's abilities to understand, encode, and process experiences that are associated with events that are relatively benign, familiar, and easily understood, on the one hand, and those that are novel, not well understood, and stressful, on the other. As will be discussed below, prior knowledge and stress are both associated with remembering, but the linkages are complex, such that the correlations are sometimes positive and sometimes negative. The key point, however, is that our impressions of children's memory skills can differ substantially as they are linked to features of the event being remembered.

Given that children do not retrieve and report everything that has been encoded and stored in memory, the context in which memory is probed is critically important for children's remembering (Ornstein, 1991; Ornstein & Myers, 1996). Assessment contexts can differ considerably in terms of the supports for information retrieval that they provide, thus affecting the conclusions we reach about children's memory capabilities. Most fundamentally, optimal performance depends on the child and the interviewer having shared expectations about just what it means to provide information about a previous experience. If, for example, a child assumes that an adult interviewer is already knowledgeable about the event under discussion, he or she may not provide a complete report. In addition, the physical characteristics of the context in which a child is interviewed can also affect information retrieval and the content of a child's memory report. To illustrate, settings vary considerably in the extent to which they contain environmental cues that can reinstate the original context in which an event was experienced and thus enhance recall. Most importantly, the nature of the questions that are posed to a child have a dramatic effect on retrieval and reporting and thus on the "cognitive diagnosis" that we make about his or her abilities. For example, as discussed above, there are clear age differences in the extent to which children can respond effectively to open-ended memory probes, with younger children providing reports that are less complete than those of older children. Including more specific yes-no types of probes can facilitate the performance of younger children, but the practice carries with it some interpretive problems because these probes can be answered correctly 50% of the time. Finally, it is important to note that suggestive interviews – driven by an interviewer's assumptions or biases concerning the nature of the experience being discussed – can lead to considerable distortion in the accuracy of children's reports.

From the vantage point of this account of context specificity, we emphasize that the memory findings discussed above reflect children's memory performance under ideal conditions. For example, in the Baker-Ward et al. (1993) study, the target event was a familiar experience – a visit to the doctor for a well-child check-up – that contained a few stressful features but was for the most part a comfortable experience. Moreover, the assessment took place in a neutral setting, and not the examination room, precisely because they examiners did not want features of the context to prompt the children. Further, these examiners went to great lengths to make sure that the children understood the nature of the interview process and they worked hard to carry out the assessment in a neutral, but supportive manner. Specifically, the questions concerning features of the physical examination – as well as activities that did not occur in the check-up – were posed in a direct, straightforward manner, rather than with the more coercive approaches that are documented in studies of child suggestibility (Ceci & Bruck, 1995; Bruck & Ceci, 1999; Bruck, Ceci, & Principe, 2006).

This brief review establishes that young children can provide extensive reports of their experiences under circumstances involving familiar events, little distress, and supportive interviewing. However, children providing legal testimony are almost certainly describing experiences that differ in critical regards from most analog events that are explored in the cognitive development literature. In the following section, we examine several important contextual factors that are likely to affect children's accounts.

Contextual Factors that Influence Performance

Given these demonstrations of context specificity in expressions of children's memory skills, it is essential to expand the discussion to distinguish between two different contexts that are critical for the assessment of children's abilities – the setting in which an event is initially experienced and encoded and the setting in which a child is interviewed (formally or informally) and a report is obtained. In this regard, it is important to emphasize that forensic interviewers (and memory researchers, in investigations involving naturally occurring experiences) have no control over the conditions of encoding, whereas they do have control over the nature of the conversation or interview that provides the setting for retrieval and reporting. Thus, prior knowledge and stress, mentioned above, reflect aspects of the encoding context over which we have no control, whereas the behavior of the interviewer can definitely be controlled and standardized. Each of these broad contextual factors is discussed below, but it is also necessary to discuss the effect of temporal delays on children's performance.

For the most part, children's autobiographical memory is not assessed immediately, but rather after a considerable period, and what happens in the delay between experiencing an event and providing an account of the experience affects recall performance considerably. Moreover, within the legal setting, at least two different delays are important: the first being between the experience and an initial report, and the second being between the initial report (disclosure) and a final report in court or some other legal venue. Importantly, these intervals are rarely "empty," but rather are filled with conversations and informal interviews, all of which can affect final performance. The events that take place in these intervals typically have not been controlled, although it is important to try to exercise as much control as possible. We examine the impact of these delay intervals below, between our treatment of the encoding and retrieval contexts.

The Encoding Context

With the exception of research involving experimenter-provided experiences, we cannot control the nature of the context in which autobiographical experiences are encoded, but it is nonetheless important for us to know as much as possible about this setting.

Knowledge and Understanding

It has long been established that what an individual knows has a considerable impact on what he or she is able to remember (see Bjorklund, 1985; Chi & Ceci, 1987; Ornstein & Haden, 2002; Ornstein & Naus, 1985). Decades of research indicate that prior event-related knowledge facilitates the encoding, storage, retention, and retrieval of experiences over time (Ornstein, Shapiro, Clubb, Follmer, & Baker-Ward, 1997; Nelson, 1986), but also knowledge can be seen as a double-edged sword in that it can lead to errors in delayed recall when the events being remembered differ from knowledge-driven expectations (e.g., Leichtman & Ceci, 1995; Ornstein et al., 1998).

Perhaps the most important determinant of the encoding of an experience in memory is the extent to which it is understood as it unfolds (Ornstein et al., 1997). When children can make sense of what they are experiencing, they are able to attend more fully to the key features of the event and to encode them more completely than would otherwise be the case. Importantly, there is considerable agreement that understanding can be driven by endogenous influences "within" the child, such as expectation, which, in turn is linked to the deployment of attention as an event unfolds. To illustrate, what a child already knows about a routine physical examination can influence seriously the extent to which individual components of a medical check-up are encoded and placed in memory (Clubb, Nida, Merritt, & Ornstein, 1993; Ornstein et al., 1997). Similarly, developmental changes in children's underlying knowledge are associated with corresponding differences in children's remembering (e.g., Ornstein et al., 2006). Importantly, understanding can also be fostered by exogenous influences, such as adult-child interchanges that help children make sense of what is being experienced. For example, mother-child conversations during a novel experience can impact understanding, thereby increasing encoding and subsequent remembering (e.g., Haden, Ornstein, Eckerman, & Didow, 2001).

Encoding and remembering can thus be seen as knowledge-driven constructive processes. As such, knowledge clearly has positive effects on children's memory, and in the legal context it especially important for investigators, clinicians, and attorneys to be aware of what a child witness understands about the events that have (presumably) been experienced. If a young child has little prior knowledge of a class of events (including those related to sexual abuse), then there is every reason to believe that she or he will not understand completely what is unfolding when a specific instantiation of that event class is experienced. Under these conditions, a coherent representation will not be established in memory. On the other hand, if a child has great knowledge of a class of events, then another type of problem may result and that concerns a difficulty with differentiating among specific instances of the class. For example, if a child has repeatedly been victimized sexually, then she or he may have established a strong "script" (Nelson, 1986) for abuse, but be unable to distinguish between specific episodes of abuse.

Stress and Emotion

The effect of stress during encoding on the subsequent recall of an event is a salient issue in basic research on children's memory and its development that is of profound importance for considerations of children's ability to provide testimony in legal settings. Decades of research on the impact of stress on the completeness and accuracy of child's accounts of forensically relevant experiences indicate that the stress-recall relation is complex, involving multiple levels of analysis from the physiological to the psychological, as well as a process that continues after the event is experienced. Nonetheless, the research supports a number of conclusions that are can inform the practice of clinical and forensic psychology.

First, it is clear that children can provide extensive information about their experiences within the context of highly stressful events. Research has documented children's high levels of recall, including open-ended recall, for their experiences with natural disasters (e.g., Bauer, Burch, Van Abbema, & Ackil, 2008; Fivush, Sales, Goldberg, Bahrick, & Parker, 2004), emergency medical treatment (see Peterson, 2015), and invasive radiological procedures (e.g., Goodman, Quas, Batterman-Faunce, Riddlesberger, & Kuhn, 1994). Further, children's accounts of such stressful events remained detailed even years after the events transpired. Moreover, children appear to provide *more* information about highly stressful events than they do about experiences associated with little distress. For example, Ornstein, Merritt, and Baker-Ward (1995) compared children's accounts of a fluoroscopy procedure involving urinary catheterization (Merritt, Ornstein, & Spicker, 1994) with another group of children's reports of a routine pediatric examination (Baker-Ward et al., 1993) and found higher levels of recall, especially in response to open-ended questions, for the highly stressful event.

Second, the abundant evidence that children can provide extensive accounts of stressful experiences, however, does *not* support a conclusion that stress enhances memory. Indeed, higher levels of stress are sometimes associated with *lower* levels of recall. In their investigation of children's memory for a painful medical procedure, Merritt et al. (1994) reported that although the children provided extensive reports of the event, the young patients who demonstrated greater stress, in comparison to those with lower levels of stress, reported less information. Peterson (2010) also reported an inverse relation between stress at encoding and the accuracy of children's reports of a traumatic injury, although the effect was present only at an initial interview. Hence, although children generally remember more stressful types of events better than less stressful events, children who demonstrate higher levels of stress within the context of a particular event may recall less information than their less-aroused peers report.

Third, this apparent contradiction may arise from the comparison of events that differ with regard to the inclusion of emotion as well as levels of arousal. Negative emotions, especially fear and anxiety, frequently accompany stressful experiences. In contrast to research on the association between stress and recall, the linkage between emotion at the time of the encoding of an event and subsequent recall for the experience reflects a consensus. Children as well as adults recall events associated with emotion better than they remember neutral occurrences (Fivush et al., 2006). Experiences involving negative emotions are particularly memorable, presumably because they are more informative and hence attending to them has adaptive significance. Adults show this *negativity bias* in a variety of tasks, and it appears to be present throughout development (Vaish, Grossman, & Woodward, 2008). The negativity bias is especially apparent when both the sympathetic branch of the autonomic nervous system and the hypothalamic-pituitary-adrenal (HPA) axis are activated, presumably because of connections to the limbic system (see Quas, Castro, Bryce, & Granger, 2018). Stimulation of the amygdala and hippocampus results in the deployment of greater attention to emotional information, and subsequently, better consolidation of emotional material. The comparison of a routine pediatric check-up with an anxiety-producing diagnostic procedure thus confounds emotional salience and stress level. Although children generally recall more emotional events better than they remember less emotional experiences, high levels of stress within the context of a particular type of event can disrupt memory performance. Fivush and colleagues (Fivush, Bohanek, Marin, & Sales, 2009) emphasize the importance of the level of stress in understanding its effect on recall, concluding, "at high levels of stress, recall may become compromised" (p. 167). This interpretation is consistent with the classic Yerkes-Dodson law (1908), which postulates a curvilinear relation between arousal and performance for difficult tasks, with the highest level of performance occurring at moderate levels of arousal.

Fourth, psychologists once assumed that we remember unexpected, highly distressing events (e.g., learning about the death of a public figure) through special memory mechanisms, resulting in highly detailed, veridical representations of such experiences (e.g., Brown & Kulik, 1977). In contrast, continuing research has established that memories for highly salient events are subject to the same types of reconstruction and errors that characterize memory for more everyday events (see Winograd & Neisser, 1992). Notably, a carefully controlled investigation of young adults' memory for the terrorist attacks of September 11 and a personal event occurring at the same time documented inconsistencies in the recall of both events over time, although the participants' confidence in their memory for the tragic but not the everyday event remained high (Talarico & Rubin, 2003). We do not form indelible representations of intense experiences; we just think we do.

Finally, experiencing stress when an event unfolds can initiate behavioral responses that affect the sequence of information processing. One important influence involves the deployment of attention (see Christianson, 1992). Notably, during encoding, participants under stress are likely to focus on the central components of an event, defined as information associated with the source of arousal. Consequently, they may direct less attention to peripheral event components, which are unrelated to this source. The contents of the individual's memory for the event are likely to reflect this focus. An extreme example of heightened attention to central information is the "weapon focus effect," observed in children as well as adults (Fawcett, Peace, & Greve, 2016). This effect describes individuals' focus on sources of danger, limiting the attention they can direct to other aspects of the event as it unfolds. This direction of attention would likely have beneficial effects on recall for at least some central event components, but at the same time could have detrimental results on memory for peripheral items. Further, both during and after the event transpires, individuals' responses to coping with stressful experiences can affect memory, as discussed in the section below on individual differences.

The Delay Interval

From the perspective articulated above, memory representations of an experience can be modified considerably as a result of both the passage of time and what happens in that time. The representations of both children and adults are readily modified, but those of young children are particularly problematic.

The Effects of Intervening Experiences

There is an extensive literature on the ways in which children's memory can be modified over time. One major determinant of changes in memory over time is exposure to experiences that are similar to an event that is being remembered, but nonetheless differ somewhat from it. To illustrate, consider, an extension of the Baker-Ward et al. (1993) study of children's memory for the details of a visit to the doctor, discussed above. Principe,

Ornstein, Baker-Ward, and Gordon (2000) examined the memory of young children for the details of a physical examination, both immediately after the check-up and after a delay of 12 weeks. The researchers observed considerable forgetting over the delay, but they were especially interested in the impact of different types of intervening on delayed recall. Halfway through the interval (at six weeks after the doctor's visit), some children received an additional interview about their check-up, whereas others viewed a video of another child receiving a physical examination, and others returned to the pediatrician's office for some unrelated memory assessments. In comparison to a control condition, the findings were that the children who had received an additional interview or who had observed the videotape showed elevated recall in response to open-ended questions at the 12-week interview. Importantly, however, a different picture emerged when we consider the children's responses to questions about activities that had not been in included in the physical examinations. For example, the 5-year-olds in Principe et al.'s sample who had viewed the video midway through the delay interval evidenced a significant reduction in the percentage of correct rejections, that is, in their abilities to say "no" to questions about things that simply did not happen during the check-ups. Indeed, these children correctly rejected only half of these items, performing at the level of chance, whereas the children in the other groups correctly rejected 81% of the items about actions that did not occur.

The findings of Principe et al. (2000) indicate intervening experiences that are similar in some ways can have both positive and negative effects on children's retention over the course of long delays. In terms of the negative impact of similar events on delayed performance, it seems likely that the 5-year-olds who viewed the video may have been confused as to the "sources" of their information, as these children made some spontaneous intrusions in their open-ended recall of features of physical examinations that were included in the video but were not present in their actual check-ups. Moreover, the data suggest that passage of time and exposure to the video altered the memory representations of the 5-year-olds in this condition. In addition to the clear impact of "external" events on delayed remembering, it is important to note that some intervening events are "internal" in that they may take place within the individual (Ornstein & Haden, 2002). Typically, these endogenous factors involve interplay between memory representations for an event and an individual's general knowledge about similar events. For example, memory for a specific event may be modified over time because of the spontaneous operation of knowledge-driven constructive processes that serve to fill gaps in memory that arise with the passage of time (e.g., Myles-Worsley, Cromer, & Dodd, 1986; Ornstein et al., 1998). Consistent with the confusion experienced by Principe et al.'s (2000) participants who viewed the video, memory modification on the basis of both external events and internal activities may result from difficulties with differentiating between the sources of information. There is a rich literature on source monitoring – including differentiating between external sources, as well as between internal and external sources – and on the memory errors that result from these errors in the differentiation process (e.g., Foley, 2014; Johnson, Foley, Suengas, & Raye, 1988). In most situations, these types of memory errors are of no consequence, but they are of critical importance in the legal context when the task is that of assessing the accuracy of the statements of a witness (Zaragoza & Lane, 1994).

The Effects of Conversation

In addition to the external and internal events that can modify the memory of an earlier experience, one major class of "intervening events" has to do with conversations with others (e.g., parents, peers, therapists), as these discussions hold great potential for shaping children's understanding and beliefs, and thus the "story" that comes to be told later in more formal interviews. As is the case with prior knowledge, discussed above, conversations with parents after an experience can be seen as a double-edged sword that can have both positive and negative effects on children's remembering. When a child understands a particular experience, conversations with a parent can facilitate subsequent remembering because of the embedded opportunities for rehearing key elements and also for building linkages between the experience and the self (e.g., Fivush, Haden, & Reese, 2006; Pipe, Sutherland, Webster, Jones, & La Rooy, 2004; Lawson, Rodriguez-Stein, & London, 2018). However, opportunities for changing a child's memory representation can be seen in situations in which the child may not thoroughly understand an event as it unfolds. Under these conditions, conversations with a parent can facilitate that child's understanding of the experience and in the process change the memory. More specifically, an event that had been encoded on the basis of imperfect understanding as it transpired can come to be reframed as a result of that conversation, with the event essentially being re-encoded in memory. Thus, even conversation that has a positive effect (i.e., of improving understanding) results in a change in the underlying memory representation.

Moreover, parent-child conversations that are based on an adult's incomplete understanding of the experience – or worse, a biased perspective, as, for example, can readily be seen in the midst of some child custody disputes – can have deleterious effects on a child's memory (e.g., Lawson et al., 2018). Conversations in which an adult provides incorrect or erroneous information about an event that a child experienced have the potential to result in considerable distortion, as the child's understanding shifts in the direction of the adult's, and the representation in memory is modified considerably (e.g., London, Bruck, & Melnyk, 2009; Principe, DiPuppo, & Gammel, 2013; Principe et al., 2017). Similar – and even more dramatic – effects can be seen in the ways in which preschoolers can be influenced by conversations with their peers. For example, children's memory reports of the details of a staged archeological dig at school in which they participated can be influenced by their conversations with friends who took part in a more complete version of the event, even to the point of claiming to have observed things that only their peers had witnessed (Principe & Ceci, 2002). Preschoolers' accounts of staged experiences even be distorted by exposing children to rumors about a plausible event that did not take place (Principe, Kanaya, Ceci, & Singh, 2006; Principe & Schindewolf, 2012). Collectively, these results demonstrate that event-related details provided by parents and peers within conversations can inadvertently inform children's own reports and lead to the creation of narratives that are entirely false.

In addition to these conversations, it is necessary to consider the impact of interactions with therapists on children's later memory for the experiences being discussed. Given what is known about the operation of the memory system – especially the role of conversation and the possibility of reframing experiences as information in memory storage is retrieved and re-encoded – it is important to be concerned about the ways in which encounters with clinicians may result in changes in children's memory (see, e.g., Lynn, Lock, Loftus, Krackow, & Lilienfeld, 2003). These issues have been raised in the context of discussions of cases (e.g., the Little Rascals trials in North Carolina in the early 1990s) in which some preschoolers who had allegedly been abused by their teachers were subjected to multiple sessions with clinicians prior to appearing in court, as well as in treatments of the recovered/false memory controversy. Although there has not been a great deal of research on this topic, Goodman, Goldfarb, Quas, and Lyon (2017) reported that counseling during a child sexual abuse prosecution was associated with improved memory after delays of 10 to 16 years for the details of abused-related information. Still, a great deal needs to be learned about the potential impact of conversations with clinicians on subsequent memory, as there are no studies in which changes in children's initial accounts of an experience are evaluated over time, as a function of whether or not they interacted with clinicians during the delay interval. Moreover, it seems highly likely that there are clear differences in the consequences of forensic interviews versus continuing therapy and of experiences with clinicians who hold different views regarding the guilt or innocence of the alleged perpetrators.

It is now commonly accepted practice to make forensic interviews as short and unbiased as possible, making use of standardized research-based interview tools, such as the NICHD protocol (Lamb, Orbach, Hershkowitz, Esplin, & Horowitz, 2007) because of an understanding of the need to avoid distorting a child's memory. Yet contrast these forensic procedures with on-going therapy sessions (as in the Little Rascals case) in which the clinicians held strong beliefs concerning the guilt of the teachers and day care owners. Because of its importance, research on this topic is urgently needed.

Some Complications in the Legal System

Of course, any discussion of intervening events and conversations during the "delay interval" becomes immensely complicated in the context of the legal system. This is because multiple memory-relevant experiences – including medical examinations, meetings with social workers and attorneys, and formal interviews – typically take place prior to a formal "telling of the tale" in court. Thus, in effect, the distinction drawn here between the encoding and retrieval contexts is an artificial one because there are multiple opportunities for retrieval prior during the interval between the key experience to be remembered and the court proceedings. As such, even though interviewing will be discussed below in the treatment of the retrieval context, it is important to point out here that children's memory representations can be altered substantially *during the delay interval* and hence before the final interview in court.

Of key concern are the problematic ways in which interviewers may interact with children: (1) interviewing in a highly suggestive manner (Garven, Wood, Malpass, & Shaw, 1998; Peterson & Bell, 1996), sometimes invoking peer pressure to induce a child to report what is expected or desired (Principe & Ceci, 2002); (2) establishing a stereotype (usually negative) about a central figure in the event being discussed, especially when combined with suggestive interviews (Leichtman & Ceci, 1995; Memon, Holliday, & Hill, 2006); (3) posing the same questions to a child repeatedly, both within one interview and across many interviews (Bjorklund, Bjorklund, Brown, & Cassel, 1998; Cassel, Roebers, & Bjorklund, 1996; Poole & White, 1991); (4) asking repeatedly, over the course of weeks, whether a specified event took place, when in fact it never occurred (Ceci, Huffman, Smith, & Loftus, 1994); (5) interviewing with anatomically detailed dolls and related types of props (Greenhoot, Ornstein, Gordon, & Baker-Ward, 1999; Poole, Bruck, & Pipe, 2011); (6) exposing to rumors about a plausible event that did not take place (Principe et al., 2006; Principe & Schindewolf, 2012).

The Retrieval Context

In contrast to the encoding context, and to some extent the delay interview, the interviewer is able to control some – but not all – aspects of the retrieval context by the nature of the questions that are posed. Thus, for example, training in appropriate techniques for interviewing children (e.g., the NICHD child interview protocol; see Lamb et al., 2007) can result in supportive interviews that are non-suggestive and minimize the stressful aspects of the interview process. Training can also ensure that interviewers are aware of the consequences of children's limited understanding of the interview process. However, no training regimen can completely eliminate the stress experienced by a child when she or he is asked to remember the details of a stressful or painful experience (see Pantell and AAP Committee on Psychosocial Aspects of Child and Family Health, 2017). In addition, it is difficult for even a skilled interviewer to deal with the consequences of a child's changing knowledge and understanding of an earlier experience. Further, the interviewer has no control over the timing of a child's initial disclosure. These issues are discussed below.

Initial Disclosure

The child's initial report of an episode of possible maltreatment may occur within the context of everyday interactions with parents or other caregivers. Such disclosures may occur shortly after the alleged actions transpired or after an extended delay, and the action or object that prompted the report may be difficult to discern. Moreover, these statements are often likely to be difficult to interpret. Preschoolers and even early elementary school children may lack the vocabulary needed to clearly reference body parts or interactions involving touch and may not differentiate appropriate caregiving and inappropriate contact. Further, especially when events occurred without adult scaffolding of the child's comprehension and connections among components of the event, young children's narratives often lack coherence and may be hard to follow (see Brubacher et al., 2019). Key elements, including temporal concepts and an actor's intentionality, may not yet be available to young children, potentially introducing further ambiguity. Understandably, caregivers are unlikely to respond calmly and carefully to such disclosures. The adult's inevitable emotional reaction and urge to protect the child can create a situation in which inconsistent information is conveyed through leading questions, the child's statements and the adult's contributions are confused, and the presence of maltreatment is accepted as a certainty rather than a possible explanation (see Lawson et al., 2018).

The Impact of Knowledge and Understanding at Retrieval

As indicated above, knowledge-driven understanding of an event as it unfolds is a major determinant of what gets encoded in memory. When a child experiences an event that he or she does not understand, it is difficult to establish a coherent representation in memory. Thus, in terms of encoding, knowledge (both prior and acquired) has a clear positive influence on memory performance. However, it is also the case that under certain conditions knowledge can lead to errors in memory performance. This negative effect of knowledge can be observed after a delay in which some of the details of an experience have been forgotten and constructive knowledge-driven processes lead to errors in memory reports. Thus, for example, by the time that memory is assessed after a delay, errors in remembering may be observed, including the omission or distortion of information that is inconsistent with the child's basic knowledge, as well as the intrusion of information that is consistent with such knowledge, but nonetheless is incorrect (Ornstein & Haden, 2002; Ornstein et al., 1998).

Given the well-documented impact of knowledge on remembering, it is also important to consider the mnemonic consequences of changes in a child's understanding over time, that is, over the interval between initial encoding and delayed memory assessment delay. This is especially relevant within the context of the legal system, as these delays are often very long and may be associated with both the decay of initial representations as well as increases in understanding of the activities being remembered. Ross (1989) called attention to this complex matter, suggesting that changes in knowledge can prompt constructive processes that that bring about a reworking of earlier memories in ways that are congruent with current understanding. To support this perspective, Ross described a series of studies that illustrate the ways in which current beliefs, attitudes, and knowledge can work to shape the recollections of adults about events that they have experienced.

Consistent with Ross's (1989) point of view, Greenhoot (2000) reported an experiment in which 5- and 6-year-olds were led to develop an understanding about a particular child who was characterized as being either a bully or prosocially oriented. With this knowledge manipulation in place, the participants then were presented with a story involving the ambiguous actions of this child (the protagonist) that could be interpreted in different ways, depending on the perspectives established through the knowledge manipulations. As expected, the children's recall was highly constructive in that they typically went far beyond the literal information provided in the story, such that their reports often were filled with "errors" – inferences, distortions, and intrusions – that were consistent with the social knowledge about the protagonist that they had received. With this recall "on record," Greenhoot then established a second knowledge manipulation, approximately a week later, through which the participants received additional information about the social motives of the protagonist. Importantly, for some children the new information was consistent with the impressions received earlier, whereas for others it was inconsistent. Following the provision of this new information about the protagonist, the participants' memory of the original stories was again assessed, and, importantly, the data revealed that the children's recall of the details changed and was consistent with the second knowledge manipulation.

Greenhoot's findings provide support with children for Ross' (1989) view that changes over time in underlying knowledge can lead to reconstructive modifications of children's memory representations on the basis of now-current understanding. Going beyond demonstrations of knowledge-driven processes, even those showing that knowledge can fill in the "gaps" of what can be remembered (e.g., Ornstein et al., 1998), the findings of Ross (1989) and Greenhoot (2000) illustrate the ways in which knowledge changes over time can result in the restructuring of earlier memories on the basis of current understanding.

Stress at Retrieval/Interviewer Support

As indicated above, stress experienced as an event unfolds can have a profound effect on encoding and the establishment of a representation in memory. Importantly, in addition to stress experienced at the time of encoding, stress associated with the retrieval of information that is represented in memory can impact various aspects of a memory report. There are at least two partially overlapping ways in which a child can experience stress as he or she retrieves information about previously experienced events. First, it must be recognized that contents of some memories may be embarrassing or painful, and under these conditions a child may not be motivated to retrieve the details and, especially, express them publicly in the form of a verbal report. Second, when dealing with these difficult memories – or even with others that are not stressful – the support and scaffolding provided by the interviewer is of paramount importance. A skilled interviewer can facilitate a child's retrieval and reporting, whereas an unskilled interviewer can turn an interview into a stressful experience, amplifying any stress that is associated with the experience being discussed. Moreover, at worst, an interviewer who questions a child in an inappropriate and biased manner can turn an interview into an interrogation, leading a child to modify his or her account of the experience and sometimes to the construction of a false report.

Interview guidelines often recommend creating a supportive interview context to mitigate the potential impact of stress on children's remembering. Supportiveness is reflected in behaviors such as making eye contact, using the child's name, responding with empathy and reassurance, building simple rapport, and providing feedback that is not contingent on the content of children's responses. It is believed to communicate to children that they are cared for by the interviewer and thereby reduce the emotional states and irrelevant thoughts that interfere with children's cognitive processing. Unsupportive behaviors or the lack of supportiveness, on the other hand, may do the opposite. They likely inhibit children from reporting their experiences, promote denial, or foster the unwavering acceptance of interviewers' suggestions by children (Saywitz, Wells, Larson, & Hobbes, 2019).

Research on interview practices reveals a complex linkage between supportiveness and children's reports of past experiences. The effects of interviewer support on children's free recall are often non-significant; however, research reliably demonstrates that children make fewer errors in response to non-leading and suggestive questions when interviewed in a supportive rather than non-supportive environment (Saywitz et al., 2019). Furthermore, supportiveness may be particularly important for certain groups of children. The effect of interviewer support on children's memory performance is strongest for children who are uncooperative or reluctant (Hershkowitz, Orbach, Lamb, Sternberg, & Horowitz, 2006), have poor executive functioning (Peter-Hagene, Bottoms, Davis, & Nysse-Carris, 2014), display heightened physiological reactions to stress (Quas, Bauer, & Boyce., 2004), or show a history of insecure attachments (Peter-Hagene et al., 2014).

Supportiveness is also particularly helpful for children who are under a great deal of stress. For example, Quas and Lench (2007) measured the heart rate of 5- and 6-year-old children during interviews about a fear eliciting video clip and found that when children were questioned in an unsupportive context (i.e., the interviewer did not build rapport, maintain eye contact, smile, or provide any encouragement or feedback), higher heart rates were associated with decreases in accuracy of children's memory reports. Yet, similar patterns were not observed for children who were interviewed in a supportive context. Heart rate was unrelated to the accuracy of memory reports when children were recipients of interviewer support. This finding reveals the role that stress plays during children's retrieval of memories and highlights the importance of a supportive interview context for children's memory performance, especially among young children (Davis & Bottoms, 2002).

One additional component of a supportive interview context stems from an interviewer's awareness of young children's limited understanding of just what is involved in an interview. In addition to the importance of using appropriate child-level language, it is essential to recognize that young children may not understand the give-and-take as an interview progresses (e.g., Bjorklund et al., 1998; Cassel et al., 1996; Lamb & Brown, 2006). For example, when a question is repeated, a young child may assume that he or she simply didn't provide the correct answer and so will change the response that was given. It is also important to realize that under some conditions, young children may feel that it is more important to conform to the expectations of an adult authority figure than to report what was experienced (Ceci, Ross, & Toglia, 1987).

Interviews and Interviewer Bias

As indicated above, during the delay interval a child may experience a range of interactions – with law officers, hospital personnel, social workers and psychologists, and attorneys – that can be viewed as "interviews." Whether or not the delay interval is filled with these types of interactions, as a case is assembled and prepared for trial a child is most definitely interviewed on multiple occasions, and the goal of each of these encounters is to encourage the retrieval and reporting of information concerning the "target" event that is to be remembered. In addition to issues of support for the child, just discussed, a range of issues arise when considering the ways in which interviewers attempt to elicit information.

Of course, the goal of the interviewer should be to pose questions in a neutral manner so as to prompt a child's recall, without distorting it to fit the bias or beliefs of the individual asking the questions. It is now well understood that leading and misleading questions have the potential to distort a child's recollections, but it is nonetheless important to indicate clearly that there are many suggestive interviewing techniques that go beyond the use of such questions (Garven, Wood, Malpass, & Shaw, 1998). Importantly, an interview does not have to include leading questions for it to be highly suggestive. Suggestive techniques include the use of: (1) repeated specific questions (some of which may, in fact, be leading) both within an interview and across a series of interviews (Bjorklund et al., 1998); (2) repeated interviews that focus on the alleged event or events (Ceci, Huffman, Smith, & Loftus, 1994); (3) implicit or explicit threats, bribes, and rewards (Garven, Wood & Malpass, 2000); and (4) stereotype induction (e.g., telling a child that the suspected perpetrator "does bad things" to many children) (Leichtman & Ceci, 1995; Memon et al., 2006). It is also the case that being questioned by an authority figure, such as a doctor or police officer, can increase the likelihood that a child will make statements that are consistent with that older individual's beliefs (Tobey & Goodman, 1992).

Two other suggestive interview techniques must be mentioned: the use of anatomically detailed dolls and drawings as aids for remembering. Given young children's limited language skills, it seems intuitively reasonable to use nonverbal props to help children report details of past experiences. In this regard, dolls and drawings have previously been used by professionals to ask sexually abused children about how and where they were touched, but, as Poole et al. (2011) indicate, research carried out over the last 25 years has done little to confirm interviewers' beliefs in the appropriateness of these aids for disclosure and remembering. In research on (nonabused) children's memory for medical experiences involving touching, the use of dolls (albeit not anatomically detailed dolls) as retrieval aids did not facilitate the performance of 3-year-olds, although that of older children improved (Gordon, Ornstein, Nida, Follmer, Crenshaw, & Albert, 1993). The use of body diagrams – simple line drawings to represent the child – did not improve younger children's performance (Poole & Bruck, 2012). Moreover, when both dolls and medical props were used to enable children to act out the details of their physical examinations, correct recall increased, but incorrect responses also rose dramatically, especially for younger children (Greenhoot et al. 1999).

A good explanation for the failure of dolls to improve the performance of young children is that the children often have difficulty using the doll because they are unable to relate to it as both a toy and as a representation of the self (DeLoache & Marzolf, 1995; DeLoache, 2000). Further, even among children for whom representational issues are not problematic, difficulties may arise because of the stimulus properties of anatomically detailed dolls. Indeed, attention to the dolls' body parts and sexualized play can be observed even among children who were not sexually abused (Bruck, Ceci, & Francoeur, 2000). All in all, although it is possible that using dolls and drawings as props will be associated with increases in correct recall, it is also the case that they are linked to increased errors (Salmon, 2001). Thus, the use of anatomically correct dolls can also result in false reports, especially when they are employed by biased interviewers who do not strictly follow guidelines for their use (see Bruck et al., 2000; Salmon, 2001).

Two other features of suggestive interviewing are important to note. First, a major factor in determining how suggestive an interview may be is the bias that an interviewer may have concerning the facts of a case. This bias can readily be seen in interviewers who hold a priori beliefs about the occurrence of certain events, and these beliefs can influence the entire architecture of the interview. As such, interviewer bias often results in the use of one or more of the suggestive interview techniques mentioned above and, more generally, in interviews that are structured so as to obtain confirmatory evidence for these beliefs without any consideration of plausible alternative hypotheses. Importantly, an interviewer does not have to be deliberately motivated to seek information that supports his or her position. Indeed, the effects of interviewer bias can be observed, even when there is no deliberate intent to be suggestive. For example, if an interviewer gains an understanding (or misunderstanding) of something that (may have) happened to a child from a previous interview with an adult, that understanding can have a direct effect on the questions that the interviewer poses to the child, as well as his or her interpretation of the answers. Second, even though each of the suggestive techniques outlined above can be associated with error, the likelihood of eliciting false statements increases dramatically when several suggestive techniques are employed in combination. Under these conditions, salience of the bias of a single interviewer or a group of interviewers who share the same perspective is increased, and performance decreases (see Bruck et al., 2006; Ceci & Bruck, 1995).

Individual Difference Variables Affecting Children's Memory Performance

In this final section, we briefly examine some characteristics of children that are relevant for understanding their memory for details of events that they have experienced. These features of the child can impact both the way in which events are interpreted as they unfold and the subsequent reports of these experiences. Our selection of individual difference characteristics is not comprehensive, but it does reflect the state of the current literature and to some extent the factors to which we have devoted attention in our own research.

Approach to Coping

As discussed above, stress as an event transpires typically triggers behavioral responses that affect the deployment of attention and hence the subsequent processing of information about the experience. These reactions involve both automatic and controlled responses that can be seen as attempts to cope with the situation at hand. Notably, these behavioral responses may promote either engagement with the stressful event as it unfolds and the accompanying emotional reactions, or disengagement (Compas, Campbell, Robinson, & Rodriguez, 2009). Tactics involving engagement, or *approach-oriented coping*, include seeking information or social support, whereas behaviors associated with disengagement, or *avoidant-oriented coping*, include minimizing the impact of the experience and attempting to escape. It makes sense that these alternative coping responses – largely because they involve quite different opportunities for encoding an event, maintaining a memory, or strengthening a representation – would have divergent effects on memory (Compas et al., 2009). However, despite extensive research on children's coping, there have been relatively few investigations of the effects of coping behaviors on recall and resistance to suggestibility. A dissertation project carried out by Lee (2011) at the University of North Carolina at Chapel Hill is a notable exception.

Lee examined the ways in which children coped with a minor dental operative procedure and their subsequent memory for the components of this treatment. She focused on linkages between children's reports of their approaches to coping and their later recall and found that information seeking was positively associated with recall performance. Further, Lee observed that this information seeking strategy accounted for a significant amount of unique variance in the children's recall, even when age and parental preparation were statistically controlled. It seems possible that children who seek information during and after an event unfolds may be able to form more interconnected event representations (e.g., involving more causal linkages between event components) than their peers who use other coping strategies, and that these interconnected cognitive structures protect and extend their memories. Lee (2011) also found that avoidance-based coping was associated with fewer rejections of misleading questions at a delayed interview. This result could reflect a weakening memory representation over time, resulting in greater difficulty in distinguishing present and absent event components (see Baker-Ward, et al. 1997).

Attachment

Attachment theory (Bowlby, 1969) posits that infants form persistent schemas or *internal working models* (IWMs) that represent the availability and supportiveness of their caregivers and serve as frameworks for understanding relationships over time. In some respects, variability across young children in their IWMs can be reflected in the different coping styles that they employ as they deal with stressful experiences involving attachment figures. As such, these IWMs serve as the foundation for differing attachment orientations (or categories) that support alternative approaches to processing information regarding important social interactions. Dykas and Cassidy (2011) theorized that children with IWMs representing secure relationships with caregivers accurately process and openly discuss negative as well as positive social information relevant to their interactions with attachment figures. In contrast, they argued that children with insecure IWMs would be associated with biased or defensive encoding of information regarding relationships with attachment figures.

Although there is little research on the relations among children's attachment categories and their memory for distressing events, Chae and colleagues (Chae et al., 2018) recently examined differences in 3- to 5-year-olds' memory of their experiences in the Strange Situation (a somewhat distressing, structured observation involving a series of separations and reunions with the parent) as a function of differences in the children's attachment security. Consistent with expectations derived from Bowlby's (1969) theory, they found that higher (vs. lower) scores on a measure of attachment security were associated with more (vs. less) accurate recall of experiences in the Strange Situation. Further, as the authors predicted, attachment security and distress during the Strange Situation interacted, such that higher levels of distress were related to greater resistance to false suggestions among children with higher but not lower scores on attachment security. The authors discuss this result as possibly reflecting the greater ability of more vs. less securely attached children to regulate negative emotions when aroused.

Temperament

Memory researchers have long assumed that temperament, the child's characteristic behavioral style (Thomas, Chess, & Birch, 1968), would help to explain differences in children's reports of salient personal experiences (e.g., Gordon et al., 1993). Although there is variability among researchers concerning the components of temperament, a widely used measure, the Martin (1988) Temperament Assessment Battery for Children conceptualizes temperament in terms of six dimensions: activity, adaptability, approach/withdrawal, emotional intensity, distractibility, and persistence. From our perspective, it seems reasonable to expect that some of these dimensions – especially approach/withdrawal – would directly affect the child's interview performance. Consistent with this expectation, Merritt et al. (1994) found that children's tendency to approach others and to adapt to new situations positively predicted their open-ended recall of components of an invasive radiological procedure. However, linkages between aspects of temperament and recall performance are not consistently found (e.g., Burgwyn-Bailes, Baker-Ward, Gordon & Ornstein, 2001).

Two factors – the child's age and type of memory assessment – are likely to influence the likelihood that characteristics of children's temperament are linked with their recall performance. In terms of age, school-age children have had extensive experience in structured learning settings, and as such have had many guided opportunities to learn to regulate their own behavior. Consequently, older children, in comparison with their younger peers, are likely to adjust their behavior to meet the demands of interviews and other assessments, regardless of their characteristic behavioral style (see Gordon et al., 2001). Regarding the assessment, the impact of some features of temperament on children's reports may vary as a function of characteristics of the reporting context. For example, Greenhoot et al. (1999) reported that 3-year-old children who were rated by their parents as having more difficulty with task persistence were more likely than other children to adopt a response set when interviewed with a verbal protocol, but not when the memory assessment involved the re-enactment of the event with props (Greenhoot et al., 1999). The way in which an interview is carried out, while always important, may be of greatest importance among young children who are especially slow-to-warm up or highly distractible.

Suggestibility

Interest in identifying individual differences in suggestibility has been long-standing and continuing (for reviews, see Quas, Qin, Schaaf, & Goodman, 1997; Bruck & Melnyk, 2004; Klemfuss & Olaguez, 2020). The extensive resulting literature supports a few conclusions and provides a number of directions for future research. In this section, we examine the evidence for cognitive and social influences on susceptibility to suggestion. We omit from further consideration two predictors of suggestibility – attachment and temperament – because these factors are examined in elsewhere in this chapter.

Generally consistent results document the influence of age and IQ on children's suggestibility. In a recent investigation, Gudjonsson and colleagues (Gudjonsson, Vagni, Maiorano, & Pajardi, 2016) presented over a thousand children and adolescents (age 7 to 16) with a version of a standardized assessment of suggestibility, the Gudjonsson Suggestibility Scale 2 (GSS 2: Gudjonsson, 1997), which involves the recall of a story before and after exposure to misleading questions. Not surprisingly, suggestibility deceased with age. In addition, although children with intellectual disabilities are more suggestible than their typically developing peers (see Klemfuss & Olaguez, 2018), there is extensive evidence that IQ scores in the normal range are not significantly related to suggestibility (e.g., Gudjonsson et al., 2016). In addition, Gudjonsson et al. (2016) further report that although girls in comparison to boys recalled more information, no gender differences in suggestibility (as assessed with the GSS2) emerged. This pattern of findings with regard to gender was also reported by Bruck and Melnyk (2004) in their review of the field.

Researchers have explored additional sources of individual differences in suggestibility, although the literature is relatively sparse. For example, Bruck and Melnyk (2004) reviewed six studies that examined the relation between creativity and suggestibility and reported that each investigation provided some evidence indicating that children who were judged to be more creative were more susceptible to suggestion than their peers who were seen as less creative. The linkage between creativity and suggestibility, however, has not been the topic of continuing investigation (see Klemfuss & Olaguez, 2018). Another hypothesized predictor of suggestibility is *traditional parenting* style, defined in terms of the extent to which children's parents emphasize obedience to authority (see Schaefer & Edgerton, 1984). In this regard, Burgwyn-Bailes et al. (2001) found that a measure of traditional parenting predicted children's suggestibility concerning the details of emergency room treatment, above and beyond the effects of age and receptive language. In addition, although both theory of mind (the understanding of mental states) and executive function (the regulation of attention) have been examined as possible influences on suggestibility, associations have been inconsistently observed (Bruck & Melnyk, 2004; Klemfuss & Olaguez, 2018).

Given the relatively large number of investigations incorporating individual difference variables, it is rather surprising that these predictors are infrequently and inconsistently associated with measures of suggestibility. As discussed by Ornstein and Elischberger (2004), this pattern may reflect the low frequency with which different combinations of individual difference variables and measures of suggestibility appear in the literature. It is also the case that many investigations are atheoretical, with individual difference measures included for exploratory purposes. Additional research testing a priori predictions with large sample sizes is clearly needed.

Language Abilities

Because interviewers rely on children's abilities to comprehend spoken questions (receptive language) and to respond verbally (productive language), language development is inherently involved in understanding children's changing capabilities in providing information about what they have experienced or observed. Receptive language abilities may be particularly important in children's responses to suggestive questioning, which often involves more complex syntax (embedded clauses, tag questions) than does open-ended or closed probes.

Although measures of vocabulary are not generally associated with suggestibility, significant relations between performance on a comprehensive language assessment battery and resistance to suggestive questioning are consistently reported (see Bruck & Melnyk, 2004). Further, experimental evidence suggests that simplifying the language comprehension demands of questions can increase rates of correct rejections of queries about event components that did not occur. To illustrate, Imhoff and Baker-Ward (1999) presented preschoolers with a classroom science activity – reading about volcanoes and creating an eruption in a model volcano – and compared performance between groups of children who had been interviewed with two different protocols. Both protocols included the same yes-no questions, but a developmentally more appropriate version was designed to be especially well-suited to preschoolers' receptive language skills. In comparison to the standard protocol, this version presented the questions in a shorter format, avoided embedded clauses and definite articles, and used transitional sentences to structure the interview. The children interviewed with the simplified protocol, in comparison to those interviewed with the standard protocol, demonstrated higher rates of resistance to misleading questions as well as more correct responses to direct questions.

It is important to note that variation in language skills appears to be more important for younger than older children's recall, presumably because most older children have acquired the level of language competence needed to participate fully in verbal interviews. In their investigation of children's memory for emergency room treatment, Burgwyn-Bailes et al. (2001) found that scores on a standardized receptive language assessment predicted total recall among the younger but not the older participants in their sample of 3- to 4-year-old children. Similarly, in Imhoff and Baker-Ward's (1999) study, the use of simplified interview protocols enhanced the memory performance among 3-year-old children, in contrast to 5-year-old participants.

Recent research further indicates that individual differences in children's narrative skills may be important for assessing the likelihood that a memory will be retained over time. Narrative coherence – as seen in children's accounts that include the context in which an event occurred, present the actions in chronological order, and develop the narrative theme (Reese et al., 2011) – has been shown to predict the persistence of memories over extended periods of time among children and younger adolescents (Peterson et al., 2014). Further, Brown, Brown, Lewis, and Lamb (2018) found that the narrative coherence of 7–11-year-olds' initial accounts of a classroom experience predicted aspects of their reports (e.g., overall accuracy and correct responses to leading questions) two years later. They concluded that younger children and older children with intellectual disabilities need guidance in constructing coherent accounts of their experiences. Moreover, narrative practice using an everyday event may be useful in preparing children to report their forensically relevant experiences (Lyon, 2014).

Addressing Individual Differences

Relatively stable differences across children in their socio-emotional (e.g., attachment) and cognitive (e.g., intellectual disability) characteristics can have a direct impact on their recall and suggestibility in reporting personally-experienced events. More often, however, individual differences in these characteristics act in conjunction with other features of the child (e.g., age) and context (e.g., the specificity of the interview questions). For example, supportive and effective interviewing is particularly important in working with children who are especially anxious or shy. It is also the case that different aspects of the child's socio-emotional and cognitive make-up may exert their greatest effects at alternative points in the child's protracted experience in the legal system. For instance, it is possible that executive function is particularly important at delayed interviews, when memory fades and the recall task becomes more difficult. Consequently, clinicians may find it helpful to consider the possible differing effects of individual difference factors on the encoding of information, on the possible reinstatement of a memory as well as interference with that memory, and also on the resulting memory report.

Conclusions and Recommendations

Understanding the information provided by a child witness necessitates knowledge regarding memory and its development. As discussed throughout this chapter, memory is not an objective, indelible record of an experience that can be directly accessed with the right questions. Rather, it must be understood as a dynamic process, affected by a range of experiences from the event being remembered through the later report of the occurrence (e.g., Ornstein et al., 1992). Consequently, the task of the clinician is to examine in detail the circumstances under which target events were encoded, focusing on children's knowledge and understanding of the actions they observed or experienced and their emotional reactions. The absence of some aspects of the experience from the child's report should be interpreted within this context. Similarly, because the status of information in memory changes over time, the experiences that intervened between the occurrence of the event and the report must be carefully assessed. The clinician should explore possibilities for memory contamination from naturally occurring experiences such as everyday conversations or repeated exposure to similar events, and from encounters within legal or medical systems that could convey suggestions or stereotypes.

The circumstances under which the children report their experiences provide additional sources of information for understanding the accuracy and completeness of the children's accounts. The degree of social support provided by interviewers (Saywitz, et al., 2019), the developmental appropriateness of the questions (Imhoff & Baker-Ward, 1999), and the types of prompts and props used in the interview (Greenhoot et al., 1999; Poole et al., 2011; Gordon et al., 1993) are well-established influences on retrieval and reporting.

Developmental changes are likely to affect each sequence in the flow of information in memory. Although it is well-established that at least under favorable conditions, children as young as 3 can provide useful reports about personal experiences, age-related changes in the extent of information provided are robust (Fivush, 2011; Gordon et al., 2001; Reese et al., 2011; Baker-Ward et al., 1993). Development in multiple domains, including source monitoring and language, contribute to the child's representation of the target events (Foley, 2014; Johnson et al., 1988; Zaragoza & Lane, 1994; Gordon et al., 1993; Burgwyn-Bailes et al., 2001). Assessment of the child's developmental status and knowledge in relevant domains can provide useful information in planning for an effective interview and in interpreting the child's account (Ornstein & Haden, 2002; Ornstein et al., 1998; Ross, 1989).

In addition, differences among children in socio-emotional and cognitive characteristics may contribute to the child's provision of information. Several of the individual difference factors examined in this chapter – notably, coping style (Lee, 2011), attachment (Chae et al., 2018), and temperament (Merritt et al., 1994) – may influence the children's experiences of stressful events, as well as their performance in the interview setting. The possible impact of these factors should be included in the assessment of the encoding context. With regard to children's interview performance, the accommodation of many characteristics of the individual child can be accomplished simply through interview practices that are almost universally beneficial. These approaches include the use of developmentally appropriate language, the establishment of rapport and a shared understanding of the purpose of the interview, the provision of social support, sensitivity to the child's physical comfort, and avoidance of unnecessary direct questions, and other techniques that are known to increase suggestibility (see Lamb et al., 2007; Lyon, 2014; Saywitz et al., 2019).

Recommendations to address the extended process of remembering and to understand the developmental and individual characteristics of children who provide testimony apply to expert witnesses as well as clinicians and forensic examiners. An important role for expert witnesses is to provide a developmental perspective on a child's report. For example, the inclusion of little spontaneously provided information may make a child less credible, whereas information provided in response to open-ended questions is more likely to be accurate (Gordon & Follmer, 1994). Similarly, a limited understanding of narrative conventions may lead to questions regarding the accuracy of a young witness' report, but these concerns are likely to be resolved when typical developmental changes are referenced.

A final word of caution is necessary. The research on which we base our conclusions does not – and ethically could not – provide a complete analog for the types of events children are called on to report in legal settings. Although some of the investigations we discuss involve highly stressful medical procedures (notably, Merritt et al., 1994), they were sanctioned by the adults in the children's lives and administered in response to the young patients' needs for services. Moreover, the interviews administered in our own research were conducted by experienced examiners who were skilled in working with children and who followed protocols that were designed to avoid coercion or suggestion among the young respondents. Hence, the depiction that we provide of young children's capabilities in reporting personally-experienced events is likely to represent the positive end of a continuum of memory performance.

References

Aktar, S., Justice, L. V., Morrison, C. M., & Conway, M. A. (2018). Fictional first memories. *Psychological Science, 29*, 1612–1619. doi:10.1177/0956797618778831

Alaggia, R., Collin-Vezina, D., & Lateef, R. (2017). Facilitators and barriers to child sexual abuse (CSA) disclosures: A research update. *Trauma, Violence, & Abuse, 20*, 260–283. https://doi.org/10.1177/1524838017697312

Baker-Ward, L., Gordon, B. N., Ornstein, P. A., Larus, D. M., & Clubb, P. A. (1993). Young children's long-term retention of a pediatric examination. *Child Development, 64*, 1519–1533. doi:10.1111/j.1467-8624.1993.tb02968.x

Baker-Ward, L., Ornstein, P. A., & Principe, G. F. (1997). Revealing the representation: Evidence from children's reports of events. In P. van den Broek, P. Bauer, & T. Borg (Eds.), *Developmental spans in event comprehension and representation: Bridging fictional and actual events* (pp. 79–107). Hillsdale, NJ: Lawrence Erlbaum Associates.

Bauer, P. J. (1996). What do infants recall of their lives? Memory for specific events by one-to two-year-olds. *American Psychologist, 51*, 29–41. doi:10.1037/0003-066X.51.1.29

Bauer, P. J., Burch M. M., Van Abbema, D. L., & Ackil, J. K. (2008). Talking about twisters. In. M. L. Howe, G. S. Goodman, & D. Cicchetti (Eds.), *Stress, trauma, and children's memory development: Neurobiological, cognitive, clinical, and legal perspectives* (pp. 204–235). Oxford: Oxford University Press.

Bauer, P. J., Hertsgaard, L. A., & Dow, G. A. (1994). After 8 months have passed: Long-term recall of events by 1-to 2-year-old children. *Memory, 2*, 353–382. doi:10.1080/09658219408258955

Bjorklund, D. F. (1985). The role of conceptual knowledge in the development of organization in children's memory. In C. J. Brainerd & M. Pressley (Eds.), *Basic processes in memory development* (pp. 103–142). New York: Springer. doi:10.1007/978-1-4613-9541-6_3

Bjorklund, D. F., Bjorklund, B. R., Brown, R. D., & Cassel, W. S. (1998). Children's susceptibility to repeated questions: How misinformation changes children's answers and their minds. *Applied Developmental Science, 2*, 99–111. doi:10.1207/s1532480xads0202_4

Bowlby, J. (1969). *Attachment and loss, vol. 1: Attachment.* London: The Hogarth Press and the Institute of Psycho-Analysis.

Brainerd, C. J., & Ornstein, P. A. (1991). Children's memory for witnessed events: The developmental backdrop. In. J. Doris (Ed.), *The suggestibility of children's memory* (pp. 10–20). Washington, DC: American Psychological Association. doi:10.1037/10097-002

Brown, D. A., Brown, E.-J., Lewis, C. N., & Lamb, M. E. (2018). Narrative skill and testimonial accuracy in typically developing children and those with intellectual disabilities. *Applied Cognitive Psychology, 32*, 550–560. doi:10.1002/acp.3427

Brown, R., & Kulik, J. (1977). Flashbulb memories. *Cognition, 5*, 73–99. doi:10.1016/0010-0277(77)90018-x

Brubacher, P., Glisic, U., Roberts, K. P., & Powell, M. (2011). Children's ability to recall unique aspects of one occurrence of a repeated event. *Applied Cognitive Psychology, 25*, 351–358. doi:10.1002/acp.1696

Brubacher, S. P., Peterson, C., La Rooy, D., Dickinson, J. J., & Poole, D. A. (2019). How children talk about events: Implications for eliciting and analyzing eyewitness reports. *Developmental Review, 51*, 70–89. doi:10.1016/j.dr.2018.12.003

Bruck, M., & Ceci, S. J. (1999). The suggestibility of children's memory. *Annual Review of Psychology, 50*, 419–439. doi:10.1146/annurev.psych.50.1.419

Bruck, M., & Melnyk, L. (2004). Individual differences in children's suggestibility: A review and synthesis. *Applied Cognitive Psychology, 18*, 947–996. doi:10.1002/acp.1070

Bruck, M., Ceci, S. J., & Francoeur, E. (2000). Children's use of anatomically detailed dolls to report genital touching in a medical examination: Developmental and gender comparisons. *Journal of Experimental Psychology: Applied, 6*, 74–83. doi:10.1037/1076-898X.6.1.74

Bruck, M., Ceci, S. J., & Principe, G. F. (2006). The child and the law. In K. A. Renninger, I. E. Sigel, W. Damon, & R. M. Lerner (Eds.), *Handbook of child psychology: Child psychology in practice* (pp. 776–816). Hoboken, NJ: John Wiley & Sons.

Burgwyn-Bailes, E., Baker-Ward, L., Gordon, B. N., & Ornstein, P. A. (2001). Children's memory for emergency medical treatment after one year: The impact of individual difference variables on recall and suggestibility. *Applied Cognitive Psychology, 15*, S25–S48. doi:10.1002/acp.833

Cassel, W. S., Roebers, C. E., & Bjorklund, D. F. (1996). Developmental patterns of eyewitness responses to repeated and increasingly suggestive questions. *Journal of Experimental Child Psychology, 61*, 116–133. doi:10.1006/jecp.1996.0008

Ceci, S. J., & Bruck, M. (1995). *Jeopardy in the courtroom: A scientific analysis of children's testimony.* Washington, DC: American Psychological Association. doi:10.1037/10180-000

Ceci, S. J., Huffman, M. L. C., Smith, E., & Loftus, E. F. (1994). Repeatedly thinking about a non-event: Source misattributions among preschoolers. *Consciousness and Cognition, 3*, 388–407. doi:10.1006/ccog.1994.1022

Ceci, S. J., Ross, D. F., & Toglia, M. P. (1987). Suggestibility of children's memory: Psycholegal implications. *Journal of Experimental Psychology: General, 116*, 38–49. doi:10.1037/0096-3445.116.1.38

Chae, Y., Goodman, M., Goodman, G. S., Troxel, N., McWilliams, K., Thompson, R., Shaver, P. R., & Widaman, K. F. (2018). How children remember the strange situation: The role of attachment. *Journal of Experimental Child Psychology, 166*, 360–379. doi:10.1016/j.jecp.2017.09.001

Chi, M. T., & Ceci, S. J. (1987). Content knowledge: Its role, representation, and restructuring in memory development. In H. W. Reese (Ed.), *Advances in Child Development and Behavior* (vol. 20) (pp. 91–142). New York: Academic Press. doi:10.1016/S0065–2407(08)60401–2

Christianson, S. Å. (1992). Emotional stress and eyewitness memory: A critical review. *Psychological Bulletin, 112*, 284–309. doi:10.1037/0033-2909.112.2.284

Clubb, P. A., Nida, R. E., Merritt, K., & Ornstein, P. A. (1993). Visiting the doctor: Children's knowledge and memory. *Cognitive Development, 8*, 361–372. doi:10.1016/S0885–2014(93)80006-F

Compas, B. E., Campbell, L. K., Robinson, K. E., & Rodriguez, E. M. (2009). Coping and memory: Automatic and controlled processes in adaptation to stress. In J. A. Quas & R. Fivush (Eds.), Series in affective science. *Emotion and memory in development: Biological, cognitive, and social considerations* (pp. 121–141). New York: Oxford University Press. doi:10.1093/acprof: oso/9780195326932.003.0005

Connolly, D. A., Coburn, P. I., & Chong, K. (2017). Twenty-six years prosecuting historic child sexual cases: Has anything changed? *Psychology Public Policy, & Law, 23*, 166–177. doi:10.1037/law0000121

Davis, S. L., & Bottoms, B. L. (2002). Effects of social support on children's eyewitness reports: A test of the underlying mechanism. *Law and Human Behavior, 26*, 185–215. doi:10.1023/A:1014692009941

DeCasper, A. J., & Spence, M. J. (1986). Prenatal maternal speech influences newborns' perception of speech sounds. *Infant Behavior and Development, 9*, 133–150. doi:10.1016/0163-6383(86)90025-1

DeLoache, J. S. (2000). Dual representation and young children's use of scale models. *Child Development, 71*, 329–338. doi:10.1111/1467-8624.00148

DeLoache, J. S., & Marzolf, D. P. (1995). The use of dolls to interview young children: Issues of symbolic representation. *Journal of Experimental Child Psychology, 60*, 155–173. doi:10.1006/jecp.1995.1036

Dykas, M. J., & Cassidy, J. (2011). Attachment and the processing of social information across the life span: Theory and evidence. *Psychological Bulletin, 137*, 19–46. doi:10.1037/a0021367

Fawcett, J. M., Peace, K. A., & Greve, A. (2016). Looking down the barrel of a gun: What do we know about the weapon focus effect? *Journal of Applied Research in Memory and Cognition, 5*, 257–263. doi:10.1016/j.jarmac.2016.07.005

Fivush, R. (2011). The development of autobiographical memory. *Annual Review of Psychology, 62*, 559–582. doi:10.1146/annurev.psych.121208.131702

Fivush, R., Bohanek, J. G., Marin, K., & Sales, J. S. (2009). Emotional memory and memory for emotions. In O. Luminet & A. Curci (Eds.), *Flashbulb memories: New Issues and new perspectives* (pp. 163–184). New York: Psychology Press.

Fivush, R., Haden, C. A., & Reese, E. (2006). Elaborating on elaborations: Role of maternal reminiscing style in cognitive and socioemotional development. *Child Development, 77*, 1568–1588. doi:10.1111/j.1467-8624.2006.00960.x

Fivush, R., Sales, J. M., Goldberg, A., Bahrick, L., & Parker, J. (2004). Weathering the storm: Children's long-term recall of Hurricane Andrew. *Memory, 12*, 104–118. doi:10.1080/09658210244000397

Foley, M. A. (2014). Children's memory for source. In P. J. Bauer & R. Fivush (Eds.), *The Wiley handbook on the development of children's memory* (pp. 427–452). Hoboken, NJ: Wiley-Blackwell.

Garven, S., Wood, J. M., & Malpass, R. S. (2000). Allegations of wrongdoing: The effects of reinforcement on children's mundane and fantastic claims. *Journal of Applied Psychology* (2000), *85*, 38–49. doi:10.1037/0021-9010.85.1.38

Garven, S., Wood, J. M., Malpass, R. S., & Shaw III, J. S. (1998). More than suggestion: The effect of interviewing techniques from the McMartin Preschool case. *Journal of Applied Psychology, 83*, 347–359. doi:10.1037/0021-9010.83.3.347

Goodman, G. S., Goldfarb, D., Quas, J. A., & Lyon, A. (2017). Psychological counseling and accuracy of memory for child sexual abuse. *American Psychologist, 72*, 920–931. doi:10.1037/amp0000282

Goodman, G. S., Quas, J. A., Batterman-Faunce, J. M., Riddlesberger, M. M., & Kuhn, J. (1994). Predictors of accurate and inaccurate memories of traumatic events experienced in childhood. *Consciousness and Cognition, 3*, 269–294. doi:10.1006/ccog.1994.1016

Goodman, G. S., Quas, J., Batterman-Faunce, J., Riddlesberger, M., & Kuhn, J. (1997). Children's reactions to and memory for a stressful event. *Applied Developmental Science, 1*, 54–75. doi:10.1207/s1532480xads0102_1

Gordon, B. N., & Follmer, A. (1994). Developmental issues in judging the credibility of children's testimony. *Journal of Clinical Child Psychology, 23*, 283–294. doi:10.1207/s15374424jccp2303_6

Gordon, B. N., Baker-Ward, L., & Ornstein, P. A. (2001). Children's testimony: A review of research on memory for past experiences. *Clinical Child and Family Psychology Review, 4*, 157–181. doi:10.1023/A:1011333231621

Gordon, B. N., Ornstein, P. A., Nida, R., Follmer, A., Crenshaw, M., & Albert, G. (1993). Does the use of dolls facilitate children's memory of visits to the doctor? *Applied Cognitive Psychology, 7*, 459–474. doi:10.1002/acp.2350070602

Greenhoot, A. F. (2000). Remembering and understanding: The effects of changes in underlying knowledge on children's recollections. *Child Development, 71*, 1309–1328. doi:10.1111/1467-8624.00230

Greenhoot, A. F., Ornstein, P. A., Gordon, B. N., & Baker-Ward, L. (1999). Acting out the details of a pediatric check-up: The impact of interview condition and behavioral style on children's memory reports. *Child Development, 70*, 363–380. doi:10.1111/1467–8624.00027

Gudjonsson, G. H. (1997). *The Gudjonsson suggestibility scales manual.* Hove: Psychology Press.

Gudjonsson, G. H., Vagni, M., Maiorano, T., & Pairdi, D. (2006). Age and memory-related changes in children's immediate and delayed suggestibility using the Gudjonsson Suggestibility Scale. *Personality and Individual Differences, 102*, 25–29. doi:10.1016/j.paid.2016.06.029

Haden, C. A., Ornstein, P. A., Eckerman, C. O., Didow, S. M. (2001). Mother-child conversational interactions as events unfold: Linkages to subsequent remembering. *Child Development, 72*, 1016–1031. doi:10.1111/1467-8624.00332

Hershkowitz, I., Orbach, Y., Lamb, M. E., Sternberg, K. J., & Horowitz, D. (2006). Dynamics of forensic interviews with suspected abuse victims who do not disclose abuse. *Child Abuse & Neglect, 30*, 753–769. doi:10.1016/j.chiabu.2005.10.016

Imhoff, M. C., & Baker-Ward, L. (1999). Preschoolers' suggestibility: Effects of developmentally appropriate language and interviewer supportiveness. *Applied Developmental Psychology, 20*, 407–429. doi:10.1016/S0193-3973(99)00022-2

Johnson, M. K., Foley, M. A., Suengas, A. G., & Raye, C. L. (1988). Phenomenal characteristics of memories for perceived and imagined autobiographical events. *Journal of Experimental Psychology: General, 117*, 371–376. doi:10.1037/0096-3445.117.4.371

Klemfuss, J. Z., & Olaguez, A. P. (2020). Individual differences in children's suggestibility: An updated review. *Journal of Child Sexual Abuse, 29*, 158–182. doi:10.1080/10538712.2018.1508108

Lamb, M. E., & Brown, D. A. (2006). Conversational apprentices: Helping children become competent informants about their own experiences. *British Journal of Developmental Psychology, 24*, 215–234. doi:10.1348/026151005X57657

Lamb, M. E., Orbach, Y., Hershkowitz, I., Esplin, P. W., & Horowitz, D. (2007). A structured forensic interview protocol improves the quality and informativeness of investigative interviews with children: A review of research using the NICHD Investigative Interview Protocol. *Child Abuse & Neglect, 31*, 1201–1231. doi:10.1016/j.chiabu.2007.03.021

Lawson, M., Rodriguez-Steen, L., & London, K. (2018). A systematic review of the reliability of children's event reports after discussing experiences with a naïve, knowledgeable, or misled parent. *Developmental Review, 49*, 62–79. doi:10.1016/j.dr.2018.06.003

Lee, S. (2011). Children's memories of a stressful dental procedure: Effects of stress and individual differences on remembering. Unpublished doctoral dissertation, The University of North Carolina at Chapel Hill.

Leichtman, M. D., & Ceci, S. J. (1995). The effects of stereotypes and suggestions on preschoolers' reports. *Developmental Psychology, 31*, 568–578. doi:10.1037/0012–1649.31.4.568

London, K., Bruck, M., & Melnyk, L. (2009). Post-event information affects children's autobiographical memory after one year. *Law and Human Behavior, 33*, 344–355. doi:10.1007/s10979-008-9147-7

Lynn, S. J., Lock, T., Loftus, E. F., Krackow, E., & Lilienfeld, S. O. (2003). The remembrance of things past: Problematic memory recovery techniques in psychotherapy. In S. O. Lilienfeld, S. J. Lynn, & J. M. Lohr (Eds.), *Science and pseudoscience in clinical psychology* (pp. 205–239). New York: Guilford Press.

Lyon, T. D. (2014). Interviewing children. *Annual Review of Law and Social Science, 10*, 73–89. doi:10.1146/annurev-lawsocsci-110413-030913

Mack, A., & Rock, I. (1998). *Inattentional blindness*. Cambridge, MA: MIT Press.

Marsh, E. J., & Roediger, H. L. (2013). Episodic and autobiographical memory. In A. F. Healy, R. W. Proctor, & I. B. Weiner (Eds.), *Handbook of experimental psychology* (2nd ed., vol. 4, pp. 472–494). New York: John Wiley & Sons.

Martin, R. P. (1988). *The temperament assessment battery for children*. Brandon, VT: Clinical Psychology Publishing.

Memon, A., Holliday, R., & Hill, C. (2006). Pre-event stereotypes and misinformation effects in young children. *Memory, 14*, 104–114. doi:10.1080/09658210500152641

Merritt, K. A, Ornstein, P A., & Spiker, B. (1994). Children's memory for a salient medical procedure: Implications for testimony. *Pediatrics, 94*, 17–23. doi:10.1002/(SICI)1099-0720(199712)11:7<S87::AID-ACP556>3.0.CO;2-Z

Morris, G., Baker-Ward, L., & Bauer, P. J. (2010). What remains of that day: The survival of children's autobiographical memories across time. *Applied Cognitive Psychology, 24*, 527–544. doi:10.1002/acp.1567

Myles-Worsley, M., Cromer, C. C., & Dodd, D. H. (1986). Children's preschool script reconstruction: Reliance on general knowledge as memory fades. *Developmental Psychology, 22*, 22–30. doi:10.1037/0012-1649.22.1.22

Nelson, K. (1986). *Event knowledge: Structure and function in development*. Hillsdale, NJ: Lawrence Erlbaum Associates.

Ornstein, P. A. (1991). Commentary: Putting interviewing in context. In J. Doris (Ed.), *The suggestibility of children's recollections* (pp. 147–152). Washington, DC: American Psychological Association. doi:10.1037/10097-000

Ornstein, P. A., & Elischberger, H. B. (2004). Studies of suggestibility: Some observations and suggestions. *Applied Cognitive Psychology, 18*, 1129–1141. doi:10.1002/acp.1081

Ornstein, P. A., & Haden, C. A. (2002). The development of memory: Toward an understanding of children's testimony. In M. L. Eisen, J. A. Quas, & G. S. Goodman (Eds.), *Personality and clinical psychology series. Memory and suggestibility in the forensic interview* (pp. 29–61). Mahwah, NJ: Lawrence Erlbaum Associates.

Ornstein, P. A., & Myers, J. T. (1996). Contextual influences on children's remembering. In K. Pezdek & W. P. Banks (Eds.), *The recovered memory debate* (pp. 211–223). San Diego: Academic Press.

Ornstein, P. A., & Naus, M. J. (1985). Effects of the knowledge base on children's memory strategies. In H. W. Reese (Ed.), *Advances in child development and behavior* (vol. 19) (pp. 113–148). New York: Academic Press. doi:10.1016/S0065-2407(08)60390-0

Ornstein, P. A., Baker-Ward, L., Gordon, B. N., Pelphrey, K. A., Tyler, C. S., & Gramzow, E. (2006). The influence of prior knowledge and repeated questioning on children's long-term retention of the details of a pediatric examination. *Developmental Psychology, 42*, 332–344. doi:10.1037/0012-1649.42.2.332

Ornstein, P. A., Baker-Ward, L., & Naus, M. J. (1988). The development of mnemonic skill. In M. Weinert & M. Perlmutter (Eds.), *Memory development: Universal changes and individual differences* (pp. 31–50). Hillsdale, NJ: Lawrence Erlbaum Associates.

Ornstein, P. A., Gordon, B. N., & Baker-Ward, L. (1992). Children's memory for salient events: Implications for testimony. In M. L. Howe, C. J. Brainerd & V. F. Reyna (Eds.), *Development of long-term retention* (pp. 135–158). New York: Springer-Verlag. doi:10.1007/978-1-4612-2868-4_4

Ornstein, P. A., Larus, D. M., & Clubb, P. A. (1991). Understanding children's testimony: Implications of research on the development of memory. In R. Vasta (Ed.), *Annals of Child Development* (vol. 8) (pp. 145–176). London: Jessica Kingsley Publishers.

Ornstein, P. A., Merritt, K. A., & Baker-Ward, L. (1995, July). Children's recollections of medical experiences: Exploring the linkage between stress and memory. In J. Parker (Chair), *Eyewitness memory: Effects of stress and arousal upon children's memories.* Symposium paper presented at the meeting of the Society for Applied Research in Memory and Cognition, Vancouver, Canada.

Ornstein, P., Merritt, K. A., Baker-Ward, L., Furtado, El., Gordon, B. N., & Principe, G. F. (1998). Children's knowledge, expectation, and long-term retention. *Applied Cognitive Psychology, 12,* 387–405. doi:10.1002/(SICI)1099-0720(199808)12:4<387::AID-ACP574>3.0.CO;2-5

Ornstein, P. A., Shapiro, L. R., Clubb, P. A., Follmer, A., & Baker-Ward, L. (1997). The influence of prior knowledge on children's memory for salient medical experiences. In N. Stein, P. A. Ornstein, B. Tversky, & C. J., Brainerd (Eds), *Memory for everyday and emotional events* (pp. 83–112). Hillsdale, NJ: Lawrence Erlbaum Associates. doi:10.4324/9781315799421

Pantell, R. H., and AAP Committee on Psychosocial Aspects of Child and Family Health. (2017). The child witness in the courtroom. *Pediatrics, 139,* e20164008. doi:10.1542/peds.2016-4008

Peter-Hagene, L., Bottoms, B. L., Davis, S. L., & Nysse-Carris, K. L. (2014, March). *Social support effects on children's suggestibility after one year.* Poster presented at the meeting of the American Psychology-Law Conference, New Orleans, LA.

Peterson, C. (2002). Children's long-term memory for autobiographical events. *Developmental Review, 22,* 370–402. doi:10.1016/S0273-2297(02)00007-2

Peterson, C. (2010). 'And I was very very crying': Children's self-descriptions of distress as predictors of recall. *Applied Cognitive Psychology, 24,* 909–924. doi:10.1002/acp.1636

Peterson, C. (2015). A decade later: Adolescents' memory for medical emergencies. *Applied Cognitive Psychology, 29,* 826–834. doi:10.1002/acp.3192

Peterson, C., & Bell, M. (1996). Children's memory for traumatic injury. *Child Development, 67,* 3045–3070. doi:10.1111/j.1467-8624.1996.tb01902.x

Peterson, C., Morris, G., Baker-Ward, L., & Flynn, S. (2014). Predicting which childhood memories persist: Contributions of memory characteristics. *Developmental Psychology, 50,* 439–448. doi:10.1037/a0033221

Pillemer, D. B. (1998). What is remembered about early childhood events?. *Clinical Psychology Review, 18,* 895–913. doi:10.1016/S0272-7358(98)00042-7

Pipe, M. E., Sutherland, R., Webster, N., Jones, C., & Rooy, D. L. (2004). Do early interviews affect children's long-term event recall? *Applied Cognitive Psychology, 18,* 823–839. doi:10.1002/acp.1053

Poole, D. A., & Bruck, M. (2012). Divining testimony? The impact of interviewing props on children's reports of touching. *Developmental Review, 32,* 165–180. doi:10.1016/j.dr.2012.06.007

Poole, D. A., & White, L. T. (1991). Effects of question repetition on the eyewitness testimony of children and adults. *Developmental Psychology, 27*(6), 975–986. doi:10.1037/0012-1649.27.6.975

Poole, D. A., Bruck, M., & Pipe, M. E. (2011). Forensic interviewing aids: Do props help children answer questions about touching? *Current Directions in Psychological Science, 20,* 11–15. doi:10.1177/0963721410388804

Principe, G. F., & Ceci, S. J. (2002). "I saw it with my own ears": The effects of peer conversations on preschoolers' reports of nonexperienced events. *Journal of Experimental Child Psychology, 83,* 1–25. doi:10.1016/S0022-0965(02)00120-0

Principe, G. F., & Schindewolf, E. (2012). Natural conversations as a source of false memories in children: Implications for the testimony of young witnesses. *Developmental Review, 32,* 205–223. doi:10.1016/j.dr.2012.06.003

Principe, G. F., Cherson, M., DiPuppo, J., & Schindewolf, E. (2012). Children's natural conversations following exposure to a rumor: Linkages to later false reports. *Journal of Experimental Child Psychology, 113,* 383–400. doi:10.106/j.jecp.2012.06.006

Principe, G. F., DiPuppo, J., & Gammel, J. (2013). Effects of mothers' conversation style and receipt of misinformation on children's event reports. *Cognitive Development, 28,* 260–271. doi:10.1016/j.cogdev.2013.01.012

Principe, G. F., Kanaya, T., Ceci, S. J., & Singh, M. (2006). Believing is seeing: How rumors can engender false memories in preschoolers. *Psychological Science, 17,* 243–248. doi:10.1111/j.1467-9280.2006.01692.x

Principe, G. F., Ornstein, P. A., Baker-Ward, L., & Gordon, B. N. (2000). The effects of intervening experiences on children's memory for a physical examination. *Applied Cognitive Psychology, 14,* 59–80. doi:10.1002/(SICI)1099-0720(200001)14:1<59::AID-ACP637>3.0.CO;2-4

Principe, G. F., Trumbull, J., Gardner, G., Van Horn, E., & Dean, A. M. (2017). The role of maternal elaborative structure and control in children's memory and suggestibility for a past event. *Journal of Experimental Child Psychology, 163*, 15–31. doi:10.1016/j.jecp.2017.06.001

Quas, J. A., & Lench, H. C. (2007). Arousal at encoding, arousal at retrieval, interviewer support, and children's memory for a mild stressor. *Applied Cognitive Psychology, 21*, 289–305. doi:10.1002/acp.1279

Quas, J. A., Bauer, A., & Boyce, W. T. (2004). Physiological reactivity, social support, and memory in early childhood. *Child Development, 75*, 797–814. doi:10.1111/j.1467-8624.2004.00707.x

Quas, J. A., Castro, A., Bryce, C. I., & Granger, D. A. (2018). Stress physiology and memory for emotional information: Moderation by individual differences in pubertal hormones. *Developmental Psychology, 54*, 1606–1620. doi:10.1037/dev0000532

Quas, J. A., Qin, J., Schaaf, J., Goodman, G. S. (1997). Individual differences in children's and adults' suggestibility and false memory. *Learning and Individual Differences, 9*, 359–390. doi:10.1016/S1041-6080(97)90014-5

Reese, E., Haden, C. A., Baker-Ward, L., Bauer, P., Fivush, R., & Ornstein, P. A. (2011). Coherence of personal narratives across the lifespan: A multidimensional model and coding method. *Journal of Cognition and Development, 12*, 424–462. doi:10.1080/15248372.2011.587854

Ross, M. (1989). Relation of implicit theories to the construction of personal histories. *Psychological Review, 96*, 341–357. doi:10.1037/0033-295X.96.2.341

Rovee-Collier, C. (1997). Dissociations in infant memory: Rethinking the development of implicit and explicit memory. *Psychological Review, 104*, 467–498. doi:10.1037/0033-295X.104.3.467

Salmon, K. (2001). Remembering and reporting by children: The influence of cues and props. *Clinical Psychology Review, 21*, 267–300. doi:10.1016/S0272-7358(99)00048-3

Saywitz, K. J., Wells, C. R., Larson, R. P., & Hobbs, S. D. (2019). Effects of interviewer support on children's memory and suggestibility: Systematic review and meta-analyses of experimental research. *Trauma, Violence, & Abuse, 20*, 22–39. doi:10.1177/1524838016683457

Schaefer, E. S., & Edgerton, M. (1984). Parent and child correlates of parental modernity. In I. E. Sigel (Ed.), *Parental belief systems: The psychological consequences for children* (pp. 287–318). Hillsdale, NJ: Lawrence Erlbaum Associates.

Stolzenberg, S. N., & Lyon, T. D. (2013). Evidence summarized in attorney's closing arguments predict acquittals in criminal trials of child sexual abuse. *Child Maltreatment, 19*, 119–129. doi:10.1177/1077559514539388

Stolzenberg, S. N., & Lyon, T. D. (2014). How attorneys question children about the dynamics of sexual abuse and disclosure in criminal trials. *Psychology, Public Policy, and Law, 20*, 19–30. doi:10.1037/a0035000

Talarico, J. M., & Rubin, D. C. (2003). Confidence, not consistency, characterizes flashbulb memories. *Psychological Science, 14*, 455–461. doi:10.1111/1467-9280.02453

Thomas, A., Chess, S., & Birch, H. G. (1968). *Temperament and behavior disorders in children*. New York: New York University Press.

Tobey, A. E., & Goodman, G. S. (1992). Children's eyewitness memory: Effects of participation and forensic context. *Child Abuse & Neglect, 16*, 779–796. doi:10.1016/0145-2134(92)90081-2

Vaish, A., Grossmann, T., & Woodward, A. (2008). Not all emotions are created equal: The negativity bias in social-emotional development. *Psychological Bulletin, 134*, 383–403. 10.1037/0033–2909.134.3.383

Winograd, E., & Neisser, U. (Eds.) (1992). *Emory symposia in cognition, 4. Affect and accuracy in recall: Studies of 'flashbulb' memories*. New York: Cambridge University Press. doi:10.1017/CBO9780511664069

Yerkes, R. M., & Dodson, J. D. (1908). The relation of strength of stimulus to rapidity of habit-formation. *Journal of Comparative Neurology and Psychology, 18*, 459–482. doi:10.1002/cne.920180503

Zaragoza, M. S., & Lane, S. M. (1994). Source misattributions and the suggestibility of eyewitness memory. *Journal of Experimental Psychology: Learning, Memory, and Cognition, 20*, 934–945. DOI:10.1037/0278-7393.20.4.934

4 Navigating Tricky Waters

Understanding and Supporting Children's Testimony about Experiencing and Witnessing Violence

Deborah Goldfarb, Hana Chae, and Laura Shambaugh

When Aaron Fraser's mother, Bonnie Haim, disappeared in 1993, Aaron found himself in the middle of a storm of legal interventions. Police officers instituted a criminal action to investigate his mother's disappearance and potential murder. He was the focus of a child welfare proceeding to decide whether he should be removed from his father's care (Burke & Associated Press, 2019; Sanchez & Smith, 2019). Later, Aaron's father's parental rights would be terminated, and Aaron would be adopted, presumably as part of a family court process. Aaron is not the only child attempting to navigate the tricky waters of multiple legal proceedings; numerous other children, either because of harm committed against them directly (described herein as direct victimization) or witnessing harm committed against someone that they love (described herein as indirect victimization), find themselves caught in a confluence of legal proceedings.

These various proceedings (family law, child protection/dependency, criminal) carry different evidentiary requirements, sanctions, and interventions. Often these potentially conflicting standards and practices are applied all at the same time and to the same child, as was the case with Aaron. Questions arise as to how well children can remember certain types of prior events, including being victimized directly, such as a sexual or physical assault, or indirectly, through seeing a loved one attacked or even murdered. Differences in legal questions, the purpose of the testimony, and the standard used to judge the testimony raise important theoretical and applied questions about how best to understand and respond to children's testimony in these varying settings. These various legal proceedings, differences in legal questions, purpose of testimony, and standards used to judge testimony create "tricky waters" for any child or any professional working with children in legal contexts.

Aaron's story has a very sad conclusion that highlights the need for us to better help children who witness violence. In the original criminal investigation, then 3-year-old Aaron told a child welfare investigator that "Daddy shot mommy" and that "My daddy could not wake her up" (Burke & Associated Press, 2019; Sanchez & Smith, 2019). Bonnie Haim's car and purse were later discovered at a motel near the airport, but she was never heard from again. Her husband claimed that they had fought and that she subsequently left the home.

Aaron was later adopted by the Fraser family, but he still had access to the home he had lived in with his biological mother (The Florida Times-Union, 2019). Decades later, while renovating his childhood backyard as an adult, Aaron discovered his mother's body. An investigation followed, and his father was charged with her murder. Aaron's father was ultimately sentenced to life in prison. This case is a particularly tragic example of what happens when children witness the assault or murder of one of their caregivers, particularly by another loved one. As children move between the various courts, their testimony may be lost or shunted aside, or they may not receive developmentally appropriate forensic interviews and clinical supports.

DOI: 10.4324/9780429397806-5

Hoping to shed further light on how to respond to these complex and devastating cases, as well as highlight the many ways children interact with the legal system, this chapter reviews potential theoretical and applied research applicable to cases where children are directly and/or indirectly victimized. Specifically, we first review research on trauma and psychopathology. We then discuss whether and how trauma impacts children's abilities to accurately recall and testify about events. Children's typical memory development is thoroughly covered in Chapter 3 of this book. As such, we do not discuss here memory's typical development but suggest the reader refer to Chapter 3. The research on trauma, psychological impact, and the impact on memory lead to an exploration of interventions for children who testify in legal proceedings and discuss research on how they may help improve testimonial accuracy and emotional responses to testifying. Finally, we conclude the chapter and propose future research that can help children navigate these difficult and tricky proceedings.

Overview of Trauma and the Possible Impact of Trauma on Memory Functioning

The focus of this section is on the role that trauma plays in children's abilities to accurately testify in the courtroom. In covering this issue, we first discuss the rates of occurrence of trauma in the United States. Next, we discuss the impact of trauma and victimization both on psychological impairment associated with trauma and psychopathology. Also reviewed is the impact of these psychological implications of trauma on memory abilities. Finally, we end with a discussion on memory for historic child sexual abuse, including briefly reviewing the relation between age and memory in general.

Childhood Trauma Rates in the United States

A substantial number of children directly experience trauma ever year within the United States. For instance, some studies find that 37.3% of children report having experienced a physical assault during the past year, and 15.2% report being maltreated by a caregiver (Finkelhor, Turner, Shattuck, Hamby, & Kracke, 2015). In 2015, there were approximately 4.0 million referrals of child maltreatment, receipt of information that a child might be experiencing harm, involving approximately 7.2 million children (U.S. Department of Health and Human Services, Administration for Children and Families, Administration on Children, Youth and Families, Children's Bureau, 2017). Approximately 2.2 million of these referrals were investigated or otherwise responded to by child protective services.

Although the rates for indirect violence vary depending on the study, they are, as with direct victimization, unacceptably high. For instance, one study found that one-quarter of children in the United States had witnessed some form of violence, and 9.8% of these cases involved violence within the home (Finkelhor, Turner, Ormrod, & Hamby, 2009). A different survey revealed that 57.7% of the surveyed children had been exposed to violence during the preceding year – further, 1 in 10 children reported being exposed to this form of violence on five or more occasions within that year (The National Survey of Children's Exposure to Violence (NatSCEV), 2011; see Finkelhor et al., 2015; Smith & Farole Jr., 2009; Truman & Morgan, 2014). The type of exposure varied widely, with 23% of the sample having witnessed violence within their family unit or living community, and 16.9% of children having been exposed to a community assault (e.g., hearing gunshots, seeing another person shot, theft, or bomb threat; see Finkelhor et al., 2015).

Children who are directly victimized are all too frequently also indirectly victimized. More than half of children who were exposed to interpersonal violence were also maltreated in their lifetime, while only 11.2% of children were maltreated in the absence of exposure to interparental violence (Hamby, Finkelhor, Turner, & Ormrod, 2010). This overlap often makes it difficult disentangle psychological impacts unique to one versus another type of violence. And, irrespective of the type of violence experienced, these traumas have a number of deleterious sequalae, which we discuss in this next section.

Psychological Impacts of Victimization

Children who have experienced victimization often reveal increased rates of both internalizing and externalizing behaviors. Victimized children are almost 4.5 times more likely to experience internalizing behaviors than non-victimized children (Turner, Finkelhor, & Ormrod, 2006), with traumatized girls reporting higher internalizing of trauma than boys (Baldry & Winkel, 2004; Bourassa, 2007). Internalizing behaviors may include depression, anxiety, withdrawing from peers or others, trouble sleeping, and somatic complaints (Achenbach, 1991; Nicholson, Chen, & Huang, 2018; Schiff et al., 2014). Children who exhibit internalizing behaviors also have a detrimental self-view and often report low self-compassion (e.g., being unkind to themselves in a challenging situation; Barlow, Turow, & Gerhart, 2017). These behaviors may develop, in part, from children suppressing negative emotions (e.g., anger) as they lack coping strategies to deal with them (Zeman, Shipman, & Suveg, 2002).

Both directly and indirectly victimized children may also exhibit externalizing behaviors, including outbursts of negative emotions (e.g., anger, aggression), hostility, and delinquent behaviors (Eisenberg, Spinrad, & Eggum, 2010; Kim & Cicchetti, 2010; Zeman et al., 2002). Children who were directly victimized are nearly four times more likely to display externalizing behaviors compared to non-victimized children (Barlow et al., 2017; Dodge, Pettit, Bates, & Valente, 1995; Shields & Cicchetti, 1998; Shipman & Zeman, 2001; Turner et al., 2006). Children with externalizing behaviors often display poor coping mechanisms for anger such as slamming doors or speaking harshly to others (Zeman et al., 2002).

Witnessing and experiencing interpersonal violence (IPV) may be particularly dire for children (Silverman & Gelles, 2001). These children are more likely to display both internalizing and externalizing behaviors as opposed to children who experience neither or only one type of trauma (Bourassa, 2007; Hughes, Parkinson, & Vargo, 1989).

Potential Psychopathologies in Victimized Children

In addition to exhibiting more internalizing and externalizing behaviors, child victims may also experience increased rates of psychopathology (Mehta et al., 2013; Merrill, Thomsen, Sinclair, Gold, & Milner, 2001; Springer, Sheridan, Kuo, & Carnes, 2007). This is true irrespective of whether children experience direct maltreatment or indirect harm through witnessing IPV (Camacho, Ehrensaft, & Cohen, 2012; Graham-Bermann, Castor, Miller, & Howell, 2012; Izaguirre & Calvete, 2015; Levendosky, Huth-Bocks, Semel, & Shaprio, 2002). Many children who experience trauma also receive a psychological diagnosis either in childhood or later in adolescence (see Dvir, Ford, Hill, & Frazier, 2015), and it is not uncommon for children with trauma to be diagnosed with more than one mental health disorder (e.g., a combination of depression and anxiety disorder, O'Sullivan, Watts, & Shenk, 2018).

Unfortunately, these psychological impacts can last for decades (Hahm, Lee, Ozonoff, van Wert, 2010; Jardim et al., 2018; Springer et al., 2007). For instance, Hahm and colleagues (2010) reported that young women (age 18–27) who were sexually and physically abused as children disclosed having had either suicidal thoughts or suicidal attempts three to four times more often than women who did not experience such abuse. In addition, Jardim and colleagues (2018) found that individuals (age 60 or older) who were maltreated as children were at higher risk of suicide than non-victimized individuals later in their life, even after controlling for differences in geriatric depression. As the most common psychopathologies in those who have experienced trauma are depression, PTSD, and disassociation (O'Sullivan et al., 2018), each of them is discussed in turn below.

Depression

Among child victims, depression is the most common trauma-related psychopathology (Eisen, Goodman, Qin, Davis, & Crayton, 2007; Goodman, Bottoms, Rudy, Davis, & Schwartz-Kenney, 2001; Hussey, Chang, & Kotch, 2006; Moylan et al., 2010; Trent et al., 2019). The relation between trauma and depression continues into adulthood with childhood trauma relating to later adult depression (Lowe et al., 2016, Xie et al., 2018). The DSM-5 (American Psychiatric Association, 2013) defines major depressive disorder as exhibiting five or more depressive symptoms (e.g., feeling sad, empty, or hopeless, loss of interest or pleasure) most of the day for at least a 2-week period. To receive a diagnosis, these individuals must not be able to meet their daily responsibilities due to the symptoms (e.g., unable to focus at work or school). The consequences of depression can be quite severe for some individuals; depression is associated with an increased risk of suicide in adolescence and in adulthood (APA, 2013; Hadland, Marshall, Kerr, Montaner, & Wood, 2012; Souza, Molina, Azevedo da Silva, & Jansen, 2016).

Posttraumatic Stress Disorder (PTSD)

The DSM-5 (APA, 2013) defines PTSD as exhibiting intrusion symptoms (e.g., nightmares, flashback), persistent avoidance (e.g., avoidance of traumatic memories), or negative alterations in cognitions (e.g., inability to remember traumatic events, feeling detached from others) for more than a month. These symptoms must be persistent and interfere with individuals' daily functioning. Children who have experienced victimization are more likely to develop a diagnosis of PTSD than non-victimized children (Barlow et al., 2017; Chae, Goodman, Eisen, & Qin, 2011; Eisen et al., 2007; Ehring & Quack, 2010; Graham-Bermann et al., 2012; Levendosky et al., 2002; Moylan et al., 2010; Trent et al., 2019) and those who have experienced trauma are also more likely to be diagnosed with PTSD in adulthood than those who have not (Lowe et al., 2016; Mehta et al., 2013; Van Voorhees, Dedert, Calhoun, Brancu, Runnals, & Beckham, 2012). Children who have experienced trauma and display symptoms of PTSD may also have decrements in emotion regulation, with the children with the most severe symptoms of PTSD displaying lower quality emotion regulation strategies (Chae et al., 2011; Ehring & Quack, 2010; Hahm et al., 2010; Shepherd & Wild, 2014).

Numerous factors increase the likelihood of being diagnosed with PTSD after trauma. Children who have witnessed IPV in the home are at a higher risk to develop PTSD when they experience further victimization (e.g., nonsexual assault by a family member or someone the child knows after the initial victimization), as compared to children who have not been exposed to the additional trauma (Graham-Bermann et al., 2012). Additionally, self-blame and self-shame are believed to increase the risk of developing PTSD (Uji, Shikai, Shono, & Kitamura, 2007). Findings about children involved in various forms of domestic violence are provided in greater details in Chapter 11.

Dissociation

Childhood trauma also increases the likelihood to develop dissociative symptoms (Chae et al., 2011; Valentino, Cicchetti, Rogosch, & Toth, 2008). Hulette and colleagues (2008) found that having experienced multiple traumatic events (e.g., being a victim of sexual and physical abuse) was associated with more severe dissociation than having single or fewer traumatic events. According to the DSM-5 (APA, 2013), there are two types dissociative symptoms: loss of touch with reality or self, and loss of the ability to retrieve information or to regulate psychological functions. Children with trauma may use dissociation, including isolating traumatic information from their awareness, to avoid thinking about unpleasant experiences (Becker-Blease, Freyd, & Pears, 2004).

The psychological impacts of trauma can negatively impact children's later ability to testify on the stand, including their ability to accurately remember the traumatic event at issue and their emotional reactions to the courtroom. We next review the research on trauma and memory.

Effect of Trauma on Memory: What Role Does Trauma Play in Children's Memory for Traumatizing Events?

Children who are victims of child abuse or who witness interpersonal violence may be called to act as a witness in legal proceedings. This includes, but is not limited to, testifying during investigations or at trial. When children testify, they are asked to provide information about their memory of what they saw and heard, much like adult eyewitnesses. Over the past several decades research has shown that children, under the right conditions, can provide accurate and legally diagnostic information (see Chapter 3).

When questioning children, however, one must always be cognizant of their heightened suggestibility as compared to older peers and adults (see Chapter 3). In response to such concerns, numerous developmentally appropriate interview protocols have been developed (London & Ceci, 2012; Poole, Brubacher, & Dickinson, 2015; Saywitz, Lyon, & Goodman, 2017; Sternberg, Lamb, Davies, & Westcott, 2001). These protocols build upon the research showing the important relation between question format and children's ability to provide accurate testimony. In general, studies show that children produce fewer commission errors (i.e., statements that something happened when it did not) in response to free recall/open-ended questions (e.g., "Tell me everything that happen" or wh- questions, see Andrews, Ahern, Stolzenberg, & Lyon, 2016 for a review) as compared to closed-ended questions (Klemfuss, Quas, & Lyon, 2014). Most interview protocols thus begin with a period of open-ended questions and only sparingly use closed-ended questions, and never misleading ones.

Children who are forensically interviewed will frequently be asked to remember traumatizing or highly emotional events. Although concerns exist that traumatizing events may be more difficult to recall than less traumatizing events (Deffenbacher, Bornstein, Penrod, & McGorty, 2004), some research suggests that negative or traumatizing events are more accurately remembered than neutral memories (Nairne, Pandeirada, & Thompson, 2008; McGaugh, 2018). Empirical support for the relation between stressful events and heightened recall has been shown across a variety of stressful events: hurricanes, tornadoes, and accidents and medical procedures (Ackil, Van Abbema, & Bauer, 2003; Bauer, Burch, Van Abbema, & Ackil, 2007; Goodman, Quas, Batterman-Faunce, Riddlesberger, & Kuhn, 1997; Peterson, 2012; Sales, Fivush, Parker, & Bahrick, 2005). In general, the children in these studies are better able to recount their memories for stressful events than for less stressful or traumatizing situations.

In addition to the traumatic nature of the event, children asked to recall traumatizing events in legal settings are likely to have experienced trauma themselves. As noted above, such negative experiences can have a cascade of potential mental health symptoms and diagnoses. One question still under inquiry, however, is the role that trauma plays in children's ability to serve as an eyewitness. Many individuals have posited that trauma has a detrimental effect of memory. Trauma in childhood can relate to poorer performance on verbal recall, attention, emotion regulation, and working memory tasks, as well as intelligence tests (Barlow et al., 2017; Bücker et al., 2012; Eisen et al., 2007; Gross, 2002; Richards & Gross, 2006).

Not all studies, however, find that trauma leads to memory impairment. Indeed, researchers have reviewed the data on trauma and memory and have posited that one must take a more nuanced view of the relation between the two; that any understanding of memory and trauma must also consider, amongst other items, the nature of the trauma, the information to be remembered, the child's own psychopathology, and the context under which the child is being questioned (Goldfarb, Goodman, Larson, Gonzales, & Eisen, 2017; Goodman, Quas, & Ogle, 2010; Goodman, Goldfarb, Quas, Narr, Milojevich, & Cordon, 2016).

One example of the complex relation between trauma, psychopathology, and memory can be found in a study conducted by Chae and colleagues (2011). There, children took part in a neutral event, a beanbag game, that occurred as part of a forensic abuse evaluation (Chae et al., 2011). Although there were no differences in memory performance between the maltreated and nonmaltreated children, children with increased levels of dissociative symptoms and higher trauma symptomology had poorer memory performance. Thus, it was not trauma itself that predicted ability to accurately remember the event, but the relation between trauma and psychopathology that revealed predictive power.

Relatedly, children who have experienced maltreatment sometimes reveal improved memory abilities for certain topics. Eisen and colleagues (2007) interviewed the same children from the Chae et al. (2011) study but, instead of discussing a neutral event, the children were interviewed about a forensic medical examination. The children who had experienced physical and sexual abuse were less likely to omit abuse-related information in their memory interview than children who had not experienced such harm. It may be that children who had previously experienced harm attended to abuse-related information more or that those events were more salient to their sense of self. Thus, it may be impossible to draw a simple conclusion between trauma and memory and, instead, one must also consider the nature of the topic being recalled.

Adults' Abilities to Recall Trauma Experienced as Children

Sometimes adults are called to testify about trauma they experienced decades ago as children. Delays in pursuing criminal or civil litigation of sexual abuse are quite common as children (and adults) are often hesitant to disclose the assault; although the rates vary, some studies find that as few as one-third of children initially tell someone else about the abuse (London, Bruck, Ceci, & Shuman, 2005). An understanding of these adults' abilities to accurately testify requires an appreciation of the role that time and trauma play in such memories.

In general, people tend to forget things with the passage of time. However, time can be helpful with respect to memory inasmuch as it marks development from birth into childhood. Older children are generally more accurate storytellers as they are better at providing more comprehensive, detailed, and accurate responses during memory interviews than are younger children (Eisen et al., 2007; Goodman et al., 2001; McWilliams, Harris, & Goodman, 2014; see also Chapter 3). These trends, however, are not absolute and children sometimes display memory accuracy that is similar to, if not better than, adults (Goldfarb & Mindthoff, 2020; Goodman & Schwartz-Kenney, 1992; Otgaar, Howe, Merckelbach, & Muris, 2018). For instance, when the topic to be recalled is one in which the children have greater expertise than the adults (e.g., chess or cartoons), children's memory disadvantage disappears or can be reversed (Chi, 1978; Lindberg, 1980). Adults are also more amenable to suggestions of association, falsely remembering that sleep was included in a list of sleep-related words, than children (Otgaar, Howe, Brackmann, & van Helvoort, 2017; Otgaar et al., 2018; Brainerd, Reyna, & Holliday, 2018; see also Ceci, Fitneva, & Williams,

2010). Adults' increased knowledge base may create a memory trap in that they have a greater ability to draw connections between the stated and unstated words and, as such, are more likely to falsely include the unstated words.

Similarly, the passage of time does not degrade the quality of all memories equally. One simply needs to attempt to evoke memories of a high school graduation versus an unremarkable Tuesday in high school to see that some memories persist. Indeed, both children and adults are often able to recall events, including traumatizing events, years, if not decades, after they occurred. One such type of event recalled by individuals in forensic settings is what has been termed Historic Child Sexual Abuse (Connolly & Read, 2006). In Historic Child Sexual Abuse cases, victims, frequently adults, are asked to recall sexual assaults that they experienced decades prior. Previously, claims of sexual assault were unable to be pursued if they were not brought in a timely manner, as they were frequently barred by the statute of limitations (a legal deadline by which claims must be made; Goldfarb, Goodman, Larson, Eisen, & Qin, 2019). Recently, however, legal reforms have allowed for such claims to be brought irrespective of the delay to prosecution or litigation (Connolly & Read, 2006; Goldfarb et al., 2019).

Research reveals that adults can accurately recall traumatizing events decades later. For instance, in one study, adults were interviewed about a forensic medical examination that they experienced 20 years prior (Goldfarb et al., 2019). When asked about the medical examination 20 years later, around half of the participants accurately disclosed that they had their genitals touched or examined as children (Goldfarb et al., 2019). Thus, many of the adults in this sample were able to remember this sensitive event decades later.

That is not to say that these older events are perfectly recalled. Indeed, as one would expect with the passage of time, details, particularly those that are peripheral (vs. central) to the event, fade (Bauer et al., 2016; Fivush, McDermott Sales, Goldberg, Bahrick, & Parker, 2004; Peterson, 2012; Van Abbema & Bauer, 2005). And, age at the time of the event often plays a role, particularly if children were younger than three at that time.

Most of the studies thus far have focused on children's and adults' abilities to either remember events that they themselves directly experienced, such as sensitive medical examinations, emergency room visits, or natural disasters. Fewer studies, however, have analyzed children's abilities to remember witnessing trauma experienced by others that they love, as would be the case in prosecutions of decades-old murder cases, such as the Bonnie Haim case. Additional work comparing direct and indirect victimization is necessary to understand potentially differential reactions to these cases. Irrespective of the nature of the claim, courts must empathetically respond to children testifying to these issues in a developmentally appropriate manner.

Encouraging Accurate Testimony by Children

Children have a long history of testifying in the United States. In 1895, the United States Supreme Court allowed a 5-year-old child to provide eyewitness testimony in the case of his father's murder (*Wheeler v. United States*, 1895). Fast-forward 124 years, and more than 100,000 child witnesses currently testify in court annually (Fansher & del Carmen, 2016). An even larger number of children's statements are involved in cases that do not reach trial, either because of a plea agreement or another dispositional procedure (Walsh et al., 2008).

Children may be called to testify at different points of the trial process. In a recent survey of prosecutors, 36.8% had cases where child maltreatment victims testified in preliminary hearings; another 25.5% of prosecutors reported that their child victims testified in sentencing hearings, and an additional 33.2% reported working with child victims who testified in other types of proceedings such as a competency hearing, grand jury, or deposition (Cross & Whitcomb, 2017). Although not every confirmed case of abuse requires the child's testimony, it still leaves a number of children testifying every year.

Understanding how testifying impacts the tens of thousands of children who are called to the witness stand each year is important. It is through this understanding that legal practitioners can work to ensure that our justice system can balance fair prosecution of the defense, while also protecting children from further traumatization due to their legal involvement. This section addresses issues relevant to child witness testimony. Specifically, it covers the potential emotional impact of testifying on children that can occur in some (but not all) cases, accommodations available to child witnesses (and possible opposition to the use of such accommodations), and factors affecting the way jurors perceive courtroom testimony given by children. In raising these accommodations, we hope to provide potential methods through which may decrease the likelihood that the highly emotional event of testifying does not lead to ongoing psychopathology.

Impact of Testifying on Children

Testifying about an emotionally charged event, under oath, in a courtroom is a potentially highly stressful experience. Indeed, children report that taking the witness stand is the most stressful aspect of criminal involvement for them (*Maryland v. Craig*, 1990; Quas & McAuliff, 2009). The primary fear induced by testifying in court is speaking in the presence of the defendant (Hobbs et al., 2014), although being embarrassed about crying, unable to answer questions, being "screamed at," or going to jail are also reported as concerns (Pantell, 2017; Sas, Hurley, Austin, & Wolfe, 1991). The level of fear varies between child witnesses, with children whose allegations involve family members (Goodman et al., 1992; Pitchal, 2008) and girls (compared to boys) expressing greater negativity about facing the defendant (Hobbs et al., 2014).

The emotional impact of testifying may be particularly pernicious for children who testify on repeated occasions. Elmi, Daignault, and Hébert (2018) interviewed 344 children, ranging in age from 6 to 14, who were all part of an ongoing legal proceeding and were also receiving services at a children's advocacy center. The children's overall mental health scores improved immediately after the initial advocacy center assessment – that is, the negative effects of taking part in a legal proceeding were ameliorated by therapeutic services. However, amongst children who testified more than once, levels of distress were actually higher two years following the initial assessment. These children (compared to those who testified once or not at all) were more likely to exhibit higher scores on measures of depression, anxiety, avoidance, PTSD, and hypervigilance. The authors argued that this emphasizes the importance of ongoing intervention for children after interaction with the legal system: Initial therapy is helpful, but its benefits may not be as long lasting as assumed for children who must repeatedly appear in court.

Exposure to repeated interviews is also associated with a negative perception of the helpfulness of the criminal justice system (Tedesco & Schnell, 1987), increased distress (Berliner & Conte, 1995), and increased mental health problems (Quas et al., 2005). In a longitudinal study of children who testified in sexual abuse prosecutions, Quas et al. (2005) found that repeated testimony during childhood was linked to an increase in mental health problems. In fact, the highest prevalence of mental health problems existed in children who gave repeated testimony regarding cases of especially severe abuse.

Unfortunately, undergoing more than one interview about a crime or alleged abuse event is commonplace for child witnesses – children typically testify more than once during an investigation (Malloy, Lyon, & Quas, 2007). In fact, sexually abused children give an average of four formal interviews (such as with law enforcement, or medical or mental health professionals) and two informal interviews (such as with caregivers or relatives); these interviews all occur before children even take the stand in court (see Malloy et al., 2007). As with testifying in court, these repeated interviews can be highly stressful for children.

Child Advocacy Centers (CACs) have arisen in response to the call to decrease the trauma of legal proceedings, including repeated interviews, for children. CACs attempt to coordinate the many legal actors involved in criminal prosecutions of crimes against children, police, prosecutors, child protection workers, physicians, and mental health workers. The goal is to increase cooperation and minimize the number of interviews children undergo; this, in turn, is thought to decrease the intrusion and pressure on the child (Connell, 2009; Jackson, 2012; Newman, Dannenfelser, & Pendleton, 2005). Having trained interviewers discuss the alleged trauma with the children, just once, also, hopefully, increases the quality of the interviews. Interviewers trained in developmentally appropriate techniques can work to avoid suggestive questioning while meeting the children at their developmental stage. Indeed, research reveals that CACs decrease children's fear in response to interviews (Jones, Cross, Walsh, & Simone, 2007).

An additional factor contributing to possible stress or distress experienced by children during interviews or courtroom testimony are attorney-questioning tactics. This is especially true during cross-examination, where one potential goal is to discredit the witness (Weiss & Berg, 1982; Zydervelt, Zajac, Kaladelfos, & Westera, 2017). Questions asked during cross-examination are often leading, challenge the witness's credibility, and asked in a linguistically complex manner (Evans, Stolzenberg, & Lyon, 2017; Klemfuss, Cleveland, Quas, & Lyon, 2017; Zajac, Gross, & Haye, 2003; Zydervelt et al., 2017). Badgering, subtle (or blatant) intimidation, and misleading questions have been linked to decreased response accuracy in both adults and children (Carter, Bottoms, & Levine, 1996; Zajac, O'Neill, & Hayne, 2012).

Such questioning may be particularly difficult for children, whose cognitive abilities may affect how they experience the trial process, and the subsequent testimony that they provide (Quas & McAuliff, 2009). For instance, children are often not prepared developmentally for the linguistically foreign legal system (Walker, 1993), which may diminish their understanding of the information provided. Further, the format of these questions may tap into children's increased tendency to succumb to such suggestive interviewing tactics (Chae et al., 2011).

Accommodations for Child Witnesses

Given that the courtroom testimony experience can be confusing and distressing for youth, researchers and legal practitioners have worked to develop procedures and safeguards that help to lessen possible stress faced while on the stand. These resources and accommodations are designed to alleviate stress associated with taking the stand, and to improve memory accuracy (Bruck, Ceci, & Hembrooke, 1998; Fansher & del Carmen, 2016; McAuliff, Nicholson, Amarilio, & Ravanshenas, 2013). For the purposes of this chapter, child witness testimony accommodations are broken down into those available before trial, and those that may be utilized during trial.

Before Trial

Developmentally Appropriate Competence Assessment and Oath

Courts have struggled with determining when children are competent to testify. In the past, children below a certain age (usually 10 or 12) were presumed incompetent to testify and, prior to appearing in court, had to prove testimonial competency (Myers, 1996).

This was the case for the child witness in *Wheeler*. He was initially questioned about his ability to tell the difference between a lie and a truth. During his *voir dire*, he confirmed that he understood the delineation between the two, and that if he were to tell a lie, "the bad man would get him" (*Wheeler v. United States*, 1895, p. 524). Further, he had promised his mother on the morning of the trial that he would "tell no lie" (p. 524). In the *Wheeler* case, the Supreme Court ruled that the child witness's testimony should not be thrown out because, although few would think of calling such a young person to testify, "there is no precise age which determines the question of competency" (p. 524). Rather, the court stated that the child's testimonial competency could be determined by his "[intelligence], [understanding] of the difference between truth and falsehood, and the consequences of telling the latter, and also what was required by the oath he had taken" (p. 525).

Universal competency exam requirements for children have generally decreased or diminished over the past 175 years. Most state laws today establish a minimum age of competence, often 10 or 12 but some states set it as high as 14, at which children are presumed able to testify; children under the age of competence must take part in a competence hearing. For instance, Federal Rules of Evidence Rule 601 presumes competence for all witnesses, and thus it is up to individual judges, *sua sponte* (on their own) or by motion of the parties, to determine whether assessments are necessary in a particular case.

Although the rules have changed as to the presumption of competence, the needle has not really moved as to how competence is assessed. Today, as in the *Wheeler* case, a primary focus of a testimonial competency determination is whether children demonstrate awareness of the difference between a lie and the truth, as well as a promise not to lie, and an understanding of the consequences of lying (Goldfarb, Goodman, & Lawler, 2015). Whether children can differentiate the boundaries between truth and a lie may depend, in part, on how such comprehension is assessed. Children can identify a statement as right or wrong starting as early as two years of age (Lyon, Quas, & Carrick, 2013). A majority of preschoolers can reasonably define a lie (Talwar, Lee, Bala, & Lindsay, 2002; 2004): when asked, between 57 and 76% of 3-year-olds, and well over 80% of older children (4–7), correctly identified a lie in an experimental procedure.

One way that courtrooms can help bolster children's understanding is by changing the nature of the test from free recall to recognition. Children are often better at *identifying* statements as truth or lies compared to *defining* a "truth" versus a "lie" is (Bussey, 1992; Lyon et al., 2013). Many courts test children's abilities to identify truths and lies by providing examples of true and untrue statements and asking the children to label them. For instance, judges might ask child witnesses whether their judicial robes are rainbow or black in color. They then ask the children whether it would be a truth or a lie if they stated that the robes were rainbow. Presuming that judges are not wearing rainbow colored robes, stating that this was a lie would show children's abilities to recognize untruths while still accounting for their developmental differences.

Although children may have the ability to lie and understand that they should not lie, an important question for competence assessments is whether the promise to tell the truth (not to lie) has any effect. Empirical research supports the use of such promises as they do, indeed, decrease children's rates of lying (Lyon & Dorado, 2008). Such promises are even more effective at promoting accuracy when the consequences of veracity are made apparent to children. This can happen through children discussing the positive (vs. negative) consequences of telling the truth, such as how it will make others feel (Talwar, Arruda, & Yachison, 2015), or witnessing another person experience positive consequences for truth telling and negative consequences for lying (Engarhos, Shohoudi, Crossman, & Talwar, 2019). Thus, in the *Wheeler* case, the child witness may have benefited not from focusing on the bad man that would get him if he told a lie, but rather on how his mother would have been proud if he worked to tell the truth. Similarly, he may have benefited from pre-trial preparation, another accommodation used frequently with the child witnesses of today.

Pre-trial Preparation

Pre-trial preparation can be obtained through a number of different methods (Cross & Whitcomb, 2017). Prosecutors report that they frequently provide children with a physical tour of the courtroom or a coloring book informing them about the legal process. Irrespective of its format, the primary goals of pre-trial resources are to help prepare children psychologically and emotionally for giving testimony, and to familiarize them with court proceedings (Quas & McAuliff, 2009; McAuliff et al., 2013). In order to ensure that children's trial participation goes as smoothly as possible, children should have an understanding of why they are involved with a case, who the other players are (e.g., attorneys, judges, etc.), and how the trial process works (Quas & McAuliff, 2009). To avoid the possibility of witness contamination, pre-trial preparation usually focuses on children's procedural understanding rather than the specifics of his or her case (Nathanson & Saywitz, 2015).

Children who are informed about the procedural aspects of the legal system may benefit in a multitude of ways: legal knowledge may help improve their communication ability during interviews (Goodman et al., 1992; Nathanson & Saywitz, 2003) and to reduce anxiety (Goodman et al., 1997). For example, one study found that increased legal knowledge (as measured by children's responses to questions about court, courtroom personnel, and the consequences of telling a lie or the truth in court) was associated with lower levels of distress regarding prospective testimony in 5–8-year-olds (see Goodman et al., 1998).

Confusion as to the various legal actors' roles can undermine children's ability to testify coherently. Children are typically interviewed by both prosecution and defense attorneys during the course of trial proceedings. Uncertainty as to the difference between the two parties may render children confused about why both sides are asking similar or repeated questions. This may lead to an assumption that answers given to the initial attorney were incorrect, resulting in omissions, inconsistencies, or inaccuracies in reporting (Quas & McAuliff, 2009). Knowing that repeated questions are a normal part of the trial process may reduce the likelihood that children attribute this repetition to being incorrect, thus reducing the likelihood that they will change their answers.

The type and intensity of pre-trial preparation can range from anything as informal as courtroom tours to as formal as trainings that focus on increasing children's testimonial accuracy (i.e., how to address attorneys' questions; Saywitz & Snyder, 1996). One example of a pre-trial training program is the Kids' Court School (KCS) in Las Vegas, Nevada. Pre-trial preparation for KCS consists of two separate sessions where the children cover three specific components: (1) legal knowledge education, (2) stress inoculation training, and (3) mock trial participation (Nathanson & Saywitz, 2015). Legal knowledge education includes the presentation of concepts like crime, investigation, evidence, accused, and law with analogies that draw parallels to the children's lives. In this way, the concepts should seem more relevant and be easier to apply to individual children's circumstances. Children also learn about the roles and functions of different courtroom players (e.g., the jury, judge, prosecuting and defense attorneys, bailiff, and witnesses).

During stress inoculation training, children learn breathing techniques and positive self-talk, as these may be utilized during trial to help reduce anxiety experienced while testifying (Nathanson & Saywitz, 2015). After the knowledge and stress trainings, children participate in a mock trial where they take turns playing the roles of judge and witness. The role-playing allows the children to experience direct- and cross-examination, interruptions, and objections (reflective of an actual trial).

Trial preparation may have a multitude of benefits for young witnesses, including increased knowledge of court procedures, helping them deal with anxiety related to their abuse and to testifying, and facilitating them in telling their story competently while on the stand (Peterson, Rolls Reutz, Hazen, Habib, & Williams, 2019; Sas et al., 1991). Nathanson and Saywitz (2015) evaluated outcomes of the Las Vegas KCS. They found that children's pre-trial anxiety decreased significantly following program attendance. In addition, children who participated in a similar pre-trial program were perceived as more prepared for giving a statement than children who did not undergo such preparation (Sas et al., 1991). Thus, it seems that empirical research does lend support to pre-trial preparation. Ideally, pre-trial preparation would work in concert with specific accommodations offered during the trial itself to make child witnesses' courtroom experience as painless as possible.

During Trial

In addition to pre-trial preparation, courts often offer social support and witness accommodations during the trial. Courts may be hesitant to institute certain accommodations for child witnesses out of concern that they may unduly bias jurors in favor of the victim (Myers, 1996; Quas & McAuliff, 2009). Below we review a handful of potential during-trial accommodations and the research as to the impact on the children, the defendants, and the juries.

Support Persons

Traditionally, courts expected witnesses to "go it alone" (Myers, 1996), but many states have now made exceptions for children to have support persons as part of the legal proceedings (Conn. Gen. Stat., 2018, title 54, § S 54–86g(b)(2); Delaware Code, 2019, title 11, §3514(b) (d); Idaho Code, 2019, § 19–3023; N.Y. Exec. Law, 2016, § 642-a 6; U.S. Code, 2019, title 18, § 3509(i)). For instance, in 1974, the Child Abuse Prevention and Treatment Act (CAPTA) conditioned receipt of federal funds for the prevention of child abuse and neglect on their providing support persons for children involved in child welfare cases. Support persons may be an attorney, guardian *ad litem* appointed by the state, a friend, family member, or "any individual who contributes to the well-being of the child" (Quas & McAuliff, 2009, p. 91).

One way that courts may ensure that children have a support person is through the provision of a victim advocate; victim advocates are assigned to help the children throughout the criminal proceeding (McAuliff et al., 2013; Whitcomb, Shapiro, & Stellwagen, 1985). Not only will the advocate provide emotional support, but they will also aid in some of the pre-trial preparation discussed above – for instance, by explaining the procedures to the children, and sometimes working with the children and their families in the logistics of getting to trial. The degree to which the support person has a role in trial proceedings may vary by state (McAuliff et al., 2013); some states restrict interactions between the child and the support person while the child is giving his or her testimony (e.g., Hawaii), whereas others allow the person to accompany and remain in close proximity to the child during testimony (e.g., Idaho, California; see McAuliff & Kovera, 2002).

The presence of a support person may help reduce children's suggestibility (Bottoms, Quas, & Davis, 2007), help children cope with trauma (Spaccarelli & Kim, 1995), and facilitate their answering attorney questions (Goodman et al., 1992). Some argue that no courtroom reform is more important than permitting a child witness to be accompanied by a supporting adult (Myers, 1996). Prosecutors similarly rate these procedures favorably and say they use them frequently, with over 72.4% of prosecutors reporting having used a victim advocate and 62.1% reporting having used another support person (Cross & Whitcomb, 2017; Goodman, Quas, Bulkley, & Shapiro, 1999).

One potential downside of such support persons is that jurors may view child witnesses who testify with a support person sitting next to them as less credible than those who testify without such a support (McAuliff, Lapin, & Michel, 2015). Additional research is needed on this issue to understand the mechanisms and potential methods to help ameliorate concerns about the presence of a support person when a child testifies.

Support Animals

Some states allow certified support dogs to accompany child witnesses when they take the stand (see Ariz. Rev. Stat 2019 §§ 11–1024, 13–4442; Ark. Code 2016 § 16–43–1002; California, Connecticut: Public Act 2017 No. 17–185; Fla. Stat. 2019 § 92.55). These dogs are specially trained to provide emotional support in a courtroom setting. Approximately 43.9% of prosecutors have reported using a therapy or comfort animal before trial and 17.2% report using support animals for child witnesses during trial. The use of emotional support dogs has been linked to a reduction in tension associated with testifying in open court, and protection of the welfare of vulnerable witnesses (Dellinger, 2009). In addition, presence of an emotional support animal may reduce blood pressure and anxiety, and increase feelings of self-worth (O'Neill-Stephens, 2006).

Videotaped Testimony

Under some limited circumstances, a videotaped statement (e.g., an interview conducted with law enforcement or a deposition taken by the attorneys) may be shown to the judge or jury at trial in place of live testimony (Kan. Stat. Ann., 2018, § 22–3434; Ky. Rev. Stat., 2013, § 421.350). According to the NCPCA (2006), at least 17 states allow for children's testimony to be presented in some form of videotape.

Using recorded interviews, rather than live testimony, is a rare accommodation, as few as 3.4% of prosecutors report having used this accommodation (Cross & Whitcomb, 2017). One reason for this is because, short of an exception to the hearsay clause, is its potential infringement on a defendant's 6th amendment right to confrontation (*Craig v. Maryland*, 1990; *Crawford v. Washington*, 2004) and right to due process (Myers, 1987). If videotaped statements are used, some states require that the defendant be present during the videotaping to help ensure that defendants' right to confrontation is not undermined (e.g., Tenn. Code, 2018, § 24–7–117). Countries that do not grant defendants the right to confrontation exercise greater ability to use videotaped testimony (such as Canada, England, New Zealand, Scotland, and most of Australia; Davies & Noon, 1991; Flin, Kearney, & Murray, 1996; Shrimpton, Oates, & Hayes, 1996).

Research findings regarding the effects of videotaped testimony on jurors are mixed – some studies suggest that perceptions of child witnesses' credibility do not change (Landström & Granhag, 2010; Swim, Borgida, & McCoy, 1993), whereas others show that mock-jurors may find children less confident, honest, believable, and convincing when they testify via a pre-recorded tape (Goodman et al., 2006; Landström, Granhag, & Hartwig, 2007).

In countries such as New Zealand, videotaped statements are commonly truncated – that is, edited such that jurors are only shown portions of the child's taped testimony containing the core allegations (i.e., the primary charges being brought against the defendant; Mahoney, McDonald, Optican, & Tinsely, 2010). Anderson and colleagues (2016) evaluated how the truncation of child witness testimony affected jurors' perceptions of the child's testimony and the defendant's culpability. The majority of mock-jurors believed the core allegation to be true even when the testimony was not truncated and additional, less-plausible allegations were present. These findings stand in contrast to similar research that has been done with the plausibility of adult witness allegations (e.g., Peace et al., 2015). Researchers posited that perhaps participants in their study were sensitive to the fact that the children in the hypotheticals were questioned using best-practices techniques, and not leading or suggestive questions. As a result, they may have found no reason not to believe the child witnesses. Thus, although jurors may be correct in appreciating children's vulnerability when poor interviewing practices are utilized, they may also make incorrect assumptions about children's accuracy in the absence of such practices.

Closed-Circuit Television, or "Live Link" Testimony

When using closed-circuit television (CCTV), a child witness answers questions via a television monitor rather than doing so in open court. This allows jurors to observe the witness's testimony in real-time, but the child is protected from possibly having to face the defendant. Sometimes both attorneys and the defendant will be in the room with the child, while the judge and jurors remain in the courtroom; other times, only the attorneys will be with the child and the defendant remains in the courtroom with the judge and jurors. In still other cases, the child is alone in a separate room, and direct and cross-examination is done entirely via CCTV (Quas & McAuliff, 2009).

In the United States, the Supreme Court has required that the court must make a finding that it was necessary to protect the child in this case before CCTV can be used (*Maryland v. Craig*, 1990). The judge cannot rely on the general harm suffered from testifying about difficult subjects but must conduct an individualized assessment of the case in which the CCTV request is made. Although it has been approved by some legislation (NCPCA, 2006) and the Supreme Court (*Maryland v. Craig*, 1990), it is rarely utilized by prosecutors (Cross & Whitcomb, 2017; Grearson, 2004). It is, however, more widely used outside of the United States, including in England (Davies & Noon, 1991).

In countries that more frequently implement this accommodation, its use has been linked to a perception of reduced witness stress (Cashmore, 1992) and increased ease of testifying (Murray, 1995). CCTV has also been associated with an increased ability to answer direct questions, as well as fewer omission errors to suggestive questions (Goodman et al., 1998) and does not necessarily increase conviction rates (Ross et al., 1994).

Use of CCTV is not without consequences. Jurors who watch a child testify via CCTV view the witness as being less credible than when the child appears and testifies in person (Goodman et al., 1998). Indeed, jurors who saw a child witness provide her testimony in open court were more likely to return guilty verdicts than those who saw the child witness testify either via CCTV or from behind a protective shield (Ross et al., 1994). Nonetheless, neither the credibility of the defendant nor of the child witness were differentially impacted. This suggests that use of testimony accommodation may not always put the defendant at a greater risk of being convicted and that CCTV may sometimes lower the rates of conviction.

Summary of Direct and Non-Direct Testimonial Aids

In some cases of alleged child abuse, a victim-witness elects to formally testify against their offender, whether it be via direct or non-direct means. If the witness chooses to provide direct testimony in court, they may be afforded some form of accompaniment, such as the presence of a support person or animal. Utilizing support entities has been linked to reduced suggestibility on the stand, better quality responses to attorney-questioning, and reduction in anxiety regarding the court appearance. However, the use of support persons or animals may also reduce jurors' perceptions of the witness's credibility.

If the witness chooses to provide non-direct testimony, they may do so via videotape or CCTV. Using CCTV to provide testimony may reduce anxiety regarding provision of testimony and facilitate answering direct questions. However, CCTV may reduce perceptions of the witness's credibility and, in some cases, impact juror verdicts. Thus, generally speaking, both direct and non-direct testimonial aids provide important benefits to vulnerable child witnesses, but also present some limitations that should be taken into account when such aids are being considered for use.

Juror Perceptions of Child Testimony

Although testimonial aids for children have utility, it is important to remember that they are not used in all cases. Under some circumstances, children may provide testimony in open court without assistance. Thus, it is important to understand how jurors perceive child testimony on a more global level. Owing perhaps to stereotypes about children's immaturity and naivety, some jurors enter the courtroom with skepticism towards child testimony (Goodman, Golding, & Haith, 1984). Other jurors, however, find child witnesses to be just as, or sometimes even more, credible than adult witnesses (Ross, Jurden, Lindsay, & Keeney, 2003). Jurors' perceptions of child witnesses play a large role in determining case outcomes and are, as such, vitally important to the prosecution of any case of child maltreatment (Leippe, Eisenstadt, Rauch, & Seib, 2004).

One factor that may influence jurors' perceptions is the age of the testifying child. As discussed above, children's abilities to provide more detailed and potentially diagnostic memories increase with age while their suggestibility generally decreases. Given that they are less mature than adults, younger witnesses may be more likely to exhibit behaviors that lower people's perceptions of credibility (e.g., lack of confidence, low status, or powerless speech style; Deffenbacher, 1980; Miller & Burgoon, 1982; Wells, Ferguson, & Lindsay, 1981). That, coupled with the fact that adults tend to believe that younger children have poorer memories and can be easily manipulated (Goodman et al., 1984), may lead jurors to perceive younger children (e.g., preschoolers) as being less credible than older children (e.g., those in middle school) and adults (Goodman, Golding, Hegleson, Haith, & Michelli, 1987).

Studies do indeed find that younger children are sometimes rated as less credible compared than older children and adults (Allison, Lindsay, & Ross, 2006; Goodman et al., 1987). Nonetheless, eyewitness age does not always produce significant differences in ratings of the defendant's degree of guilt. Of interest, however, eyewitness testimony was the primary evidence used to rate guilt of the defendant when an adult witness provided this testimony. But when eyewitness testimony was provided by a child, the testimony given by additional (circumstantial) witnesses became more important. Researchers concluded that eyewitness age alone may not directly affect jurors' perceptions of a defendant, but it may affect the extent to which they need corroboration from other sources.

Not all studies find that age predicts perceptions of credibility. More recently, Cleveland and Quas (2016) evaluated adults' sensitivity to the impact of children's development on their ability to accurately report abuse. Age of the child witness (6 vs. 11) did not affect the credibility of their testimony in a sexual abuse trial. Children who were more confident in their testimony, however, were rated as being more credible than children who were less sure (Cleveland & Quas, 2016). In terms of accuracy, children who were confident were believed to be more accurate than those who were not confident.

The authors concluded that participants in this study penalized children for being unsure about the temporal details of abuse (by returning fewer guilty verdicts), and displayed insensitivity to developmental trajectories for how children describe temporal information (Wandrey, 2013). Specifically, jurors tended to believe that younger children were more likely to be accurate regarding temporal details than were older children. Nonetheless, research suggests that with age, children may become more aware that they are unsure of the answer to temporal questions (and thus may answer accordingly). Although they are being more honest by doing so, it may cause jurors to view their reports more negatively. Thus, it may be important for legal practitioners to make jurors aware of these developmental trends.

Children's role in the case, whether they are testifying as the victim of abuse or a witness of it, may also affect the extent to which they are believed by jurors (Bottoms & Goodman, 1994; Nikonova & Ogloff, 2005). More specifically, when children are testifying as victims, jurors are more likely to consider a possibility of fabrication and as a result, perception of credibility are influenced by the child's earnestness (Bottoms & Goodman, 1994). Conversely, when the children are testifying as bystanders, believability is influenced by whether they seem to have the required levels of cognitive functioning to produce accurate testimony (Luus, Wells, & Turtle, 1995). Indeed, mock-jurors are more likely to find a defendant guilty when a child witness testifies as a bystander than as a victim-witness (Holocomb & Jacquin, 2007).

In addition to serving as an eyewitness as to violence perpetrated against others, children may also be asked to serve as an alibi witness, perhaps providing a defense for a parent or another loved one. In general, alibi evidence is often believed by jurors to be deceptive (Allison, Jung, Sweeney, & Culhane, 2014). This may especially be true when the alibi witness has a previous relationship to the defendant as he or she may be more motivated to lie on the defendant's behalf (Olson & Wells, 2004). At the same time, however, children are commonly thought to be more honest compared to adults (Connolly, Price, & Gordon, 2010) – some people have even considered children incapable of deception (Nunez, Kehn, & Wright, 2011).

Research on children as alibi witnesses is somewhat limited and the effects of age are mixed. For instance, Fawcett and Winstanley (2019) exposed mock-jurors to a fictitious murder trial transcript that contained testimony from a child witness who was either 8, 12, or 16 years of age. The only significant predictor of perceptions of the child witness was the level of displayed confidence: the high-confidence alibi witness was perceived as more reliable, honest, and accurate (Fawcett & Winstanley, 2019). Neither the age of the child witness nor his level of confidence had a significant effect on mock-jurors' trial verdicts, nor did their perceptions of the defendant. The authors concluded that in cases of indirect testimony (such as with alibi witnesses), increasing the witness's confidence in his or her statement may be vitally important for encouraging jurors to interpret the statement positively.

Dahl and Price (2012) investigated how an alibi witness's age (6 or 25 years of age) and relationship to the defendant (son or neighbor) impacted jurors' beliefs about the alibi's credibility and the defendant's guilt. Overall, jurors believed that the child alibi witness was more credible than the adult alibi witness and were less likely to convict the defendant. This study is in line with prior work finding that jurors often believe that children will be more honest in comparison to adults. For a consensus to be reached from these mixed results, future research should analyze the mechanisms underlying credibility of children's alibi statements and consider potential rationales for differences in the findings.

Although adults tend to believe children are more honest than adults, how good are jurors are detecting when children are not telling the truth? People are generally not very good lie detectors: performing at approximately chance accuracy (around guessing) whether the liar is a child or an adult (Bond & DePaulo, 2006; Edelstein, Luten, Ekman, & Goodman, 2006; Johnson et al., 2017). A recent meta-analysis, however, revealed a slightly different trend. Overall, it appeared that adults performed slightly above chance in detecting lies (Gongola, Scurich, & Quas, 2017). Thus, adults' own assessments may not be the most reliable indicator of children's veracity and, instead, the legal system might be better served by the institution of some of the reforms discussed above.

Conclusions

Considerable work has been done over the past few decades on children's abilities to serve as witnesses in the courtroom. This work has shown that all too many children in the United States experience harm and some of these children will subsequently experience increased levels of psychopathology. Although trauma alone does not necessarily decrease the accuracy of children's recall, there is evidence that increased trauma symptomology may negatively impact their ability to recall.

Children who experience trauma may also be asked to testify on the stand about said traumas. Research reveals that children can and do accurately testify about acts perpetrated against them. Testifying, particularly repeatedly or with the defendant present, can be a stressful experience for children. There are, however, numerous mechanisms that can be used to reduce the stress, including victim advocates and pre-trial preparation. Supporting children who testify in this way can help reduce further traumatization and help bring criminal cases to resolution.

When we provide children with supports, we must also be cognizant of the impact that these supports have on jurors' perceptions of child witnesses. Some aids, including testifying via CCTV, decrease jurors' beliefs that the child is a credible witness. Relatedly, jurors are also skeptical of child witnesses who show uncertainty in their responses, despite the fact that this uncertainty may reflect children's careful consideration of their testimony and increased cognitive abilities. These two trends lead us to argue that lawyers and jurors must be made aware of the developmental trends found in the research and the impact of that work on cases involving child witnesses.

Although the research conducted thus far has helped researchers and legal practitioners gain a better understanding of how children interact with the trial process, there is still a great deal to be done. Arguably one of the biggest obstacles to studying the impact of trauma on child witnesses is doing so empirically – researchers cannot conduct true experiments (i.e., involving random assignment) on maltreatment or trauma to determine causality. The majority of the observations made are based on naturalistic observation or individual court cases. Given that there are large variations in abuse cases (i.e., the nature of the abuse, the severity, individual differences in coping with trauma, etc.), it can be difficult – or impossible – to tease apart true causal relationships.

Nonetheless, incredible research within analogous situations for trauma, including medical events, and important intervention work within courtroom settings has been conducted. Researchers should continue exploring ways to use empirical science to determine the relative effectiveness of various courtroom accommodations, as well as the longitudinal effects of providing courtroom testimony. As the long-term effects of testifying are clarified, researchers should also work to develop additional accommodations for particularly young witnesses to help reduce adverse effects. Together, we can help children like Aaron Fraser and ensure that legal interventions help children navigate the "tricky waters" of the legal system rather than causing further harm.

References

Achenbach, T. M. (1991). *Manual for the child behavior checklist/4–18 and 1991 profile.* University of Vermont, Department of Psychiatry.

Ackil, J. K., Van Abbema, D. L., & Bauer, P. J. (2003). After the storm: Enduring differences in mother—child recollections of traumatic and nontraumatic events. *Journal of Experimental Child Psychology, 84*(4), 286–309.

Allison, M., Jung, S., Sweeney, L., & Culhane, S. E. (2014). The impact of illegal alibi activities, corroborator involvement and corroborator certainty on mock juror perceptions. *Psychiatry, Psychology and Law*, *21*, 191–204.

Allison, M., & Lindsay, R., & Ross, D. (2006). Age-related expectations of child witness credibility. *Modern Psychological Studies*, *11*, 37–48.

American Psychiatric Association. (2013). *Diagnostic and statistical manual of mental disorders* (5th ed.). American Psychiatric Pub.

Anderson, L., Gross, J., Sonne, T., Zajac, R., & Hayne, H. (2016). Where there's smoke, there's fire: The effect of truncated testimony on juror decision-making. *Behavioral Sciences & the Law*, *34*, 200–217.

Andrews, S. J., Ahern, E. C., Stolzenberg, S. N., & Lyon, T. D. (2016). The productivity of wh-prompts when children testify. *Applied Cognitive Psychology*, *30*, 341–349. https://doi.org/10.1002/acp.3204

Ariz. Rev. Stat 2019 §§ 11–1024, 13–4442

Ark. Code 2016 § 16–43–1002

Baldry, A. C., & Winkel, F. W. (2004). Mental and physical health of Italian youngsters directly and indirectly victimized at school and at home. *International Journal of Forensic Mental Health*, *3*(1), 77–91.

Barlow, M. R., Turow, R. E. G., & Gerhart, J. (2017). Trauma appraisals, emotion regulation difficulties, and self-compassion predict posttraumatic stress symptoms following childhood abuse. *Child Abuse and Neglect*, *65*, 37–47. https://doi.org/10.1016/j.chiabu.2017.01.006

Bauer, P. J., Burch, M. M., Van Abbema, D. L., & Ackil, J. K. (2007). Talking about twisters: Relations between mothers' and children's contributions to conversations about a devastating tornado. *Journal of Cognition and Development*, *8*(4), 371–399.

Bauer, P. J., Stark, E. N., Ackil, J. K., Larkina, M., Merrill, N., & Fivush, R. (2016). The recollective qualities of adolescents' and adults' narratives about a long-ago tornado. *Memory*, 1–13. https://doi.org/10.1080/09658211.2016.1180396

Becker-Blease, K. A., Freyd, J. J., & Pears, K. C. (2004). Preschoolers' memory for threatening information depends on trauma history and attentional context: Implications for the development of dissociation. *Journal of Trauma and Dissociation*, *5*(1), 113–131. https://doi.org/10.1300/J229v05n01_07

Berliner, L., & Conte, J. R. (1995). The effects of disclosure and intervention on sexually abused children. *Child Abuse and Neglect*, *19*, 371–384.

Bond, C., & DePaulo, B. (2006). Accuracy of deception judgments. *Personality and Social Psychology Review*, *10*, 214–234.

Bottoms, B. L., & Goodman, G. S. (1994). Perceptions of children's credibility in sexual assault cases. *Journal of Applied Social Psychology*, *24*, 702–732.

Bottoms, B. L., Quas, J. A., & Davis, S. L. (2007). The influence of the interviewer-provided social support on children's suggestibility, memory, and disclosures. In M. E. Pipe, M. Lamb, Y. Orbach, & A. C. Cederborg (Eds.), *Child sexual abuse: Disclosure, delay, and denial* (pp. 135–157). Mahwah, NJ: Lawrence Erlbaum Associates Publishers.

Bourassa, C. (2007). Co-occurrence of interparental violence and child physical abuse and its effect on the adolescents' behavior. *Journal of Family Violence*, *22*(8), 691–701.

Brainerd, C. J., Reyna, V. F., & Holliday, R. E. (2018). Developmental reversals in false memory: Development is complementary, not compensatory. *Developmental Psychology*, *54*, 1773–1784. http://dx.doi.org/10.1037/dev0000554

Bruck, M., Ceci, S., & Hembrooke, H. (1998). Reliability and credibility of young children's reports: From research to policy and practice. *American Psychologist*, *53*(2), 136–151.

Bücker, J., Kapczinski, F., Post, R., Ceresér, K. M., Szobot, C., Yatham, L. N ... & Kauer-Sant'Anna, M. (2012). Cognitive impairment in school-aged children with early trauma. *Comprehensive Psychiatry*, *53*(6), 758–764.

Burke & Associated Press. (2019, April). Son of Florida woman who disappeared in 1993 testifies in father's murder trial. *NBC News*. Retrieved from https://www.nbcnews.com

Bussey, K. (1992). Lying and truthfulness: Children's definitions, standards, and evaluative reactions. *Child Development*, *63*, 129–137.

California, Connecticut: Public Act 2017 No. 17–185

Camacho, K., Ehrensaft, M. K., & Cohen, P. (2012). Exposure to intimate partner violence, peer relations, and risk for internalizing behaviors: A prospective longitudinal study. *Journal of Interpersonal Violence, 27*(1), 125–141.

Carter, C. A., Bottoms, B. L., & Levine, M. (1996). Linguistic and socioemotional influences on the accuracy of children's reports. *Law and Human Behavior, 20*, 335–358.

Cashmore, J. (1992). The use of closed-circuit television for child witnesses in the ACT. Sydney, New South Wales: Australian Law Reform Commission

Ceci, S. J., Fitneva, S. A., & Williams, W. M. (2010). Representational constraints on the development of memory and metamemory: A developmental—representational theory. *Psychological Review, 117*, 464–495. http://dx.doi.org/10.1037/a0019067

Chae, Y., Goodman, G. S., Eisen, M. L., & Qin, J. (2011). Event memory and suggestibility in abused and neglected children: Trauma-related psychopathology and cognitive functioning. *Journal of Experimental Child Psychology, 110*(4), 520–538. https://doi.org/10.1016/j.jecp.2011.05.006

Chi, M. T. H. (1978). Knowledge structures and memory development. In R. S. Siegler (Ed.), *Children's thinking: What develops?* (pp. 73–96). Hillsdale, NJ: Erlbaum.

Cleveland, K., & Quas, J. (2016). Adults' insensitivity to developmental changes in children's ability to report when and how many times abuse occurred. *Behavioral Sciences & the Law, 34*, 126–138.

Conn. Gen. Stat., 2018, title 54, § S 54–86g(b)(2)

Connell, M. (2009). The Child Advocacy Center model. In K. Kuehnle & M. Connell (Eds.), *The evaluation of child sexual abuse allegations: A comprehensive guide to assessment and testimony* (pp. 423–449). Hoboken, NJ: John Wiley & Sons.

Connolly, D. A., & Read, J. D. (2006). Delayed prosecutions of historic child sexual abuse: Analyses of 2064 Canadian criminal complaints. *Law and Human Behavior, 30*(4), 409–434.

Connolly, D. A., Price, H. L., & Gordon, H. M. (2010). Judicial decision-making in timely and delayed prosecutions of child sexual abuse in Canada: A study of honesty and cognitive ability in assessments of credibility. *Psychology, Public Policy and Law, 16*, 177–199.

Crawford v. Washington, 541 U.S. 36 (2004).

Cross, T., & Whitcomb, D. (2017). The practice of prosecuting child maltreatment: Results of an online survey of prosecutors. *Child Abuse & Neglect, 69*, 20–28.

Dahl, L., & Price, H. (2012). He couldn't have done it, he was with me!: The impact of alibi witness age and relationship. *Applied Cognitive Psychology, 26*, 475–481.

Davies, G. M., & Noon, E. (1991). *An evaluation of the live link for child witnesses.* London: Home Office.

Deffenbacher, K. A. (1980). Eyewitness accuracy and confidence: Can we infer anything about their relationship? *Law and Human Behavior, 4*, 243–260.

Deffenbacher, K. A., Bornstein, B. H., Penrod, S. D., & McGorty, E. K. (2004). A meta-analytic review of the effects of high stress on eyewitness memory. *Law and Human Behavior, 28*(6), 687–706.

Delaware Code, 2019, title 11, §3514(b)(d)

Dellinger, M. (2009). Using dogs for emotional support of testifying victims of crime. *Animal Law Review, 15*, 1–20.

Dodge, K. A., Pettit, G. S., Bates, J. E., & Valente, E. (1995). Social information-processing patterns partially mediate the effect of early physical abuse on later conduct problems. *Journal of Abnormal Psychology, 104*(4), 632–643. https://doi.org/10.1037/0021-843X.104.4.632

Dvir, Y., Ford, J. D., Hill, M., & Frazier, J. A. (2015). Childhood maltreatment, emotional dysregulation, and psychiatric comorbidities. *Harvard Review of Psychiatry, 22*(3), 149–161. https://doi.org/10.1097/HRP.0000000000000014.Childhood

Edelstein, R., Luten, T., Ekman, P., & Goodman, G. (2006). Detecting lies in children and adults. *Law and Human Behavior, 30*, 1–10.

Ehring, T., & Quack, D. (2010). Emotion regulation difficulties in trauma survivors: The role of trauma type and PTSD symptom severity. *Behavior Therapy, 41*(4), 587–598. https://doi.org/10.1016/j.beth.2010.04.004

Eisen, M. L., Goodman, G. S., Qin, J., Davis, S., & Crayton, J. (2007). Maltreated children's memory: Accuracy, suggestibility, and psychopathology. *Developmental Psychology, 43*(6), 1275–1294.

Eisenberg, N., Spinrad, T. L., & Eggum, N. D. (2010). Emotion-related self-regulation and its relation to children's maladjustment. *Annual Review of Clinical Psychology, 6*, 495–525.

Elmi, M., Daignault, I., & Hébert, M. (2018). Child sexual abuse victims as witnesses: The influence of testifying on their recovery. *Child Abuse and Neglect, 86*, 22–32.

Engarhos, P., Shohoudi, A., Crossman, A., & Talwar, V. (2019). Learning through observing: Effects of modeling truth-and lie-telling on children's honesty. *Developmental Science*, e12883.

Evans, A., Stolzenberg, S., & Lyon, T. D (2017). Pragmatic failure and referential ambiguity when attorneys ask child witnesses "do you know/remember" questions. *Psychology, Public Policy, and Law, 23*, 191–199.

Fansher, A., & Del Carmen, R. (2016). "The child as witness": Evaluating state statutes on the court's most vulnerable population. *Children's Legal Rights Journal, 36*(1), 1–45.

Fawcett, H., & Winstanley, K. (2019). Children as alibi witnesses: the effect of age and confidence on mock-juror decision making. *Psychiatry, Psychology and Law, 25*, 957–971.

Federal Rules of Evidence, Rule 601

Finkelhor, D., Turner, H., Ormrod, R., & Hamby, S. (2009). Violence, abuse, and crime exposure in a national sample of children and youth. *Pediatrics, 124*, 1411–1423.

Finkelhor, D., Turner, H., Shattuck, A., & Hamby, S. (2015). Prevalence of childhood exposure to violence, crime, and abuse: Results from the national survey of children's exposure to Violence. *JAMA Pediatrics, 169*, 746–754.

Fivush, R., McDermott Sales, J., Goldberg, A., Bahrick, L., & Parker, J. (2004). Weathering the storm: Children's long-term recall of Hurricane Andrew. *Memory, 12*, 104–118. https://doi.org/10.1080/09658210244000397

Fla. Stat. 2019 § 92.55

Flin, R., Kearney, B., & Murray, K. (1996). Children's evidence: Scottish research and law. *Criminal Justice and Behavior, 23*, 358–376.

Florida Times-Union (2019). The disappearance of Bonnie Haim: Missing in 1993 and unearthed by son in 2014, her husband's trial begins Monday. Retrieved from www.firstcoastnews.com

Goldfarb, D., & Mindthoff, A. (2020). Often but not always: When does age at the time of event predict memory for sexual violence? In J. D. Pozzulo, E. Pics, & C. Sheahan (Eds.), *Memory and sexual misconduct: Psychological research for criminal justice* (pp. 71–99). New York: Routledge.

Goldfarb, D., Goodman, G. S., Larson, R. P., Eisen, M. L., & Qin, J. (2019). Long-term memory in adults exposed to childhood violence: Remembering genital contact nearly 20 years later. *Clinical Psychological Science, 7*, 381–396. https://doi.org/10.1177/2167702618805742

Goldfarb, D., Goodman, G. S., Larson, R. P., Gonzalez, A., & Eisen, M. L. (2017). Putting children's memory and suggestibility in their place: An analysis considering person, topic, and context. In H. Otgaar & M. L. Howe (Eds.), *Finding the truth in the courtroom: Dealing with deception, lies, and memories* (pp. 137–162). New York: Oxford University Press.

Goldfarb, D., Goodman, G., & Lawler, M. (2015). Children's evidence and the Convention on the Rights of the Child: Improving the legal system for children. *Child-Friendly Justice: A Quarter of a Century of the UN Convention on the Rights of the Child*. 85–109. doi:10.1163/9789004297432_010

Gongola, J., Scurich, N., & Quas, J. (2017). Detecting deception in children: A meta-analysis. *Law and Human Behavior, 41*, 44–54.

Goodman, G. S., & Schwartz-Kenney, B. M. (1992). Why knowing a child's age is not enough: Influences of cognitive, social, and emotional factors on children's testimony. In H. Dent & R. Flin (Eds.), *Wiley series in the psychology of crime, policing and law. Children as witnesses* (pp. 15–32). Oxford: John Wiley & Sons.

Goodman, G. S., Bottoms, B. L., Rudy, L., Davis, S. L., & Schwartz-Kenney, B. M. (2001). Effects of past abuse experiences on children' s eyewitness memory. *Law and Human Behavior, 25*(3), 269–298.

Goodman, G. S., Golding, J. M., & Haith, M. M. (1984). Jurors' reaction to child witnesses. *Journal of Social Issues, 40*, 139–156.

Goodman, G. S., Myers, J. E. B., Qin, J., Quas, J. A., Castelli, P., Redlich, A. D., & Rogers, L. (2006). Hearsay versus children's testimony: Effects of truthful and deceptive statements on jurors' decisions. *Law and Human Behavior, 30*, 363–401.

Goodman, G. S., Quas, J. A., & Ogle, C. M. (2010). Child maltreatment and memory. *Annual Review of Psychology*, *61*(1), 325–351. https://doi.org/10.1146/annurev.psych.093008.100403

Goodman, G. S., Quas, J. A., Bulkley, J., & Shapiro, C. (1999). Innovations for child witnesses: A national survey. *Psychology, Public Policy, and Law*, *5*, 255–281.

Goodman, G. S., Goldfarb, D. A., Quas, J. A., Narr, R. K., Milojevich, H., & Cordon, I. M … (2016). Memory development, emotion regulation, and trauma-related psychopathology. In D. Cicchetti (Ed.), *Developmental psychopathology* (pp. 555–590). New York: Wiley.

Goodman, G., Golding, J., Helgeson, V., Haith, M., & Michelli, J. (1987). When a child takes the stand: Jurors' perceptions of children's eyewitness testimony. *Law and Human Behavior*, *11*, 27–40.

Goodman, G., Quas, J., Batterman-Faunce, J., Riddlesberger, M., & Kuhn, G. (1997). Children's reactions to and memory for a stressful event: Influences of age, anatomical dolls, knowledge, and parental attachment. *Applied Developmental Science*, *1*, 54–75.

Goodman, G., Taub, E., Jones, D., England, P., Port, L., Rudy, L., & Prado, L. (1992). Testifying in criminal court: Emotional effects of child sexual assault victims. *Monographs of the Society for Research in Child Development*, 57(229). https://pubmed.ncbi.nlm.nih.gov/1470193/

Goodman, G., Tobey, A., Batterman-Faunce, J., Orcutt, H., Thomas, S., Shapiro, C., & Sachsenmaier, T. (1998). Face-to-face confrontation: Effects of closed circuit-technology on children's eyewitness testimony and jurors' decisions. *Law and Human Behavior*, *22*, 165–203.

Graham-Bermann, S. A., Castor, L. E., Miller, L. E., & Howell, K. H. (2012). The impact of intimate partner violence and additional traumatic events on trauma symptoms and PTSD in preschool-aged children. *Journal of Traumatic Stress*, *25*(4), 393–400. https://doi.org/10.1002/jts.21724

Grearson, K. (2004). *Proposed Uniform Child Witness Testimony Act: An Impermissible Abridgement of Criminal Defendants' Rights*, 45 B.C.L Rev. 467. http://lawdigitalcommons.bc.edu/bclr/vol45/iss2/5

Gross, J. J. (2002). Emotion regulation: Affective, cognitive, and social consequences. *Psychophysiology*, *39*(3), 281–291. https://doi.org/10.1017/S0048577201393198

Hadland, S. E., Marshall, B. D. L., Kerr, T., Qi, J., Montaner, J. S., & Wood, E. (2012). Suicide and history of childhood trauma among street youth. *Journal of Affective Disorders*, *136*(3), 377–380. https://doi.org/10.1016/j.jad.2011.11.019

Hahm, H. C., Lee, Y., Ozonoff, A., & van Wert, M. J. (2010). The impact of multiple types of child maltreatment on subsequent risk behaviors among women during the transition from adolescence to young adulthood. *Journal of Youth and Adolescence*, *39*(5), 528–540. https://doi.org/10.1007/s10964-009-9490-0

Hamby, S., Finkelhor, D., Turner, H., & Ormrod, R. (2010). The overlap of witnessing partner violence with child maltreatment and other victimizations in a nationally representative survey of youth. *Child Abuse & Neglect*, *34*(10), 734–741.

Hobbs, S., Goodman, G., Block, S., Oran, D., Quas, J., Park, A., Widaman, K., & Baumrind, N. (2014). Child maltreatment victims' attitudes about appearing in dependency and criminal courts. *Children and Youth Services Review*, *44*, 407–416.

Holocomb, M., & Jacquin, K. (2007). Juror perceptions of child eyewitness testimony in a sexual abuse trial. *Journal of Child Sexual Abuse*, *16*, 79–95.

Hughes, H. M., Parkinson, D., & Vargo, M. (1989). Witnessing spouse abuse and experiencing physical abuse: A "double whammy"?. *Journal of Family Violence*, *4*(2), 197–209.

Hulette, A. C., Fisher, P. A., Kim, H. K., Ganger, W., & Landsverk, J. L. (2008). Dissociation in foster preschoolers : A replication and assessment study. *Journal of Trauma and Dissociation*, *9*(2), 173–190. https://doi.org/10.1080/15299730802045914

Hussey, J., Chang, J. J., & Kotch, J. (2006). Child maltreatment in the United States: Prevalence, risk factors, and adolescent health consequences. *Pediatrics*, *118*, 933–942.

Idaho Code, 2019, § 19–3023

Izaguirre, A., & Calvete, E. (2015). Children who are exposed to intimate partner violence: Interviewing mothers to understand its impact on children. *Child Abuse and Neglect*, *48*, 58–67. https://doi.org/10.1016/j.chiabu.2015.05.002

Jackson, S. (2012). Results from the Virginia Multidisciplinary Team Knowledge and Functioning Survey: The importance of differentiating by groups affiliated with a child advocacy center. *Journal Children and Youth Services Review*, *34*, 1243–1250.

Jardim, G. B. G., Novelo, M., Spanemberg, L., Gunten, A. von, Engroff, P., Nogueira, E. L., & Neto, A. C. (2018). Influence of childhood abuse and neglect subtypes on late-life suicide risk beyond depression. *Child Abuse and Neglect*, *80*, 249–256. https://doi.org/10.1016/j.chiabu.2018.03.029

Johnson, J. L., Hobbs, S. D., Chae, Y., Goodman, G. S., Shestowsky, D., & Block, S. D. (2017). "I didn't do that!" Event valence and child age influence adults' discernment of preschoolers' true and false Statements. *Journal of Interpersonal Violence*, 1–9. https://journals.sagepub.com/doi/abs/10.1177/0886260517736276

Jones, L., Cross, T., Walsh, W., & Simone, M. (2007). Do children's advocacy centers improve families' experiences of child sexual abuse investigations? *Child Abuse & Neglect*, *31*, 1069–1085.

Kan. Stat. Ann., 2018, § 22–3434

Kim, J., & Cicchetti, D. (2010). Longitudinal pathways linking child maltreatment, emotion regulation, peer relations, and psychopathology. *Journal of Child Psychology and Psychiatry*, *51*(6), 706–716. https://doi.org/10.1111/j.1469-7610.2009.02202.x

Klemfuss, J. Z., Cleveland, K., Quas, J., & Lyon, T. (2017). Relations between attorney temporal structure and children's response productivity in cases of alleged child sexual abuse. *Legal Criminology and Psychology*, *22*, 228–241.

Klemfuss, J. Z., Quas, J. A., & Lyon, T. D. (2014). Attorneys' questions and children's productivity in child sexual abuse criminal trials. *Applied Cognitive Psychology*, *28*, 780–788. https://doi.org/10.1002/acp.3048

Ky. Rev. Stat., 2013, § 421.350

Landström, S., & Granhag, P. A. (2010). In-court versus out-of-court testimonies: Children's experiences and adults' assessments. *Applied Cognitive Psychology*, *24*, 941–955.

Landström, S., Granhag, P. A., & Hartwig, M. (2007). Children's live and videotaped testimonies: How presentation mode affects observers' perception, assessment and memory. *Legal and Criminological Psychology*, *12*, 333–347.

Leippe, M. R., Eisenstadt, D., Rauch, S. M., & Seib, H. M. (2004). Timing of eyewitness expert testimony, jurors' need for cognition, and case strength as determinants of trial verdicts. *Journal of Applied Psychology*, *89*, 524–541.

Levendosky, A. A., Huth-Bocks, A. C., Semel, M. A., & Shaprio, D. (2002). Trauma symptoms in preschool-age children exposed to domestic violence. *Journal of Interpersonal Violence*, *17*(2), 150–164.

Lindberg, M. A. (1980). Is knowledge base development a necessary and sufficient condition for memory development? *Journal of Experimental Child Psychology*, *30*, 401–410. https://doi.org/10.1016/0022-0965(80)90046-6

London, K., & Ceci, S. J. (2012). Competence, credibility, and reliability of children's forensic reports: Introduction to special issue on child witness research. *Developmental Review*, *32*, 161–164.

London, K., Bruck, M., Ceci, S. J., & Shuman, D. W. (2005). Disclosure of child sexual abuse: What does the research tell us about the ways that children tell? *Psychology, Public Policy & Law*, *11*, 194–226. http://dx.doi.org/10.1037/1076-8971.11.1.194

Lowe, S. R., Quinn, J. W., Richards, C. A., Pothen, J., Rundle, A., Galea, S ... Bradley, B. (2016). Childhood trauma and neighborhood-level crime interact in predicting adult posttraumatic stress and major depression symptoms. *Child Abuse and Neglect*, *51*, 212–222. https://doi.org/10.1016/j.chiabu.2015.10.007

Luus, C. A. E., Wells, G. L., & Turtle, J. W. (1995). Child eyewitnesses: Seeing is believing. *Journal of Applied Psychology*, *80*, 317–326.

Lyon, T. D., & Dorado, J. S. (2008). Truth induction in young maltreated children: The effects of oath-taking and reassurance on true and false disclosures. *Child Abuse & Neglect*, *32*, 738–742.

Lyon, T. D., Quas, J.A, & Carrick, N. (2013). Right and righteous: Children's incipient understanding and evaluation of true and false statements. *Journal of Cognition and Development*, *14*, 437–454.

Mahoney, R., McDonald, E., Optican, S. L., & Tinsley, Y. (2010). *The Evidence Act 2006: Act & analysis* (2nd ed.). Wellington, NZ: Thomson Reuters.

Malloy, L., Lyon, T. D., & Quas, J. A. (2007). Filial dependency and recantation of child sexual abuse allegations. *Journal of the American Academy of Child and Adolescent Psychiatry*, *46*, 162–170.

Maryland v. Craig, 497 U.S. 836 (1990).

McAuliff, B. D., & Kovera, M. B. (2002). The status of evidentiary and procedural innovations in child abuse proceedings. In B. L. Bottoms, M. B. Kovera, & B. D. McAuliff (Eds.), *Children, social science, and the law* (pp. 412–445). New York: Cambridge University Press

McAuliff, B. D., Lapin, J., & Michel, S. (2015). Support person presence and child victim testimony: believe it or not. *Behavioral Sciences & the Law, 33*(4), 508–527.

McAuliff, B., Nicholson, E., Amarilio, D., & Ravanshenas, D. (2013). Supporting children in U.S. legal proceedings: Descriptive and attitudinal data from a national survey of victim/witness assistants. *Psychology, Public Policy, and Law, 19*, 98–113.

McGaugh, J. L. (2018). Emotional arousal regulation of memory consolidation. *Current Opinion in Behavioral Sciences, 19*, 55–60. https://doi.org/10.1016/j.cobeha.2017.10.003

McWilliams, K., Harris, L. S., & Goodman, G. S. (2014). Child maltreatment, trauma-related psychopathology, and eyewitness memory in children and adolescents. *Behavioral Sciences & the Law, 32*, 702–717. https://doi.org/10.1002/bsl.2143

Mehta, D., Klengel, T., Conneely, K. N., Smith, A. K., Altmann, A., Pace, T. W … Binder, E. B. (2013). Childhood maltreatment is associated with distinct genomic and epigenetic profiles in posttraumatic stress disorder. *Psychological and Cognitive Sciences, 110*(20), 8302–8307. https://doi.org/10.1073/pnas.1217750110

Merrill, L. L., Thomsen, C. J., Sinclair, B. B., Gold, S. R., & Milner, J. S. (2001). Predicting the impact of child sexual abuse on women: The role of abuse severity, parental support, and coping strategies. *Journal of Consulting and Clinical Psychology, 69*(6), 992–1006. https://doi.org/10.1037/0022-006X.69.6.992

Miller, G. R., & Burgoon, J. K. (1982). Factors affecting assessments of witness credibility. In N. L. Kerr & R. M. Bray (Eds.), *The psychology of the courtroom* (pp. 169–196). New York: Academic Press.

Moylan, C. A., Herrenkohl, T. I., Sousa, C., Tajima, E. A., Herrenkohl, R. C., & Russo, M. J. (2010). The effects of child abuse and exposure to domestic violence on adolescent internalizing and externalizing behavior problems. *Journal of Family Violence, 25*, 53–63. https://doi.org/10.1007/s10896-009-9269-9

Murray, K. (1995). *Live television link: An evaluation of its use by child witnesses in Scottish criminal trials.* Edinburgh: Scottish Office, Central Research Unit.

Myers, J. E. B. (1987). *Child witness law and practice.* New York: Wiley Law Publications.

Myers, J. E. B. (1996). A decade of international reform to accommodate child witnesses. *Criminal Justice and Behavior, 23*, 402–422.

Nairne, J. S., Pandeirada, J. N. S., & Thompson, S. R. (2008). Adaptive memory: The comparative value of survival processing. *Psychological Science, 19*(2), 176–180.

Nathanson, R., & Saywitz, K. (2003). The effects of the courtroom context on children's memory and anxiety. *The Journal of Psychiatry and Law, 31*, 67–98.

Nathanson, R., & Saywitz, K. (2015). Preparing Children for Court: Effects of a Model Court Education Program on Children's Anticipatory Anxiety. *Behavioral Sciences and the Law, 33*, 459–475.

National Center for Prosecution of Child Abuse. (2006). *Legislation regarding the use of closed-circuit television testimony in criminal child abuse proceedings.* www.ndaa.org/pdf/ncpca_statute_tv_testimony_may_06.pdf.

Newman, B., Dannenfelser, P., & Pendleton, D. (2005). Child abuse investigations: Reasons for using child advocacy centers and suggestions for improvement. *Child & Adolescent Social Work Journal, 22*, 165–181.

Nicholson, J. V., Chen, Y., & Huang, C. C. (2018). Children's exposure to intimate partner violence and peer bullying victimization. *Children and Youth Services Review, 91*, 439–446. https://doi.org/10.1016/j.childyouth.2018.06.034

Nikonova, O., & Ogloff, J. R. P. (2005). Mock jurors' perceptions of child witnesses: The impact of judicial warning. *Canadian Journal of Behavioural Science, 37*, 1–19.

Nunez, N., Kehn, A., & Wright, D. (2011). When children are witnesses: The effects of context, age and gender on adults' perceptions of cognitive ability and honesty. *Applied Cognitive Psychology, 25*, 460–468.

N.Y. Exec. Law, 2016, § 642-a 6

Olson, E. A., & Wells, G. L. (2004). What makes a good alibi? A proposed taxonomy. *Law and Human Behavior, 28*, 157–176.

O'Neill-Stephens, E. (2006). Courthouse canines reach out to those in need. King Co. B. Assn., http://kcba.org/scriptcontent/KCBA/barbulletin/archive/2006,-11-article8.cfm

O'Sullivan, D., Watts, J., & Shenk, C. (2018). Child maltreatment severity, chronic substance abuse, and disability status. *Rehabilitation Psychology, 63*(2), 313–323. https://doi.org/10.1037/rep0000196

Otgaar, H., Howe, M. L., Brackmann, N., & van Helvoort, D. H. (2017). Eliminating age differences in children's and adults' suggestibility and memory conformity effects. *Developmental Psychology, 53*, 962–970. http://dx.doi.org/10.1037/dev0000298

Otgaar, H., Howe, M. L., Merckelbach, H., & Muris, P. (2018). Who is the better eyewitness? Sometimes adults but at other times children. *Current Directions in Psychological Science, 27*, 378–385. https://doi.org/10.1177/0963721418770998

Pantell, R. (2017). The child witness in the courtroom. *Pediatrics, 139*, 1–9.

Peace, K. A., Brower, K. L., & Rocchio, A. (2015). Is truth stranger than fiction? Bizarre details and credibility assessment. *Journal of Police and Criminal Psychology*, 30, 38–49. https://doi.org/10.1007/s11896-014-9140-7

Peterson, C. (2012). Children's autobiographical memories across the years: Forensic implications of childhood amnesia and eyewitness memory for stressful events. *Developmental Review, 32*(3), 287–306.

Peterson, L., Rolls Reutz, J. A., Hazen, A. L., Habib, A., & Williams, R. (2019). Kids and teens in court (KTIC): A model for preparing child witnesses for court. *American Journal of Community Psychology, 65*(1–2), 35–43.

Pitchal E. (2008). Where are all the children? Increasing youth participation in dependency proceedings. *U.C. Davis Journal of Juvenile Law & Policy, 12*, 233–264.

Poole, D. A., Brubacher, S. P., & Dickinson, J. J. (2015). Children as witnesses. In B. L. Cutler & P. A. Zapf (Eds.), *APA handbook of forensic psychology, vol. 2: Criminal investigation, adjudication, and sentencing outcomes* (pp. 3–31). American Psychological Association.

Quas, J., & McAuliff, B. (2009). Accommodating child witnesses in the criminal justice system: Implications for death penalty cases. In R. Schopp, R. Wiener, B. Bornstein, & S. Willborn (Eds.) *Mental disorder and criminal law: Responsibility, punishment, and competence* (pp. 79–102). New York: Springer.

Quas, J. A., Goodman, G. S., Ghetti, S., Alexander, K., Edelstein, R., Redlich, A., Cordon, I., & Jones, D. P. H. (2005). Childhood sexual assault victims: Long-term outcomes after testifying in criminal court. *Monographs of the Society for Research in Child Development, 70*(280). https://www.jstor.org/stable/3701439?seq=1

Richards, J. M., & Gross, J. J. (2006). Personality and emotional memory: How regulating emotion impairs memory for emotional events. *Journal of Research in Personality, 40*, 631–651. https://doi.org/10.1016/j.jrp.2005.07.002

Ross, D. F., Hopkins, S., Hanson, E., Lindsay R., Hazen, K., & Eslinger, T. (1994). The impact of protective shields and videotape testimony on conviction rates in a simulated trial of child sexual abuse. *Law and Human Behavior, 18*, 553–556.

Ross, D. F., Jurden, F. H., Lindsay, R. C. L., & Keeney, J. M. (2003). Replications and limitations of a two-factor model of child witness credibility. *Journal of Applied Social Psychology, 33*, 418–431. doi:10.1111/j.1559-1816.2003.tb01903.x

Sales, J. M., Fivush, R., Parker, J., & Bahrick, L. (2005). Stressing memory: Long-term relations among children's stress, recall and psychological outcome following hurricane Andrew. *Journal of Cognition and Development*, 6(4), 529–545.

Sanchez, R., & Smith, T. (2019). Bonnie Haim case: Husband found guilty of killing her in 1993, burying body in backyard. *CNN Wire*. www.localnews8.com.

Sas, L., Hurley, P., Austin, G., & Wolfe, D. (1991). *Reducing the system-induced trauma for child sexual abuse victims through court preparation, assessment and follow-up* (Final Report, Project No. 4555–1–125, National Welfare Grants Division, Health and Welfare Canada). London, Canada: London Family Court Clinic.

Saywitz, K. J., & Snyder, L. (1996). Narrative elaboration: Test of a new procedure for interviewing children. *Journal of Consulting and Clinical Psychology, 64*, 1347–1357.

Saywitz, K. J., Lyon, T. D., & Goodman, G. S. (2017). When interviewing children: A review and update. In J. B. Klika & J. R. Conte (Eds.), *The APSAC handbook on child maltreatment* (pp. 310–347). Los Angeles, CA: Sage.

Schiff, M., Plotnikova, M., Dingle, K., Williams, G. M., Najman, J., & Clavarino, A. (2014). Does adolescent's exposure to parental intimate partner conflict and violence predict psychological distress and substance use in young adulthood? A longitudinal study. *Child Abuse and Neglect, 38*(12), 1945–1954. https://doi.org/10.1016/j.chiabu.2014.07.001

Shepherd, L., & Wild, J. (2014). Emotion regulation, physiological arousal and PTSD symptoms in trauma-exposed individuals. *Journal of Behavior Therapy and Experimental Psychiatry, 45*(3), 360–367. https://doi.org/10.1016/j.jbtep.2014.03.002

Shields, A., & Cicchetti, D. (1998). Reactive aggression among maltreated children: The contributions of attention and emotion dysregulation. *Journal of Clinical Child Psychology, 27*(4), 381–395.

Shipman, K. L., & Zeman, J. (2001). Socialization of children's emotion regulation in mother-child dyads: A developmental psychopathology perspective. *Development and Psychopathology, 13*, 317–336. https://doi.org/10.1017/S0954579401002073

Shrimpton, S., Oates, R., & Hayes, S. (1996). The child witness and legal reforms in Australia. In B. L. Bottoms & G. S. Goodman (Eds.), *International perspectives on child abuse and children's testimony: Psychological research and the law.* Thousand Oaks, CA: Sage.

Silverman, A., & Gelles, R. J. (2001). The double whammy revisited: the impact of exposure to domestic violence and being a victim of parent to child violence. *Indian Journal of Social Work, 62*, 305–327.

Smith, E. L., & Farole, D. J. (2009). Profile of intimate partner violence cases in large urban counties. In *US Department of Justice, Bureau of Justice Statistics.*

Souza, L. D. de M., Molina, M. L., Azevedo da Silva, R., & Jansen, K. (2016). History of childhood trauma as risk factors to suicide risk in major depression. *Psychiatry Research, 246*, 612–616. https://doi.org/10.1016/j.psychres.2016.11.002

Spaccarelli, S., & Kim, S. (1995). Resilience criteria and factors associated with resilience in sexually abused girls. *Child Abuse and Neglect, 19*, 1171–1182

Springer, K. W., Sheridan, J., Kuo, D., & Carnes, M. (2007). Long-term physical and mental health consequences of childhood physical abuse: Results from a large population-based sample of men and women. *Child Abuse Neglect, 31*(5), 517–530. https://doi.org/10.1016/j.chiabu.2007.01.003

Sternberg, K. J., Lamb, M. E., Davies, G. M., & Westcott, H. L. (2001). The memorandum of good practice: Theory versus application. *Child Abuse & Neglect, 25*(5), 669–681.

Swim, J., Borgida, E., & McCoy, K. (1993). Videotaped versus in-court testimony: Is protecting the child witness jeopardizing due process? *Journal of Applied Social Psychology, 23*, 603–631.

Talwar, V., Arruda, C., & Yachison, S. (2015). The effects of punishment and appeals for honesty on children's truth-telling behavior. *Journal of Experimental Child Psychology, 130*, 209–217.

Talwar, V., Lee, K., Bala, N., & Lindsay, R. (2002). Children's conceptual knowledge of lying and its relation to their actual Behavior: Implications for court competence examinations. *Law and Human Behavior, 4*, 395–415.

Talwar, V., Lee, K., Bala, N., & Lindsay, R. (2004). Children's lie-telling to conceal a parents' transgression: Legal implications. *Law and Human Behavior, 28*, 411–435.

Tedesco, J. F., & Schnell, S. V. (1987). Children's reactions to sex abuse investigation and litigation. *Child Abuse and Neglect, 11*, 267–272.

Tenn. Code, 2018, § 24–7–117

Trent, E. S., Viana, A. G., Raines, E. M., Woodward, E. C., Storch, E. A., & Zvolensky, M. J. (2019). Parental threats and adolescent depression: The role of emotion dysregulation. *Psychiatry Research, 276*, 18–24. https://doi.org/10.1016/j.psychres.2019.04.009

Truman, J. L., & Morgan, R. E. (2014). Nonfatal domestic violence, 2003–2012. In *US Department of Justice, Bureau of Justice Statistics.*

Turner, H. A., Finkelhor, D., & Ormrod, R. (2006). The effect of lifetime victimization on the mental health of children and adolescents. *Social Science & Medicine, 62*, 13–27. https://doi.org/10.1016/j.socscimed.2005.05.030

U.S. Code, 2019, title 18, § 3509(i)

U.S. Department of Health and Human Services, Administration for children and Families, Administration on Children, Youth, and Families, Children's Bureau, 2017

Uji, M., Shikai, N., Shono, M., & Kitamura, T. (2007). Contribution of shame and attribution style in developing PTSD among Japanese university women with negative sexual experience. *Archives of Women's Mental Health, 10,* 111–120.

Valentino, K., Cicchetti, D., Rogosch, F. A., & Toth, S. I. (2008). True and false recall and dissociation among maltreated children: The role of self-schema. *Development and Psychopathology, 20*(1), 213–232. https://doi.org/10.1017/S0954579408000102

Van Abbema, D., & Bauer, P. (2005). Autobiographical memory in middle childhood: Recollections of the recent and distant past. *Memory, 13,* 829–845. https://doi.org/10.1080/09658210444000430

Van Voorhees, E. E., Dedert, E. A., Calhoun, P. S., Brancu, M., Runnals, J., & Beckham, J. C. (2012). Childhood trauma exposure in Iraq and Afghanistan war era veterans: Implications for posttraumatic stress disorder symptoms and adult functional social support. *Child Abuse and Neglect, 36,* 423–432. https://doi.org/10.1016/j.chiabu.2012.03.004

Walker, A. (1993). Questioning young children in court: A linguistic case study. *Law and Human Behavior, 17,* 59–81.

Walsh, W., Lippert, T., Cross, T., Maurice, D., & Davison, K. (2008). How long to prosecute child sexual abuse for a community using a children's advocacy center And two comparison communities? *Child Maltreatment, 13,* 3–13.

Wandrey, L. (2013). *"How many times did he do this to you?" Attorneys' temporal questions during child sexual abuse trials.* (Doctoral dissertation). Retrieved from ProQuest. (Publication No. 3565436)

Weiss, E., & Berg, R. (1982). Child psychiatry and law: Child victims of sexual assault: Impact of court procedures. *Journal of the American Academy of Child Psychiatry, 21,* 513–518.

Wells, G. L., Ferguson, T. J., & Lindsay, R. C. L. (1981). The tractability of eyewitness confidence and its implications for triers of fact. *Journal of Applied Psychology, 66,* 688–696.

Wheeler v. United States, 159 US 523 (1895).

Whitcomb, D., Shapiro, E. R., & Stellwagen, L. D. (1985). *When the victim is a child: Issues for judges and prosecutors* (U.S. Dept. of Justice NCJ-97664). Washington, DC: U.S. Government Printing Office.

Xie, P., Wu, K., Zheng, Y., Guo, Y., Yang, Y., He, J ... Peng, H. (2018). Prevalence of childhood trauma and correlations between childhood trauma, suicidal ideation, and social support in patients with depression, bipolar disorder, and schizophrenia in Southern China. *Journal of Affective Disorders, 228,* 41–48. https://doi.org/10.1016/j.jad.2017.11.011

Zajac, R., Gross, J., & Hayne, H. (2003). Asked and answered: Questioning children in the courtroom. *Psychiatry, Psychology and Law, 10,*199–209.

Zajac, R., O'Neill, S., & Hayne, H. (2012). Disorder in the courtroom? Child witnesses under cross-examination. *Developmental Review, 32*(3), 181–204.

Zeman, J., Shipman, K., & Suveg, C. (2002). Anger and sadness regulation: Predictions to internalizing and externalizing symptoms in children. *Journal of Clinical Child and Adolescent Psychology, 31*(3), 393–398. https://doi.org/10.1207/S15374424JCCP3103_11

Zydervelt, S., Zajac, R., Kaladelfos, A., & Westera, N. (2017). Lawyers' strategies for cross-examining rape complainants: Have we moved beyond the 1950s? *British Journal of Criminology, 57,* 551–569.

Part Two

Assessment

5 Assessment

Methods, Measures, Protocols, and Report Writing

S. Margaret Lee

Assessing children involves flexibility, nuance and complexity. When an evaluator first meets a child, they must informally assess the child's language level, their comprehension, their cognitive development, and their understanding of the process. They must then be ready to adjust the types of questions asked and the specific vocabulary most likely to be understood by the specific child. Assessing adults requires some rapport in the evaluation process, it is critical when assessing children. By providing a "child-friendly" environment, establishing rapport and constantly adjusting how the interviewing and formal testing proceeds we are likely to obtain the most reliable information.

When assessing children for forensic purposes, the flexibility, nuance and complexity must be combined with interviewing techniques that include standardization and are research-based. The development and refinement of the forensic child interview originated in the child sexual abuse allegations that exploded in the 1980s, in daycare and school settings. Those allegations were assessed by clinicians who utilized the clinical tools available at that time. Regrettably, the interviewing resulted in contaminations, the likely implantation of false memories and the conviction of several daycare providers, whose convictions were later overturned. Fortunately, however, this led to the development of a considered, research-based approach to interviewing children in forensic settings aimed to obtaining accurate and reliable information.[i] Overtime, protocols and refinements occurred with the emergence of more standardized interview protocols.[ii] Although the developed protocols were, initially, specifically applied to sexual abuse allegations, the underpinnings for interviewing children in a forensic setting have proven useful for a variety of situations. Thus, whether we are asking children about sexual abuse or their experiences in the family or whether their parents are influencing them, it is good practice to assess narrative abilities and practice narrating events. It is also good practice in interviews to move from very broad questioning, asking expansive questions to more specific questions, avoiding the use of language or ideas that the child him or herself has not introduced to finally, perhaps, asking few limited, closed ended questions that could potentially distort the child's responses (see Chapter 10 for case material involving sexual abuse allegations).

Additional intricacies arise when assessing children in forensic settings. Many of the situations that bring children into the legal system involve difficult and/or traumatic experiences. Trauma can impact memory (see Chapter 4) and can significantly influence the child's interactional style. Traumatized children may dissociate when triggered, may be avoidant and shut down or the opposite, may become flooded when talking about their experiences. For some thoughts about assessing children who are constricted, the reader is referred to Chapter 9 where Dr. Levy discusses some strategies. Thus, the evaluator must assess the impact of trauma on the child's ability to provide information, recall events accurately and communicate all that they know.

DOI: 10.4324/9780429397806-6

Interviewers must also be conscious of informed consent. With most older adolescents and adults of average intelligence, the evaluator explains the purpose of the evaluation, how the obtained data will be used and disseminated and the limits to confidentiality. With adults this is quite straightforward and easy to determine if they have understood. With children, it is the responsibility of the evaluator to explain these concepts to their clients, which requires adjusting the concepts and language to fit the child's cognitive and linguistic level. The child must then be able to demonstrate their correct understanding of the explanation (see Chapter 15 for a case example with an older adolescent with Intellectual Disability). It is also important to recognize that children may need to be reminded of the parameters of the situation numerous times. After explaining to a child that the information given to the evaluator will be shared with their parents, it is not infrequent that a young child, in the middle of an interview, will say, "don't tell my Mom."

The unique requirements of assessing children involve a number of levels of assessment, numerous steps to assure accuracy in the process and the assessment of multiple domains. This must be accomplished while complying with ethical standards and requires creating environments that help a child feel at ease and open to providing information.

Venues and Areas of Assessment

The complexity of assessing children is also evident in the wide range of questions posed to a forensic evaluator, depending on both the type of court, the individual case and whether the evaluation has been ordered by the court or an evaluator has been hired as a consultant for an attorney.

Children in Juvenile Court

In juvenile court, questions primarily pertain to dependency and delinquency. In dependency cases the questions before the court include: is this child safe in their home? Has there been evidence of abuse or neglect? If so, are the parents able to take advantage of reunification services offered and provide a safe environment or should parental rights be terminated and a different permanent placement be explored? Exploring these questions may also involve assessing the impact of a particular situation on a child by identifying treatment needs for the child, the parents and the family system. The evaluator may also be responsible for formulating monitoring processes that are designed to insure the future safety of the child. When there is a dependency question in juvenile court, a mental health provider (MHP) may be hired by the Department of Social Services (DSS) to perform an assessment. Alternatively, a parent's attorney or public defender may hire a MHP to assess similar questions, as an alternative or in opposition to an evaluator for DSS. The Department of Social Services is essentially tasked with making recommendations regarding a specific child or a family. As noted above, the legal questions can be broad or more specific. Has this child likely been abused, has this child experienced trauma, and if so, what are reasonable interventions and treatment goals. Chapter 6 of this volume by Dr. Barbara Mercer including cases involving out-of-home placement and Chapter 10 by Dr. Jaqueline Singer involving interviewing children in sexual abuse cases, illustrate several examples of the legal questions posed and the assessment approaches used.

A MHP's role in assessment in juvenile court includes addressing criminal forensic questions about competency and insanity, amenability to treatment, and consultation. Historically, assessment has evolved considerably from the 1960s to the present. In the 1960s, greater prioritization of procedural rights of juveniles resulting from *Kent versus the United States* and *re: Gault* (see Chapter 1 of this volume), when goals like public safety and sophistication-maturity merged with the rehabilitative domain of treatment amenability in juvenile decision-making.[iii] In the 1970s, approaches to assessment focused on legal standard and functional-legal capacities associated with these standards, resulting in development of checklists with regard to certain areas like competency to proceed.[iv] Following these developments, measurement of risk and criminogenic needs was promoted with the development of risk-need-responsivity theory that subsequently influenced development of specialized measurements of risk, need, and responsivity for juveniles.[v] The 1990s saw growth of semi-structured and specialized measures. By 2000, empirical foundations provided substance to notions of psychosocial maturity and issues like competence, *Miranda* waiver capacity, risk, treatment needs, and treatment responsivity.[vi] Contexts in which juvenile assessment occur include *Miranda* waiver, competence to stand trial, diversion, waiver and reverse waiver, post-adjudication disposition, and post-sentence civil commitment.[vii] When evaluating for treatment considerations, evaluators consider assessment of family patterns of interaction and the family system as a context for the juvenile, peer relations and their influence for the juvenile, community strengths or limitations, academic and vocational skills of the juvenile and personality functioning of the individual juvenile.[viii]

Juvenile re-sentencing evaluations are a special subset of juvenile assessment. In the *Roper, Graham and Miller* decisions (see Chapter 1 of this volume) of the U.S. Supreme Court (SCOTUS) and that same court's *Miller and Montgomery* decisions,[ix] justices for SCOTUS relied heavily upon adolescent brain science and behavioral functioning of adolescents in their conclusions and arguments. The age related reasons that juveniles should be treated differently with regard to culpability and special protection were delineated in the *Miller* decision and include the following factors. (1) Decisional: juveniles' inclination toward sensation-seeking and risk-taking resulting in errors in judgment during decision-making; (2) Dependency: juveniles' focus or reliance on those around them and the attendant difficulty in avoiding negative influences (e.g., abusive family environment, peer influence; (3) Offense context: the possible relationship of decisional and dependency factors to the juvenile's justice involvement; (4) Rehabilitation Potential: juveniles' generally greater capacity for behavioral change and (5) Legal Competency: juveniles' immature capacity for making important legal decision (e.g., *Miranda* waiver, interrogations, assisting legal counsel).[x] Since the *Montgomery* decision was relatively recently decided, there remain few standardized protocols for evaluations involving re-sentencing. However, the citations included in this chapter provide a rich source of information to evaluators on how to conduct these with the Five "*Miller*" factors as a framework.

Children in Family Court

In family court, when families dispute legal and physical custody of children, the legal question is to define the "best interest of the child" (BIC) and analyze what parenting plans and interventions are needed to address those needs. Given the broad definition of BIC and the complexity of assessing the individual family members and the family dynamic, these evaluations tend to be extensive and involve the collection of a wide range of data. The family law cases that require evaluation include allegations of child abuse, exposure to domestic violence, exposure to substance abuse, the impact of parental mental illness, among other possible allegations. Given the breadth of allegations, assessment of these issues tends to be time consuming and complex, see Chapters 10, 11 and 14. Assessments for family court are typically done by a neutral evaluator ordered by the court, such an appointment includes being the court's expert and that evaluator is provided with quasi-judicial immunity. There are specific requirements for child custody evaluators in many states, so the MHP must be aware of those requirements. Some family law cases do not require a comprehensive child custody evaluation but rather a Brief Focused Assessment (BFA) is ordered. In that case, the referral from the court will define a specific question to be addressed, such as what school the child should attend, the question of whether the child would benefit from psycho-therapy or the evaluator might be requested to assess a specific parent–child relationship. Family law cases can also involve questions about who should be considered the "parents" of a child, as discussed in Chapter 12 by Deborah Wald.

Children in Criminal Court

Children may be involved in criminal cases either as witnesses and/or victims … These situations usually involve informal or formal assessment, by attorneys with or without the aid of a mental health professional, regarding the effectiveness of the child as a potential witness and to collect evidence that will potentially be used at trial. The reader is also directed to Chapter 4 by Goldfarb et al. for understanding how child witnesses and victims can be supported when testifying in court. Child victims may be assessed to determine whether they have been traumatized and the results of this assessment may be included in the court proceedings. Given that some victims are involved in both criminal trials and civil trials related to the same events, the same evaluation may be utilized to claim damages. The questions arising in personal injury cases heard in civil court are illustrated in Chapter 9 by Dr. Amy Levy.

Children in Federal Court

There are two types of Federal Court cases that we discuss in this volume: Immigration Court and Hague Convention cases. In Hague Convention cases, the court's question is whether the child should be returned to the country of habitual residence where that jurisdiction will determine the child's best interests. There are two broad categories of questions for an evaluator in these cases: one involves evaluating the possibility of grave risk of harm should a child be returned to their country of habitual residence and the other involves ascertaining the meaning of the child's objection to the return to their country of habitual residence. That opinion needs to be assessed through the lens of the child's age and maturity, capacity to form a reasonable opinion and whether they have been unduly influenced by a parent (see Chapter 13 by Dr. Lee and Mr. Seymour.)

Immigration Court is currently in some disarray due to the shifting policies of the government, particularly in regards to potential asylum seekers from Central America. Historically, asylum seekers who alleged trauma in their country of origin could apply for asylum, including children. Evaluations would be performed to assess both the veracity of their claims and the extent of the trauma. Dr. Hass in Chapter 8 discusses assessment within this court system.

Difference between Clinical and Forensic Assessment

A seminal article by Stuart A. Greenberg and Daniel Shuman[xi] outlines many of the differences between the role of a clinician and a forensic evaluator. One major difference is the definitions of "who is the client." For a clinician, the client is the patient in their office. A clinician's role is to help the client manage their issues, improve their psychological functioning and provide appropriate treatment. Since the patient is the client, they hold the privilege. With some exceptions, what the client tells a clinician is confidential unless the client requests sharing of some or all obtained information with others. Another difference is in the fact that the clinician generally will accept the client's version of reality, without cross-checking it. Yet another is that the clinician's goal is the goal that the client identified, not another goal such as the court's need to make legal decisions.

In forensic evaluations, the person being evaluated is not the client. The client is the court or can be an attorney for the court. When an attorney hires an evaluator privately and the evaluator renders an opinion that would not be helpful to the attorney's client, that opinion can be dismissed and not used in a legal proceeding. When the court orders an evaluation, the court is the client and has the right to all information gathered in the course of an evaluation. The court is the client and imposes guidelines that can include the data collected and how results and underlying evidence will be monitored. An example is in family law where child custody evaluations are conducted by order of the court, whether that order is reached by agreement between the attorneys or not. In forensic cases, the individual does not hold the privilege, but rather an attorney or the court holds the privilege.

A major difference between clinical evaluation and forensic evaluation is the cognitive set maintained by the evaluator. As a clinician one has a supportive, accepting, empathic attitude whereas a forensic evaluator maintains a more distanced, neutral, objective and detached stance. In part, this difference is due to different processes and different goals utilized in clinical as compared to forensic evaluations. In a clinical evaluation, the client asks for the clinician's assistance in understanding their difficulties. The credibility of a clinical patient is not questioned and generally, if it is their decision to enter clinical treatment, they are motivated to feel better or otherwise change their behaviors. The response from the clinician is one of helpfulness and the setting is non-adversarial. In forensic evaluations a goal is to gather evidence that will help the court address a specific legal question. As part of that process, it is common to educate the court with regards to critical factors the court should consider in making their decision and to address how reliable and valid the collected data is. Issues of the person's credibility, possible secondary gains, motivations for either presenting in an overly favorable manner or in a manner that exaggerates difficulties are considered as data is collected and assessed. This setting can be adversarial and the evaluator maintains an evaluative, rather than completely accepting, approach and mindset.

Performing forensic evaluations requires a commitment to maintaining neutrality and objectivity regardless of one's role or by whom one is hired. Regardless of which side they are contracted by, the task of a forensic evaluator is to collect appropriate data, analyze data in an objective manner, present findings and show the analysis of findings as they relate to the psycho-legal question(s). The Specialty Guidelines for Forensic Psychologists developed by the American Psychological Association (APA)[xii] provide guidance for how to use best practice in forensic work. Maintaining neutrality in conducting forensic evaluations is sometimes difficult due to retention bias, confirmatory bias, wish to please attorneys who serve as frequent referral sources, and unrecognized influence from "group think" if engaging with attorneys and their teams.

Given the difference in roles, goals and need for different types of information, it is not surprising that therapeutic and forensic roles require different kinds of training and expertise. Although clinical and forensic evaluators may both use some of the same basic tools, such as some specific psychological tests, and general interviewing skills, the forensic evaluator maintains a more rigid approach being sure to follow standard administration procedures, noting and explaining any deviations or limitations in the administration of the testing or in the interviewing. A clinical evaluator might deviate from these standards if they believe that it will yield useful information that will help the client. If there are unintended consequences of a non-standard procedure these will likely be picked up and adjustments can be made during treatment that follows the evaluation. When forensic evaluators relax the standards of administration and interpretations, the consequences may be dire, such as loss of life or freedom, loss of access to a parent, or loss of substantial sums of money. Consequences emanating from legal decisions lead to significant scrutiny of the data collected, the process of the evaluation and the opinions offered by forensic evaluators or consultants. Given that the court is an adversarial system, the control for these procedures comes from the court and opposing attorneys. There is, therefore, the need for the evaluator to cross-reference information provided in the course of an evaluation and to verify data or information through collateral sources of information, review of documents from multiple sources and analysis of data as to congruence and non-congruence of findings.

The scope of forensic evaluations differs from clinical evaluations, which are sufficiently broad to include diagnosis, personality functioning and treatment targets meant to assist behavioral change.[xiii] Forensic evaluations address specific legal questions or issues. The complexity of these questions is variable, ranging from a specific question like "Is this individual competent to proceed?" to broadly ranging questions like those posed in family law, where an evaluator must address the relevant Best Interest of the Child (BIC) factors in a specific case, assess the validity of various allegations parents make, and recommend a parenting structure, parental decision-making responsibilities, and possible therapeutic interventions for individual family members or parents jointly. As noted in this example from family law and as is often the case for juvenile matters, forensic evaluators might address treatment needs of individuals. Generally speaking, the need for addressing treatment interventions and clinical diagnosis is less frequent in forensic criminal or personal injury civil evaluations as compared to evaluations for therapeutic matters. When, however, "the legal question is directly related to the presence of a clinical disorder," as in the case of insanity or civil commitment, "or the likely response to intervention such as treatment needs and amenability as part of criteria for juvenile transfer or reverse waiver," then there is overlap of clinical with forensic considerations.[xiv]

In some situations, diagnoses may contribute to confusion for forensic matters.[xv] In family law, diagnoses of parents are rarely provided as they are seen as weapons the other parent will use in ongoing custody disputes and are not probative. However there are exceptions. For example, in a child custody evaluation performed, the referral question included whether the mother of a toddler was suffering from a mental illness that was impairing her parenting or endangering her child. There was a finding of paranoid schizophrenia, which led her to believe that her husband was sexually abusing their child and that she and her child should perhaps escape by going to heaven. It was clear that until this condition was treated, the child was endangered.

Heilbrun and Locklair[xvi] summarize some of the principles discussed above and issues to be discussed below as it relates to forensic assessment of juveniles. "Consistent with the contemporary emphasis on empirically supported assessment and interventions in a broad array of human services, we strongly emphasize the importance of providing juvenile FMHA that is empirically driven and scientifically supported." They conclude that improvement in the area of providing juvenile FMHA along policy lines will occur if the following information is disseminated:

> the importance of structure, the necessity of legal relevance, the use of validated measures (particularly those developed specifically for application to the legal question at hand), the employment of multiple sources of information, the impartial interpretation of findings, and the communication of results in such a way that allows those reading (or hearing) to understand the basis for such conclusions.

Additionally, analysis of the data is done with an understanding that different courts have different burdens of proof that relate to the type of court, the nature of the legal issues and the degree of risk associated with the outcomes. As will be discussed by various authors in the book, whether a case is decided by the preponderance of evidence, clear and compelling evidence, or beyond a reasonable doubt is related to the specific case and venue.

Data Collection

The specific data collected will be highly dependent on the legal claim, setting or charges, and the standard of proof that applies. For example in juvenile homicide cases, where the burden of proof is beyond a reasonable doubt, the most stringent burden, data collection must involve more investigation, greater number of multiple sources, and thoroughness due to the seriousness of the crime, the evidentiary level required, and the standard of proof that applies.

In a case of child abuse allegations in family court, the child's age, the use of interview protocols and the assessment of the child's credibility and presence of or lack of possible parental influence are critical. Family court is usually "child-friendly," the child's opinion is typically entered into evidence through a child custody evaluation (CCE), interviews by GALs, or social workers who work for the court. The child's opinion is provided within the context of a family system. Cases in family court are determined by the preponderance of the evidence or clear and convincing evidence, depending on the state and issue. However, child abuse cases heard in criminal court are determined by the standard of clear and compelling evidence and are heard in an adversarial setting where the alleged victim will be a witness (see the Goldfarb et al. chapter in this volume). In a criminal child abuse matter, most evidence will be collected by the attorneys, whereas in a CCE, data collection is the responsibility of the forensic evaluator.

Given the potential serious outcomes that can be informed by forensic evaluations, the potential impact of bias on data collection and interpretation, and the complexity of many cases, it is critical in a Forensic Mental Health Evaluation (FMHE) to use multi-modal assessment. This allows for scrutinizing the reliability and validity of data from different sources. Particularly critical is finding avenues to assess reliability of data obtained through interviewing individuals. The possibility of malingering, secondary gain, and brainwashing or undue influence can be explored through the use of data from various sources. Typically, these cross-checked data sources include interviews with the other individuals involved, collateral witnesses, assessment of relationships, document and record review and formal assessment with standardized measures. For more detailed description of the types of documents and collateral informants, the reader is referred to Melton[xvii] and to Heilbrun.[xviii]

As noted earlier in this chapter and as discussed in Chapters 3, 10 and 11 of this volume, interviewing children is often central in forensic evaluations that involve children in the courts. When allegations of abuse exist, then structured, videotaped interviews using standardized interview protocols are best practice and gold standard for interviews. Videotaped interviews makes less likely the need for multiple interviews of the child that can be associated with less reliable statements by the child. The interview protocol developed by the National Institute of Child Health and Disease (NICHD) are the ones that should be used. Recorded interviews may be used in dispositions for criminal matters, dependency court or as part of a child custody evaluation. In criminal and civil court, children may be interviewed as eyewitnesses and may potentially testify at trial (see the Goldfarb et al. chapter in this volume). Such interviews may or may not be conducted by forensic mental health professionals. Mental health professionals may assist the prosecution and/or defense to interview the child witness however the child may be interviewed by prosecution and/or defense attorneys. Since there are some interviews conducted by both MHP, and attorneys that are poorly conducted and the information may be tainted by the interviewing process, in some cases mental health professionals are brought in to review the interview data and may present to the court alternative hypotheses regarding whether the child's recall should be relied up or not.

To address legal questions involving an individual child, a combination of interviewing, reviewing documents and psychological assessment with standardized measures is usually performed, in addition to interviewing collateral sources. Interviews with children require initially determining their language level, language comprehension, narrative ability and overall cognitive ability (see the Baker-Ward et al. chapter in this volume). Although somewhat determined by developmental level and age, each child interviewed requires at least an informal assessment of these areas so that the evaluator can adjust the vocabulary they use, adjust the complexity of the language used and pace questions in a manner the child can process and respond to. Unlike the more distant approach used with adults being forensically assessed, building a working relationship with a child is critical to obtaining useful data.

In the NICHD interview, an understanding is built by having the child practice producing a narrative of a recent event. Even when not doing a formal child sexual abuse interview, the technique of using narrative practice to both build rapport and as a means of assessing functioning, can be very useful. This protocol notes the importance of conveying a message to the child that the examiner is interested in "who" they are and in what they know about the situation under discussion. It is also important not to reinforce any particular piece of data by being "supportive." For example, if a child described being hit by a parent, a response like "How awful for you!" could be very problematic, especially if the child was not hit by the parent. With friendly neutrality, on the other hand, the question might be posed, "Can you tell me more about that?" It is necessary to remember that in many interviews, an evaluator asks children to discuss traumatic events. When these traumatic events include discussions of parents or loved ones, it is critical to create support for the hard work in which the child is engaging. Most of the case based chapters in this volume include commentary about interviewing children within differing legal settings and with the kind of supportive yet also evaluative approach required for forensic work.

In many cases involving children, parents will also be interviewed. In these interviews, parents can provide a historical context about their child, can discuss any observed behavior changes that have been seen in the child, can provide developmental history and noteworthy details regarding development, and can contextualize and individualize their child. For example, after a traumatic event occurred, a forensic examiner wants to know: how did the child's behavior change, what symptoms were seen, did they resolve the experience of trauma, with what specific support(s) were they able to resolve the traumatic experiences. Dr. Levy's chapter in this volume provides depth with regard to questioning these experiences of trauma.

When cases involve an assessment of the family system, usually in dependency matters or in family court, interviews with parents will be a part of the evaluation process, not just a way to gather information about the child. It is also the case that parents and care givers are interviewed in juvenile delinquency matters (see Chapter 15 in this volume). In dependency matters and family court this may include direct forensic assessment of the parents to evaluate psychological functioning and parenting skills or may be focused on understanding the interrelationships in the family and the overall system dynamic. Family relationships can be observed in naturalistic settings such as home visits or can be conducted in semi-structured ways, such as asking the parent and child to engage in a task together, plan a vacation or talk about a shared experience. The evaluation can contain more formal parent–child assessment such as using the Strange Situation as described in Chapter 7 of this volume by Attorney Alicia Jurney, which provides information about attachment relationships.

A less formal approach to obtaining attachment information is by creating situations that are likely to prompt attachment system activation, especially in young children. For a discussion of children's attachment relationship data in child custody evaluations see article by Lee, Borelli and West.[xix] Through directly observing parents and children together, an evaluator can gather data regarding both parenting skills and the nature of the attachment relationship. Qualities such as the parent's emotional attunement towards their child, their insightfulness in response to their child's behavior and over all warmth in the interactions, help the evaluator develop a deeper understanding of the quality of the relationship. Evaluators can also create opportunities to view a parent manage difficult behavior, such as cleaning up after a play interaction, and to notice how a parent interacts with a child to solve problems and to perform tasks.

In family law matters, direct observations of parent–child relationships, in addition to previously mentioned interviews, are critical to the evaluator in assessing the accuracy of a parent's perceptions about the child and about the parent–child relationship. Another source of data about the parents' perceptions is achieved through administration of behavioral checklists. These checklists can be provided to teachers, daycare providers, coaches, therapists and others who have interacted with the child to provide collateral information. In family law cases, parents sometimes have highly discrepant perceptions and beliefs about their child, the child's wishes, preferences, natural inclinations, temperament, preferred activities, and symptoms, among a host of variables. The evaluator must determine "who the child is" descriptively, must arrive at a conclusion as to whether either parent has an accurate understanding of the child and must note what parental factors contribute to a distorted view of the child. In Chapter 14 of this volume, this type of analysis is central to Dr. Calloway's understanding of a complex family engaged in a "high conflict" divorce.

Formal assessment is frequently a part of forensic evaluations, with the child and/or with parents. Traditional tests used by clinicians[xx] and specific measures developed to gather data for specific legal questions are used in forensic evaluations. This is a complex area and there is extensive literature. The reader who wishes to access this literature is referred to the APA *Handbook of Psychology and Juvenile Justice*[xxi] and Melton's comprehensive tome.[xxii] There is a distinction between forensically relevant instruments and use of traditional measures in forensic settings. If the reader is interested in pursuing more comprehensive study of these distinctions and specific tests, handbooks by Melton[xxiii] et al. and Heilbrun et al.[xxiv] and which provide details that are beyond the scope of this chapter.

Regarding traditional clinical measures, the top four measures frequently used in a forensic context include the Minnesota Multiphasic Personality Inventory-Adolescent Version (MMPI-A), Child Behavioral Checklist (CBCL), Millon Clinical Multiaxial Inventory (MCMI) and. Parenting Stress Index (PSI).[xxv] Acher[xxvi] notes that his original research on frequency of tests used in forensic evaluation was prior to the development of the Personality Assessment Inventory – Adolescent (PAI-A), which he viewed as "holds substantial potential." The Rorschach Inkblot Method continues to be a very popular measure for child custody evaluations.[xxvii] In Chapter 9 in this volume, Dr. Levy describes in depth the uses of projective testing and self-report measures, including the so called "controversy" about the use of the Rorschach Inkblot Method. For a more comprehensive coverage of forensic uses of the Rorschach when using the Rorschach Performance Assessment System R-PAS, the reader is referred to Mihura, and Meyer's handbook[xxviii] where there are chapters on Criminal Responsibility,[xxix] Violence Risk assessment,[xxx] Child Custody Evaluations,[xxxi] and Domestic Violence.[xxxii]

Organizing the Data

Given the amount of data collected in some of these evaluations and the various types of data collected, timelines on different dimensions that can be compared provide great assistance to the evaluator while analyzing data, to the reader of the resultant report and to the trier of fact. For example, there may be a developmental timeline, a timeline of assessments and interventions, and a timeline of legal events in a CCE. In developing these timelines, the evaluator can identify the source of the data, as to whether it originated from interviews, documents, collateral informants, and/or repeated child abuse interviews. Organizing data in this manner and comparing different timelines allows for analysis of and integration of information that is greatly simplified and presented visually for the reader and the trier of fact. Children are constantly changing and events can occur over several developmental stages. Thus children have different, sometimes more nuanced, understandings of events as they grow and develop different emotional, cognitive and social capacities. Timelines aid an evaluator with memory sorting and they serve to highlight relevancy of different data. Finally, timelines contribute to greater confidence in the face of scrutiny and intense cross-examination.

Report Writing

When writing a report, clearly stated legal questions, data collected, and sources of data plainly identified serve to inform any reader. Limitations to the evaluation should be unequivocally stated and any irregular procedures or those that depart from standard practice should be explained. At the beginning of an evaluation, multiple hypotheses are generated. This ensures that possible outcomes are stated and that data is collected to assist in confirming or disconfirming these alternative hypotheses. All data should be included in the report, whether or not it fits in with final conclusions. This approach is critical to the task of remaining objective and neutral, without hastily forming opinions that are based on "gut" instinct or "cherry picking" the data. After the raw data is explained, the evaluator analyzes the data with reference to the legal question(s) for the specific case. Any opinions offered, whether about the individual or family or about the ultimate question before the court, should be proffered with a statement regarding the degree of certainty of that opinion. The degree of certainty may derive from the consistency of the data and whether or not the evaluator accessed or was provided access to the data thought to be relevant. For example, if child abuse records exist, yet the court does not release them in a family law matter, this might constitute a significant limitation of the conclusions offered from the evaluation. Some disputes exist in some areas of law as to whether or not an evaluator should offer an opinion to "the ultimate issue" before the court.[xxxiii] For example, if a family law case involves a request by one parent to re-locate with the child, some evaluators analyze the pros and cons of a child relocating or remaining with the other parent without addressing the ultimate question of whether the child's best interests are better served by moving or staying. In this type of case, many judges want to know an evaluator's opinion as to the ultimate question and the reasoning underlying it, and in fact in some states, notably Illinois there is a statute requiring custody evaluation reports to include recommendations.[xxxiv] On the other hand, some scholars assert that "*mental health professionals ideally should refrain from giving opinions as to ultimate legal issues.*"[xxxv]

Testifying

Detailed discussion about testifying is beyond the scope of this book and chapter. However, a few, general comments are in order. When in court as a forensic evaluator, education to the court about the data that has been collected and its meaning will help the trier of fact address the legal questions raised in the evaluation. Testimony should closely follow a report and findings and conclusions from a report. Developing charts and tables to summarize data can be used as exhibits, as illustrations to visually present findings and conclusions, and to support testimony. This can be an effective, simple and clear way to present data. Opinions should be neutral but may be vigorously presented, as one is not defending oneself but is defending the data collected. If there are "opposing" experts, testimony by both should be professional, neutral, objective and based on the procedures used, the data collected and the nexus between the data and the opinions rendered. As is true in report writing the need to present all of the data whether or not it supports the ultimate opinion should be reported as should the limitations to the data that is being relied upon for the opinions developed. It is only through this this strict adherence to transparency, neutrality, and objectivity as recommended by various professional standards [xxxvi] that we can practice in ethical ways and be useful to the court.

Notes

i Newlin, Chris, Steele, Linda C., Camberlin, Andra, Anderson, Jennifer, Kenniston, Julie, Russell, Amy, and Stewart, Heather (2015). Child Forensic Interviewing: Best Practices. Juvenile Justice Bulletin September, U.S. Department of Justice.

ii Lamb, Michael E., Orbach, Y., Hershkowitz, I., Esplin, P.W. and Horowitz, D. (2007). Structured Forensic Interview Protocols Improve the Quality and Effectiveness of Investigative Interviews with Children: A Review of Research using the NICHD Investigative Interview Protocol. *Child Abuse and & Neglect*, Vol. 31(11–12), 1201–1231.

iii Heilbrun, K. and Locklair, B. (2016). Chapter 16: Forensic Assessment of Juveniles. In K. Heilbrun, D. DeMatteo, and N.E.S. Goldstein, Eds, *APA Handbook of Psychology and Juvenile Justice*. Washington, D.C.: American Psychological Association. https://doi.org/10.1037/14643-000.

iv Ibid., p. 345.

v Ibid.

vi Ibid., p. 346. Heilbrun, K., DeMatteo, D., King, C., and Filone, S. (2017). *Evaluating Juvenile Transfer and Disposition: Law, Science and Practice*. New York: Routledge.

vii Heilbrun and Locklair, 2016.

viii Melton, G.B., Petrila, J., Poythress, N.G., Slobogin, C., Otto, R.K., Mossman, D. and Condie, L.O. (2018). *Psychological Evaluations for the Courts: A Handbook for Mental Health Professionals and Lawyers*, 4th Edition. New York: The Guilford Press.

ix Heilbrun et al., 2017.

x Ibid., p. 242. Grisso, T. and Kavanaugh, A. (2016) in Heilbrun et al., 2017. Grisso, T. et al. (in press).

xi Greenberg, S. and Shuman, D. (1997). Irreconcilable Conflict between Therapeutic and Forensic Roles. *Professional Psychology: Research and Practice*, Vol. 28(1), 50–57. https://doi.org/10.1037/0735-7028.28.1.50.

xii Specialty Guidelines for Forensic Psychologists (2013). *American Psychologist*, Vol. 68(1), 7–19. Practice Directorate, American Psychological Association, Washington, D.C., 20002-4242. doi:10.1037/a0029889.

xiii Melton et al., 2018.

xiv Heilbrun, K., DeMatteo, D. and Goldstein, N.E.S., Eds. (2016). *APA Handbook of Psychology and Juvenile Justice*. Washington, D.C.: American Psychological Association. https://doi.org/10.1037/14643-000. Page 354.

xv Greenberg, S.A., Shuman, D.W. and Meyer, R.G. (2004). Unmasking Forensic Diagnoses. *International Journal of Law and Psychiatry*, Vol. 27(1), 1–15. https://doi.org/10.1016/j.ijlp.2004.01.001.

xvi Heibrun and Locklair, 2016.

xvii Melton et al., 2018.

xviii Heilbrun et al., 2016.

xix Lee, S. Margaret, Borelli, Jessica L. and West, Jessica L. (2011). Children's Attachment Relationships: Can Attachment Data be Used in Child Custody Evaluations? *Journal of Child Custody*, Vol. 8(3), 212–242.

xx Archer, R.P. and Wheeler, E.M.A. (2013). *Forensic Uses of Clinical Assessment Instruments*, 2nd Edition. New York: Routledge.

xxi Heilbrun et al., 2016.

xxii   Melton et al., 2018.

xxiii   Ibid.

xxiv   Heilbrun et al., 2016.

xxv   Archer, R.P. and Baum, L.J. (2016). Forensic Uses of Clinical Assessment Instruments, in K. Helibrun, Ed., *APA Handbook of Psychology and Juvenile Justice*, APA.

xxvi   Ibid., p. 427.

xxvii   Bow, James N. (2006). Review of Empirical Research on Child Custody Practice. *Journal of Child Custody*, Vol. 3(1).

xxviii   Mihura, Joni L. and Meyers, Gregory J., Eds. (2018). *Using the Rorschach Performance Assessment System*. New York: Guilford Press.

xxix   Aklin, Marvin W. (2018). Using the R-PAS in a Criminal Responsibility Evaluation. In Mihura and Meyers, 2018.

xxx   Kaakinen, Saara, Muzio, Emiliano and Saavala, Hanna (2018). In Mihura and Meyers, 2018.

xxxi   Lee, S. Margaret (2018). Using the R-PAS in Family Law Evaluations. In Mihura and Meyers, 2018.

xxxii   Kasar-Boyd, Nancy and Kennedy, Reneau (2018). Using the R-PAS in the Assessment of Psychological Variables in Domestic Violence. In Mihura and Meyers, 2018.

xxxiii   Cutler, B.L. and Zapf, P.A. (2015). *APA Handbook of Forensic Psychology*, Volume 1, p. 8. Washington, D.C.: American Psychological Association. https://doi.org/10.1037/14461-000; Brodsky, S.L. and Gutheil, T.G. (2016). *The Expert Expert Witness: More Maxims and Guidelines for Testifying in Court*, 2nd Edition. Washington, D.C.: APA. https://doi.org/10.1037/14732-049; Buchanon, Alec (2006). Psychiatric Evidence on the Ultimate Issue. *The Journal of the American Academy of Psychiatry and the Law*, Vol. 34(1), 14–21; Slobogin, C. (1989). The Ultimate-Issue Issue. *Behavioral Sciences and the Law*, Vol. 7(2), 259–266; Tippins, T. M., & Wittmann, J. P. (2005). Empirical and Ethical Problems with Custody Recommendations: A Call for Clinical Humility and Judicial Vigilance. *Family Court Review*, Vol. 43(2), 193–222.

xxxiv   750 ILCS 5/604. 10-

xxxv   Melton et al., 2018, page 17 and citation 91 for Chapter 1 for additional references and opinion.

xxxvi   APA, 2017. Ethical Principles of Psychology and Code of Conduct. Washington, D. C.: APA;

AFCC (2006). *Model Standards of Practice for Child Custody Evaluations*. Association of Family and Conciliation Courts. Madison, WI.

Part Three

Case Studies

6 Out-of-Home Care

Depending on the Kindness of Strangers

Barbara L. Mercer

> We drove to an unfamiliar destination in Manhattan ... I had no idea why we had come to this place but the adults seemed to know what was going to happen ... The woman spoke. Alexis and I would be moving into a foster home ... to live with a family that had not been yet selected. As the words sunk in, rage took over *"I'll jump off the Empire State Building"* I shouted ... *"You can't do this to me, you can't give me away if I don't want to leave."*
> (Francine Cournos, *City of One: A Memoir*, 1999, pp. 95–96)

Children who are removed from their families of origin and enter government care are part of a system called *juvenile dependency, out-of-home-care, foster care*, or as they are called in the United Kingdom, *looked-after children*. The system is the *Child Welfare System* and the agency who serves them, *Child Protective Services*. Like refugees who flee dangerous situations, these children and youth are dislocated, their links to the past, their voices and stories often lost. The reality of foster care involves navigating what Jill Doerr Berrick called *The Impossible Imperative* (2018), of supporting families of origin and protecting children and the systemic contradictions and personal turmoil this often entails; the demands it places on the court, the child welfare system, the parents, foster parents, and child. The foster care system is intended to be beneficial or even curative for a terrible situation, yet the process renders a child who is already vulnerable even more so (Gin, 2008).

Studies indicate that children in foster care are not only at greater risk for behavioral and psychological problems related to attachment, depression, and chronic post-traumatic stress reactions, but many more report difficulties in maintaining age-appropriate grade level achievement, completing high school, or finding employment (McDonald & Allen, 1996). While some youth removed from their biological parents and are raised in foster care "by the system," achieve stability, productivity, and well-being, – as did Columbia University psychiatrist Dr. Francine Cournos (in the quote above) – research has suggested that the population as a whole is highly vulnerable and in need of social policy and programs designed to support them in many aspects of their lives (Wulczyn, Brunnre, & George, 2002).

This chapter provides an overview of the Foster Care System, followed by the story (a composite of stories) of a young girl removed from her family and placed in foster care following allegations and her reported experience of neglect and abuse. The context of out-of-home-dependency is important as we think about how to improve the lives and futures of children and youth: What follows are attempts to answer: (1) What is the current scope of the U.S. foster care population as a whole? (2) What is the historical context of child welfare and child protection? (3) Where are children's voices in juvenile dependency court proceedings? (4) How has the community and practitioners' perspectives evolved on child representation and child-friendly courts. (5) What are the complex contexts involved in thinking about children in foster care? *Attachment and loyalty, child development, trauma,*

DOI: 10.4324/9780429397806-7

race and culture, reunification, and permanency planning are some of the highlights and will be reflected in the case of Ruby, a 4-year-old girl entering foster care, living in multiple placements, termination of parental rights following a contested court procedure, and ultimately adopted … ten years later.

Any Given Year

The most recent data from the Foster Care Analysis and Reporting System (U.S. Department of Health and Human Services, The AFCARS Report #25, FY2017) states that at the end of 2017, 442,995 children (roughly the population of Miami, Florida) in the United States were in foster care placements. Of this population: 44% were White, 23% were African American, 21% were Latino, 2% Native American, 8% were listed as multi-racial, 2% were "unknown" or unable to be determined. The trend from 2013 to 2017 has gradually increased each year (400,000 in 2013). The male-female difference was small. Types of placement include: 45% in non-relative foster homes, 32% in kinship (relative or family link), 7% in institutions, 5% in group homes, 5% in trial home visits with State supervision, 4% in pre-adoptive homes, 1% had run away, 1% in supervised independent living. (Child Welfare Information Gateway, 2017)

Of children entering care almost half were not old enough to attend kindergarten. In 2017, 49% of children *entering* foster care for the first time were 5 years or under, and 26% of children *entering* care were 1 year old or younger. Children had the highest risk of first foster care placement during infancy (1.09%) of all U.S. children). The median age of children entering foster care in FY 2017 was 7.7 years. Neglect and parental drug abuse comprised the highest percentage of reasons for removal. The number of children waiting for adoption for whom parental rights had been terminated was 69,125, with 123,437 waiting for adoption contingent on final parental rights termination (U.S. Department of Health and Human Services, *The AFCARS Report #25, FY2017*).

Of the 247,631 children who exited foster care in FY 2017, the *mean* time spent in foster care was 19.2 months; the median amount of time spent in foster care was 14.3 months. Nine percent of these children were in care less than one month, 15% in care for 1 to 5 months, 19% in care for 6–11 months, 44% in care for 12–35 months, 9% in care for 3–4 years, 4% in care for 5 or more years. Nearly 10,000 children exiting foster care in FY2017 had remained in foster care five or more years; however, of all the children currently in foster care, 24,838 or 6% had been in care for five years or more (U.S. Department of Health and Human Services, *The AFCARS Report #25, FY2017*).

Over half of the children in foster care at the end of FY2017 (56%) had a case plan of reunification with their parents or primary caretakers. About half the children exiting (49%) were discharged to be reunited with their parents or primary caretakers. Twenty-four percent were adopted (U.S. Department of Health and Human Services, The AFCARS Report #25, FY 2017). Adoption remained the least likely permanency outcome for children in years past. In 2004–2005, about four years following placement in care, 16% of the children were adopted, primarily Caucasian children who had placed in foster care at or near birth (Berrick, 2009, *Take me Home*, p. 59). The higher percentage of reunification cases may reflect the policy priorities and hopefully the existence of increasing support services to parents.

Race and income disproportionality permeate referrals and entrance into out-of-home dependency. A study (Woods & Summers, 2016) analyzing risk of foster care placement for any U.S. child between birth and 18 predicted that African American and Native American children are at least twice and three times respectively as likely to be placed in foster care in any given year than White children. Before age 18, 5.9% of U.S. children (1 in 17) will spend time in foster care. The risk for entering foster care is 15.44% (1 in 7) of Native American children, and 11.53% (1 in 9) of African American children to enter foster care before they turn 18. Cumulative risks of foster care placement by age 18 for U.S. Children, 2000–2011, declined gradually but racial/ethnic disparities became greater (Wildeman & Emanuel, 2014).

Child Protection: An Historical Perspective

"Please Sir, I would like some more ..."
The master aimed a blow at Oliver's head with a ladle. (Charles Dickens, *Oliver Twist*, p. 15)

Children have always been vulnerable to victimization from their parents or other adults. Child removal and protection are as old as the Bible. The abandoned child has been seen in Jungian psychology as a collective archetypal problem where every child is a potential hero who must overcome frightening forces at some point in life. But the lived experience of a child who is truly abandoned is a far lonelier and less exalted one.

Fiction and sociological literature focus on the plight of children: Charles Dickens in 1839, Lloyd de Mause's *History of Childhood* (1974), John Boswell's *The Kindness of Strangers: Child Abandonment in Western Europe from Late Antiquity to the Renaissance* (1988). Charles Dickens' famous Oliver Twist was born in an almshouse, after his "unwed" mother died. At 8 years old, because he was hungry, he came forth with his bowl daring to ask for more gruel, saying; "Please, Sir, I would like some more." For that effrontery, he was placed in solitary confinement and eventually sold to abusers. As a child, when his father was sent to debtor's prison, Dickens himself was forced to work ten-hour days in a boot-blacking warehouse. When his father was finally released and his debts settled, Dicken's mother did not ask for her son's release. Dickens was never able to forgive her for this rejection (Wilson, 1970). Such experiences and emotions of abandonment, despair and loneliness, anger, and the threat of annihilation resonate for youth removed from their families throughout recorded history.

John E.B. Myers (2004) in his book *History of Child Protection in America* provides a relevant context for our current child protection policies summarized below. Myers notes that Moses was placed in a basket in the Nile to protect him against a decree of death for all Jewish boys by Pharaoh, from where he was "adopted" by Pharaoh's daughter. In A.D. 110 Roman Emperor Trajan established the first asylum for poor children, and by 787, there were *foundling* homes in Europe. At the end of the 12th century Brother Guy, a French monk, established the first Children's Aid Society for the protection, shelter, and education of destitute children.

A law in 1642 allowed child removal, although children were often placed in the "trades" as indentured servants. Almshouses and orphanages were created in the 1700s. The first orphanage was created by French Ursuline nuns in Louisiana in 1728. The first official organization, The New York Society for the Prevention of Cruelty to Children (a knowing extrapolation of the ASPCA) was created in 1875. Before this time, extreme cases of cruelty or abandonment were publicized and sporadically prosecuted. The Children's Aid Society in New York was started in 1853 by Charles Loring Brace, an advocate for placing children in foster homes rather than institutions.

Simultaneously social work as a profession was developing in the late 1800s and in the first two decades of the 20th century. Advocates for the poor in London's settlement movement (e.g., Arnold Toynbee) and in the United States (e.g., Jane Adams), aimed to *assist* people in poverty rather than criminalize them. With the increasing role of state and federal government in social services, protections from their agencies also grew.

By 1919, all states but three had juvenile courts who could (conceivably) intervene for both delinquent and dependent children, and by 1922 there were also 300 non-governmental child protection societies. FDR's New Deal and Entitlement Services and passage of the Social Security Act in the 1930s, moved toward protection of children and families. The federal government actually began providing grants to states for abuse prevention as early as 1935.

The advent of reporting laws, culminating in the Child Abuse Prevention and Treatment Act (CAPTA) of 1974, resulted in the reporting of thousands of child abuse and neglect cases. The rising numbers of children in long-term foster care resulted in the Adoption Assistance and Child Welfare Act of 1980 that required states to make "reliable efforts" to avoid removing children from parents and to have a reunification or permanency plan to either return a child home or move toward termination of parental rights. The expansion of systems resulted in controversies borne of the dilemma of balancing the disparate goals of protecting the child versus preserving the family. This led to a "child-centered" approach strongly put forth by Richard Gelles (Loseke, Gelles, & Cavanaugh, 2005) who believes protecting children is the ultimate priority. To hold both these principled roles in mind while implementing the best course of action, requires attunement to each child and family, and the ability to think in nuanced and non-binary ways.

While laws to protect children have been in place for over 100 years, the physical or sexual abuse of children and youth, the desire for profit and power through exploitation, the desperation to sell children to escape extreme poverty, or because of misdirected fervent moral beliefs, children continue to be vulnerable to significant danger. There are wide-ranging differences now in legal and cultural standards for children in different countries. In the United States, for example, parents are held accountable if they keep their children from attending school, and educators and mental health professionals can be prosecuted for failing to report child abuse. In Afghanistan, it is the opposite: it is estimated that two-thirds of girls are *prohibited* from an education and could be in mortal danger if they dare to pursue studies. "If we go to school they will kill us" (Human Rights Watch, 2017).

Also in Afghanistan, children of school age who come from low-income homes are required to work. According to the Human Rights Watch (2017), at least 25% of Afghani children between the ages of 5 and 14 work for a living, and as a result, education for both boys and girls oftentimes becomes an untenable burden (the Borgen Project, 2018).

Genital mutilation is a horrific abuse in one culture, but culturally endorsed in another. Widely disparate customs like this pose the dilemma of whether children have individual rights at all, or are they the property of their parents. A book by Mei Fong (2016) *One Child Nation: The Story of China's Most Radical Experiment*, documents pervasive child abandonment due to governmental edicts, most poignantly the death of the authors' uncle's baby who was placed in a basket at the roadside for adoption, but tragically resulted in the baby's death several days later.

Even in U.S. today, where family resources are strained, children take a role in the care of siblings and housework instead of going to school. While our country continues to struggle with how to support children and their families, we still have evolving court processes in the service of child welfare.

Children in the Court System

The purposes of the Child Welfare System, according to the California Courts, are:

- Maximum protection for children who are physically, sexually, emotionally abused, neglected or exploited, or at serious risk of abuse or neglect.

- Includes provision of services to the child and family and presumes that the best interest of the child is to remain in or be returned to the child's home or family.
- The mandate throughout is to keep a child at home, or return if detained (California Courts, 2017).

Every state has its own variation of a child protection law that follows a federal guideline from the Federal Child Abuse Prevention and Treatment Act CAPTA (1974), the Social Security Entitlement Act (1961), and the Title IV-(E) Act (1980). In the State of California, the Central California Appellate Proceeding says that in order to initially remove a child – during the initial detention hearing, which must take place within three days of physical removal – the burden of proof is on the social services agency to show by prima facie evidence (WIC§300 Code) that there is substantial danger to the physical or emotional health of the child and that there are no reasonable means to protect the child without removal. (*Prima facie* evidence is "that which suffices for the proof of a particular fact, until contradicted and overcome by other evidence" [In re: Raymond G., 1991].) At this time, social workers explore other relatives and important connections that should be included in the process.

In California, there are three successive court hearings in dependency cases: *Detention Hearing, Jurisdiction Hearing*, and *Disposition Hearing*. While prima facie evidence is the burden of proof required for initial removal, a "preponderance of evidence," a more stringent standard of evidence is required for Jurisdictional Evidence. This means that, under the California Welfare Code 300, the court has to determine if there is a preponderance of evidence (WIC §355; 358) to formally retain in the child in jurisdiction based on the truth of the allegations, although the court must consider any submission from the parents or guardians who may disagree, dispute, or contest the allegations.

In conjunction with the jurisdiction hearings, whether the child is returned to the family or removed into agency custody, social services can utilize a Child and Family Team (WIC §16501(a) (4)) to engage the child, family, extended family, and treatment and educational persons to identify family strengths and weaknesses and work towards a positive outcome in the case plan. This can also help toward reunification if the disposition is to not return the child (California Courts, 2017).

Even if removal is determined to be the course of action, a reunification plan is mandated, unless the court finds, by clear and convincing evidence, to "Bypass" a reunification plan. (A bypass can occur, for example, if the parent has a history of chronic substance abuse and failed treatment, the parent or guardian does not wish the child returned, the parent has abducted the child or sibling, *or* the sole parent is incarcerated or institutionalized.) To *formally remove* the child and proceed toward a new placement disposition, the court must prove by "clear and convincing evidence" that there would be substantial danger to the physical and emotional well-being of the child and that there is no reasonable means to protect the child without removal. The burden of proof then shifts to the parent (or child) to produce evidence to the contrary. The goal is to protect the child, not to punish the parent.

Time Frames for Juvenile Dependency Process

A court must order reunification services to the child, mother, father, or guardian. If reunification does not occur Child Welfare must have a plan for "achieving legal permanence."

The timeline for reunification begins at the time of initial removal from the home. The proscribed time frame in a reunification plan is one year. This can be extended to 18 months if the parent needs more time, or 24 months if returning home is fairly certain and the parent needs time for further rehabilitation, treatment, or housing supports. For children under 3, the time for review can be as short as six months from the date of the dispositional hearing, and in any case no later than one year after the date of the child's entry to foster care the date of the jurisdictional hearing (WIC §§ 362.5 and 361.21). For children under 3 the services can be extended to 18 months from initial removal, if there is a substantial probability of return within the extended period or the parent was not provided reasonable services; or 24 months if the court finds it to be in the child's best interest, and with a substantial probability of return.

At each permanency review for a child in long-term foster care, the court must consider permanency planning options, *including* return to the home of the parent. The social service agency is not required to prove the parent unfit at each status review; rather, the burden will have shifted to the parent to prove (by a preponderance of evidence) that circumstances have changed, and that return would be in the child's best interest. If there is clear and convincing evidence that the child is likely to be adopted, parental rights can be terminated at any of these review points. This happens much sooner with young children, as "young children are most vulnerable to the effects of maltreatment, and both maltreatment and involvement in the child welfare system's impact on development, can have life-long implications" (Judicial Council of California/Office of Administration: A Dependency Quickguide Dogbook, 2011). The six-month review for children three years or younger conveys the developmental urgency of the situation to those involved in the case plan and recognizes the need for a permanent family.

Many states and counties have programs for at-risk pregnant women and parents with children ages zero to three at risk of losing custody. These front-end services are valuable in their support of the mandate to preserve families and support families with drug dependency, mental illness, or financial and environmental stresses. These services depend on government priorities, and need for federal, state, or county financial support. Children older than three may fall under a similar developmental vulnerability rubric, but may remain longer in foster care without a permanency plan if they continue to have multiple placements, behavioral and emotional struggles, or difficulty in finding appropriate long-term homes.

Child Advocacy and Representation

Under the federal Child Abuse Prevention and Treatment Act (CAPTA, 1988), every child detained into state custody must be appointed an attorney counsel and a *guardian-ad-litem* (who can be the appointed lawyer or a Court Appointed Special Advocate – CASA-) (WIC §326.5; 44 U.S.C.§5106 et. seq.). The appointed counsel has the responsibility to gain knowledge of the case, by interviewing the child and witnesses, and of the child's needs in order to represent the "child's best interests" and make recommendations to the court. The counsel must interview children four and older to hear and communicate their wishes. However, the child's expressed wish may be directly contrary to the attorney's view of the child's safety (In re: *Alexis W.*, 1999; In re: *Kristin B.* 2008). The attorney is the holder of the child's privilege with regard to psychotherapy and physician information. The parent likewise is permitted but not required to retain representation at all stages of the proceedings.

Since dependency is child-focused, the court must allow the child, if the child desires, to address or be present at the court, or speak privately in court chambers to the judge. A child 10 years of age or older must be notified of the right to attend the hearing. It is crucial in a "child friendly" court atmosphere to explain the process to children in a developmentally appropriate and responsive way. Children can also provide testimony if they are willing and able. The child can testify in chambers away from the parent's presence and a potentially intimidating formal court setting.

Child-Responsive Courts

According to the U.N. Convention on the Rights of the Child (UNCRC), children's views of their circumstances should be taken into account. Article 12 states: "Children shall be provided the opportunity to be heard in any judicial and administrative proceedings affecting the child, either directly, or through a representative or an appropriate body" (UN Committee on the Rights of the Child. *General Comment No. 12, The right of the child to be heard* [Geneva: Author, 2009]).

But what does it mean to be *heard?* Are courts considered *child-friendly?* How do courts vary as child-responsive settings across varying systems?" Children can potentially feel empowered or disempowered by a court process that can be confusing and chaotic or alternately validating of their feelings (Gal & Duramy, 2015; Weisz et al., 2011).

Guidelines for the implementation of U.N. Article 12 suggest nine conditions that are necessary to fulfill participation rights for children (U.N. Committee on the Rights of the Child, General Comment 12 [2009], #134). These include processes that are (1) transparent and informative; (2) voluntary; (3) respectful; (4) relevant; (5) inclusive; (6) supported by training; (7) safe and sensitive to risk; (8) accountable; and (9) child-friendly.

A fascinating study was conducted looking at an international perspective on child-responsive courts (Berrick, Dickens, Poso, & Skivenes, 2018), where court policies were reviewed in the United States (California), the United Kingdom (England), Finland, and Norway, by asking participating judges in each country to write about the following topics:

1　Children's right to express their views is followed well in my country's (state's) courts.
2　Care order proceedings are conducted in a child-sensitive time frame.
3　The courts offer a child-friendly environment.
4　The courts use child-friendly language.
5　Statements by children are collected in a child-friendly manner.
6　"Children's rights" serve as the paramount frame for decision making in care order proceedings.

Child-friendly language is conversation that matches a child's developmental age, hopefully free of technical words or jargon. A child-friendly environment can be anything from the ability of a judge to speak with a child in chambers to a comfortable, well-designed waiting room with art supplies, a child's support person, or an invitation to view the courtroom in advance.

According to the authors, California judicial respondents were "more likely than respondents in other countries to endorse the ideas that children had a right to express their views, that judicial proceedings were responsive to children's sense of time, that the courts offered a child-friendly environment, and used child-friendly language." Interestingly, in the Child Rights International Network (2016) ranking, California is 52nd in the child-sensitive rankings.

The authors posit that perhaps the positive attitude of California judges about their courts' child-friendly approach reflect concerted efforts in recent years (post-ranking) to train judges, encourage the advocacy of a few vocal judicial leaders, and provide legislative clarification about children vis-à-vis the court. California is also recognized across the nation as one of the few states that legislates an "indirect" voice for the child through an assigned attorney. Compared to California courts in previous years, judicial settings are probably much more child-responsive than they used to be. Nevertheless, it is important to bear in mind that dependency proceedings in California and many states in the U.S. are normally very brief events. According to one study of California juvenile courts, the median duration of dependency hearings in California is between 10 and 15 minutes (Administrative Office of the Courts, 2005); thus, not the optimal opportunity for meaningful youth participation ("California Juvenile Dependency Court Improvement Program Reassessment" [San Francisco, Ca: Center for families, children, and the court, Administrative Office of the Courts, 2005]).

In that sense, training for the judicial decision makers is essential, along with the other changes identified above for achieving child-responsive courts. One of the challenges for delivering such training is that it must be consistent with the principles of judicial independence and sensitive to the particular circumstances of each case (Berrick et al.).

In the past decade training projects have been implemented in California to promote understanding and collaboration among judges and treatment teams including importantly foster parents and therapists. Judges will benefit from knowing more about the mental health and emotional/behavioral struggles of children and youth in foster care; and mental health providers will benefit from understanding more about the workings of the juvenile courts.

Programs for Child Participation

Children rarely appear in court in their own behalf in child dependency cases. Child testimony is more likely to happen when allegations of sexual abuse are investigated, and more likely to occur in judges' chambers. Children's wishes in placement decisions are typically communicated through social workers, child lawyers, and child advocates. The burden on social workers is especially stressful as they are responsible for gathering and sorting through information from all parties in order to write a report for the court. The creation of multi-disciplinary child advocacy agencies (e.g., East Bay Children's Law Offices in Alameda County, California) has focused on increasing representation and voice for children in a wide range of child cases. Judges, notably in Alameda County in California, prefer to protect children from open court testimony. Not only is testifying in court intimidating for a child, but the child's situation related to their home is fraught with turmoil and nuanced problems. A parent may request for their child to testify if they think that the child may be more truthful to a judge than to their social worker. One California lawyer from the East Bay Children's Law Offices reports that out of approximately 300 of her dependency cases, there have been only two or three times when a child has been asked to testify, and then *only* in the judge's chambers. She has *never* had a child testify in open court in a dependency case (Liz Aleman, Personal Communication, 2019). This striking statistic underscores the complex and difficult issue of child testimony and voice in the legal system.

Children's desires are almost never easy or uncomplicated. Longing and loyalty to parents and home are strong, and advocates are tasked with recommending the best plan forward for the child given the circumstances. Collaboration with the child, the social worker, treating therapist, and family members is essential. States and participating counties have developed programs in the last several years to facilitate effective programs to carry out the international and federal mandate to include children in the systemic process. This mandate is often undermined by stressing immediate placement, and by the reality that children's status does not grant them control of what happens to them.

One such program in the state of California in collaboration with several participating counties called Safety Organization Practice (California Courts, 2017) is a prevention and family-focused approach that aims to coordinate the ways information is gathered, shared, and presented with professionals and with the courts. A method adopted to elicit participation from young children is derived from projects called The Safety House (Parker, 2008) or the Three Houses Tool, both from Australia (Weld, 2008). These tools can be utilized by social workers and child advocates to listen to children draw or talk about their level of safety, their worries, and hopes in a way that can help in potential reunification processes and placement decisions, and shared with judges and other team members. The ultimate goal in these needed programs is to coordinate information and collaborate for more informed outcomes. Listening to children's worries and hopes can be a part of helping them hold the complexity of mixed feelings about their families and themselves. It increases transparency about the court and placement process in a way they might be better able to understand. This will not solve problems easily, will not cure parental troubles, or provide perfect placements, but it can begin to address the conflicts and paradoxes in the Child Protection System. The more financial support given to prevention and wraparound programs, the more headway we make as a society to address the underlying problem of child maltreatment and safety.

Racial and Socioeconomic Disproportionality

There may be a tendency, as participants in a system, to write about out-of-home-dependency as a discrete subject. We delve into statistics, juvenile courts, topics of attachment, trauma, reunification, often with the correlations, causes, and contexts *outside* our awareness. Researchers have begun to illuminate the precursors and correlates associated with children removed from their families in the hope of bringing more effective interventions and solutions to bear on improving the lives of children and families.

Caucasian/White children are underrepresented at a rate eight times lower than their proportion in the U.S. population as a whole and in almost every state in the country, whereas African American children are *over*represented in the child welfare system (Brevard, 2017). Brevard states that although recent efforts have been made to address the racial disproportionality, African American families are more likely to be reported, investigated, have their allegations substantiated, enter foster care, and remain there longer than White children (Brevard, 2017; Rolock, 2008). Brevard suggests that the way African American parenting behavior styles are socially constructed can influence reporting patterns and decisions made in the child welfare process. An example would be an African American cultural value about corporal discipline and the view that physical discipline can be a loving and protective way of parenting in a society where African American children can be physically targeted outside their homes (Tilmon, 2003).

Even more striking is that American Indian/Alaska Native (AI/AN) children are 2.7 times greater than their proportion in the general population to enter the system (they are .9% of children in U.S population). This underestimates the percentage of AI/AN children in foster care since one-third of the children placed in care by tribal authorities and are not included in this data set.

In an effort to show the breadth of the systemic problem and the need for intervention, a comprehensive study of investigative maltreatment reports (*whether or not substantiated*) gathered data from the National Child Abuse and Neglect Data System Child Files and Census Data from 2003 to 2014, sought to develop synthetic cohort life tables to estimate the cumulative lifetime risk for the prevalence of *reported* childhood maltreatment investigations. The researchers found that one-third (37.4%) of all U.S. children would experience a child protective services investigation by 18 years of age; that African American children had the highest lifetime prevalence of projected investigations of over half of African American children (at 53%), 32% for Hispanics, 24% for Native Americans, 10% for Asian Pacific Islanders, and 28.3% for whites (Kim, Wildeman, Jonson-Reid, & Drake, 2017).

There are further variables associated with the racial disproportionality that have been less visible, specifically socioeconomic status (SES) of families whose children enter out-of-home dependency. Child welfare data indicates that the majority of families that come to the attention of the child welfare system do so on allegations of neglect, with poverty being a major contributor (Child Welfare Information Gateway, 2017). The

National Institute of Study of Child Abuse (NIS-4, 2010) found a "powerful relationship" between socioeconomic characteristics and rates of child maltreatment referrals. Variables of family structure (e.g., single parent households), parental employment, number of children in the household, and parent's highest education were also correlated with removal rates (Sedlak & Broadhurst, 1996; Sedlak & Schulz, 2005; Sedlak et al., 2010). NIS-4 included a socioeconomic measure that defined a child as living in a low-SES family if their parents had less than a high school education, annual income of below $15,000, or household members in a poverty program. In the NIS-4 study, the census findings on median income for both Blacks and Whites improved between 2000 and 2004, but the Black children lost ground relative to White children at a faster rate, and the gap between median incomes of these racial groups increased substantially (U.S. Census Bureau, 2009). Studies show that income and indicators of poverty are among the strongest and most consistent correlates of reasons for child maltreatment, whereas increases in income levels and reductions in poverty are associated with decreases in child maltreatment risk. From this data NIS-4 suggests a causal link between income and CPS involvement. In an unpublished study on income ranges for Wisconsin families between 2012 and 2016 (Slack, Berger, & Collins, 2019), the average income in the year before a screened-in maltreatment report in Milwaukee, Wisconsin, was approximately $18,000. Additionally, in the year prior to being "screened-in" for a CPS report, 74% of families were on SNAP (Supplemental Nutrition Assistance Program, formerly known as Food Stamps) and 75% of families were on SNAP in the year prior to Out of Home Placement (Berger et al. 2014).

This research strongly suggests that economic support policies are one efficient prevention strategy and that child welfare interventions may be well served by addressing families' economic issues. Program policies and research are also addressing disproportionality in the Child Welfare System (Green, Bellinger, McRoy, & Bullard, 2016). Many studies explore and discuss the correlates of child maltreatment to race, poverty, and family and community stress; however, to receive even a screened-in referral a family must be noticed, identified as problematic, then viewed as posing a danger.

Families with high incomes and/or influence have a lesser chance of discovery, or (a greater chance) of ultimately being dismissed as not meeting the threshold of posing a significant threat to child safety. Families with financial and social resources can turn more easily to other familial or natural support networks without landing in juvenile court or the foster care system.

Children's Voices: Breaking the Glass

"I want to save her." Alex, 11 years-old

While the journey of a child through the Social Welfare System, life in foster care, and therapeutic treatment, exist side-by-side with court dates and proceedings, the two worlds often do not speak the same language. Children's voices of their experience of identity, attachment, and trauma are not easily visible, while their behaviors can be flagrantly obvious. School personnel rarely know if a student with academic, behavioral, or emotional problems has a history of removal from parents, and living in foster care, yet they know they are acting badly. Youth in foster care are usually silent and feel shame about being "fostered" and not having a "normal" family.

Children will try to forget the traumas of removal and abuse and "fit in," and say "I'm fine," until something or someone in their new family or at school triggers a powerful negative reaction. Traumatic images seep through in psychological assessment data, especially in young children whose responses are unfiltered because they have not had time to be repressed. These often gruesome and shocking images and memories can be actual, real, visceral memories mingled with the child's inner experience of trauma.

Despite the distressing nature of their words, it is critical for the therapist and assessor to hold the real impact of their trauma. Bessel van der Kolk states in his powerful book *Traumatic Stress: The Effects of Overwhelming Experience on Mind, Body, and Society* (van der Kolk, McFarlane & Weisaeth, 2007), that the willingness to engage with the raw nature of the child's traumatic material in relational context of being understood and feeling safe is what allows therapeutic healing. He stresses that if the essence of the trauma is secret, the traumatic memories, often in disquieting fragments, are more likely to prey on the traumatized person's mind. He reminds us that despite the indifferent face of suffering, humans have an innate need to find meaning in the face of trauma. He states that the "personal meaning of trauma is influenced by the social context in which it occurs" (p. 26). Trauma experts and psychoanalysts have reminded us that disturbing experiences need to be communicated to the "other" and cannot be held by one mind alone (Bion, 1975; Ogden, 2009). Therapists must at times carry the feelings and words that the child cannot bear to think about. Providing this kind of "holding environment" for overwhelming and adverse experiences is a way to build resiliency for the child (Winnicott, 1963). Anne Alvarez, a noted British psychoanalyst, working extensively with traumatized children, many in foster care, called this providing "live company" (Alvarez, 1992). These authors described this reclaiming process, rather than a reliving of the trauma, as helping the child transform over time these "bad," distressing memories into something more bearable. The following vignettes and case exploration reflect the voices of young children, in out-of-home care, related to trauma, danger, attachment, and identity. Their experience is most powerfully communicated through stories, play, and therapeutic interaction.

Trauma and Danger

When Rochelle, age 7, and her younger sister were found in their house there was drug paraphernalia and an undetonated explosive device on the site. Rochelle often had to change the diapers of her baby sibling, and her mother later told the social worker that Rochelle would often sleep with her young sibling to protect her from an abusive father. Rochelle's social worker referred her for a psychological assessment to understand the impact of her early trauma. Rochelle's responses to projective material in her psychological testing were distressing to hear and reflect the experience of her trauma: She perceived, "an evil force ... that's mixed up with a troll and a raccoon and a squirrel," a spider she associated with what she said was her memory of a man eating a spider, and ominous images of lizards eating a skeleton. "The skeleton's been buried 10 million years ... It died of a shot." Story themes from the assessment of young children reflect overwhelming fears and a dangerous and disorganized environment, evidenced by the following responses to one story card showing two young bears in a crib and an empty bed, from 3-year-old Hannah: "Everywhere there was ants all over the bed. Everything on the bed was keys, candy, glasses, and teddy bears ..." and to a subsequent story card, "Once upon a time, there was two puppies. The toilet was flowed. The black water was sticky. All the spiders were in the toilet but they can't get it out ... there's a baby and she got lost." Parents get lost or injured and can't help. "I get scared, scared, scared." She subsequently crawled under the table. When asked about the content of her nightmares, she reported, "monster eats me" or "clown kills me." During a projective drawing task, Hannah was asked to construct a picture of a house. In response, she drew a "house with eyes" and identified the house as a "scary haunted house ... there's blood dripping ... it's gonna try to eat me." In Figure 6.1 her drawing of a Person-in-the-Rain, a drawing (Verinis et al., 1974) is seen to represent a child's resources and experience of adversity (inclement weather).

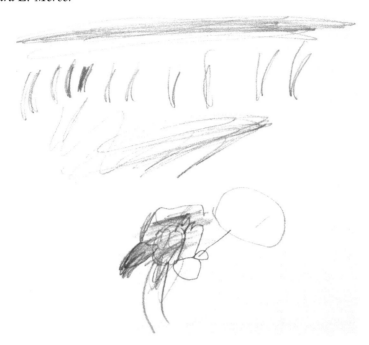

Figure 6.1 Hannah's Person-in-the Rain drawing

Four-year-old Dee drew a picture of a house that she named "The Vampire House" where a vampire lived who eats people:

> The tree is cold and the weather is cold and everybody gets cold". Vampire came out of the house. Going to bite the person and then another person and they are going to die. Her turned into a vampire. That's the black blood coming out of her head. This is the dried blood. He a messy eater. Her too.

When a story contained these strong negative emotions, Dee would shriek loudly and become frantic. At the end of one session she tried to throw up in the wastebasket. Characters in play are hungry, and must stock pile and hide food to survive. Five-year-old Noni created scenes in which young animals searched for food for their family. She stated, "The little ones are tired, but they're not gonna stop looking until they find the food." Attempts to meet these basic needs were unsuccessful when child characters faced environmental dangers without the protection of their parents. The child characters remained distressed and unready for these roles, and ultimately surrendered to their hunger and fatigue. Noni stated "the tigers gave up looking for food because there are so many predators, and the foxes gave up too because they're too tired."

In these less than protective environments, older children give a more direct voice to a need to be loyal, protect their parents and take on responsibility. Here 12-year-old Jordan said:

> It's my job to keep the adults acting right. It's my job to punish the adults when they fight and argue at home because of drugs and alcohol. I fall off my bike a lot and bump my head and miss school. There's no one to take me to the doctor when I'm sick or get hurt. I love my family very much and don't want anyone to get in trouble.

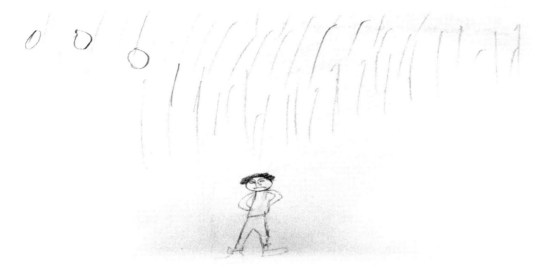

Figure 6.2 Jordan's Person-in-the-Rain drawing

Separation and Identity

Removal is another searing trauma: Alex reported he and his brother first became aware of their monster identity when they were in the police car being taken away from their mother. He has a heroic memory of wanting to break the glass in the police car to reach his mother and save her. He reported that his birth scared his mom because she realized he and his brother weren't regular babies but little monsters, and his mother couldn't know how to raise monster children. Children feel to blame for the removal which affects their sense of goodness and identity. They begin to feel that they are bad, and subsequently that they cannot depend on protection and must fend for themselves. Even self-hate and a desire for self-harm are not atypical. Another aspect to remember is that when children blame themselves they can still hold on to a notion of goodness, of a good parent. If they feel they are to blame, they still hold onto a sense of choice and agency. One boy told the following to a story card:

> This is about a boy who thought heaven was good and the devil was bad but he switched them around because his parents always told him heaven was bad and the devil was good. And then he started acting up and acting up until his parents gave him up to a foster home, and when he was 21 he went to jail and said, "I am going to kill myself to get away from me" … and when he went to heaven god said, "why do you do all these bad things?"

After the parents "die" or are lost, the children must then learn to fend for themselves with sad results:

> Their mom died when they were born and they didn't have anyone to teach them to fly. They had to depend on themselves. The father has worms and dies of heart disease. They die too because they haven't learned how to depend on themselves.

Even in a good foster home a child's sense of cultural identity is impacted. Tricia's foster mother wanted to know why Tricia was lying, cheating, and aggressive. Tricia was battling loyalties to her mother, especially in contrast to a more stable foster home. Tricia is bi-racial and says: "My Mama B is Black, I want to be Black like her."

One girl in foster care described her drawing of a girl during therapy and told what it would take for her to believe in herself after being removed from her home:

> That's a girl. She's feeling lonely in Brooklyn because her mommy and daddy leaving. Then she heard her mom singing her a song: "Things are going to be easier." So today she is happy. Her name is Sharena. I'll make her a brain. Empty at first, but every time she goes to school, she got more brain, little by little She practiced it, practiced it, practiced it, and finally she got all filled up. She knows how to spell. She wants to be a teacher.

These voices must be heard and understood by the adults since they answer some of the queries about disruptive and regressive behaviors causing stress for foster parents. These difficult behaviors will invariably resurface when a child is reunified with a biological parent, causing stress for a parent in recovery from substance abuse who is trying to survive financially, sometimes in an unsafe neighborhood.

Ruby's Voices and her History

Ruby was placed on a Child Protective Services hold upon her birth due to her positive toxicology screen for cocaine. She entered a temporary foster care placement while her mother enrolled in an outpatient substance abuse program. Family Maintenance services were ordered and Ruby was reunified with her biological mother six months later. Her mother continued to struggle with residential instability, substance abuse, and Bipolar Disorder for which she began receiving treatment. There had been an intergenerational history of psychosocial trauma, sexual abuse, and a history of involvement with Child Protective Services of many previous referrals regarding the safety and well-being of Ruby's older siblings.

Ruby's early childhood included neglect, verbal and physical abuse, witness to multiple incidences of domestic and community violence, witness to adult sexual activity, and possible sexual abuse. There were records of physical abuse by her mother, as well as alleged incidents of severe domestic violence from Ruby's father who had been part of her life until shortly before her removal. Some of the violence was allegedly perpetrated by Ruby's mother towards her father who reported that he had been stabbed and once set on fire. It was suspected that Ruby witnessed these incidents.

Ruby disclosed that she had witnessed community violence of someone putting a gun to her mother' head. There were unsubstantiated reports of sexual abuse. Ruby herself reported witnessing her mother engaging in sexual activity. She was finally removed because of neighbors reporting her crying, and even seen wandering outside alone at night. Ruby's mother could not be located following Ruby's removal. She was put in an emergency foster home for a month until she could be placed with relatives. Reports from relatives indicated that Ruby would awaken at night and attempt to light objects on fire with flames from the gas stove. This placement was brief, however, and due to apparent behavior problems, Ruby was transitioned to a non-relative foster care home.

There she had periods of inconsolable crying, patterns of indiscriminate approaches to strangers, intense separation anxiety, and experiences of auditory hallucinations. During these episodes, she would disengage and consult with her "voices." She would conference with these voices, little "Hobbits" she called them, and refer to herself in the third person, seeming dissociated from her surroundings. Ruby told her lawyer and her social worker that she did not want to return to her mother. She would alternate between yelling, as if speaking to her mother: "I don't want you here. I hate you, you're a loser!" and "I love you, I like you." This cry typifies the battling emotions of children losing their primary attachment person who has also hurt them.

Psychological Assessment

Although Ruby made substantial improvement in foster care, with respect to an absence of the most extreme behaviors, a positive response to therapy, and a beginning trust in her caregiver, she continued to struggle with emotional and behavioral problems related to the emotional impact of her early traumas. She struggled with periods of crying, sexualized play, nightmares of dogs attacking her, and nighttime terrors. When there was respite care, Ruby asked who was going to take care of her if her foster mother never came for her, or died. Ruby's mother had recently resurfaced and had phone contact with Ruby. Her mother told her she loved her and promised to take her home again.

Following contact with her mother Ruby's symptoms increased. She developed nocturnal enuresis, self-harming behavior of biting herself, flooded the bathroom floor with water, and expressed constant anxiety about her placement. The foster mother reported indiscriminate behavior towards strangers in stores, running towards the street at a family outing. She often would engage in conflicts with her foster siblings, but deny her actions even when they were observed by others.

Both her social worker and her foster mother referred Ruby to our community mental health clinic for an assessment, to understand more about her auditory hallucinations as well as the impact of her early traumas on her behaviors, and to offer treatment recommendations. At this time, when Ruby was 4 years 10 months old, her foster mother was struggling to parent Ruby, and her placement was in jeopardy. While Ruby was a bright and energetic girl, she was provocative and often threatening or trying to hit her foster mother.

One of the most difficult aspects of placing children in foster care who have been traumatized with neglect and abuse, is that their behaviors often externalize or project aspects of their suffering onto their environment and/or caretakers. Their actions of turning the abuse they have suffered into something where they have some active control is a way of (1) getting rid of unwanted, unbearable, frightening feelings related to the trauma, and (2) communicating to someone through their emotional outbursts and actions what has happened to them. "Now you know how I feel!" (Ogden, 1990). Anger is often a way of engagement. Their communications are an unconscious way of engaging a caretaker, albeit in a conflictual and off-putting way, what has happened to them, a kind of reaching out to "someone" – to the "universe" – with the hope that someone can help and contain them. As such this communication can be a vehicle for change (Ogden, 1990), either with a sturdy parent or in therapy.

Foster parents may or may not have been informed about the history of their charge. In either situation, these behaviors are annoying, challenging, often destructive, and it is difficult for any caretaker to connect the behavior to a trauma, or tolerate such behaviors. A foster parent may have their own trauma history, or perhaps harbor hope of rescuing a child who has suffered and might express gratitude for a better home, and ultimately be restored to health. These dramas happen below the level of awareness. It is human nature to subsume hurtful feelings and injurious history in order to go on with our lives. Nevertheless, these enactments impact the child and their sense of security and attachment in a new home. These scenarios are an extreme amplification of what any parent experiences when their child is challenging, dismissive, or angry. Trauma, added to the fact that this child is not one's own, pile onto the stress that is developing in foster care to potentially lead to a 7-day or 14-day notice where the child with their worldly belongings in a large garbage bag are picked up by their social worker and transported to the next locale.

One approach for providing empathy and supporting a foster parent is called Therapeutic Assessment (Finn, 2007) by involving her directly with the assessment process. The foster parents and a second clinician observe through live video feed, the child and assessor in action. Research has shown this kind of assessment can become an intervention, potentially producing a deeper understanding for the caretaker and a shift in dynamics. In utilizing this approach in Ruby's case, the hope was to shore up her placement and make their fragile bond a little stronger

Because there is frequently an inclination to let go of the child and enforce yet another foster care placement and disrupted attachment, therapists will make every effort to work with foster parents to remain steady and "hold on" while these difficult relationships are supported. Research has shown that multiple placements affect a child's ability to repair disorganized attachments and to form more secure trust in relationships. Studies indicate that multiple placement children have a distorted sense of reality and interact in new environments based on their own past traumatic histories, and will struggle to function on a daily basis. (Eshom, 2006). A simple example is when a boy at school is accidentally bumped by another boy, but believes he is being assaulted, then yells or strikes out. If this happens repeatedly, the boy may build on a belief that his peers hate him and are out to get him.

Results of the assessment revealed that Ruby was intelligent and articulate. She identified her "voices" as characters from a video she saw, but said they were no longer talked to her. She was anxious and depressed throughout the evaluation, and became despondent when she perceived any task as difficult. Other times she became irritable and withdrawn and would turn her back on the examiner.

The rejecting and demanding ways in which she related made her behaviors confusing and difficult to predict. For example, during a free play task, Ruby loudly refused the examiner's offer of assistance. She subsequently yelled, "Why aren't you helping me! I need help!" Similarly, she simultaneously rejected *and* invited verbal praise. When praise was offered by the examiner, she yelled, "Shh! Too loud!" However, when praise was *not* offered, she inquired "Why didn't you say I was excellent?" Ruby often misperceived the actions of the assessor as mocking and subsequently became upset and frustrated.

The following measures are typically given to assess a young child's emotional experience: (1) Parent Checklists: Behavior Assessment Rating Scale (BASC-2, 2004); (2) The Trauma Symptom Checklist for Young Children (Briere, 2005); (3) Puppet Sentence Completion Test (Knell & Beck, 2000); (4) Story-telling tests; (5) the MacArthur Story Stem Battery (Bretherton, Oppenheim, Emde, & the MacArthur Narrative Working Group, 2003); (6) Unstructured play session; (7) Projective Drawings.

Findings from the emotional assessment suggested that Ruby's symptoms were rooted in the adverse emotional and psychological impact of the multiple traumas that she experienced during her early childhood. Her foster mother's ratings of her emotional and behavioral problems were clinically significant across multiple areas including internalizing symptoms, externalizing behaviors, and atypical behaviors (BASC-2, 2004). Her foster mother reported that Ruby is "almost always: easily frustrated, changes moods quickly, cries easily, worries about parents, and tries to be perfect."

Results from the emotional testing suggested that Ruby became physiologically and emotionally dysregulated in response to visual or visceral reminders of her prior traumas. Her foster mother's ratings of her post-traumatic stress symptoms were clinically significant for hyperarousal. She noted that Ruby "very often: is easily startled, flinches or jumps when there is a loud noise, is tense and jumpy, and watches out for danger."

Given the extent of Ruby's trauma history, her anxious, sad, and atypical behaviors appeared related to substantial post-traumatic stress symptoms. Her trauma-related distress manifested by vacillating quickly between a highly aroused and frightened state, and becoming alternately distanced or dissociated. Ruby struggled with "re-experiencing" times from her past – that is, having thoughts and flashbacks of traumatic times. These symptoms include distressing nightmares, and repetitive anxiety-evoking play.

Ruby's hyperarousal and jumpy responses were an emotional and physiological response to perceived threat or danger. Given the context of prior trauma, her inappropriate behaviors were likely a response to the physiological survival signals that she experienced in her body. An intrusive thought or feeling unsafe likely contributed to her behavioral difficulties and others could easily misperceive her intentions as solely oppositional rather than anxious and emotionally disorganized.

During an open-ended projective task, Ruby was asked to complete sentence stems with whatever thoughts came to mind. Her responses indicated intrusive thoughts regarding her early experiences under the care of her mother. She completed the stem, "I hate ..." with *"getting hit ... it's the worse to get hit."* She completed the stem, "Mommy is so nice but *mommy doesn't be nice"* and "Mommy ... *mean."* Ruby subsequently digressed into memories of being left home alone during the night.

Ruby told of nightmares during which she was either attacked or trapped by dogs and "can't get out." Court documents indicate that her experiences of physical abuse included being hit in the head and face. Interactions with her caregiver seemed to trigger memories of prior physical abuse when faced with routine tasks. It was hard for her foster mother not to take these instances as rejection.

Ruby expressed her distress in both structured and unstructured play activities. Post-traumatic play occurs when a traumatized child engages in play that represents some aspect of the trauma in an anxiety-evoking manner. This type of play enabled Ruby to attempt to contain the flood of her feelings, at the same time to express and momentarily get rid of some of her upsetting emotions and turmoil. However, the quality of this type of play becomes repetitive and compulsive, and lacks the developmentally adaptive, relaxed play of a young child. For example, Ruby repeatedly directed the lamb puppet to "hide when she's afraid [because] the bad guy will come and eat her." After verbally assuring the puppet's safety, Ruby immediately introduced characters that attempt to "eat" the puppet. During the play observation session where Ruby was allowed to direct the play, Ruby introduced themes of moving and leaving home. She directed and attempted to pack the entire contents of the play room into boxes and suitcases. Ruby repeatedly asked the doll characters, "Are you gonna come?! Are you gonna miss me?!" and her inquiries later became, "Are you gonna be scared? Are you gonna be hungry?"

Ruby was also administered a play-based projective task during which she was asked to resolve particular story situations ranging from a child's accidental mistake (e.g., spilling juice) to a child's separation from a caregiver (MSSB, 2005). Although Ruby attempted to resolve the conflict introduced in each story stem, she became engrossed and overwhelmed by traumatic content that she either introduced or gleaned from the story stem. Themes of her play centered on a lack of a protective adult figure, vulnerability to sexual exploitation, and sexualized themes. During the next story stem, Ruby introduced an invasive and dangerous figure who "kissed the boobs and private parts" of the other characters, both adult and child doll figures. Ruby carried these themes into the subsequent story stems, became preoccupied by them, compulsively acted out sequences of sexual penetration, and was unable to transition to a new and different story. In addition, her play lacked resolution and concentrated on the unavailability of adult helper figures. Although she once attempted to introduce a helper figure who aggressively tried to fend off the dangerous figure, the helper's attempts were ultimately unsuccessful and remained vulnerable to victimization. When asked directly about possible experiences of sexual abuse, Ruby was quiet and did not answer. However, she noted that she "saw my mom and dad do that" in reference to the scenes that she had re-enacted in her play.

Feedback in the form of a letter to her foster mother emphasized Ruby's strengths as well as acknowledging her demanding and challenging behaviors. The assessor validated all the foster mother was doing to keep Ruby safe and listen to Ruby's feelings and worries. Ruby liked this home and told the social worker that she did not want to leave it. The foster mother was concerned with her potential running and destructive behaviors, as well as the ways Ruby could be alternately needy and hostile. Her psychotic symptoms appeared to be trauma based rather than genetically rooted. Despite all attempts to bolster Ruby's parent and the placement, the social worker was asked to search for a new placement a few months later. Ruby was only 5 at the time she was placed in a foster home with a distant paternal cousin.

Long-term Foster Placement and Therapy

Both placement and therapy began with a hopeful prognosis. Ruby displayed a positive attitude, a honeymoon adjustment to her new foster mother, and a strong adjustment to her school environment. There was a compatible match temperamentally and racially with this foster mother, and a potential for this to be permanent: a foster-adopt home.

It was urgent for Ruby to please her foster mother, Miss Loretta. In the first month of therapy, Ruby returned to her push/pull relationship with her new therapist. She was distrustful and sarcastic. "Why do you always wear the same outfit?" she would inquire. "You never get anything right," "You look weird," "I don't want you to play with me. You're stupid." She would try to hit her therapist, try to scare her by grabbing her keys and bringing her fist close to her face, or threaten to run away. Yet she was an avid fan of play therapy and entered into it wholeheartedly. Much of it was repetitive, emotionally upsetting play, often punitive and sadistic. She would defend her pretend home against attackers, but then immediately pack toys in a suitcase and pretend to move. Nevertheless, she was strong in school, without significant problems. Soon the honeymoon in foster care turned difficult. She left dirty underwear in the bathroom, dumped bottles of shampoo, destroyed her toys and belongings. Her sexualized behaviors resurfaced. She sat in the laps of male visitors, and she became flirtatious with her foster mother's nephew. She even became provocative with her foster mother.

The intense aggressive play was constant and unrelenting so therapy was increased to twice weekly as a way to contain her. Increased countertransference reactions are often a natural accompaniment to intense therapy that must be worked through in consultation or supervision. Her therapist felt traumatized and upset by these disorganized attachment interactions, and would feel anxious going to see her (the community funding source allowed sessions at school and at home). At the same time her therapist was afraid to speak in supervision about how hard it was. She felt ashamed, as if she were in an abusive relationship. "She put me through the ringer. She made me feel like a horrible person, like a monster. I would feel angry and get upset, trying to teach her to be more empathetic, more socially kind." After many weeks, she was able to take the risk to unpack these behaviors, seeing Ruby's *meanness* as an acting out of her past treatment, and trying to "torture" her therapist with the experience of her worst feelings. Her therapist was then able to step back and tolerate these assaults without becoming indignant or returning anger and to recognize that this was not her fault, that she was not doing something wrong. She was also able to let Miss Loretta know that she understood how hard Ruby must be to parent. These reactions experienced by foster parents and therapists are common with children who have experienced trauma.

Sorting through them honestly as normal can help detoxify the turmoil. We all hoped this wouldn't last forever. In one session, Ruby became angry and stormed out of the room, running back into the larger school building. Her therapist said, "I know you are mad but I'll be here when you come back." Another turning point was when the therapist's car broke down on the day of the session. She rented a car and drove the hour distance to Ruby's school. On this day, she was mad and having a hard time. "You're only here because you are paid to come here" she proclaimed. Her therapist replied, "Ruby, my work with you means a lot and that is what brought us together. My car broke down today and I rented a car so I could get here and not miss our session." For the first time, Ruby was able to hear this without a retort. After a year of conflict there was a shift in their relationship and Ruby's behavior in therapy. Her provocations and belligerence transformed into an exploration of her life and her sense of self. While she would still alternate between "I hate you" and "Don't leave me," she permitted her therapist play with her. They made a "Life Book" and Ruby began to record in a less compulsive way some of her past traumatic experiences: witnessing of adult sexual activity, and abandonment. They made a box to put their artwork, jewelry and crafts. Ruby wondered why her therapist wanted to save them because they "are no good like me." Her therapist replied "No, they are treasures from your life."

The foster-adopt situation was still in process. Her foster mother professed the desire to finalize this placement after two years, and to make Ruby her own child. Yet she continued to have difficulty with Ruby's behaviors. Ruby would alternately be defiant and adoring. Some dramatic incidents of sexualized behaviors came to light – including Ruby taking phone pictures of her private parts at an overnight and sending them to her friend, and a discovery that Ruby and an older nephew who often stayed at their house were engaged in sexualized play. It was even possible that Ruby had pursued and initiated these interactions. This convinced Miss Loretta that it was not safe for her family to adopt or keep Ruby. Ruby pleaded with Miss Loretta not to make her leave. Even up to the last minute and final decision, Miss Loretta had mixed feelings. She wanted to keep Ruby as her own, but at the same time, she could not keep her because of the negative effect on other family members. In making decisions about children's needs we must also understand the experience of caring foster parents who face a most difficult task.

Parental Rights and Adoption

Her social worker became the adoption person to search for a family as looking for another foster placement was undesirable. The adoption process for a child in foster care is a strange one. The social worker makes a flier with a child's photo and circulates it. Ruby is taken with other children to an adoption fair.

A family saw her profile and was interested. They asked a lot of questions. Much of Ruby's history was communicated to them, although not the last piece of acting out behavior as the details of this incident were not clear and had not been investigated. There were two week-end meetings with Ruby, an African American girl and her interracial family – a White mother and father and an African American adoptive son. There was one overnight, and adoption moved quickly. The social worker, therapist and adoptive parents all met. The family was enthusiastic, reflective, willing to have therapy, to do whatever was needed to have Ruby in their home. Miss Loretta was worried about a transracial adoption, and both the social worker and Ruby's lawyer had concerns. However, this family seemed to be optimal in other ways and motivated to acknowledge and work with issues of race.

Ruby attempted to be excited about the adoption, but underneath she was heartbroken, sad about leaving Miss Loretta, and felt abandoned. Her coping style was to be positive. She made a book with her therapist to introduce her to her new family.

In terminating parental rights before a child can be adopted, caretakers are permitted by law to contest the adoption. Ruby's biological mother filed to block the termination of her parental rights and the adoption in court. There was a court hearing at which Ruby's first therapist was subpoenaed. Calling therapists to testify in dependency hearings is becoming less prevalent because it stirs up conflicts regarding the role of the therapist to give a placement opinion, rather than remaining an emotional mainstay for the child. Often the therapist can speak informally with the social worker and lawyer about the effects of trauma, for example, without having to provide written letters or court testimony stating an opinion.

The lawyer and social worker were also subpoenaed to testify. A lawyer advocate is typically versed in the effects of trauma to be able to advocate in the child's best interest. A defense lawyer can argue that if a child has significant strengths, that this is evidence of a parent's capabilities. Ruby's social worker was called to speak about the extent of her early trauma at the time of her removal at age 4. If a parent contests an adoption, it is their burden of proof to provide a reason to halt the process. A parent can have many strengths and early attachment to their child, but still not be able to provide for their protection and well-being. The judge ruled that there was insufficient proof that her mother or any family member could reasonably parent Ruby. Even after moving and with the support of her new family, Ruby continued to visit her foster mother.

The lawyer, social worker and therapist continued meeting to discuss this plan. The adoptive mother was loving and open, yet a month or two into the move, Ruby began showing signs of sexualized behaviors. She undressed with the door open, was overly friendly with visiting family men friends, and she was provocative with her adoptive brother. He accused her of touching him. There were family meetings with Ruby's therapist and social worker. The therapist revealed to the family the extent of Ruby's past sexualizing behaviors (the full history still had not been shared with the family). Ruby had just turned 9 years old and once again there was a fear that she would not be able to sustain her placement. Her behaviors had always subsided at times but to continually resurface.

At times, she had been vilified in her placements, and again this crisis pointed to how volatile her behaviors could be. Her parents were worried, but they were willing to continue to work with Ruby's therapist, and they wanted to keep Ruby. Her new mother was often tearful and worried about keeping her. Her sexual acting out was the most troublesome. Could they take her to friends' houses? Could she stay overnight anywhere? Would she threaten the emotional stability of her new brother? Her therapist continued to link Ruby's behavior to her past trauma, and to her need to test out, in a primitive way, whether she was worth loving and keeping. Without holding her context and experience in mind, she would have been returned to the system, to the courts; all voices, all meaning, would be lost.

Her therapist worked with Ruby and her family for another year. She was making progress without further serious incidents and was doing well in school. The parents relied on the therapist for encouragement to reinforce their parenting, to give them guidance, and to aid in the interpretation of some of Ruby's more difficult behaviors. By the end of therapy Ruby would often decline her therapy session; but the mother would use her session to feel more empowered as Ruby's parent. They discussed how to help with Ruby's outbursts, and how to think about supporting Ruby's racial identity through transracial PACT camps and consultations.

One year after therapy ended, Ruby's adoptive mother called to report that Ruby had been accepted at an art school and was doing well. Ruby's was that she excited and wanted her therapist to see how well she doing although she didn't want to talk to her. After some time, the family was able to have visits with her former foster mother. When Ruby was poised to enter high school at 14 years old, her adoptive mother phoned to say that Ruby had bonded with her adopted family, was excelling in dance, and working with other students for social justice.

There is no overestimating how difficult this case was for all involved: for the social service system, the advocates, the Courts, the foster parents, the therapist, and the adoptive parents – and at the core, for Ruby. Ruby was perceived as smart but a manipulator, somewhat of a little "demon." She seemed fated for multiple foster placements, for rejection, even for sexual exploitation as she developed into adolescence. Every month her future hung in the balance. It had taken ten years of persistence, refusal to give up on her, with each person in her life contributing along the way.

The Well-Being of Children

Our children elicit in us our deepest attachments, reminding us of our own early sense of security, loss, or suffering. They are carriers of our collective future. When children enter a system, they hopefully will be safe from harm; but this removal and protection simply does not guaranty their well-being, or their ability to thrive or succeed.

Our solutions to assist children and families involved with out-of-home dependency need to be multi-layered, across systems, and most importantly, collaborative. Review of therapeutic treatment literature suggests that both reactive attachment disorders and post-traumatic stress disorders are prevalent with children in foster care (Marsenich, California Institute for Mental Health, 2002). While not all children in foster care meet the current DSM-IV criteria for PTSD, the van der Kolk contribution of a developmental trauma diagnosis (2005) does apply. Attachment disorders, specifically the category of disorganized attachment, can overlap with trauma, but extends the definition beyond the trauma itself to relational traumas of unresolved grief and mourning from abandonment (George & West, 2012). Therapeutic treatment must be trauma and culturally informed, and relational. Systemic approaches for children in "rich nations," according to UNICEF, must include children's material well-being, health and safety, education, behavior and risk, and housing and environment (UNICEF, 2013).

Many counties across the U.S. provide family permanence and maintenance services related to protective service referrals that address substance abuse treatment for parents, housing and food assistance, transportation, and income support. In other countries, considering issues of maltreatment are integral to children services and are designed to support both children and parents. Many U.S. programs depend on government funding that imposes time limits for services or requires crisis referrals that delay needed intervention. For instance, family reunification programs need to be able to support families *beyond* the initial stages. Wraparound services are crucial at every stage of the removal, foster care, and family maintenance process.

The foster care system and the mental health component need to be connected, as Francine Cournos has stated, in order to help both foster care parents and children make sense of their experience. She stresses the need to recognize the importance of recognizing the role of foster parents, who may often be viewed in functional terms, as opposed to a potential attachment person (Cournos, 2004). When reunification is a planned outcome, biological parents need to be offered services to support them in navigating the transition and finding ways to reconnect with their children and to become parents again. We must also remember that with parenthood, there is an eventual letting go process for the well-being of children. This is accentuated in the child welfare system; it can be painful and heroic.

Dependency advocacy programs rightly function in the legal representation of children and youth at *every* stage, from detention through permanency. Within the court process they identify services and advocate for policies and laws that will help insure children have a voice in decisions, in their support, and through transition programs and to the extension of foster care to 21 years old, in their ultimate independence (CA AB12, 2012). Another crucial area of training involves finding strategies to address disproportionality related to child protection – looking toward agencies in the child and family services delivery system, and judges in the judicial system (Green et al., 2016). Other programs like Transitional Age Youth Programs (TAYS), including programs for sexually exploited minors, and Independent Living Skills Programs, offer support like wraparound and skill training through groups. One unique program – Youth Advocacy Program (YAP), West Coast Children's Clinic, Oakland, California – offers training fellowships for current and former foster youth. These youth advocates attend Team Decision Meetings to give voice to issues related to foster children and youth, and to professionals. They also receive training in entering the work force.

In an effort to create greater equality and a chance for productive lives for our foster children, we must think of these rifts in children's lives and parenting tragedies as part of a larger context of locale and community (Mercer, 2016). Will life in foster care be an added trauma, "good enough," or can it be ultimately restorative? The goal is to promote the voice and agency of these children who are most often thrust out, separated too early from their sense of a secure home. We, as professionals, need to be able to hold a meaningful sense of their experience, and mirror that understanding back to them. Here is a fable written by an assessor for a youth in foster care at the end her assessment.

> This evaluator told the story of a princess named Imani from the land of Wazoo who was a dreamer, "a Wazoo dreamer is someone who holds onto their dreams for the future" she says, "when others cannot." The village celebrated and expressed their hope for Imani's future. Unfortunately, Imani is caught in a terrible storm at sea and shipwrecked, losing her parents, village, and after nearly starving, ending up on a far-away island with a strange family who had no knowledge of her gift for dreams or her princess identity. She began to doubt herself. It was not until a young man called at her from his car window: "Hey princess. You look so good. You wanna ride?" that she started to cry and recall her past. The evaluator wrote: "She tried to get close to people in hopes they would see who she really was ... she would often let people get close to her for a short time and then get scared and do something to turn them away ... How would she realize her special dreams without the help of her Wazoo family?" The story ends with a gradual memory of her abilities without offering false promises or reassurances. At the end of the session when the assessor finished reading the story, the girl said, excitedly: "How did you know? My grandmother used to call me that, Princess. You wrote that for me?" (Dara Goosby, Personal Communication, 2000)

We must continue, as professionals, parents, helpers, to listen to children's voices, that often lie beneath their behaviors, to help them find meaning in their experience (van der Kolk et al., 2007). We must be willing, as Anne Alvarez says in her book *Live Company*, to hold onto, together with the child, a vision of their wholeness, their dream of achievement, at the same time helping them believe in, voice, and embody their real power and capability to reach their potential.

Acknowledgments

Special thanks to the personal communications over the years from Tricia Fong, Brooke Guerrero, Dara Goosby, Christy Hobza, and Ryan Adams who, with heartfelt persistence, worked with children in foster care.

References

Administrative Office of the Courts. (2005). Administrative Office of the Courts, *California juvenile dependency court improvement program reassessment*. San Francisco, CA: Center for families, children, and the court, Administrative Office of the Courts 2005.

In re: Alexis W. (1999) 71 Cal. App.4th 28, 36.

Alvarez, A. (1992). *Live company*. London: Routledge.

Berger, L. M., Noyes, J. L., & Slack, K. (2014). *Understanding the link between income and child maltreatment*. Presentation at the Wisconsin Department of Children and Families/Institute for Research Learning Exchange, Madison, WI, December 4, 2014.

Berrick, J. D. (2009). *Take me home*. New York: Oxford University Press.

Berrick, J. D. (2018). *The impossible imperative*. New York: Oxford University Press.

Berrick, J. D., Dickens, J., Poso, T., & Skivenes, M. (2018). International perspectives on child-responsive courts. *International Journal of Children's Rights, 26*, 251–277.

Bion, W. R. (1975). Learning from experience. In *Seven servants: Four works* (pp. 1–105). New York: Aronson.

Borgen Project. (2018). Retrieved from: https://borgenproject.org/facts-about-girls-education-in-afghanistan/

Boswell, J. (1988). *The kindness of strangers: Child abandonment in western Europe from late antiquity to the renaissance*. Chicago: University of Chicago Press.

Bretherton, I., Oppenheim, D., Emde, R. N., & the MacArthur Narrative Working Group. (2003). Revealing the inner worlds of young children: The MacArthur Story Stem Battery and parent – child narratives. In R. N. Emde, D. P. Wolf, & D. Oppenheim (Eds.), *The MacArthur Story Stem Battery* (pp. 381–396). New York: Oxford University Press.

Brevard, K. C. (2017). *Child welfare decision-making: Does race matter?* School of Social Work, University of North Carolina Chapel Hill. ProQuest Dissertations Publishing, 2017. 10608054

Briere, J. (2005). *Trauma symptom checklist for young children (TSCYC): Professional manual*. Odessa, FL: Psychological Assessment Resources.

California Courts. The Judicial Branch of California. (2017, December 14). *Juvenile dependency law and process. Beyond the Bench 24*. Retrieved from https://www.courts.gov/documents/BTB2.

Child Abuse Prevention and Treatment Act. (CAPTA). Public Law 93–247. (1974) PL 100–294(1988).

Child Rights International Network. (2016). CRIN: Rights, Remedies & Representation: Global Report on Access to Justice for Children. Retrieved from: https://www.crin.org/

Child Welfare Information Gateway. (2019). *Foster care statistics 2017*. Washington, DC: U.S. Department of Health and Human Services, Children's Bureau.

Cournos, F. (1999). *City of one: A memoir*. New York: W. W. Norton.

Cournos, F. (2004). Parental death and foster care: A personal and professional perspective. *Journal of Infant, Child, and Adolescent Psychotherapy, 3*(3), 342–355.

De Mause, L. (1974). *History of childhood*. Lanham, MD: Rowman & Littlefield.

Dickens, C. (2009). *Oliver Twist* [first published 1837–38]. London: Penguin Books.

Eshom, J. A. (2006). *An examination of the impact of trauma in multiple placements in foster care children using the ego impairment index II on the Rorschach*. The Wright Institute. ProQuest, UMI Dissertations Publishing, 3230476.

Finn, S. E. (2007). *In our client's shoes: Theory and techniques of therapeutic assessment*. Mahwah, NJ: Lawrence Erlbaum Associates.

Fong, M. (2016). *One child nation: The story of china's most radical experiment*. Boston: Houghton Mifflin Harcourt.

Gal, T., & Duramy, B. (2015). *International perspective and empirical findings on child participation: From social exclusion to child inclusive policies*. New York: Oxford University Press.

George, C., & West, M. (2012). *The adult attachment projective picture system*. New York: The Guilford Press.

Gin, K. B. (2008). Demands on the mind for work: Fostering agency within an organization. *Journal of Infant, Child, and Adolescent Psychotherapy, 7*(2), 79–87.

Green, D. K., Belanger, B., McRoy, R. G., & Bullard, L. (Eds.). (2016). *Racial disproportionality in child welfare: Research, policy, and practice.* Washington, D.C.: CWLA Press.

Human Rights Watch. (2017). Retrieved from: https://www.hrw.org/news/2017/10/17/afghanistan-girls-struggle-education

Judicial Council of California/Administrative Office of the Courts. (2011). *A dependency quick-guide: A dogbook for attorneys representing children and parents second edition.* Cal. App 3d 1288.1299. San Francisco, CA.

Kim, H., Wildeman, C., Jonson-Reid, M., & Drake, B. (2017). Lifetime prevalence of investigating child maltreatment among U.S. children. *American Journal of Public Health, 107*(2), 274–280. doi:10.2105/AJPH,2016.303545

Knell, S. M., & Beck, K. W. (Eds.). (2000). The puppet sentence completion task. In K. Gitlin-Weiner, A. Sandgrund, & C. Schaefer (Eds.), *Play diagnosis and assessment* (pp. 704–721). Hoboken, NJ: John Wiley & Sons.

In re: Kristen B. (2008) 163 Cal. App.4th 1535.

Loseke, D., Gelles, R. J., & Cavanaugh, M. (Eds.). (2005). *Current controversies on family violence.* Thousand Oaks, CA: Sage Publications.

Marsenich, L. (2002). *Evidence-based practices in mental health services for foster youth. Report component of the CIMH Caring for Foster Youth initiative funded and supported by the Zellerbach Family Fund.* San Francisco, CA: California Institute for Mental Health.

McDonald, T., Allen, R. (1996). *Assessing the long-term effects of foster care: A research synthesis.*

Mercer, B. L. (2000, March). *Rorschach variables of children in foster care: W:M ratio, egocentricity ratio and projective metaphor.* Paper presented at the annual meeting of the Society for Personality Assessment, San Francisco, CA.

Mercer, B. L. Fong, T., & Rosenblatt, E. (Eds.). (2016). *Assessing children in the urban community.* New York: Routledge.

Myers, J. B. (2004). *A history of child protection in America.* Xlibris Corporation. Library of Congress: 2003095230.

National Child Abuse and Neglect Data System Child Files and Census Data. (2003–2014). In T. Ogden (1990), *The matrix of the mind: Object relations and the psychoanalytic dialogue.* Northvale, NJ: Jason Aronson.

Ogden, T. H. (1990), *The matrix of the mind: Object relations and the psychoanalytic dialogue.* Northvale, NJ: Jason Aronson.

Ogden, T. H. (2009). *Rediscovering psychoanalysis, thinking and dreaming, learning and forgetting.* New York: Routledge.

Parker, S. (2008). *The safety house.* Retrieved from https://www.spconsultancy.com.au.

Public Health and Welfare: 42 USC § 5106

In re: Raymond G. (1991) 230 Cal.APP.3d 964). Retrieved from: https://www.capcentral.org/juveniles/dependency.

Reynolds, C. R., & Kamphaus, R. W. (2004). *Behavior assessment system for children* (2nd ed.). Circle Pines, MN: American Guidance System.

Rolock, N. (2008). *Disproportionality in Illinois child welfare.* Urbana, IL: Children and Family Research Center.

Sedlak, A. J., & Broadhurst, D. (1996). *Third national incidence study of child abuse and neglect.* Washington, D.C.: US Department of Health and Human Services. Retrieved from https://www.childwelfare.gov

Sedlak, A. J., & Schultz, D. (2005). Racial differences in child protective services investigation of abused and neglected children. In D. Dennette, J. Poertner, M. Testa, F. Mark, & Race Matters Consortium (Eds.), *Race matters in child welfare: The overrepresentation of African American children in the system* (pp. 97–118). *Washington, DC*: Child Welfare League of America, distributed by CWLA Press.

Sedlak, A. J., Mettenburg, J., Basena, M., Petta, I., McPherson, K., Greene, A., & Li, S. (2010). *Fourth national incidence study of child abuse and neglect (NIS-4): Report to Congress.* Washington, DC: U.S. Department of Health and Human Services, Administration for Children and Families.

Sedlak, A. J., & McPherson, K., & Das, B. (2010). *Fourth national incidence study of child abuse and neglect (NIS-4). Supplementary analyses of race differences in child maltreatment rates in the NIS–4.* Washington D.C: Department of Health and Human Services. Retrieved from: https:www.acf.hhs.gov.>opre >resource>fourth national incidence study

Slack, K. S., Berger, L. M., & Collins, M. (2019). *Can improving access to economic resources prevent child maltreatment? Preliminary evidence from a randomized experiment.* Presentation at the Wisconsin-Madison Population Health Sciences Seminar, Madison, WI, April 22, 2019.

Tilmon, S. (2003). *Speaking the unspeakable: A qualitative look at discipline in African American families.* The Wright Institute. ProQuest Dissertations Publishing, 2003. 3084497.

Title IV of the Civil Rights Act of 1964, 42 U.S.C. § 2000d, et seq. Retrieved from: http://www.justice.gov/crt/about/cor/coord/titlevistat.php

U.S. Census Bureau. (2009). *Historical income tables. Table F-9. Presence and number of related children under 18 years old – families by median and mean income.* U.S. Census Bureau, Housing and Household Economic Statistics Division. Accessed 11/09 at http://www.census.gov/hhes/www/income/histinc/incfamdet.html:56. Retrieved from: https:www.acf.hhs.gov.>opre >resource>fourth national incidence study

U.S Department of Health and Services. (2018). *The AFCARS report #25.* Retrieved from: https://www.acf.hhs/gov.ch

Van der Kolk, B. A. (2005). Developmental trauma disorder. *Psychiatric Annals* (May 2005), *35*(5), 401–408.

Van der Kolk, B. A., McFarlane, A. C., & Wisaeth, L. (Eds.). (2007). *Traumatic stress: The effects of overwhelming experience on mind, body, and society.* New York: Guilford Press.

Verinis, J. S., Lichtenberg, E. F., & Henrich, I. (1974). The draw-a-person-in-the-rain technique: Its relationship to diagnostic category and other personality indicators. *Journal of Clinical Psychology, 30*(3), 407–414.

Weisz, V., Wingrove, T., Beal, S., & Faith-Slaker, A. (2011) Children's participation in foster care hearings. *Child Abuse & Neglect, 35*(4), 267–272.

Weld, N. (2008). *The 'three houses' tool.* Retrieved from https://www.partnering for safety.com

Welfare and Institutions Code §300 Dependent Children – Jurisdiction [300–304.7] *(Article 6 added by Stats. 1976, Ch. 1068.)*; 16501 (a) (4)

Wildeman, C., & Emanuel, N. (2014). *Cumulative risks of foster care placement by age 18 for U.S. children, 2000–2011. PLuS One.* (9)3 e92785. doi:10.1371/journal.pone.0092785

Wilson, A. (1970). *The world of Charles Dickens.* New York: Viking Press.

Woods, S., & Summers, A. (2016). Technical assistance bulletin. *Disproportionality rates for children of color in foster care (fiscal year 2014).* Reno, NV: National Council of Juvenile and Family Court Judges.

Winnicott, D. W. (1963). Psychiatric disorders in terms of infantile mental processes. In *The maturational processes and the facilitating environment* (pp. 230–234). Madison, CT: International Universities Press.

Wulczyn, B. K., & George, R. (2002). *Multistate foster care data archive.* Chicago, IL: University of Chicago Press.

7 Attachment Relationships for Attorneys

Using Expert Testimony to Guide the Court's Determination of Children's Best Interests in Family Court Cases

Alicia Jurney
Introduction by Ginger C. Calloway

Introduction

In 2010, when Dr. Erard and I wrote the introduction to the Special Issue on Attachment and Child Custody for *The Journal of Child Custody*, we noted that a literature search of the word "attachment" yielded 10,000 entries since 1975 to 2008. In their most recent edition of the *Handbook of Attachment: Theory, Research and Clinical Applications*, Third Edition,[1] Jude Cassidy and Phillip Shaver, Editors, note that since their 2008 Second Edition to the Handbook, the number of entries for a search of the word "attachment" has tripled, making the number 30,000 rather than 10,000, from 1975 to 2016. Clearly, the interest in and importance of attachment theory to understanding children's relationships with their caregivers, as well as the short and long-term impact of these relationships, is obviously keen and broadly of interest. Cassidy and Shaver offer further, "In the study of social and emotional development, attachment theory is the most visible and empirically grounded conceptual framework guiding today's research."[2] Cassidy and Shaver's three volumes of Handbooks are richly deep, informed and comprehensive on the subject of attachment theory and relationships. These volumes are a must for anyone seeking the most up-to-date research findings and wanting to delve into the complexity and range of attachment relationships and their connection to other behavioral, emotional, social and psychological systems.

"Whilst especially evident during early childhood, attachment behavior is held to characterize human beings from the cradle to the grave."[3] John Bowlby, Mary Ainsworth and associates are considered the pioneers and authors of early attachment theory. Bowlby defined attachment in young children as "a strong disposition to seek proximity to and contact with a specific figure and to do so in certain situations, notably when frightened, tired or ill."[4] Attachment behaviors, seeking out caregivers who provide comfort and launching out from the secure base those caregivers provide to engage in exploration, are distinguished from affectional ties, affiliation or social engagement. Cooper, Hoffman, Marvin and Powell[5] developed the notion of a "Circle of Security," shown below in Figure 7.1, that captures well and succinctly the notions basic to attachment relationships. Primary to an understanding of the significance of attachment relationships for children is the function of a caregiver or multiple caregivers to provide both a safe haven for children to anchor when tired, frightened, or confused and a secure base from which to explore once recharged by the caregiver(s) attentions and solicitations to the child's comfort and greater ease.

"How children and their caregivers organize protective proximity and contact, and how they continue to use their caregivers as a secure base for exploration remain as important during later periods of development as during the first year of life."[6] Marvin and co-authors in Cassidy and Jude note that activation of the attachment system occurs across the lifespan, in increasingly more diverse ways and becomes organized with other behavioral systems

DOI: 10.4324/9780429397806-8

Circle of Security®
Parent Attending To The Child's Needs

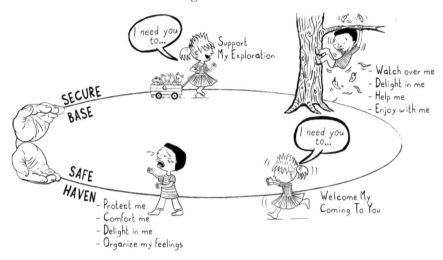

© 2016 Cooper, Hoffman, and Powell. Circle of Security International

Figure 7.1 Circle of Security

of the individual. Accordingly, their chapter, "Normative Development: The Ontogeny of Attachment in Childhood" reflects this consideration of attachment behavior in a larger context than tasks only of infancy and early childhood. In short, the child's experiences of caregiving, whether attuned or not attuned, provide a foundation for and lens through which the child perceives later relationships and a base for how the child develops into adolescence and adulthood.

In this chapter that follows, Attorney Jurney reports on a case of a young child in the dependency part of the juvenile court system involving Child Protective Services and Department of Social Services (DSS). While the judge in the matter made his decision about permanent placement based on his own experience, intuition and presumably common sense, he nevertheless ruled to allow expert testimony on the potential effects to the child if removed from the care of the adoptive parents, with whom the child had resided since birth. It bears repeating that in this matter, DSS made a recommendation to the court for placing the child in a home with half-siblings he had never met. The parental rights of the mother of these half-siblings and the child in this chapter were terminated, such that the child in this chapter never had contact with that mother and never had contact with his half-siblings. It is also worth noting that more often than not, the trier of fact in such dependency matters typically agrees with and rules in favor of DSS recommendations. Ms. Jurney has provided a fascinating look into the two experts who testified about the potential impact of removal, from the home in which he had lived since birth, to this little boy and has provided practical, valuable and concrete suggestions for examination of experts on the topic of attachment relationships. Of note also is that when DSS sought to appeal the judge's decision, the court of appeals rejected their brief and argument and concurred with the judge's decision not to remove the child. The appeals court also agreed with the judge's decision to allow expert testimony on the subject of attachment relationships.

Case Study[7]

Lawrence and Mary Ann Miller were experienced foster parents. They had been licensed for nearly ten years, and during that time, they provided temporary care for many children of all ages. The Millers were also the biological parents of a 5-year old boy, Mason. They had a good relationship with the local Department of Social Services (DSS) and made DSS aware that they were interested in adopting a child, if the opportunity arose, so Mason would have a sibling.

In October 2018, DSS notified the Millers that a woman with whom the agency had been involved previously, Erin Smith, had just given birth to baby boy named Oliver. Ms. Smith had three children older than Oliver, all of whom had been placed in foster care and adopted by non-parents after termination of her parental rights. Neither Ms. Smith nor DSS was able to determine the identity of Oliver's father. Because all of Ms. Smith's older children had been adopted after being placed in foster care and Oliver's father was unknown, DSS informed Mr. and Mrs. Miller that reunification between Ms. Smith and Oliver would likely not be successful and that DSS anticipated Oliver would be a candidate for adoption.

DSS took custody of Oliver when he was only two days old and still in the hospital where he was born. Upon being taken into DSS's custody, Oliver was immediately placed with the Millers. Mr. Miller picked Oliver up from the hospital, where he received Oliver from the DSS social worker, and brought him to the Millers' home.

Oliver quickly became part of the Miller family, and Mr. and Mrs. Miller confirmed to DSS that they were very interested in a foster-to-adopt arrangement with Oliver. Mr. Miller, who is a retired military veteran, was a stay-at-home caretaker for Oliver and Mason. The Millers took Oliver on trips to visit their family members and vacations to Disney World. They ensured that Oliver received proper medical care, stayed up at night with him when he was sick, fed him, bathed him, played with him, and acted in every meaningful way as though they were his parents. By all accounts Mr. and Mrs. Miller provided excellent care for Oliver, and he developed a close attachment bond with the Millers and Mason. By the time he was nine months old, Oliver was referring to Mrs. Miller as "mama" and Mr. Miller as "dada."

In June 2019, Richard and Karen Wilson, the adoptive parents of Ms. Smith's two middle children, Julie and Noah, reached out to Ms. Smith through Facebook to ask her if she would like to receive updates about Julie and Noah. Through Julie and Noah's caseworker with DSS in another county, Ms. Wilson learned in February 2018 that Ms. Smith was pregnant and later discovered that Oliver had been born in October 2018. Ms. Smith did not comply with the DSS reunification plan for Oliver and ultimately stopped exercising visitation with him. Although Oliver had been in a stable placement with Mr. and Mrs. Miller since he was two days old, Ms. Smith told Ms. Wilson that there was no one to take him and that she had been trying to find somewhere that would be a good place for him. Based on this information, Mr. and Mrs. Wilson appeared at a permanency planning review hearing in Oliver's case at the end of June 2019 and informed DSS that they would like to adopt Oliver.

In July 2019, DSS and Oliver's guardian ad litem (GAL) informed Mr. and Mrs. Miller that they would both be recommending[8] at a permanency planning hearing on August 2, 2019 that Oliver be removed from the Millers' home and placed for adoption with the Wilsons, and Oliver's half-siblings, whom Oliver had never met. Mr. and Mrs. Miller were shocked and did not believe that it was in Oliver's best interests to be removed from their home and placed for adoption with people who were strangers to him. Desiring to provide information to the trial court about Oliver's attachment to their family and their beliefs regarding his best interests, Mr. and Mrs. Miller hired counsel and appeared for the permanency planning review hearing on August 6, 2019.

Mr. and Mrs. Miller were not parties to Oliver's case and, as foster parents, had no legal right to intervene. They were not able to put on evidence or formally request that the court continue Oliver's placement in their home. However, the jurisdiction in which the case was filed required the court to consider the testimony of the child's caretakers to determine the placement that would be in his best interests. The court permitted Mr. and Mrs. Miller to testify and allowed their attorney to direct the examinations.

In a two-day trial that took place on 6 and August 13, 2019, the trial court heard testimony from the DSS social worker assigned to Oliver's case, Oliver's GAL, the GAL for Julie and Noah, Mr. Miller, Mrs. Miller, Mr. Wilson, and Mrs. Wilson. None of the parties presented expert testimony. DSS, Oliver's attorney advocate, and Ms. Smith, who were the only parties[9] to the case, all requested that Oliver be removed from the Millers' care and placed with the Wilsons so that he could be in the same home as his Julie and Noah, even though he had never had contact with his half-siblings. Each of the parties conceded that the Millers had provided a stable, loving, nurturing home for Oliver and that Oliver had a close attachment bond with Mr. and Mrs. Miller and Mason. The parties did not contend that Mr. and Mrs. Wilson could provide better care or a more suitable environment for Oliver – they simply argued that Oliver should be placed with the Wilsons so that he could live in the same home as his half-siblings. Because Oliver was only 9 months old at the time of the trial, the parties believed that any negative effects on him would be brief and minimal. Their arguments about the impact of Oliver's age on his ability to recover from the change in placement included the following statements:

DSS: You have to look at the age of the child. That's very important for the Court to consider. I think the GAL was correct that the bonding a child receives in his first few months is significant. But at the same time and unfortunately in this court, we are sometimes tasked with moving a child. The longer a child is in the home, the harder the transition is. This child is only nine months old.

MS. SMITH: Mr. and Mrs. Miller talked about what a loss for Oliver it would be if he were removed from their home. I don't mean this harshly, but nine months does not a lifetime make. Yes, there was bonding with this family. Even from a nine-month old's perspective, there has been bonding. The Millers have loved him and made him feel safe, but I don't think at nine months old Oliver will feel the trauma that they believe he will feel. At nine months old, changing placement would be more of a sorrow for the Millers than for Oliver. I think it's still early enough that this separation would be less traumatic on him than the rest of his life wondering why he couldn't be with his siblings.

OLIVER'S ATTORNEY ADVOCATE: You know, the unfortunate thing as an advocate for children that I have is oftentimes I get children after they have been bounced from home to home, or after they have been from relative to relative, or they live from pillar to post with family or with their parents, and they have got a number of traumas. In this case, it's early in the child's life. It would not be detrimental to Oliver to move him to the home with his half-siblings.

At the conclusion of the parties' arguments, the court orally rendered its decision to grant guardianship of Oliver to Mr. and Mrs. Miller. Acknowledging the difficulty the court had in reaching a decision about placement, the presiding judge said that he had given the case near constant thought in the intervening week between the first and second day of trial. The court expressly determined that it would not be in Oliver's best interests to be removed from the Millers' home and placed with the Wilsons. The court's explanation for its decision, in part, was as follows:

Unlike many sibling situations, Oliver has never lived with or bonded with his half-siblings, nor have they ever lived with or bonded with him. Oliver has lived for nine and a half months with the Millers. He went home from the hospital with the Millers. He has had nine and a half months to bond with the Millers. Mr. and Mrs. Miller are the only parents Oliver has ever known. Oliver is bonded with them as parents and refers to Mrs. Miller as his mother and Mr. Miller as his father. Oliver recognizes one and only one individual as his sibling, and that is the Millers' five-year-old son, Mason. The court does not find that it is in Oliver's best interests to be taken out of a safe, permanent home to place him with siblings that he does not know. The court has considered the fact that Oliver is at an age where he is not old enough to understand that his half siblings are his half-siblings, nor is he so young that he would not experience the loss of his bond with the Millers and Mason. The court is greatly concerned that there is a significant risk that Oliver would suffer irreparably if he were torn out of the only home he has known and placed in another home. The risk of emotional, mental, and psychological harm to Oliver, particularly given that he is in a safe, permanent home, is not in his best interests. Oliver should be allowed to remain in the safe, permanent home with the people that he has come to know as his parents.

The court entered a temporary order granting Mr. and Mrs. Miller immediate guardianship of Oliver and directed DSS to prepare the formal written permanency planning order from the trial. Before the permanency planning order was entered, Ms. Smith made a motion to re-open the evidence. In her motion, Ms. Smith argued that the court's decision to grant Mr. and Mrs. Miller guardianship, which made them parties to the case and put them on a path to adopt Oliver, would have a life-long impact on Oliver and that the court should not make a final decision about placement without considering expert testimony about the effect, if any, that changing placement would have on Oliver. The court granted Ms. Smith's motion and permitted Ms. Smith and Mr. and Mrs. Miller (through Oliver's attorney advocate) to present expert witness testimony about whether there would be a risk of harm to Oliver if he were removed from the Millers' home and placed with the Wilsons.

On October 29, 2019, the court re-opened the evidence and received testimony from two expert witnesses – Dr. Mallory Jones, who was tendered by Ms. Smith and qualified as an expert in clinical psychology, and Dr. Courtney Reynolds, who was tendered by Oliver's attorney advocate and qualified as an expert in child development and attachment relationships. Dr. Jones, who had worked broadly in clinical psychology but did not have significant experience in child development in general, or attachment relationships in particular, testified that because of the secure attachment relationships Oliver had with Mr. and Mrs. Miller, he was likely to have a healthy, resilient brain and unlikely to suffer any permanent damage if he were removed from the Millers' home. Dr. Jones opined that, because of the secure attachment Oliver had to Mr. and Mrs. Miller, he had a "prototype or template" for attachment relationships and would be able to "reattach" to new caregivers relatively easily. Dr. Jones further opined that Oliver, who was twelve and a half months old at the time of the hearing, was at a "sweet spot" in terms of his ability to transition to a new placement, because he had the benefit of stability and secure attachment relationships during the first year of his life, but had not yet reached the age where he had begun to develop a sense of self-identity and autobiographical memory.

Dr. Reynolds, who had devoted a significant portion of her career to child development and attachment relationships, disagreed with Dr. Best's testimony that Oliver was unlikely to suffer long-term damage if he were removed from the Millers' home. Contrary to Dr. Jones's testimony that, because of the foundation the Millers had provided, Oliver would be able to easily adjust to being placed with Mr. and Mrs. Wilson and his half-siblings, Dr. Reynolds noted that attachments are not abilities or characteristics, nor are they interchangeable; they are interactive, individual and specific. In other words, a child's attachment involves a specific person and a unique relationship with that person. Even if Oliver were placed in a loving home with his half-siblings after being removed from the Millers' home, he was developing an internal working model that he had of the Millers as his primary caregivers. He had engaged in a variety of attachment behaviors with the Millers. Dr. Reynolds explained that, even at the age of 9 to 12 months old, Oliver would be traumatized by the loss of his attachments to Mr. and Mrs. Miller and Mason and that these losses would be, from Oliver's perspective, as though the Millers had died. Rather than reducing the risk of emotional harm to Oliver, his young age could actually exacerbate the damage caused by the disruption to his relationships with the Millers. Dr. Reynolds testified that, experiencing severe trauma, such as the loss of his caregivers, when Oliver is pre-verbal could cause problems for which therapy may not be an effective intervention later on because he doesn't have the verbal ability to be able to put this loss into a context and it could become something that stays with him and affects every part of who he is.

> Although insensitive care and insecure attachment have provided most of the focus for attachment research in nonclinical populations, Bowlby was concerned with more extreme breakdowns in caregiving that we have termed "attachment disruptions." These severe or prolonged threats to a caregiver's availability or responsiveness activate defensive process and symptomatic expressions of attachment-related anger, fear, and sadness that severely compromise an individual's ability to cope with normal stressful and developmental challenges.[10]

After hearing the testimony of Dr. Jones and Dr. Reynolds, the court maintained its decision that it was in Oliver's best interests to remain with Mr. and Mrs. Miller and for the Millers to be granted guardianship of Oliver. The court was persuaded by Dr. Reynolds's testimony that Oliver would suffer some degree of trauma, from which he might never fully recover, if his relationships with the members of the Miller family were disrupted. The court remarked that, in many juvenile cases, it is necessary to remove children from their homes because the trauma they experience as a result of the loss of their caregivers is outweighed by the danger of allowing them to remain in an environment where abuse or neglect occurs. In this case, though, Oliver was in a safe, nurturing home with the only parents and sibling he had ever known, and the court was able to develop a permanent plan to keep him in that home and prevent him from experiencing the trauma of separation that so many children involved in the legal system must endure.

Attachment Relationships in Practice

The case study illustrates the importance of expert testimony in cases involving custody of young children, especially when a major change in physical custody is possible. In Oliver's case, DSS, Ms. Smith, and Oliver's attorney advocate all urged the judge to change placement and argued Oliver was so young that removing him from the Millers' home would not result in any lasting negative consequences. Despite these arguments, the judge had serious concerns about the effect of changing placement on Oliver's psychological well-being, and even without the benefit of expert testimony during the initial phase of the trial, understood that the loss of the people Oliver understood to be his parents and sibling would be traumatic for him. Because of the subjectivity of the best interests standard, another judge may have shared the opinion of the parties to Oliver's case and reached a different result. Family law practitioners have a duty to ensure that the court receives reliable information about attachment relationships and that the judge is not left to rely on common sense notions about child development, which may not be supported by the extensive research and analysis conducted by experts in these areas of psychology.

Selecting an Expert

The notes of the advisory committee on the proposed rules include the following statement regarding Rule 702 of the Federal Rules of Evidence, which governs the admissibility of expert witness: "An intelligent evaluation of facts is often difficult or impossible without the application of some scientific, technical, or other specialized knowledge. The most common source of this knowledge is the expert witness, although there are other techniques for supplying it." Federal Rule 702 provides as follows:

> A witness who is qualified as an expert by knowledge, skill, experience, training, or education may testify in the form of an opinion or otherwise if:
> a the expert's scientific, technical, or other specialized knowledge will help the trier of fact to understand the evidence or to determine a fact in issue;
> b the testimony is based on sufficient facts or data;
> c the testimony is the product of reliable principles and methods; and
> d the expert has reliably applied the principles and methods to the facts of the case.

Each state has adopted some variation of this rule. In general, an expert witness may be appointed where specialized knowledge will assist the court in understanding the evidence or making a determination regarding a disputed fact, and the expert's opinion is reliable and well founded. The psychology of child development and attachment relationships are areas in which an expert's specialized knowledge can assist a judge tasked with making a decision about child custody.

As a practical matter, when choosing an expert witness, it is typically more advantageous to select a professional who has specialized training and experience pertinent to the contested factual issue than a professional who has general training and experience in the field but lacks the qualifications that would make her a credible authority as a sub-specialist. The more narrowly tailored an expert's experience and qualifications are to the relevant factual dispute, the more weight a court is likely to give the expert's opinion. For instance, if substance abuse is an issue in the case, the opinion of a psychologist who has practiced for 20 years and devoted the majority of her practice to treating individuals recovering from substance abuse, worked at a rehabilitation clinic, and received specialized training in therapeutic techniques designed to treat recovering addicts is of more probative value to the court than the opinion of a psychologist who has practiced for the same length of time and devoted her practice to treating individuals suffering from eating disorders, but encountered substance abuse issues occasionally as a comorbidity.

If an expert has the appropriate qualifications, the requirement most likely to be attacked by a party opposing the admission of the witness's testimony concerning attachment relationships or other areas of child psychology is subsection (c). In most jurisdictions, the *Daubert*[11] standard is used to assess whether an expert's opinion is based on sound methodology that can be properly applied to the facts in issue. Under this standard, the court may consider the following non-exhaustive list of factors to evaluate the validity of the method in question:

1 whether the theory or technique in question can be and has been tested;
2 whether it has been subjected to peer review and publication;

3 its known or potential error rate;
4 the existence and maintenance of standards controlling its operation; and
5 whether it has attracted widespread acceptance within a relevant scientific community.

While the established theories and techniques used in social science fields, such as psychology, may be somewhat less precise than those used physics, chemistry, or mathematics, they are nevertheless sufficiently reliable to satisfy the requirements of *Daubert* and Rule 701.[12,13] So long as the expert has properly applied the established theories and techniques to the evidence before the court, the court should permit her to offer her opinion on the relevant facts in issue. For those seeking more information about states using *Daubert* as opposed to *Frye* standards see: https://www.expertinstitute.com/resources/insights/daubert-v-frye-a-state-by-state-comparison.

Qualifying the Witness as an Expert

The process for qualifying a witness as an expert is intended to elicit information about the expert's credentials, training, experience, and scholarly work not only to meet the technical requirements of Rule 702, but also to give the court confidence in the witness's opinion. The party seeking to qualify a witness as an expert should ask questions about the witness's educational background (including the specific topic of the witness's master's thesis and doctoral dissertation), professional licenses (including the requirements for obtaining and maintaining licensure), subspecialty training received, academic and professional speaking engagements, academic and professional publications[14] (including whether the published work was peer-reviewed), years of experience, percentage of time devoted to working in the broader field and subspecialty area, professional awards received, previous expert witness testimony (including the jurisdiction of the cases and the area(s) in which the witness was qualified as an expert), and any other subject that would tend to show the witness has expertise in the subspecialty area.

Using Oliver's case study as a hypothetical, the expert qualification portion of Dr. Reynolds's testimony might look something like this:

Q: How are you employed?
A: I'm a forensic and clinical psychologist. I have a private practice and am self-employed.
Q: How long have you been a licensed psychologist?
A: Since 1974.
Q: Please tell the court a little bit about your educational background.
A: I obtained a bachelor's degree from Kings College. I obtained a six-year master's degree in psychology from State University and a Ph.D. in clinical psychology from State University.
Q: What is your area of focus as psychologist?
A: My work now is almost exclusively forensic. I began doing forensic work in family law conducting child custody evaluations in 2000. Prior to that, I had a clinical practice in which I worked with children, families, and couples. A significant portion of my clinical practice has been devoted to co-parenting therapy, couples counseling, and treatment of children of separated and divorced parents. As my forensic work has increased, I have taken on fewer patients and my clinical work has decreased. While I still do some clinical work, most of my time is spent on custody evaluations.
Q: What kind of specialized training have you had in the areas of child development and attachment relationships?

A: My post-doctoral work included ten years that I worked with both an adult psycho-analyst, understanding more about family relationships and substance abuse disorders, and a child psychoanalyst. That work was intended to give me a foundation for doing psychotherapy with families and children. I have done 60 hours of training with, Dr. Anderson, the head of a renowned child development center learning how to conduct what's called the Strange Situation. That's a specific research technique for evaluating attachment relationships. When I first began doing child custody evaluations almost twenty years ago, I consulted with Dr. Anderson on all of my evaluations as part of my training specifically on attachment relationships to see what the attachment relationships were like between each parent and each child.

Q: Have you done any presentations or taught any courses on child development and attachment relationships?

A: Yes. I have done several presentations with Dr. Anderson and many more on my own. I've done presentations for the Association of Family and Conciliation Courts, the Society for Personality Assessment, and the American Psychological Association. I've also taught portions of the annual judges' conference at the Institute of Government on child development and attachment relationships.

Q: Have you ever written or edited any publications on child development and attachment relationships?

A: Yes. I've authored several journal articles on these topics, most of which have been peer-reviewed. I co-edited a special issue of the Journal of Child Custody on attachment relationships and child custody evaluations.

Q: Have you ever been qualified as an expert witness?

A: Yes.

Q: How many times have you testified as an expert witness in the area of child development or attachment relationships?

A: Several hundred. I've testified as an expert on these topics in this county at least twenty times. The other cases in which I testified as an expert were in other counties in this state.

After you have established the witness's qualifications to offer an expert opinion, you should move to qualify her as an expert in the relevant field and subspecialty. At this point in Dr. Reynolds's testimony, Oliver's attorney advocate would move to qualify Dr. Reynolds as an expert in child development and attachment relationships. If any of the other parties believed that Dr. Reynolds did not have the necessary knowledge, training, skill, experience, or education to be qualified as an expert in those areas, that party could object to her qualification and ask to *voir dire* the witness to bring out any deficiencies that would warrant denial of the motion to designate Dr. Reynolds as an expert.

Admitting Expert Opinion Testimony

Even if a witness is qualified as an expert in a relevant field and subspecialty area, the witness may only offer an expert opinion if it is based on sound methodology and the proper application of reliable theories and techniques to the facts of the case. In Oliver's case, the question before the court was whether Oliver, at such a young age, would suffer emotional harm and lasting trauma if he were removed from the Millers' home, which would necessarily disrupt his relationships with Mr. and Mrs. Miller and Mason. Dr. Reynolds's expertise in child development and attachment relationships allowed her to address this issue, but only after the proper foundation was laid:

Q: Dr. Reynolds, what have you done to familiarize yourself with the facts of this case?

A: I read the reports that were submitted to the court at the trial in August by DSS and Oliver's GAL. I listened to the entire audio recording of the proceedings that took place in August, which contained all of the arguments and testimony at the trial from start to finish. I also reviewed a number of journal articles on attachment relationships.

Q: You understand that the issue the court is considering today is whether an almost thirteen-month-old child, Oliver, who is the subject of this action is going to be removed from the home of his caregivers, where he has lived for his entire life, and placed with the adoptive parents of his half-siblings?

A: Yes.

Q: When you listened to the trial audio, did you hear DSS, Ms. Smith's attorney, and Oliver's attorney advocate argue that the change in placement would not significantly affect Oliver because of his young age?

A: Yes.

Q: And you were in the courtroom earlier today when Dr. Jones testified?

A: Yes.

Q: Did you hear Dr. Jones testify about her understanding of attachment relationships and opinion that Oliver's brain was healthy and resilient enough that he would fully recover and not suffer any significant harm if his placement were changed?

A: Yes.

Q: What is an attachment relationship?

A: An attachment relationship is between a specific person and a specific child. These relationships are reciprocal, interactive, and individual. You can't just take a child like Oliver and say, "Oh, he's attached, so he is going to have a good adjustment regardless of where he is placed." No, the child's attachment is to a specific person or persons. The specificity and reciprocity are important characteristics of the attachment relationship.

Q: So, it's not as though the child forms a secure attachment relationship with one caregiver and that caregiver is interchangeable with another caregiver?

A: Correct. One of the things that Dr. Anderson came up with is something called the Circle of Security. In the Circle of Security, you have the child being able to go out and then return to a safe haven for nurturance, recharging their batteries, so to speak. The child is able to go out and explore, making new relationships with other children and people, because of the kind of foundation they have received – the same caregiver, day in and day out, hundreds of times a day. That's what allows a baby to go out and form multiple relationships with playmates and temporary caregivers. The child understands that he will eventually be able to return to his primary caregiver, because that has been the child's experience. He can go to daycare everyday and form relationships with the people there, because he knows that his primary caregiver will retrieve him and take him back to the place where he knows, comfort, security, continuity, and has been cared for and loved.

Q: How would you define a secure attachment relationship?

A: Mary Ainsworth was the person who did a lot to inform us about secure relationships. What she theorized, and what came to be substantiated by research, if you have children without many problems and good parents, most of those children are going to form secure attachments. The child is little and vulnerable, but is cared for by a parent who is wiser and stronger. That's an essential relationship and what we need to survive.

Q: How soon after birth does a child start forming an attachment relationship with a caregiver?

A: There has been some research to suggest that the attachment relationship actually begins in the womb, but certainly what the bulk of the research literature says is that children start developing attachment relationships from day one.

At this point in Dr. Reynolds's testimony, after she has established her familiarity with the evidence before the court and gone over key terminology, Oliver's attorney advocate should ask Dr. Reynolds to discuss in more depth the substantiated theories on attachment relationships and techniques used to assess the quality of attachments and the effects of disrupting these relationships. It would be helpful to provide the court with copies of any journal articles, tables, or other materials that Dr. Reynolds refers to during her testimony.

Once Dr. Reynolds has laid the foundation for her opinion, it is time for her to apply the theories and techniques she described to the facts of Oliver's case:

Q: At the age of nine to ten months old, would you expect that a child has formed attachment relationships with the people he lives with?

A: Yes, absolutely. That starts happening as soon as the child is around people and they begin interacting with him. Whether it's entertaining him, feeding him, changing his diapers, putting him down at night, those interactions form relationships.

Q: What is your opinion about the consequences of removing Oliver from the Millers' home and placing him with another family?

A: For any child, any baby, who has formed attachments to specific people, loss of those attachments is like death. If you take the child away from those people, he will suffer. The experience of loss and trauma is every bit as real preverbally as it is verbally, but you don't have the cognitive or verbal skills to make sense of it. The trauma to Oliver would be very real.

Q: In addition to the short-term grief that a child would feel, could there be long-term consequences to Oliver from that kind of disruption in an attachment relationship?

A: Yes. Removal from caregivers who have become dependable, known, and bring comfort to a baby is highly traumatizing and does have long-term effects. In my experience as a clinician, in some ways it's harder to work with children who suffered losses when they were pre-verbal, because they didn't have the cognitive and verbal ability to put the loss into context. It becomes something that just kind of sticks to every part of who they are, and you can't quite pull it together in therapy. There can be consequences to their learning in school, their self-confidence, and their ability to regulate emotions. There can be a range of negative consequences.

Conclusion

Expert witness testimony is one just one part of a child custody case, but it can be critical to the court when a case involves complex issues. One role of experts is to educate the trier of fact. Judges in family court make decisions that have the ability to forever change the lives of the children involved in the legal system – for better or worse. These are not matters to be taken lightly, and each decision should be made with the benefit of all the information necessary to understand the impact that possible outcomes could have on those children the legal system is intended to protect.

Notes

1. Cassidy, J. and P. R. Shaver (2016). Handbook of Attachment: Theory, Research and Clinical Applications, Third Edition. New York: The Guilford Press, page x.

2. Ibid, p. x.
3. J. Bowlby (1979, p. 129) in Cassidy and Shaver (2016), p. 273.
4. J. Bowlby (1969/1982, p. 371) in Zeanah, C.H., L.J. Berlin and N.W. Boris (2011). "Practitioner Review: Clinical Applications of Attachment Theory and Research for Infants and Young Children." *Journal of Child Psychology and Psychiatry, 52:8*, pp. 819–833.
5. Cooper, G., K. Hoffman, R. Marvin and B. Powell (1999) in C. Zeanah (2009). Handbook of Infant Mental Health, Third Edition. New York: Guilford Press.
6. R.S. Marvin, Britner, P.A. and B.S. Russell in Cassidy and Shaver (2016), p. 274.
7. The case study is based on an actual abuse, neglect, and dependency case filed by DSS in juvenile court. To protect the privacy of those involved, the jurisdiction is not identified, aliases are used, and the dates of events have been changed.
8. In this jurisdiction, a statute known as the Foster Child's Bill of Rights required first priority to be given to placement in a home with siblings. The statute was likely intended to preserve existing sibling relationships, not to require a child to be removed from a stable placement to be placed with siblings he has never met. Oliver's case is an example of the devastation that can occur when a statute is mechanically, rather than thoughtfully, applied.
9. DSS was never able to identify Oliver's father, so he was not a party to this proceeding.
10. Koback, R., K. Zajac and S. D. Madsen. "Attachment Disruptions, Reparative Processes and Psychopathology: Theoretical and Clinical Implications." In Cassidy, J. and P. Shaver (2016), Handbook of Attachment, Third Edition. New York: Guilford Press, p. 36. Casanueva, C., M. Dozier, S. Tueller, M. Dolan, K. Smith, M. B. Webb, T. Westbrook and B.J. Harden (2014). "Caregiver Instability and Early Changes among Infants Reported to the Child Welfare System." *Child Abuse and Neglect, 38:3*, pp. 498–509.
11. This standard was established by the United States Supreme Court in *Daubert v. Merrell Dow Pharms., Inc.*, 509 U.S. 579 (1993).
12. For cases in which a witness was qualified as an expert in an area of psychology and permitted to offer an opinion, *see Sneed v. Sneed*, 820 S.E.2d 536 (2018) (child custody evaluation methodology held to be sufficiently reliable for the psychologist who conducted the evaluation to offer an expert opinion on custody); *In re E.C.L.*, 278 S.W.3d 510, 512 (Tex. App. 2009) (setting out a framework to determine whether a technique or theory in a "soft science" field is sufficiently reliable); *Robb v. Robb*, 687 N.W.2d 195 (Neb. 2004) (psychologist permitted to offer an opinion on child custody even though he had not conducted a full custody evaluation where "his techniques were established and recognized in the profession of psychology, that they were peer reviewable, and that he had formed opinions to a reasonable degree of psychological certainty"); *In re Lauren P.*, 2004-Ohio-1656 (witness qualified and permitted to testify as an expert in psychology with a specialty in parenting and custody issues).
13. For a case in which the appellate court found that a witness was improperly permitted to testify as an expert and that admission of her testimony was prejudicial error, *see Giannaris v. Giannaris*, 960 So. 2d 462, 470 (Miss. 2007) (social worker based her expert opinion on unrecorded sessions with the child, a five-week training course, and her instincts).
14. It is a good idea to read and be familiar with your expert witness's publications. If the witness has previously taken a position that could be construed as contrary to his position in your case, you should be prepared to address that seeming inconsistency.

8 Considerations when Working with Central American Immigrant Children in the Legal System

Giselle A. Hass

Immigrant children addressed in this chapter refer to children who were born in another country but migrated to the United States (U.S.). A child may have traveled to live in the U.S. with both or only one parent, a sibling, grandparent, or another relative, a stranger like a friend or neighbor of the family, or may have entered the U.S. alone, often with peers or strangers. Some of these children entered the U.S. by plane, by boat, by bus, private cars, or walking. Some immigrant children reach the border patrol offices or customs officers in ports of entry with or without proper documents to enter and live in the U.S., and many cross inconspicuously to the U.S. without being inspected by border patrol. Some children may come to join relatives who live in the U.S. and who may be undocumented themselves. Other children may come with legal papers to stay in the U.S. where they live with U.S. citizen parents, siblings, or foster parents who sponsored them. Some children come to the U.S. with a tourist visa and then overstay their visit. When immigrant children do not have a permit to enter the U.S., they often surrender themselves voluntarily to border patrol which allows them to apply, with help, for asylum, or other immigration relief measure to stay in the U.S. Other times they try to apply later, sometimes years after arriving, for legal papers to stay in the U.S. In general terms, children tend to come to the U.S. to escape from unbearable conditions in their native country, to try to build a new life for themselves and help the family they left behind or reunite with parents or relatives who already live here.

Immigrant children who come to the U.S., just as all human beings, have rights, whether they have or do not have legal papers to enter and stay in the US. Children are covered by the United Nations Convention on the Rights of Children, which has established that actions concerning children shall have the best interest of the child as a primary consideration (UNICEF, 1989). Given these human rights recommendations, it should be expected that the best interest of the child becomes a primary consideration when making decisions about them and that decision-makers find the best way to help the children they work with claim those rights, since children may lack that knowledge, autonomy and know-how to claim them themselves (Thronson, 2002). This does not mean that they do not know what is in their best interest. Children's own voice and decisions need to be recognized as they exercise a best-interest judgment when they chose to leave their country and migrate to secure protection and a viable life (Bhabha, 2014). However, in real life children's rights are usually ignored or violated and even when they act on their own behalf, immigrant children are by and large left unprotected.

Because of the complex and intersecting issues that affect immigrant children, those who need to address children's matters in the courts of law of the U.S. want to be well informed about the specific considerations that immigrant children require regarding their psychological and emotional needs. When a mental health professional provides services to immigrant or refugee clients, whether they are recent arrivals or they have resided

DOI: 10.4324/9780429397806-9

in the host country for a long time, it is critical to understand these individuals' own world and experiences to better serve their needs (American Psychological Association [APA], 1998). A working model that takes into consideration how the cultural, individual, familial, community and societal factors interact in a reciprocal manner to shape the risks and protective factors that affect immigrants and refugees is appropriate and useful to all professionals who work with immigrant children.

This chapter will discuss issues relevant to the work with immigrant children who come to the attention of the courts in the U.S. The information presented here is based on immigrant children from Central America, which at the present time is the most pressing and alarming humanitarian crisis in the U.S. However, these considerations are applicable to children from other countries who present with similar circumstances and social context. Mental health practitioners, policy makers, border officials, law enforcement, and staff from social service, non-profit and religious organizations who interact with immigrant children and their families will benefit from this information in order to provide the tailored care that immigrant children need.

Current Socio-Political State for Immigrant Children in the U.S.

Immigrant children who are already in the U.S. were estimated in 2017 to be 2.2 million (12%) out of 18.2 million children born of at least one immigrant parent (Chishti, Pierce, & Telus, 2019). Although both Obama and Trump's administrations have implemented aggressive policies to prevent irregular immigration, many unaccompanied children have continued to make the journey to the U.S. Between October 2018 and February 2019, the U.S. Border Patrol apprehended more than 136,000 minor children and adults travelling as family units and about 27,000 unaccompanied children along the Southwest border. These numbers in only five months predict that in 2019 there will be a significant increase over the numbers from Fiscal Year 2018 (107, 200 family units and 50,000 unaccompanied children). Immigrant children constitute a significant portion of our youth population in the U.S.

Unfortunately, certain policies of the U.S., particularly of late, demonstrate a profound lack of understanding about immigrant children and families generally and trauma specific needs. Recent government decisions about immigration are based on a "Zero Tolerance" policy, and include practices such as the border wall, separation of parents and children, detention of immigrant parents and children, indefinite detention of children in overcrowded, unsanitary, and neglectful detention facilities, asylum bans, stricter rules for granting asylum, mass raids of immigrant workers, crackdown on "Sanctuary Cities," and the "Remain in Mexico" policy. These practices are devastating for the immigrants and refugee communities, and lead to the fragmentation of families, traumatization of parents and children, and creation of panic (APA, 2018). The social, economic, and emotional impact of these inhumane policies and practices have a long and lasting reach in both the immigration policies of the U.S., the racist and anti-immigrant attitude that they sow in our society, and the trauma suffered by immigrants who arrive to the U.S., their families, and their communities.

Immigrant Children in the Legal System

There has been some enlightening in the way courts address children and their needs over the past 100 years. Purportedly, the legal system takes an interest in providing protection to children that come in contact with the courts, including educating and rehabilitating them instead of punishing them when they have committed a crime. Most courts have provisions specific to children, in recognition that courts are places for adults to resolve disputes in a litigious forum which is intimidating to children who, in most cases, are not developmentally prepared to be fully informed participants. Changes such as the establishment of Juvenile and Family Courts, providing children with Guardian Ad Litem, Court Appointed Special Advocate (CASA) or Children's Attorneys, and specific rules about children's appearance in court and testimony have been developed (Thronson, 2002). These provisions try to offer participation to the children but still fall short of considering children's needs and demands, or what has been recognized as the Best Interest of the Child doctrine (UNICEF, 1989). Rather, these tools have most often increased the children's vulnerability, risk exposure and identity as a victim (Thronson, 2002).

Children nationals of the U.S. or immigrants are at a disadvantage when facing the legal system for any reason without guidance or representation. Children do not have the knowledge or experience to represent themselves or their needs in a manner that the legal system can understand or utilize. In fact, immigrant children have their rights consistently trampled when they come to the U.S. unaccompanied but also when they arrive to the U.S. with immigrant parents, and when they live with immigrant parents due to the myths surrounding undocumented immigration status, racial stereotypes, and uninformed developmental and cultural values. Immigration status in and outside immigration proceedings often disregard the child's voice, fails to reliably evaluate their situation, or focus on their needs.

Venues and Roles

Legal, judicial, and mental health professionals will inevitably come in contact with an immigrant child in the course of their professional practice at one point or another. Children may be in family, juvenile, dependency, immigration court, and even criminal court as an interested party, victim, collateral informant, defendant, or testifying witness. Additionally, an immigrant child may come to play a role in a contested custody case in which a parent is an immigrant and had a child born outside the U.S. or has adopted a child born in another country. In juvenile criminal court an immigrant child may come to our attention after being accused of an offense or misdemeanor, or a statutory violation. In child protective services, we may encounter an immigrant child when he or she is the victim of abuse, incest, neglect, or other type of intra-family maltreatment or out of family violence, abuse, or trafficking. In immigration court we may come into contact with an immigrant child when they apply for asylum, special immigrant status, or other immigration relief measure, or if we provide therapeutic services in immigration detention.

Immigrant children who have suffered much injustice, hardship, and abuse often suffer from psychological conditions that would make their participation in their legal cases very challenging (see Chapter 4). They may have significant difficulty recalling and retelling their stories of victimization, they may be too afraid to speak up on their own behalf, or they may have experienced abusive authority figures and therefore not trust them. Indeed, their trauma symptoms may interfere with their ability to testify or to raise their concerns and needs. These issues may require adaptations, accommodations, psychotherapy, or psychoeducation. Children may avoid psychotherapy because it is not culturally sanctioned and because they may have other pressing needs that appear to them more practical. This does not mean that they do not need some type of intervention to assist with the healing and improve daily functioning.

While the situation may place immigrant children into a dependent role vis à vis the encounter with the legal system, they are also capable of opinions, insight, and search for meaning in their lives. Most of all, they are the experts about their own world. In fact, research has shown that even while suffering from psychological symptoms, children's competency to participate in legal procedures may be appropriate. What was found to interfere with meaningful participation was lack of legal knowledge and some basic knowledge such as understanding and appreciating their rights and the legal proceedings (Viljoen & Roesch, 2005: Grisso, 2003),

What may interfere with the ability of an immigrant child to raise their voice and be heard in the legal system is also at the level of the interpersonal encounter. If children-adult relationships are characterized by their power hierarchy, immigrant children interactions with legal and mental health professionals have an even greater power differential. The opportunities for a lapse in empathy, compassion, respect, and engagement on the part of the professional as an authority figure are numerous. There is also a risk of assuming a condescending attitude that robs the immigrant child of meaningful participation, pushes them further into a victim role, and disempowers them.

Although immigrant children have rights and usually the judgment to participate in their own behalf, it falls on the shoulders of the professionals to be mindful that these children may not have someone else actively protecting them or they may not know themselves what actions or decisions may violate their rights. Because many immigrant children have been raised in a cultural context where they have been prematurely compelled into adult responsibilities and autonomy, they may behave in pseudo-mature ways in their day-to-day functioning. Therefore, they may not be aware or feel entitled to having the rights, protection, and security designed for children. Subsequently, during their immigration process as undocumented children, they may not know that there are legal and social benefits they have a right to claim. At the same time, the immigrant's child participation on decisions that affect his or her life and future can be empowering.

An Ecological and Intersectional Framework when Working with Immigrant Children

An appropriate framework to understand the nested level of dangers that vulnerable groups like children, women and LGBT individuals from Central America face is the Ecological Model (Bronfenbrenner, 1979). Through the ecological model we understand that child development occurs within the context of the complex systems of relationships in his or her environment and that this influence is reciprocal. The impact on the child of the risks and protective factors within the family, community, and society is particularly relevant because children are not autonomous and are being developmentally shaped at the most fundamental level of brain architecture and developmental maturation. Bronfenbrenner's four levels include child's own biology, immediate family, community environment, and the larger society, which are in turn named micro, meso, exo, and macro systems.

A second and complementary perspective is the Intersectional theory (Crenshaw, 1989), which explains how diverse identities interact to magnify marginalization in society. This means that for children who meet more than one diversity status (such as poverty, gender, ethnic diversity, sexual orientation, class, disability, etc.) their exposure to marginalization, invisibility, and discrimination is multiplied (Purdie-Vaughns & Eibach, 2008).

Introduction to the Background of Immigrant Children

The Motivations for and Impact of Migration

Those arriving at the U.S. border are being depicted as "illegal immigrants" by the media and/or for political purposes. However, crossing an international border for asylum is not illegal and an asylum seeker's case must be heard, according to U.S. and international laws (Thronson, 2002). Asylum is a protective measure that applies to someone who is seeking international protection from dangers in his or her home country. In most cases, these undocumented immigrant children have fled their country of origin because of prolonged social or political conflict, social and individual violence or persecution, abuse and neglect, combined with conditions of stark poverty.

The criteria for qualifying for asylum is a well-founded fear of living in their country of origin. Historically, asylum seekers must apply for protection in the country of destination. This means that children seeking asylum must apply when they arrive at or cross the U.S. border. This policy has been recently changed by current U.S. government policies, which require that immigrants apply in Mexico or Guatemala and wait there for the results of their application. Mexico and Guatemala have complex social and political problems and pose diverse risks and challenges for immigrant children who receive no services and have no means to earn a living while waiting there. Hence, this policy places immigrant children and families in an unresolvable conundrum.

For children, there is also a unique form of immigration relief, Special Immigrant Juveniles Status (SIJS), which is a form of humanitarian immigration process that provides a path for legal status and continued safety for children who are unable to be reunited with one or both parents due to abuse, abandonment, neglect, or a similar basis under state law (USCIS, n.d.). Immigrant children who do not fulfill criteria for asylum or SIJS, sometimes have suffered experiences that qualify them for other immigration relief measures and which include a path to lawful permanent residency for children who qualify. These include T-visas for victims of trafficking, U-visas for victims of a crime that happened once they were in the U.S., and Violence Against Women Act (VAWA) immigration protections for children who have been abused by a parent or step-parent who is a U.S. citizen or lawful permanent resident (Fitzpatrick & Orloff, 2016). There is also Deferred Action for Childhood Arrivals (DACA), which temporarily suspends deportation to minors with unlawful presence in the U.S. after being brought to the country as children (USCIS, n.d.). In order to apply for any of these forms of immigration protection, the child needs to be helped through a process of developing an affidavit or providing testimony before an immigration judge in which they retell their history of the abuse or crime victimization.

Immigrant children from the Northern Central American triangle (Guatemala, Honduras, and El Salvador) perceive their situation to be so dire that unless they escape, immense suffering or premature end to their lives will be certain. According to a study by UNHCR (2014), migrants from Central America leave their countries for the following reasons: long-standing family separations and desire for reunification, community-based insecurity, including gang violence and ineffective institutional supports, lack of available caregivers, physical, emotional, and sexual abuse, social deprivation, escape from the threat of human smuggling, trafficking, and corruption, hopes for better education and work opportunities, and misunderstanding of U.S. immigration policy (i.e., having unrealistic expectations of obtaining legal status quickly and easily) (Baily, 2017; Kennedy, 2014; Rosenblum, 2015). Most of these immigrant children were born in chronic stark poverty, which cannot be minimized in its role regarding aggravating adversity and destroying hope for the future (Hulme & Shepherd, 2003).

Factors at the individual, family, community, and social level combine to make it nearly impossible for many children in the Northern Central American triangle to have a normal life and a semblance of an adequate future for themselves. At the macro, exo, meso, and micro levels the grim picture of some developing countries is characterized by extreme levels of violence as well as social and economic inequities, weakened and impoverished governments that lack the resources and will to protect their population (Geneva Declaration,

2015), and the dominant presence of non-state actors such as gangs, transnational organized crime, and drug-trafficking (United Nations Office on Drugs and Crime, 2012). These social ills are the result of civil unrest, economic stagnation, social inequities, and political and economic corruption that dates to historical events, at times including damaging intervention and exploitation from the U.S. and other developed countries. To this set of adversities, we must add the climate changes that have led to floods, draught, earthquakes, and hurricanes, which have devastated entire regions for living and working.

The U.S. is directly linked to much of the instability in the Northern Central American triangle countries through decades of intervention. For instance, the U.S. has exploited this region to protect their own political and economic interests in agricultural goods and cheap labor (Eguizábal, Ingram, Curtis, Korthuis, Olson, & Phillips, 2015). During the 1980s many Central American immigrants sought asylum in the U.S. due to the civil wars in the region. The young people or children of immigrants who felt disenfranchised became recruited by gangs from Los Angeles. Beginning in 1996, many gang members were repatriated to their countries in the Northern Central American triangle, where they continued their affiliation and criminal activities (Seelke, 2016). U.S. led efforts to curb drug-trafficking in Mexico and the Caribbean led the trade to relocate to Central America, further empowering the regional and transnational gangs (UNODC, 2012). Adding to the supremacy of gangs is the fact that U.S. policies have not properly restricted the trafficking of American firearms from the U.S. into Mexico and Central America (Eguizábal et al., 2015). This increased lawlessness as the government's law enforcement is no match for strongly organized and powerful gangs. The gangs' escalating violence and social dominance exposes children to the terror of murders, kidnapping, and extortion in their families and communities. Additionally, children are prey of intimidation, forced recruitment, and physical or sexual assault by gang members.

El Salvador and Guatemala rank first and second respectively in rates of homicide against children and adolescents globally (UNICEF, 2014). The U.N. Office on Drugs and Crime, (UNODC, 2012) found that Honduras had the world's highest per-capita homicide rate in 2012, at 90.4 homicides per 100,000 people. El Salvador was fourth in the world, with a rate of 41.2 homicides per 100,000 people, and Guatemala was fifth, with a rate of 39.9 homicides per 100,000 people. To put these numbers into context, consider that the war-ravaged Democratic Republic of the Congo, from which nearly half a million refugees have fled, has a homicide rate of 28.3 homicides per 100,000 people. Other countries in Central America, such as Costa Rica, have 8.5 homicides per 100,000 people and Nicaragua, 11.3 homicides per 100,000 people.

This violence is particularly alarming for the manner in which it targets vulnerable groups. For instance, El Salvador and Guatemala rank first and second respectively in rates of homicide against children and adolescents globally (UNICEF, 2014) and the rates of femicide, the intentional killing of women because they are females, in El Salvador, Guatemala, and Honduras are up to five times higher than overall homicide rates in the majority of Northern, Western, and Southern European countries (Geneva Declaration, 2015). Femicides are only the end of a constellation of violence against women and girls in countries with this problem. Women and girls are also frequently harassed and attacked in public, and suffer from gang and intimate partner violence and rape. Women and girls in these countries are also victims of trafficking, economic crimes, and psychological abuse (UNHCR, 2014). Both intra-family and intimate partner violence are widespread and go on with impunity in most instances (Geneva Declaration, 2015). Added to this domestic violence is the violence against women and girls perpetrated by gangs and other armed criminal groups, and the fact that trafficking of women and children for forced labor and sex is a serious concern in all three countries (USDS, 2016).

In addition, there are structural factors in many countries that, at the economic, political, and cultural level prioritize economic prosperity over social well-being. There are high levels of inequity and inequality in Latin America as the distribution of wealth is concentrated among very few, and the gap with the rest of the population tends to be extremely large. People with multiple factors of disadvantage are at a higher risk of poverty and limitations in their ability to access education, remunerated jobs, housing, food, and health and social services. Developing countries concentrate resources in large cities. This situation limits resources to minority, immigrants, and poor populations that live in other areas, and leads to their discrimination and exclusion (Castro, Savage & Kaufman, 2015). Even basic services such as water and sanitation are unequally distributed, with a Pan American Health Organization (PAHO) study asserting that in 2010, water and sanitation in Latin America was the millennium development goal most off-track among PAHO goals (Mújica, Haeberer, Teague, Santos-Burgoa, & Galvão, 2015). Within this perspective, the exploitation of human work and human bodies for economic gain becomes normalized, and the struggle for survival of vulnerable groups is ignored.

While challenges and risk are present in many communities even in developed countries, for children in the Northern Central American triangle the potential for traumatic situations and threats to their lives are magnified. The helplessness born out of the social security and quality of life rate differentials, and lack of resources and government protection is a powerful force as to why some children from the Northern Central American triangle countries are fleeing to neighboring countries despite their entrenched family heritage and attachment links, the enormous natural beauty of the country, their cultural richness, and love for their land. People do not uproot themselves from their life and history lightly and the fact that immigrants from the Northern Central American triangle decide to risk their lives in a perilous journey is a testament to their desperation.

Pre-immigration Development and Risks for Children

Prenatal and Infancy Periods

Immigrant children's biological and social background may be disadvantaged from the earliest stages of development during the prenatal, newborn, and infancy periods. Children are born carrying the weight of historical trauma and their parents' fear for their newborn's safety, life, and future in such uncertain and dangerous environments. A fetus and infant's development are intimately linked to the family and caregivers' own factors of risk and social context. For instance, when a mother is exposed to violence, whether personally or in her community, the fetus' growth may be impacted by: (a) reduction in blood flow to the uterus and fetus at increased levels of maternal stress; (b) transplacental transport of maternal hormones; and (c) stress-induced release of placental CRH to the intrauterine environment (Mulder, Robles de Medina, Huizink, Van den Bergh, Buitelaar, & Visser, 2002). This exposure impacts brain and nervous system development and has been linked to subsequent development of disorders. Similarly, if a mother suffers from health problems whether due to genetics, drug, or alcohol abuse, food scarcity, or lack of medical care during pregnancy, the fetus's development could be impacted (Forray, 2016; Noonan, Corman, Schwartz-Soicher, & Reichman, 2013). For instance, low birth weight, nervous system immaturity due to pre-term delivery, and medical complications resulting from lack of medical care during pregnancy and childbirth are potential risks for the fetus and lead to long-term problems.

The community and social context of mothers in the Northern Central American triangle is not only plagued by both family and community violence, and stark poverty as described earlier, but also poor health services. According to the U.S. Center for Disease Control and Prevention (CDC, 2017) physician density in El Salvador, Guatemala, and Honduras is insufficient to adequately meet the primary health care needs of their society when using the World Health Organization standard of 23 healthcare workers per 10,000 population. Physician population density is of approximately 1.6 physicians per 1,000 population in El Salvador, 0.93 in Guatemala and 0.37 in Honduras. El Salvador, Guatemala, and Honduras do not have national newborn screening programs for life threatening, treatable medical conditions (CDC, 2017). Worse yet are the health services in rural areas or for people of lower socioeconomic status or indigenous background (Garcia Ramirez, 2018).

Newborns and infants may be at risk of abandonment, irregular adoptions, neglect due to poverty, stress, or cultural values such as disliking the child's gender. There are cultural values that are problematic, such as erroneously believing that infants and young children are not aware of their environment and would not remember victimization. Given this attitude, some caregivers are careless about the toxic situations a child is exposed, or abuse a child as if there were no lasting consequence.

Early Childhood

During early childhood, children from the Northern Central American triangle are at risk of violence by primary caregivers and other family members, as well as by the violent social environment in which they live. Children can become victims during domestic violence incidents directed to a parent, or they may become abused in retaliation against their mothers or fathers. Children who were left with other caregivers when their primary caregiver migrated, may be at risk of abuse or neglect. Parents of children with disabilities suffer from high levels of stress that may result in abusive or neglectful behaviors when other contextual factors are in confluence (Pinheiro, 2006). Poverty in the family may lead to inability to properly meet physiological needs, lack of early stimulation or education for the children, lack of medical or other important services, use of inappropriate caregivers or leaving a child unsupervised. Living with chronic poverty also disadvantage the proper development of a child and may lead to the family prioritizing economic generating activities instead of stimulation and schooling for the children.

While the process of parent-child attachment starts at the prenatal period, it is during a child's 0 to 3 years period that this process becomes vital to both the child and mother's emotional well-being. It has been said that rhythm of caregiver and child dyad "sets the tone of the care giving-receiving patterns affecting the quality of care for child survival and development" (Bernard van Leer Foundation, 2010, p. 15). Maternal mental health is also impacted by the bonding with their child and determines the quality and continuum of care for young children. Family and community support to the mother and baby are essential to the safety and well-being of this parent-child relationship. Living in an environment that is unsafe, depriving, hostile, and depressive impact the emotional quality of this attachment process.

Family migration tends to occur in stages, with parents migrating first and sending for their children later. Children left behind in the home country may experience disruptions in attachment bonds. Sometimes, a child may have several caregivers before they were able to migrate to join a parent in the receiving country. Attachment disturbances and loss of a caregiver have been linked to behavior in which a child reverts to earlier ways of functioning and behaving, and are risk factors for depression, attachment problems, and problems in the social, emotional, cognitive, and motor development of a child (Sroufe, 2005).

Living in a violent community or exposed to the social problems that were described earlier surely meet criteria for high risk of experiencing toxic stress and traumatic incidents.

Toxic stress occurs when children experience prolonged, strong, or frequent adversity, such as physical, emotional, or sexual violence, or chronic neglect, without adequate adult support. When children are exposed to chronic traumatic experiences and toxic stress, especially during their early years of development, they are at risk of developing neuropsychological and neurobiological changes that may lead to developmental delays, stress-related health problems, and complications to learn and develop their intellectual potential (Lupien et al., 2009; Shonkoff, Boyce, & McEwen, 2009).

Middle Childhood

As children grow, their risk of being victimized increases because they expand their social circle and begin to exercise their new-found independence. Dangers both inside and outside the home augment. Research has found that the period between 5 and 9 years as being more at risk of experiencing violent punishment (Dietz, 2002). In Central American countries, cultural values related to gender roles and children's behavior may become more rigid and stereotyped for children in this age range. In the Latino culture, physical punishment is justified as discipline because caregivers often endorse an authoritarian style of parenting. While Latino families are loving and supportive with their children, they also emphasize good manners, respect and pride following collectivistic and familism values (Fontes, 2008). Parents with lower levels of education, greater stresses, and lower resources are at greater risk of insensitive discipline despite being loving and caring with their children.

The world that opens to children in middle childhood in the streets, churches, and schools represent opportunities for both enrichment and victimization if the environment is unsafe and the community surveillance is inefficient. Children may be exposed to bullying, sexual harassment, and violence from peers or strangers with its consequent negative impact. For instance, school violence may lead to compromised attendance, lower academic results, and higher drop-out rates (Glew, Fan, Katon, Frederick, Rivara, & Kernic, 2005).

Late Childhood and Adolescence

The risks of victimization for children in this age group are exponentially multiplied for children who live in the Northern Central American triangle as they become more independent and socially aware. However, this new attitude does not protect them, and for children who have a history of abuse and neglect, facing new risks and adversity may be retraumatizing and aggravating of their vulnerability. Children at this age may be vulnerable to engaging in risky behaviors either for exploration or in search of something to alleviate their suffering, such as drinking liquor, using drugs, having unprotected and unsafe sex, or exploring alternative lifestyles which places them at risk of victimization (UNICEF, 2009).

In the Northern Central American countries, children at this stage are vulnerable to gang, cartel, military, or paramilitary recruitment (American Immigration Council, AIC, 2015). Children are targeted by gangs and threaten that, if they do not join, they or a family member would be killed. At the same time many children are abused by police for suspected gang membership even when that is not the case (Baily, 2017). Children not only are vulnerable of being forcefully recruited but also, some children who have suffered from neglect and deprivations may voluntarily seek in gang membership a place to belong and feel protected.

It is also during this period when children in the Northern Central American triangle may have to voluntarily or involuntarily join the workforce to help their families. A world they may need to navigate without much help, resources, or skills and that exposes them to different types of risks. When there are no legal labor options, children may be coerced into servitude or prostitution. The message many times for these children is that they need to earn their living. Often, they are thrust into adult responsibilities at home including primary caregiving responsibility for siblings and relatives, excessive housework, and joining parents in their respective jobs (for instance, cleaning houses, agriculture, etc.) in a manner that is not developmentally appropriate.

Children of these ages are vulnerable of different forms of sexual and gender violence as their gender, sexuality, and sexual identity processes are more prominent in their lives and development. Girls may be at risk of sexual abuse or sexual violence, early marriage, and unwanted pregnancies. In Honduras, El Salvador, and Guatemala, an overwhelming majority of women who reported child sexual abuse indicated that it happened before age 11 (Speizer, Goodwin, Whittle, Clyde, & Rogers, 2008). Girls and boys of non-conforming sexual orientation or gender identity may become the target of violence and discrimination in countries where toxic masculinity tends to prevail in sexual and gender norms (UNHCR, 2012).

The Immigration Journey and Resettlement

The traumatic experiences during the time children lived in their country of origin happened within a specific place, time, psychosocial, cultural, and political conditions within their family, community, and country. In many situations, children fled their country because they did not find protection, support, and rescue from violence and neglect in their families and communities. But after fleeing from such horrific situations, they may encounter a similarly hostile and dangerous environment. Immigrant children must face two other sources of stress and potential traumatic experiences: journey and resettlement.

Children make the journey to the U.S. usually with minimal or no money, safe social supports, or resources. They may have to take dangerous means of transportation that threaten their physical safety, work every segment of the trip to obtain food and provisions to go on, and rely on strangers for orientation and help. During this time, they usually have little or no contact with a benevolent person who could guide, warn, protect, and inform them, and thus they may become vulnerable to exploitation and abuse. Without good options to make the journey to the U.S., children may turn to smugglers or traffickers. Girls and boys may be exploited sexually, subjected to sexual or labor trafficking, they may be used as drug mules, they may be kidnapped for ransom, they may be abused, assaulted, and killed.

Children who endure or escape from these dangers and arrive to the U.S. border encounter other victimization and exploitation. They are detained in unsanitary and deplorable conditions for long periods, are sometimes placed in isolation, they are treated with discrimination. They may not be protected from abuse or bullying, nor provided legal help, and may be forced to return to their countries of origin. They will sometimes be interrogated several times in a hostile manner and asked to provide evidence of the persecution they suffered but which they may not have. Although many children have legitimate asylum claims, they do not have the knowledge, information, evidence, or resources to claim their rights and present their case.

Even after successfully gaining legal entry in the U.S. the problems of the immigrant child continue to increase. Services for immigrant children who have been released from detention, whether they join relatives or enter the foster care system, are dependent on a number of factors. These factors include availability of bilingual services in the town where the child lives, capacity of the responsible adult to arrange and take the child for services, availability of funds to pay for those services, and other such practical concerns. These services, when found, may also suffer from lack of sensitivity, cultural-appropriateness, language fitness, and may not cover the child's individual needs. There is the risk of neglecting the psychological needs of the child due to poorly informed policies and practices based on erroneous or absent notions of trauma, resiliency, and development. Sometimes there is an assumption that immigrant children automatically enter a safe environment after being released from detention, when the reality is that for immigrant children the complexities of integration into a new life carries numerous risks.

In 2014, it was reported that in about 15% of cases a family member was not identified for reunification with the immigrant child and between 5 to 35% cases the sponsors were unavailable or unsuitable to take custody of the immigrant child (Byrne & Miller, 2012). These children are then placed in long-term foster care, group homes, or secure residential programs for the rest of the length of their immigration cases, which may take several years (Crea, Lopez, Taylor, & Underwood, 2017; Roth & Grace, 2015). After release from detention, children are provided with minimal or no support services, which increases the risk that reunifications or placements fail and children suffer multiple placements, more abandonment, maltreatment, and neglect (Webster, Barth, & Needell, 2000).

For children who reunite with their family, they may encounter stresses such as poverty, and limited social supports and economic resources for their integration. These immigrant children may have to heal the lengthy separation from their parents, or even lack prior relationship with their parents altogether, while mourning separations from family members who, in their home countries, took on a caregiving role. Their family receiving them in the host country may not be intact or have new members. Foster and residential placements may present their own risks as well (Baily, 2017).

Immigrant children face barriers in education, health care, and social insertion in U.S. society. They may encounter racism and exclusion in schools, community, and families (Ramos & Marrero, 2015). The healing and development of a new identity with awareness of their rights and entitlements is complicated by their developmental needs of going to school while learning a new language, often making up for past inadequate schooling, and learning the cultural and social nuances of the new country. All these stressors may exacerbate the impact of past trauma (Perreira & Ornelas, 2013).

Immigrant children from groups that have multiple minority identities such as indigenous, religious and ethnic minorities within their own culture, and LGBTQ youth are at risk of further abuse, exploitation, and discrimination in the host country (United Nations High Commissioner for Human Rights, UNHCHR, 2012).

Traumatic Stress Reactions of Immigrant Children

Kaiser Permanente conducted a groundbreaking study about traumatic experiences in childhood and its impact on individual's health risk behaviors and disease. The Adverse Childhood Experiences (ACEs), has brought to light that damaging childhood experiences are direct basic causes of morbidity and mortality in adult life (Felitti et al., 1998). Specifically, adverse childhood experiences have a dose – response relationship with many health problems. As researchers followed participants over time, they discovered that a person's cumulative ACEs score had a strong, graded relationship to numerous health, social, and behavioral problems throughout their lifespan, including substance use disorders. Furthermore, many problems related to ACEs tend to be comorbid or co-occurring, which speeds up the processes of disease and aging, and compromise immune systems.

One of the basic mechanisms by which this connection has been explained is that abuse and ongoing adversity in childhood leads to a chronic state of fight, flight, or freeze. Research has recently shown that when inflammatory stress hormones flood a child's body and brain, they alter the genes that oversee our stress reactivity, re-setting the stress response to "high" for life. This increases the risk of inflammation, which manifests later in life in cancer, heart disease, autoimmune diseases, and others (Liu, Wang, & Jiang,

2017). These issues have not been fully studied with immigrant children, but an extrapolation can be done from the information on the toxic stresses to which they are exposed.

Inherent in the fact that they arrive to the U.S. in order to escape from an unsafe environment is the fact that immigrant children have been victims of traumatic experiences. In fact, research studies have found that as many as 25% unaccompanied children immigrants have experienced extreme traumatic experiences such as witnessing the killing of a parent, living on the streets, or being kidnapped; and approximately two-thirds have experienced four or more distinct traumatic events (Huemer, 2009).

The impact of trauma is not confined to the psychiatric diagnosis of post-traumatic stress disorder (PTSD), anxiety, depression, dissociation, or other diagnoses. Rather, harm of trauma to a child or adolescent is long-lasting and widespread at the biological, cognitive, emotional, and social development, particularly when the trauma is continuous or long-term (McFarlane, 2010; Pechtel & Pizzagalli, 2010). Immigrant children with histories of abuse, violence, and neglect are more likely to be psychologically and physiologically vulnerable, develop psychopathology, disorders of personality, and in some cases suffer from developmental delays (Anda et al., 2006).

Research suggests that biological development of the brain– particularly certain aspects of the brain related to cognition, memory, and executive functioning – are highly vulnerable to stress and trauma (Pechtel & Pizzagalli, 2010). Many of these areas of the brain are connected to higher-order, complex skills such as decision-making, executive function and inhibition, and these processes continue to develop well into the mid 20s (Steinberg & Cauffman, 2009). Because brain development goes well into early adulthood, revictimization after migration will compound the harm already suffered from pre-migration traumatic experiences.

Understanding Vulnerability and Resilience in Immigrant Children

While immigrant and refugee children present a multilayered case of challenges, the reality is that many immigrant children became vulnerable due to the conditions and situations in their lives and these are not necessarily internal irreparable flaws. Some studies have reported exceptional children's resilience in the midst of unspeakable victimization and hardship. Even while living in environments that consistently abuse them, many children can develop important social values and competencies (Boyden & Cooper, 2007). Even while suffering from psychological effects from trauma, many children continue to function in major life and developmental domains (educationally, socially, vocationally, etc.) with hope, determination, and self-reliance.

While living in the middle of severe risks and traumatic experiences, children usually also experience positive events embedded within an emotionally rich culture. The Latino culture possesses factors of empowerment and resilience that are passed on to the children from very early ages. Traditions, and the generational, and historical heritage of the Latin American peoples are strong and a source of pride, identity, and existential meaning. Stutman, Baruch, Grotberg, and Rathore (2002) summarized the cultural elements of Latino culture that foster resilience. Central among those factors are loyalty and attachment to family, collectivism, respect for authority, and warmth in interpersonal relationships. For instance, the passionate and affectionate way in which they meet, greet, celebrate, and honor each other provides a strong foundation for attachment ties and social support. Strong multigenerational family structures and relationships, which includes not only blood relatives but also other emotionally meaningful adults (e.g., benevolent teachers, religious individuals, neighbors and helpers), are protective factors for Latino youth (Gunnestad, 2006). Latino children will be inclined to seek out fellowship, cooperation, and extended meaningful and protective networks throughout their lives due to the primacy of connections fostered culturally since they were very young. Latino children are also taught the value of having practical skills, the beauty and meaning of artistic and creative expressions, and the need to have a spiritual practice. These experiences are not only cultural expressions, but they also carry the underlying values and norms that are a foundation of the children's ways of thinking and behaving. Developmentally, children are primed to dream about their future and experience hope, courage, and optimism. Understanding the nature of these factors of resilience for Latino immigrant children leads to the knowledge of the environmental modifications and interventions that would carry them through healing, finding meaning from their past, and adapting to their new reality.

Case Example

Melvin: When the Bough Breaks

I encountered Melvin,[1] a 14-year-old from Honduras who migrated by himself crossing the border two years earlier, when he was ordered to undergo a psychological evaluation in Family Court, where I worked as a forensic psychologist. This branch of the court deals with families and children, particularly regarding issues such as child maltreatment, child abuse, intimate partner violence, custody, and guardianship. Melvin was a ward of the court because he had no parents, or guardian, and lived in foster care.

Melvin's mother was a gang member who had no knowledge of who Melvin's father was and she was killed when Melvin was less than a year old. Melvin was informally adopted by an older couple who used violent physical discipline and, by age 7, forced Melvin to earn money to pay for his maintenance instead of attending school. Melvin sold fruit in buses and on the streets. Reportedly, his adoptive father punished him severely when he did not bring money home because he could not sell enough. While his adoptive mother was kind and gentle, she never stood up to protect Melvin. After Melvin was kicked out by his adoptive father at age 11, he lived on the streets and sold knick-knacks. At 12, he was recruited by a gang but a week later he failed the gang initiation by refusing to hurt a person. He reported that the gang leader beat him up and told him to go far away while pointing a gun to his head, and said that if he saw him again, he would kill him "for having played them."

Melvin made the trip to the U.S. by himself with $50 in his pocket. Melvin reported that the journey involved significant physical hardship. He fell from the Death Train in Mexico losing consciousness and suffering cuts, extreme bruising and swelling to the point that he required nursing attention from Good Samaritans who are present around the train tracks to help immigrants. Melvin said that while crossing the border between Mexico and the U.S, he got lost in the dessert. He had to return to Mexico and later he tried to cross again by following other people. After crossing the border, he was detained by immigration officers. After interviewing Melvin, officials determined that Melvin could not return to his home country due to safety concerns and that Melvin should be resettled in a program for unaccompanied alien children.

Melvin was placed in a foster home and he went to school. Melvin enjoyed living with his foster family and tried to please his foster parents, his teachers loved him, he made many friends, and played soccer in his free time. Melvin called his foster parents, "Mom and Dad," and his foster siblings, "sisters and brothers." Melvin refused to engage in therapy and since he appeared to be doing well in all settings, the issue was not pressed by his case manager. In this case, while it is important to consider the child's wishes, sometimes emotional support can be provided by using other approaches and close observation for his response to the challenges he was facing and potential triggers. Children with a long history of emotional trauma are vulnerable even though they may not always show it. Melvin started having some academic difficulties at school and expressed his desire to quit school and work instead. This attitude is not unusual due to the premature thrust into adulthood that Melvin experienced. However, with the support of his new caregivers he began to understand that he was still a child and he needed to accept developmentally appropriate activities. After being with his foster family for over a year, he was put in a respite home because his foster family was going away on vacation and could not bring him since he did not have a stable immigration status to leave the country. Melvin then made a suicide attempt by taking a large amount of someone else's sleeping pills and had to be hospitalized. All the people around him were very surprised at this turn of events.

The psychological evaluation that I conducted was designed to assess Melvin's psychological functioning in order to provide the treatment that could better fit his needs. Although he was still a young adolescent, Melvin was on a path to independent living and this suicidal gesture could put a stop to such plan. When I interviewed Melvin, he shined by his optimism, cleverness, energy, and drive. He denied current symptoms of trauma, depression, or anxiety but acknowledged that at the time of his suicidal gesture, he felt overwhelmed by sadness, grief, and despair but did not know why. An in-depth assessment showed that the chronic abuse, neglect, and abandonment he suffered during sensitive years left a psychological picture congruent with complex trauma, which he had tried to fiercely suppress. It was easy to see how Melvin's charm, streets smarts, strengths, and resilience caused professionals who evaluated him earlier to neglect his psychological scars until he showed that when triggered, he was incapable of pulling himself together. It is not hard to miss signs of trauma in many children who, despite a history of abuse and neglect, show a robust ability to protect themselves, cope with a challenging environment, attach to new parental figures, and work to improve themselves.

The assessment revealed that the trigger for Melvin's suicide attempt was the threat of losing the new-found family where he had found a sense of belonging, protection, and identity. Melvin's purpose when fleeing his country was his basic need for a loving family. The UN Convention on the Rights of the Children has declared that "for the full and harmonious development of his or her personality, [children] should grow up in a family environment, in an atmosphere of happiness, love and understanding" (UNICEF, 1989, Preamble, p. 2). The threat to this basic human need for attachment which he had finally started to obtain after much adversity was enough to topple the sturdy drive he had shown to face life's adversities, move beyond suffering to overcome his situation, and the conviction that he could be the architect of his life. The psychological evaluation in this case demonstrated the need for prompt attention to the complex mental health issues of immigrant children. Mapping Melvin's psychological fragility and resilience when he arrived to the U.S. could have identified that a major trigger was the fear to be alone again if a traumatic experience happened. Timely psychological assessments can alleviate unnecessary suffering and potentiate the benefits of providing a safe haven to a traumatized child.

Conclusions

This chapter aimed to provide professionals working with immigrant children in the legal system some understanding of the issues that they may encounter. This information may help professionals become more effective, sensitive, and knowledgeable. Immigrant children are likely to experience physical, sexual, and/or psychological abuse prior to the immigration, during the immigration journey, and/or after their arrival to the U.S. Many of these children continue to experience social discrimination, rejection, and limited resources and opportunities after living in the U.S. for many years, due to the social discrimination and socioeconomic conditions they have within our society as minorities. These experiences are life-changing and understanding these issues and its reach is integral to a professional's ability to tailor services to immigrant children's needs and facilitate traumatic growth.

Practical Points

- Professionals working with immigrant children within the framework of legal and judicial processes may want to engage in diverse and constant efforts to familiarize themselves with ethnic groups, cultures, and issues different than their own, particularly those of the immigrant children they work with. Most importantly, a curious self-examination of personal biases, attitudes, and assumptions will help professionals understand how these affect their interaction with immigrant children.
- Professionals may want to consider the diverse areas in which immigrant children need to be socialized to understand their own human and civil rights and be provided with opportunities to assert their rights.
- Professionals may want to utilize a trauma-informed and culturally sensitive approach in all interactions with immigrant children including interviews, preparation, and adaptations to the children's testimony, recommendations, decision-making process, etc.
- Professionals should strive to consider protective factors (i.e., cultural values, extended family and community relationships, resilience, etc.) when working with immigrant children in the context of the legal system in order to empower the children, provide opportunities for their meaningful participation, and avoid revictimization.
- Professionals must have an awareness of the stress of multiple stigma in the lives of immigrant children, and the discrimination and barriers immigrant children face in the U.S. regarding access to services, opportunities, and support, and take this into consideration when making recommendations or offering opinions.
- Professionals should ensure that immigrant children's 'Best Interests' are being served and children have a meaningful opportunity to participate in decisions and plans that affect their lives and future.

Note

1. A pseudoname

References

American Immigration Council. (2015). *A guide to children arriving at the border: Laws, policies and responses.* Retrieved from: http://immigrationpolicy.org/sites/default/files/docs/a_guide_to_children_arriving_at_the _border_and_the_laws_and_policies_governing_our_response.pdf

American Psychological Association. (1998). *APA resolution on immigrant children, youth and families.* Retrieved from http://www.apa.org/about/policy/immigrants.aspx

American Psychological Association. (2018). *Letter to President Trump.* Retrieved from: https://www.apa.org/advocacy/immigration/separating-families-letter.pdf

Anda, R. Felitti, V. J., Bremner, J. D., Walker, J. D., Whitfield, C., Perry, B. D. ... & Giles, W. H. (2006). The enduring effects of abuse and related adverse experiences in childhood: A convergence of evidence from neurobiology and epidemiology. *European Archives of Psychiatry and Clinical Neuroscience, 256*(3), 174–186.

Baily, C. D. R. (2017). *Investigating the mental health needs of unaccompanied immigrant children in removal proceedings: A mixed-methods study* (Doctoral dissertation). Retrieved from: https://academiccommons.columbia.edu/catalog/ac:206906

Bernard van Leer Foundation. (2010). *Setting our agenda on early learning, violence and physical development: Early childhood matters.* The Hague: Bernard van Leer Foundation. Retrieved from: https://bernardvanleer.org/app/uploads/2017/10/Setting-our-agenda-on-early-learning-violence-and-physical-environment7baf.pdf

Bhabha, J. (2014). *Child migration and human rights in a global age.* Princeton, NJ: Princeton University Press.

Boyden, J., & Cooper, E. (2007). *Questioning the power of resilience: Are children up to the task of disrupting the transmission of poverty?* Chronic Poverty Research Center, Working Paper 73. Retrieved from: http://www.chronicpoverty.org/uploads/publication_files/CP_2006_Boyden_Cooper.pdf

Bronfenbrenner, U. (1979). *The ecology of human development.* Cambridge, MA: Harvard University Press.

Byrne, O., & Miller, E. (2012). *The flow of unaccompanied children through the immigration system: A resource for practitioners, policy makers, and researchers.* Retrieved from Vera Institute of Justice website: https://storage.googleapis.com/vera-web-assets/downloads/Publications/the-flow-of-unaccompanied-children-through-the-immigration-system-a-resource-for-practitioners-policy-makers-and-researchers/legacy_downloads/the-flow-of-unaccompanied-children-through-the-immigration-system.pdf

Castro, A., Savage, V., & Kaufman, H. (2015). Assessing equitable care for Indigenous and Afrodescendant women in Latin America. *Revista Panameña de Salud Pública, 38*(2), 96–109.

Center for Disease Control and Prevention. (2017). *Immigrant refugee health: Central American health profile.* Retrieved from: https://www.cdc.gov/immigrantrefugeehealth/pdf/central-american-health-profile.pdf

Chishti, M., Pierce, S., & Telus, H. (2019). *Spike in unaccompanied child arrivals at US-Mexico border proves enduring challenge.* Migration Policy. Retrieved from: https://www.migrationpolicy.org/article/spike-unaccompanied-child-arrivals-proves- enduring-challenge.

Crea, T. M., Lopez, A., Taylor, T., & Underwood, D. (2017). Unaccompanied migrant children in the United States: Predictors of placement stability in long term foster care. *Children and Youth Services Review, 73,* 93–99. https://doi:10.1016/j.childyouth.2016.12.009

Crenshaw, K. (1989). Demarginalizing the intersection of race and sex: A Black feminist critique of antidiscrimination doctrine, feminist theory and antiracist politics. *University of Chicago Legal Forum, 140,* 139–167. Retrieved from https://philpapers.org/rec/CREDTI

Dietz, T. L. (2002). Disciplining children: Characteristics associated with the use of corporal punishment and non-violent discipline. *Child Abuse & Neglect, 24*(12), 1529–1542.

Eguizábal, C., Ingram, M. C., Curtis, K. M., Korthuis, A., Olson, E. L., & Phillips, N. (2015). *Crime and violence in Central America's northern triangle: How U.S. policy responses are helping, hurting and can be improved.* Retrieved from the Woodrow Wilson Center website: https://www.wilsoncenter.org/publication/crime-and-violence-central-americas- northern-triangle-how-us-policy-responses-are

Felitti, V. J., Anda, R. F., Nordenberg, D., Williamson, D. F., Spitz, A. M., Edwards, V., Koss, M. P. & Marks, J. S. (1998). Relationship of childhood abuse and household dysfunction to many of the causes of death in adults: The Adverse Childhood Experiences (ACE) study. *American Journal of Prevention Medicine, 14*(4), 245–258. Retrieved from: http://www.iowaaces360.org/uploads/1/0/9/2/10925571/relationship_of_childhood_abuse _and ... _1998.pdf

Fitzpatrick, M., & Orloff, L. (2016). Abused, abandoned, or neglected: Legal options for recent immigrant women and girls. *Journal of Law and International Affairs, 614.* Retrieved from: https://elibrary.law.psu.edu/jlia/vol4/iss2/12

Fontes, L. A. (2008). *Child abuse and culture: Working with diverse families.* New York: Guilford.

Forray, A. (2016). Substance use during pregnancy. Retrieved from: https://www.ncbi.nlm.nih.gov/pmc/articles/PMC4870985/

Garcia Ramirez, J. A. (2018). *These are the five health challenges facing Latin America.* Retrieved from WEB website: https://www.weforum.org/agenda/2016/06/these-are-the- 5-health-challenges-facing-latin-america/

Geneva Declaration. (2015). *The global burden of armed violence.* Retrieved from: http://www.genevadeclaration.org/measurability/global-burden-of-armed violence/global-burden-of-armed-violence-2015.html

Glew, G. M., Fan, M., Katon, W., Frederick P., Rivara, F. P., & Kernic, M. A. (2005). Bullying, psychosocial adjustment and academic performance in elementary school. *Archives of Pediatric and Adolescent Medicine, 159*, 1026–1031.

Grisso, T. (2003). *Evaluating competencies: Forensic assessments and instruments* (2nd ed.). New York: Kluwer Academic/Plenum Press.

Gunnestad, A. (2006). Resilience in a cross-cultural perspective: How resilience is generated in different cultures. *Journal of Intercultural Communication, 1*, 1–29.

Huemer, J., Karnik, N., Voelkl, S., Granditsch, E., Dervic, K., Friedrich, M., & Steiner, H. (2009). Mental health issues in unaccompanied refugee minors. *Child and Adolescent Psychiatry and Mental Health, 3*(13). doi:10.1186/1753–2000-3-13.

Hulme, D., & Shepherd, A. (2003). Conceptualizing chronic poverty. *World Development, 31*(3), 403–423.

Kennedy, E. (2014). *No childhood here: Why Central American children are fleeing their homes.* Retrieved from American Immigration Council website: https://www.americanimmigrationcouncil.org/research/no-childhood-here-why-central- american-children-are-fleeing-their-homes

Liu, Y. Z., Wang, Y. X., & Jiang, C. L. (2017). Inflammation: The common pathway of stress-related diseases. *Frontiers in Human Neuroscience, 11*, 316. https://doi.org/10.3389/fnhum.2017.00316

Lupien, S. J., McEwen, B. S., Gunnar, M. R., & Helm, M. (2009). Effects of stress throughout the lifespan on the brain, behavior and cognition. *Nature Reviews Neuroscience, 10*(6), 434–445.

McFarlane, A. C. (2010). The long-term costs of traumatic stress: Intertwined physical and psychological consequences. *World Psychiatry, 9*(1), 3–10.

Mújica O. J., Haeberer, M., Teague, J., Santos-Burgoa, C., & Galvão, L. A. C. (2015). Health inequalities by gradients of access to water and sanitation between countries in the Americas, 1990 and 2010. *Revista Panameña de Salud Pública, 38*(5), 347–54.

Mulder, E. J. H., Robles de Medina, P. G., Huizink, A. C., Van den Bergh, B. R. H., Buitelaar, J. K., & Visser, G. H. (2002). Prenatal maternal stress: Effects on pregnancy and the (unborn) child. *Early Human Development, 70*(1–2), 3–14.

Noonan, K., Corman, H., Schwartz-Soicher, O., & Reichman, N. E. (2013). Effects of prenatal care on child health at age 5. *Maternal Child Health Journal, 17*(2), 189–199. doi:10.1007/s10995-012-0966-2

Pechtel, P., & Pizzagalli, D. A. (2010). Effects of early life stress on cognitive and affective function: An integrated review of human literature. *Psychopharmacology, 214*(1), 55–70.

Perreira, K. M., & Ornelas, I. (2013). Painful passage: Traumatic experiences and post-traumatic stress among immigrant Latino adolescents and their primary caregivers. *International Migration Review, 47*(4), 976. Retrieved from: https://www.ncbi.nlm.nih.gov/pmc/articles/PMC3875301/pdf/nihms529682.pdf

Pinheiro, P. S. (2006). *World report on violence against children: UN Secretary-General's study on violence against children.* Geneva: United Nations. Retrieved from: https://resourcecentre.savethechildren.net/node/2999/pdf/2999.pdf

Purdie-Vaughns, V., & Eibach, R. P. (2008). Intersectional invisibility: The distinctive advantages and disadvantages of multiple subordinate-group identities. *Sex Roles, 59*, 377–391. doi:10.1007/s11199-008-9424-4

Ramos, M., & Marrero, G. (2015). *Unaccompanied immigrant youth in New York: Struggle for identity and inclusion. A participatory research study.* Vera Institute of Justice. Retrieved from: http://archive.vera.org/sites/default/files/resources/downloads/unaccompanied-youth-nyc-technical.pdf

Rosenblum, M. R. (2015). *Unaccompanied child migration to the United States: The tension between protection and prevention.* Retrieved from the Migration Policy Institute website: https://www.migrationpolicy.org/research/unaccompanied-child-migration-united-states-tension-between-protection-and-prevention

Roth, B. J., & Grace, B. L. (2015). Falling through the cracks: The paradox of post-release services for unaccompanied child migrants. *Children and Youth Services Review, 58*, 244–252. http://dx.doi:10.1016/j.childyouth.2015.10.007

Seelke, C. L. (2016). *Gangs in Central America* (CRS Report No. RL34112). Retrieved from Congressional Research Service website: https://fas.org/sgp/crs/row/RL34112.pdf

Shonkoff, J. P., Boyce, W. T., & McEwen, B. S. (2009). Neuroscience, molecular biology, and the childhood roots of health disparities: Building a new framework for health promotion and disease prevention. *Journal of the American Medical Association, 301*(21), 2252–2259.

Speizer, I. S., Goodwin, M., Whittle, L., Clyde, M., & Rogers, J. (2008). Dimensions of child sexual abuse before age 15 in three Central American countries: Honduras, El Salvador and Guatemala. *Child Abuse and Neglect, 32*(4), 455–462.

Sroufe, A. L. (2005). Attachment and development: A prospective, longitudinal study from birth to adulthood. *Attachment and Human Development, 7*(4), 349–367.

Steinberg, L., Cauffman, E., Woolard, J., Graham, S., & Banich, M. (2009). Are adolescents less mature than adults? Minors' access to abortion, the juvenile death penalty, and the alleged APA "flip-flop." *American Psychologist, 64*(7), 583–594. Retrieved from: http://psych.colorado.edu/~mbanich/p/steinberg2009_are_adolescents.pdf

Stutman, S., Baruch, R., Grotberg, E., & Rathore, Z. (2002). *Resilience in Latino youth.* Working Paper, Institute for Mental Health Initiatives. Washington DC: The George Washington University

Thronson, D. B. (2002). Kids Will Be Kids? Reconsidering conceptions of children's rights underlying immigration law. *Ohio State Law Journal, 63*, 979–1016.

United Nations Children's Fund. (1989). *Convention on the rights of the child.* Retrieved from United Nations Office of High Commissioner for Human Rights website: http://www.ohchr.org/en/professionalinterest/pages/crc.aspx

United Nations High Commissioner for Refugees. (2012). Born free and equal: Sexual orientation and gender identity in international human rights law. Retrieved from: https://www.ohchr.org/Documents/Publications/BornFreeAndEqualLowRes.pdf

United Nations High Commissioner for Refugees. (2014). *Children on the run: Unaccompanied children leaving Central America and Mexico and the need for international protection.* Retrieved from: http://www.unhcr.org/en-us/children-on-the- run.html?query=children%20on%20the%20run

United Nations Children's Fund (UNICEF) (2014). *Hidden in plain sight: A statistical analysis of violence against children.* New York: UNICEF. Retrieved from: https://data.unicef.org/resources/hidden-in-plain-sight-a-statistical-analysis-of-violence- against-children/

United Nations Office on Drugs and Crime (UNODC). (2012). Transnational organized crime in Central America and the Caribbean: A threat assessment. Retrieved from: https://www.unodc.org/documents/data-and-analysis/Studies/TOC_Central_America_and_the_Caribbean_english.pdf

United States Citizenship and Immigration Services. (n.d.). *Policy manual.* Retrieved from: https://www.uscis.gov/policy-manual/volume-6-part-j

United States Department of State. (2016). Trafficking in persons report. U.S. Department of State: Washington, DC. Retrieved from: https://2009-017.state.gov/documents/ organization/258876.pdf

Viljoen, J. L., & Roesch, R. (2005). Competence to waive interrogation rights and adjudicative competence in adolescent defendants: Cognitive development, attorney contact, and psychological symptoms. *Law and Human Behavior, 29*(6). doi:10.1007/s10979-005-7978-y

Webster, D., Barth, R. P., & Needell, B. (2000). Placement stability for children in out-of-home care: A longitudinal analysis. *Child Welfare, 79*(5), 614–632.

9 Adolescent Post-Traumatic Stress Disorder in the Civil Arena

Amy Levy

Introduction

Despite living and breathing civil lawsuits the last decade of my professional life, when my toddler daughter and I were hit by a car while walking across the street, the last thing on my mind was a lawsuit. When trauma hits, the immediate sensations to those who remain conscious are terror and pain. Later, questions of survival linger long after they have been answered as one's sense of vulnerability is now forever in the spotlight. My daughter was physically and emotional injured, but she would survive and my husband and I would get her the help she needed. Financial remuneration for her became a consideration as part of the necessity to cover medical expenses and as a means to provide for associated challenges she will encounter in her future. If the system of medical care in the U.S. were different, perhaps we would not have engaged her in the civil legal process. As my husband, a French native, is quick to remind me, it is not an obvious consideration for many in European countries. But as an American, the process seems inevitable. Why is that? And what does it mean to involve a child in a lawsuit alleging trauma? For the purposes of this chapter, the focus will be on adolescent plaintiffs, whose memory of the alleged trauma is typically more robust, and whose personal investment in the lawsuit may be greater.

Brief History of Personal Injury Cases in the U.S.

The atmosphere of civil litigation in the United States today is not what it was 100 years ago. To begin with, the cultural perception of filing a civil lawsuit has changed from a hostile and inappropriate act, certain to stigmatize the plaintiff, to an understandable and inevitable course of action following a personal injury (Sugarman, 2000). Perceptions of personal injury attorneys have changed as well. While "ambulance chasers" still exist, they are not necessarily the first image that comes to mind. Such associations are being replaced by those of impressive litigators taking on tobacco companies, toxic spills, sexual abuse in the clergy, sexual harassment in the entertainment industry, pharmaceutical companies in the opioid epidemic, and a variety of other generally understood wrongs in our society. Further, mental health professionals today receive less scorn and criticism for expert witness testimony than previously (Melton et al., 2018). Criticisms of mental health professional's behavior on the stand, most notably the 1980s and 1990s high profile publications of Jay Ziskin and David Faust, which argued that clinical opinions did not meet standards of validity or reliability sufficient to be used as evidence in court, spurred decades of vigorous research and self-examination. As a result, mental health professionals are now increasingly better trained, and with roles more clearly defined, to take the stand as expert witnesses (Melton et al., 2018).

As the stigma against filing a civil lawsuit recedes, engagement in the process may increasing appeal to plaintiffs from a psychological perspective. Sugarman notes that

DOI: 10.4324/9780429397806-10

filing a lawsuit allows victims to transfer questions of blame for their predicament away from themselves and onto another and offers a sense of comfort in battling evil and seeking justice (Sugarman, 2000). For those who have genuinely suffered, the process of litigation may also engender powerful feelings of agency that usefully counteract the shame and weakness that usually accompanies trauma. On the other end of the spectrum, darker motives exist as well. A paved entryway to tort litigation may appeal to those who are driven by greed, vengeance, narcissism, paranoia, and other preexisting mental illness. A myriad of cases lies in between. For those living without health care and working two-to-three jobs to feed and educate a growing family, a slip-and-fall in Walgreens, or rear-end with someone better off may literally be "a lucky break."

The tort system is rooted in the idea of "fault," with liability depending upon whether the harming party is to blame for the physical or emotional harm (Melton et al., 2018). The litigant must demonstrate that the injury was the result of negligence, defamation, and/ or intentional. If their claim is substantiated in court, the plaintiff receives financial compensation for the injury. Tort damages are set by a jury to compensate all damages resulting from the wrongdoing, including pain and suffering, loss of consortium, and mental anguish (Melton et al., 2018).

Throughout most of the 20th century, psychological injuries were not compensable outside of physical injuries. In the past few decades, this has changed and compensation for emotional injuries alone is allowed in the U.S (Kane & Dvoskin, 2011). In order to be granted pecuniary compensation, the litigant must demonstrate that psychological injury equals measurable loss or impairment. Compensation is then granted to restore the litigant to their pre-incident condition or make the person "whole" (Erard & Evans, 2017).

Other legal avenues of compensation for mental injury exist as well. Discrimination claims based on the Americans with Disabilities Act and the Fair Housing Act, sexual harassment under Title VII of the Civil Rights Act, and other work-related litigation may also involve psychological injury claims (Melton et al., 2018).

The Mental Health Expert Witness

In order to receive an award for what in legal parlance is called, "emotional damages," it is the plaintiff's burden to prove that they have sustained damages. In other words, the plaintiff must satisfactorily present evidence of their mental loss or impairment in an objective and verifiable manner. The plaintiff, as well as the defense, retain mental health experts to examine the plaintiff and the evidence presented in order to reach "expert opinions" about whether or not the alleged wrongdoing gave rise to diagnosable impairments or categorical losses.

Attorneys that contact potential experts usually begin with a brief summary of the case and overall estimate of the timeframe for the litigation. In that initial contact, several questions are addressed: Will the expert be available to conduct an exam, and participate in deposition and trial testimony in the anticipated timeframe? Does the expert's training and experience qualify them to work on this particular case? Are there any conflicts of interest (relationships to the plaintiffs, defendants, or their attorneys) that would compromise the expert's judgment or create a dual role? The expert will consider the case and whether there are personal elements that would limit their ability to be objective. For example, an expert with a close family member who was injured by police may find a police brutality claim emotionally triggering. Alternately, an expert might be unduly influenced if retained by attorneys for their favorite celebrity.

Experts have a legal and ethical duty to strive toward fair and impartial thinking in the formation of their opinions. However, in practice, experts may find themselves siding with whoever has retained them. We are generally compassionate people and when our help is sought, we may emotionally align with those who need us. This may involve unrecognized slips in judgment that lend greater weight to the viewpoint of the retaining side. Additionally, it is compelling to establish positive working relationships with attorneys and satisfied customers are return customers. Especially in forensic work, it is essential to be alert to and acknowledge one's potential biases.

My way of navigating this understandable, yet dangerous, undertow is to assume that the emotional injury narratives presented by both sides are likely to be overstated so as to drive their point. The expert's role at times then becomes to locate the truth in the middle. Though attorneys are sometimes disappointed when our formulations do not match their own, I find that most often, they are compelled by the force of an honest appraisal and adjust their legal strategies accordingly. Despite our best intentions to reach the truth, no human thought is purely objective. Given the inevitable blind spots, it is also prudent to return repeatedly to the facts of the case, to present ones thinking in consultation groups and/or to have colleagues read over our reports and discuss our opinions with us.

Experts tasked with evaluating for psychological injury strive to establish an understanding of the individual's baseline functioning prior to the event and to then compare that with their functioning immediately following the event and in subsequent years. This is best achieved through careful consideration of three primary categories of information: (1) records, (2) interviews, and (3) standardized testing.

Records include medical, academic, and employment records if applicable. The records are carefully reviewed with an eye toward potential changes in the plaintiff's functioning and general condition around the time of the event and in the months and years that follow. For children and adolescents, a dip in academic performance or attendance is particularly useful to note, as are changes in health such as frequent illness or infections that would suggest a compromise in the immune system or a psychosomatic reaction.

Interviews of the plaintiff and family members offer the plaintiff and witnesses to the alleged injury an opportunity to articulate what changes they have noticed since the incident. Plaintiffs recount their version of events and describe the injuries they believe they have suffered. It is an opportunity for the mental health professional to ask questions and observe behaviors that help to establish how veritable the claim is, as well as to gather a more nuanced understanding of how the alleged injury has affected the adolescent's life and functioning. In particular, it is critical for experts to investigate whether trauma or mental illness was present prior to the alleged incidents leading to the tort action.

Psychological Testing

Following this collection of data, psychologists who are asked to conduct an evaluation of the plaintiff typically administer psychological tests. The utility of psychological testing lies in the fact that the administration and scoring of psychological measures is standardized and objective, and the interpretation of results is based upon research findings in both normal and clinical populations. Therefore, psychological tests can fortify and lend credibility to and/or present alternative hypotheses for the data gathered in an in-depth clinical interview and review of records. There are three primary types of tests that psychologist will use to evaluate psychological functioning: questionnaires and self-report inventories, self-report-based test with validity scales, and performance-based tests.

Self-report testing is limited by dependence on what people are able and willing to report about themselves (Erard & Evans, 2017). In a legal setting, where litigants have strong incentives to advocate for the seriousness of their alleged injuries and to place themselves in a positive light, some will exaggerate or malinger their symptoms. There is therefore, limited justification for using questionnaires, self-report inventories, or any other self-report-based test that does not include measures to check for over-endorsement, under endorsement and/or feigning. Clinical scales for these types of instruments present the conditions they are measuring in a transparent manner, allowing the plaintiff to endorse symptoms of the condition. The results are tabulated and the final number is used as an indication of whether and to what degree the person is suffering from the condition measured by the instrument. The problem with such a method for legal settings is that it assumes that the litigant will be honest. Experts who rely on these instruments run the risk of being "attacked" on the witness stand and portrayed to the jury as naïve and unscientific in their approach to the evaluation without a thorough understanding of response style.

Self-report tests with validity scales are applicable in legal contexts. Prominent examples of these tests include the Minnesota Multiphasic Personality Inventory-2 (MMPI-2), Minnesota Multiphasic Personality Inventory-Adolescent Version (MMPI-2-A) and as well as the Minnesota Multiphasic Personality Inventory–2–Restructured Form (MMPI-2-RF) and Minnesota Multiphasic Personality Inventory-Adolescent-Restructured Form (MMPI-A-RF). Other frequently used self-report inventories include the Personality Assessment Inventory (PAI) and the Personality Assessment Inventory for Adolescents (PAI-A).

The MMPI and the PAI measure the plaintiff's subjective assessment of their complaints and functioning and then compares their scores with those of others. This allows the psychologist performing the exam to understand how closely the plaintiff's responses align with responses of those in a previously identified group, such as depressed adolescents. Items reported by truly depressed adolescents may not always appear to be about depression, therefore, the meaning on the face of some items may be misleading for those motivated to exaggerate or to deny symptoms. Further, the MMPI and PAI have validity scales that recognize efforts to exaggerate or minimize symptoms. Validity scales aid psychologists in determining if the scores achieved in the clinical scales should be treated with caution due to evidence of on the one hand exaggeration, or due to understatement of symptoms on the other hand. At times, validity scales measuring exaggeration are elevated not by deception, but by a "cry for help." There are score ranges that help to facilitate this distinction, so that a score beyond a specific standard deviation above the mean is highly unlikely to be due to a "cry for help." When the score falls in a more ambiguous range, the expert will need to make a clinical judgment using data from other scales, comparison of the litigant's scores on different tests, as well as behavioral observations of the subject during the evaluation, to reach a determination regarding response style.

Performance-based tests such as the Rorschach Ink Blot test do not rely on personal endorsement of items and rather measure how people behave, or "perform," when given the task of organizing ambiguous stimuli such as ink blot cards. Another example of a performance measure is an individually administered intelligence test. For both intelligence tests and the Rorschach, a sample of the subject's behavior is obtained. That behavior is scored according to strict and standardized rules that are summated into categorical descriptions.

The Rorschach has met with some criticism as an instrument for forensic use. Initially, the methods of administration and scoring were viewed as lacking rigorous standards of reliability and validity. With nearly one-thousand meta-analyses and multimethod assessment studies combined, the Comprehensive System (CS) emerged during the 1960s and 1970s as a robust scoring system that later met the legal standards for admissibility in court (Gacono, Evans, & Viglione, 2002; Hilsenroth & Stricker, 2004); Society for Personality Assessment, 2005).

In 2011, a newly developed scoring system, the Rorschach Performance Assessment System, or R-PAS, came into use.[1] The R-PAS builds on the decades of research on the CS in peer-reviewed publications. The R-PAS system refined the various findings produced from decades of use of the CS. Subsequently, exchanges between the developers of R-PAS and

Rorschach critics who questioned the applicability of the norms and the empirical support for the interpretation of the test variables (Wood, Nezworski, & Stejskal, 1996; Lilienfeld et al., 2000; Meyer & Archer, 2001) took place in the Psychological Bulletin, a publication of the American Psychological Association (APA). The Psychological Bulletin has long been recognized by psychologists in the U.S. as a "premier" publication of the APA.

In 2013, Mihura et al. published the results of their systematic evaluation of peer-reviewed Rorschach validity literature for the 65 main variables in the CS system in the *Psychological Bulletin*. An exchange in the *Psychological Bulletin* between Mihura et al. and the Rorschach's staunchest critics, Wood, Lilienfeld, Garb, and Nezworski ensued over the next several years. In their 2015 response, Wood et al. lifted their previous recommendation for a moratorium on the use of the Rorschach in clinical and forensic settings. Wood et al. now agreed that there was sufficient evidence to trust that 14 Rorschach variables were related to cognitive ability/impairment and thought disorder (Wood et al., 2015). Wood et al. then ran a new meta-analysis that included unpublished dissertations, "correlations instead of semipartial correlations" and used Rorschach International Norms (Wood et al., 2015).

Following their meta-analysis, Wood et al. agreed that Mihura et al.'s 2013 meta-analysis accurately reflected the published literature, but argued that Mihura et al.'s exclusion of unpublished studies generated "substantial overestimates" of validity for some Rorschach scores. Wood et al. concluded that Mihura et al.'s evidence was insufficient to justify using the CS measure for noncognitive characteristics (Wood et al., 2015). Mihura et al. retorted that Wood et al.'s procedures contradicted their own standards and recommendations for research, and repeatedly led to substantially lower effect sizes. Further, Mihura et al. found "... numerus methodical errors, data errors, and omitted studies" (Mihura et al., 2015, p. 1). They showed how many of Wood et al.'s conclusions were "based on a narrative review of individual studies and post hoc analyses rather than their meta-analytic findings" (Mihura et al., 2015). Mihura et al. challenged Wood et al.'s exclusive use of dissertations to test publication bias, and ultimately determined that the conclusions reported in Wood et al. 2015 were not reliable.

The numerous systematic reviews and meta-analyses of the CS's validity, most notably Mihura et al.'s, and exchanges with critics have consistently shown validity and general acceptance for the Rorschach's procedures and features (Meyer, Viglione, Mihura, Erard, & Erdberg, 2011; Erard & Evans, 2017), and established the Rorschach a psychometrically sound and researched-based system.

Many features of the R-PAS make it well-suited to forensic evaluations and especially to evaluation of psychological injury in personal injury cases.[2] The Rorschach shows strength as a measure of neuropsychological factors in children (Meyer, 2016), and may be useful in evaluating children in brain injury cases. The Rorschach is effective in assessing for trauma as the moderately stressful test situation coupled with the ambiguous and sometimes dark cards may stimulate flashbacks during the evaluation (Van der Kolk & Ducey, 1989; Erard, 2012; Viglione et al., 2012; Erard & Evans, 2017).

Performance-based tests are particularly valuable as the individual taking the test is not aware of how the information they are offering will be scored or interpreted. Not having a sense of control over the outcome of the test leads some to respond candidly, others to respond in a guarded manner, for fear of what they might reveal about themselves, and others still to attempt to influence the data by offering responses that they believe are consistent with the population they wish to imitate. For example, if an adolescent taking the Rorschach wishes to present as traumatized, they may offer imagery that is particularly dramatic (Sewell, 2008). This will yield a score for dramatic content that is above what is expected and will raise a red flag for the psychologist conducting the assessment.

The remaining scores on the Rorschach, as well as the adolescent's performance on other tests, will help the clinician to interpret the meaning of the dramatic content as reflecting feigning, exaggeration, or genuine trauma. With trauma, scores having to do with mental control and reality testing, as well as high degrees of stress, are typically elevated along with dramatic content (Viglione, 2012).

A forensic evaluator will consider all sources of data, including Rorschach and other test data in addition to information obtained through record review and behavioral observations. This inclusion of multiple sources of data characterizes and distinguishes forensic from clinical evaluations and work. For a discussion of the guidelines governing the Forensic examiner, see the "Specialty Guidelines for Forensic Psychology" (2011), see Appendix 1 at the end of this volume.

Guarded Adolescents

Children tend not to think in terms of monetary compensation for their pain and suffering. Therefore, when you encounter a child in a personal injury matter you are also encountering a parent or guardian with significant investment in pleading the case. That will often be an influencing factor in the child's presentation. With older adolescents, whose appreciation for financial reward is already well developed, their own fantasies about what will help their case and their personal investment in it, will also affect what they say and do during the examination.

Adolescents may be reluctant to speak during psychological evaluations. Contributing factors include the formality of the setting, the unfamiliarity of evaluator and whatever positive or negative feelings have been communicated to the adolescent about the evaluator, lack of sincere investment in the lawsuit, as well as reluctance to discuss an event that was upsetting or traumatic.

As an example, Charlie witnessed his aunt being hit by a car when he was 13. Four years later, when I met with him for an evaluation, he was noticeably guarded. He avoided eye contact and gave brief and faint responses. Therefore, I did not rush the process, giving him time to get used to me and the setting. After explaining my role as a defense expert and the purpose of the exam, I used direct and open-ended questions and explained that I was interested in learning about his experiences and feelings, whatever they may be. I encouraged him to take breaks as needed. Eventually he disclosed that he was no longer troubled by memories of the accident. Intrusive mental images and dreams of what he observed had stopped 8 to 12 months following the accident. He passed the intersection where the accident occurred almost daily on his way home from school and did not feel compelled to avoid it. Rather, what bothered him in the years that followed the accident and into the present was the way his aunt's subsequent disability affected his mother and by extension, his entire family. Because his mother was busy taking care of his aunt, she was frequently tired and had less energy for Charlie and his siblings. Further, the long and drawn out lawsuit was a stress on the family. Depositions were scheduled and rescheduled and his personal schedule felt in constant disruption as a result. He was starting to wonder if "the money" would ever come and ultimately, he just wanted it to be "over with."

As another example, when she was 16, Helen witnessed her father getting non-fatally shot during a hold-up in his business. Two years later, I was retained by the plaintiff's attorney to conduct an evaluation. Like Charlie, Helen was extremely guarded. Her answers were curt and she displayed no signs of emotion. Unlike Charlie, however, my attempts to put her at ease had little impact. She doggedly kept her answers to a minimum and maintained an internal focus so that every time I asked her a question it seemed to interrupt some private conversation she was having. Helen reported spending most of her time studying in her bedroom or playing team volleyball. She revealed nightmares three to five times a week. Her test results were all consistent with one another and reflected acute post-traumatic stress disorder with intrusive experiencing and high levels of defensive avoidance.

I understood Helen's presentation in the evaluation to be a direct reflection of how she was coping with the trauma of seeing her father shot. By keeping her mind and body in constant use during the day, she was effectively suppressing the trauma she had not emotionally processed. However, at night, when these defenses were not available, the terror and pain would break through.

Charlie's initial reluctance to engage in the interview seemed to be a direct result of the pressure he was feeling to perform in the evaluation and to present a story that would "get the money" for his family. Though Charlie had some initial trauma symptoms, his psyche had repressed the trauma in a healthy fashion as time passed. In Helen's case, she had PTSD and was not in therapy as she needed to be. She was pushing thoughts of what happened out of her awareness, or "suppressing" them, but suppression of trauma leads only to its continued re-emergence. Her withdrawal and avoidance in the interview was a protective stance against feeling traumatized all over again.

Adolescence and Trauma

Trauma shatters a sense of safety and personal cohesion. In addition to leaving victims with post-traumatic stress symptoms, when trauma affects children, if untreated, it derails or upends healthy development. Adolescence generally spans from ages 12 to 19 and is characterized by a rush of hormones and budding sexuality (Becker, Daley et al., 2003), as well as a search for identity (Erikson, 2013). Experimentation and risk taking characterize this period of life as adolescents try out different roles and learn where their personal limits are. They are working to define the boundaries between their parents and themselves (Hales & Yudofsky, 2003). Because of this increased openness to new life experiences, and search for personal identity via experimentation, they may inadvertently be at increased risk of experiencing trauma.

Case Presentation: Kathy[3]

A 21-year-old Latina female, Kathy, filed a civil action for damages against her former gymnastics coach, Mark, and the gymnastics organization that employed him. In her complaint she alleged childhood sexual abuse starting when she was 14 years old and lasting 2 years, intentional infliction of emotional distress against Mark, and negligence against the organization and its founder. Kathy also sued the organization for vicarious liability based on Mark's acts of sexually abusing her, and based on the founder's negligence in not protecting her.

A psychiatrist and I were hired by the plaintiff's attorney as mental health experts for the plaintiff. Our first task was to conduct an Independent Medical Examination or IME[4] The word "independent" implies not that the expert has not been retained by a single side, but rather that the clinician has not been involved in care and treatment of the plaintiff (Erard & Evans, 2017). Though she filed her lawsuit several years earlier, Kathy did not present for the IME until she was 20 years old. Long spans of time such as these are often involved in legal proceedings, and highlight the importance of the work of Baker-Ward, Ornstein, & Taylor in this volume in offering professionals an understanding of children's memory.

By the time of the IME, Kathy was living with her 8-month-old daughter and her boyfriend, who was not the baby's father. They all resided in her father's home with her father, her father's girlfriend, as well as two of Kathy's half-siblings. Kathy was not working and planned to attend a local community college. Her primary complaint was drug addiction. She had just reached six months sobriety.

Her parents never married and conceived Kathy when they were both in high school. Kathy grew up primarily with her mother. She did well in grade and middle school and was engaged in gymnastics, a sport her father – a coach for a local gymnastics organization – introduced her to. Kathy maintained regular weekend contact with her father throughout her early childhood and recalls feeling angry and pushed out when he and his girlfriend at that time became pregnant.

When Kathy was 11 years old, her father introduced Kathy to Mark, the perpetrator. Mark was 26 years old, and a friend of her father's as they were both gymnastic coaches. She came to know Mark through meets, and remembers him making comments to her such as "You're looking good out there." Kathy noted that his emphasis was always "on the wrong words." She also remembered how he observed a hole in her leotard and commented that he would take better care of her than her father did.

When Kathy was 13, her mother became pregnant and relocated with Kathy's stepfather. Kathy then began acting up at school, not attending classes and letting her grades slip. As a reaction to the changes at home, she recalls trying on the identity of a black gangster and living the "street life." She recalled going to see a horror film one evening with her father, his girlfriend, and Mark. During the film, Mark gave Kathy sips of alcohol that he concealed in his shirt and comforted her during scary moments in the film by holding her hand and bringing her legs over his lap. She felt that the contact was "wrong," but reassured herself that they were "just cuddling."

Kathy moved in with her father shortly after she turned 14 in order to change schools and thereby become more involved with gymnastics. At the time, she identified as bisexual, presented as gay, and began a relationship with a girl, all of which Mark took notice of.

During a post-gymnastics meet at her home where people were drinking, Mark left the group to find Kathy in her bedroom on the phone with her girlfriend. He retreated, but approached Kathy again later in the evening to inquire if she was "still gay." When she told him that she was, he pulled her hips to his and said, "You must hate me." Kathy promised him that she did not, and Mark kissed her. She let the kiss last a moment before pushing him away. Mark asked her not to tell her father. The next morning, Kathy shared what had happened with her stepmother. Her stepmother said that she would speak to Kathy's father, but judging by her father's true reaction when he learned of the abuse, Kathy is confident that her stepmother never informed him. Feeling at fault for the kiss, Kathy broke up with her girlfriend. A few days later, she made a suicide attempt with alcohol and ibuprofen. She wrote in her journal that she "messed up by making Mark want to kiss her."

Over the next couple of months, Kathy avoided Mark. She began dressing in baggy clothing, stopped wearing makeup, ate a lot of junk food and gained 15 pounds. Her grades dropped and she went into academic probation, which prohibited her from participating in gymnastics. She withdrew from her friends and family and began smoking marijuana. During this time, Kathy wrote a poem in which she described herself as a "sinner among saints." She suffered over having enjoyed the kiss and letting it linger and felt confused about whether or not she was gay.

Sometime later, at another gymnastics community party at her home, Mark appeared drunk and "passed out." Once the others were asleep, he went into Kathy's bedroom and provided her with alcohol. Over the course of several weeks, Mark continued this pattern and introduced her to a game called "nervous" where each person touches the other increasingly close to their genitals asking every time, "does this make you nervous?" Mark escalated the sexual touching and an early attempt at oral sex led Kathy to push him away. She liked his nighttime visits and found herself thinking a lot about him. She began drinking when alone and selling watered down liquor at school to earn money to buy weed.

Their drinking escalated and Mark continued to push sexual boundaries. After several weeks, Kathy agreed to intercourse.

Mark began to insist that Kathy ask to have intercourse. She found herself begging and crying to have sex with him, and felt horrible about herself and her growing need for him. As her feelings intensified, Mark turned cold toward her. A few times he left the gymnastics party without coming to her room. As he withdrew, Kathy found his phone number on her father's phone and called him compulsively. Mark agreed to see her, but only if she would perform specific sexual acts. She also came to learn that he was 29 years old, and not 20 as he had led her to believe. She tried numerous times to end the relationship, but breaks in their contact made her feel that she was "having a nervous breakdown." She would then reach out, only to be rejected. Once she would begin to get over him, Mark would reappear for another sexual encounter.

When she was 16, Kathy began dating an age-appropriate boyfriend. Learning of this, Mark rented a hotel room and persuaded Kathy to cheat on her boyfriend with him. Following sex, Mark left her showering in the hotel room. Though she planned to turn her attention to her steady boyfriend, Kathy began fighting at school and was arrested for shoplifting.

During her senior year of high school, Kathy's father found her diary left in the living room and read about her relationship with Mark. Her father called the police and they set up a scene using Kathy as bait to arrest Mark. After Mark was arrested, Kathy felt confused about her identity and morals. She felt guilty for "getting him arrested" and confused as others insisted that Mark "got himself arrested." She wondered if she was good and weak, or bad and powerful.

Kathy was blacklisted by the gymnastics community for her role in Mark's arrest. In response, she moved to New York City with a girlfriend and began using hydrocodone, which she stole from her grandmother. It made her feel warm and tingly and stopped her from thinking about the case and the hostility she was experiencing from the gymnastics community. Kathy began working nights as a stripper. She enjoyed the club scene, and in particular liked seeing people looking at her. Her drug use expanded to oxycontine, heroine, and methedrine. Kathy began having cardiac arrhythmias and made another suicide attempt with an overdose of Trazodone. She was hospitalized on a 72-hour hold.

Six months into her pregnancy, Kathy realized she was pregnant. Her daughter was born 14 months after her New York City suicide attempt. At risk of losing her daughter over her drug use, Kathy felt motivated to reach sobriety. At the time of the IME, Kathy was in a year-long drug treatment program and seeing a therapist.

Anticipating her day in court and seeing Mark again, Kathy noted, "I know it wasn't real love, but I still worry about how I'll look to him." She wondered if he would hate her or think she was pretty. Kathy complained of violent nightmares, biting her boyfriend during sleep, and – since getting sober – night terrors. She had panic attacks when she thought of Mark and the approaching trial that would bring them face to face.

She reported many avoidant behaviors such as not getting off the freeway near his house, as well as other areas that she associated with him including the cinema where they saw the horror movie. Since her sobriety, she lost her sex drive and felt "gross" during sex. Once while she and her boyfriend were having sex, Kathy felt overwhelmed by anger and attacked him physically.

Psychological Testing

I administered three psychological tests to Kathy and their findings were all consistent with one another. This consistency increases the likelihood that they were giving an accurate picture of her mental state. Across the board her tests reflected sexual abuse trauma and post-traumatic stress reaction. Kathy's scores on the Trauma Symptom Inventory – 2, a self-report test with validity scales, showed a post-traumatic stress disorder with multiple sexual concerns including unwanted sexual thoughts or feelings. Kathy's MMPI-2 profile corresponded with profiles of others who have reported a background of early sexual abuse and violation of trust due to sexual trauma. Kathy's MMPI-2 profile suggested that her subsequent sexual relationships and behaviors may be marked by chronic problems and perversions. She may be inclined to overt sadomasochism and adrenaline, rush-seeking behaviors such as shoplifting and problematic sexual encounters or promiscuity – all to counteract the numbed-out or "dead" feeling that is typically present after abuse.

On the Rorschach, Kathy's perceptions of the cards were replete with graphic sexual themes such as girls with legs spread, lap dances, and a "drippy penis." At the end of the test administration, she confided that she felt embarrassed by her responses. She had "tried to see normal stuff." Her R-PAS scores suggest that she is intelligent with a capacity to think well and to experience empathy. Her Rorschach responses also suggest a good sense of awareness and purposefulness, but due to the disruptive force of trauma in her psyche, she was susceptible to states of confusion, paranoia, and unpredictability as well as problems thinking clearly and seeing things accurately. This combination of cognitive impairment with content specific traumatic imagery is consistent with responses suggesting PTSD on the Rorschach (Viglione et al., 2012).

Case Outcome

Kathy's trial ended with an award of several million in damages against Mark. She appealed this judgment arguing for additional damages due to her from the gymnastics organization. This appeal was rejected and the original judgment affirmed.

Case Discussion

Sexual offenders typically "groom" their child victims and their victims' families. Grooming functions to: establish trust with the child and the adults who protect that child, secure access to and isolate the victim, and control and conceal the sexually abusive relationship (Pollack, 2015). Mark's grooming behaviors involved building confidence with Kathy's family by spending time with her father socially and by frequently sleeping over when he had had too much to drink. Mark established a bond with Kathy's father, as well as respect among those in the gymnastics community. In so doing, he reduced the likelihood that others would notice the abuse, and that Kathy would be believed if she were to disclose it. Though her father did believe her, the gymnastics community initially boycotted Kathy and sided with Mark.

Mark manipulated Kathy into becoming a "cooperating participant." Common in grooming, turning the child into a cooperating participant functions to reduce the likelihood that the child will disclose the abuse, and increases the chances that the child will repeatedly return to the abuser (Pollack, 2015). Internally, it confounds the child's sense of agency and free will. Externally, it distorts the public's perception of the child's volition as well.

It is not uncommon that victims like Kathy are betrayed first by the offender and second by the community surrounding the pair. Since 2017, the #MeToo movement against sexual abuse and sexual harassment of woman has gained momentum and generated increased support for female victims. With the advent of online communities, social media, and the "cancel culture," which turns a perpetrator into a pariah, women as a group have recently begun to feel supported in speaking out. This is a positive development, but the ostracization of those who are abused remains a problem. While the #MeToo movement has mobilized a turn in the direction of hearing and believing victims, there is still work to be done in understanding and stopping the tendency to blame the victim.

With reference to Erik Erikson's, theory of development, adolescence falls in the stage of "identity versus identity diffusion" (Erikson, 2013). During this time, adolescents are working to develop a sense of self and to explore their sexual and occupational identities through a questioning of their values, beliefs, and goals. If all goes well during this phase of development, they achieve the virtue of "fidelity" and gain the capacity to commit to and accept others even when there are ideological differences. Failure to move through this phase leads to "role confusion" or uncertainty about themselves and their place in society. In cases of extreme and/or prolonged trauma, some adolescents may form Dissociative Identity Disorder, a condition in which the personality is essentially divided up into distinct identities without integration. A more frequent reaction of traumatized adolescents at this juncture of development, however, is a premature closure of identity formation (Figley, 1985). Developmental effects include difficulties with emotional regulation and the establishment of positive self-esteem. Disturbance in emotion regulation caused by trauma also leads to increased psychopathologies, such as anxiety disorder, depression, and post-traumatic stress disorder (Amstadter, 2008; Ehring, Tuschen-Caffier, Schnulle, Fischer, & Gross, 2010; Goldfarb, 2020).

When trauma accumulates over years, children will seek to emotionally deaden themselves from "the blows" and may build defenses such as denial, dissociation, and numbing to cope with prolonged trauma (Lenor Terr, 1990; Briere, 2006). The easiest and most dependable numbing agents of course are drugs and alcohol. Drug and alcohol use function first as a means of self-medicating to offset depression and shame, and later, if untreated, lead to problems with brain development and addiction (Mayhew, Flay, & Mott, 2000). There is some evidence in Kathy's primitive thinking that her development may have been stunted by the trauma and drug use.

The impact of Mark's controlling abuse and torture is unending. Prolonged sexual and emotional abuse such as Kathy experienced generates a myriad of emotional and developmental catastrophes. Striking as it did during the phase of her development in which identity formation was the goal, she was vividly confused about hers. Kathy articulated the crux of her identity confusion: am I powerful and bad, or weak and good?

When Mark entered her life, she was a young adolescent. Her sense of identity exploration had just begun, and it was primarily in the realm of gymnastics, where she was discovering her physical abilities and changing female body. As Mark entered the arena, one could argue that her explorations became more rapid and extreme. She played with the identities of a gangster girl and a lesbian. These natural avenues of exploration were quickly shutdown, however, as he reoriented her focus onto him and onto gauging her self-worth through his inconsistent sexual interest in her.

In the sadistic, abusive relationship that developed, Kathy did not learn to regulate her emotions and to form a steady sense of positive self-regard, both of which might have helped her to rebound when Mark finally broke it off. Instead, when the relationship ended, she began using drugs and looking to patrons in strip clubs to achieve a sense of value through the sexual excitement that she could incite in them. Such behaviors are common among adolescents with post-traumatic stress disorder that is the result of sexual trauma. Research shows that long-term effects of childhood sexual abuse in girls includes later sexual preoccupation, younger age for first voluntary intercourse, and higher rates of teen pregnancy (Noll, Trickett, Putnam, 2003).

Kathy was ostracized by the gymnastics community, which complicated her view of herself as problematic, and weakened her resources for emotional healing as she lost the social support system on which she had depended for a sense of belonging, positive self-esteem, and identity.

At the time of our evaluation, Kathy had a new and appealing identity as a mother and she was excited by its potential to transport her away from pain and addiction. However, years of abuse are not erased with a single birth. Kathy's lifecare plan partitioned funds for psychotherapy and psychiatric treatment, which she desperately needed. Unfortunately, there was no trust fund in place to ensure that Kathy would necessarily engage in mental health treatment.

Conclusion

Litigation of mental injury is a relatively new and developing area of law that offers remuneration for an adolescent's psychological loss or impairment following an alleged wrongdoing. Simultaneously, it has the potential to exacerbate injury when the process becomes excessively adversarial, prolonged, or when parties engage unprofessionally. In cases where the child is coerced by family members into the process or is otherwise less than sincerely engaged, it may also prove detrimental.

Mental health expert witnesses are retained by each side to assist the trier of fact. The psychological evaluation of adolescents with post-traumatic stress claims is a complex undertaking. For the examiner, it involves numerous tasks including learning the facts of the case, meticulous evaluation of the adolescent's attitude toward the litigation and their truthfulness, an understanding of the impacts of trauma on an adolescent's behaviors and course of development, the acquisition of thorough interview and valid and reliable test data, as well as active monitoring and attending to the evaluator's own biases.

At the outset of this chapter, I posed the question, "What does it mean to involve a child in a lawsuit alleging trauma?" Though the question may have been addressed from a concrete vertex, the psychological implications bear further thought. Remaining in litigation for years can create an identity for the child as "that child to whom that bad thing happened" (G. Calloway, personal communication, July 8, 2020). The child's sense of self becomes interwoven with the narrative of injury, and the task of forging a life apart from the incident is mired.

My personal and professional experience with the topic has led me to the conclusion that litigation often serves to insert a child into a parental dynamic. Further, the meaning of the lawsuit for the child may be inseparable from the meaning for the parents. Kathy's father's anger at the fact that someone he had brought into his daughter's life had so viciously damaged theirs made him an active participant in the case. His narrative danced constantly with hers and in my impression both confused and redirected her way of processing the experience. On an extreme end of the spectrum are cases of Factitious Disorder Imposed on Another (formerly termed Munchausen's by proxy), where were it not entirely for a parent's narrative of injury, the child would not believe that anything was wrong with them. While the parent's influence on the child's experience can be positive, negative, or too nuanced and complex to quantify, it may always be there, sometimes paving the child's path to a law office, and at times affecting their mindset for the litigation as well as their recovery.

Notes

1. The system was developed by Gregory J. Meyer, Joni L. Mihura, Donald J. Viglione, Robert E. Erard, Philip Erdberg, and Fabiano K. Miguel.
2. It provides a check against exaggerated or minimized symptom presentation, generates evidence regarding implicit traits and behavioral tendencies, uses internationally applicable reference, and has improved non-patient adult and children's norms as compared with the Comprehensive System (Erard, 2012; Erard & Evans, 2017).
3. Though the case is in the public domain, I have made efforts to disguise the parties involved.

4. IMEs are examinations conducted by mental health clinicians at the request of a third party, usually lawyers, in response to legal questions, such as whether or not an alleged assault engendered mental injuries.

References

Amstadter, A. (2008). Emotional regulation and anxiety disorders. *Journal of Anxiety Disorders*, *22*, 211–221.

Becker, D. F., Daley, M., Green, M. R., Hendren, R. L., et al. (2003). Trauma and adolescence II: The impact of trauma. *Adolescent Psychiatry, 27*, 165–200.

Briere, J. (2006). Dissociative symptoms and trauma exposure. *The Journal of Nervous and Mental Disease, 194*, 78–82.

Ehring, T., Tuschen-Caffier, B., Schnulle, J., Fischer, S., & Gross, J. J. (2010). Emotion regulation and vulnerability to depression: Spontaneous versus instructed use of emotion suppression and reappraisal. *Emotion, 10*, 563–572.

Erard, R. E. (2012). Expert testimony using the Rorschach assessment system in psychological injury cases. *Psychological Injury and Law, 5*, 122–134.

Erard, R. E., & Evans, B. F. (Eds.). (2017). *The Rorschach in multimethod forensic assessment: Conceptual foundations and practical applications*. New York: Routledge.

Erikson, E. H. (2013). *Identity and the life cycle* (rev. ed.). New York: W. W. Norton & Company.

Figley, C. R. (Ed.). (1985). *Trauma and its wake: The study and treatment of post- traumatic stress disorders*. New York: Brunner/Mazel.

Gacono, C. B., Evans, F. B. III, & Viglione, D. J. (2002). The Rorschach in forensic practice. *Journal of Forensic Psychology Practice, 2*(3), 33–54.

Goldfarb, D. (2020). Navigating tricky waters: Understanding and supporting children's testimony about experiencing and witnessing violence. In G. Calloway & M. Lee (Eds.), *A handbook of children in the legal system: A guide for forensic and mental health practitioners*. New York: Routledge.

Hales, R. E, & Yudofsky, S. C. (2003). *The American psychiatric publishing textbook of clinical psychiatry* (4th ed.). Arlington, VA: American Psychiatric Publishing.

Hilsenroth, M. J., & Stricker, G. (2004). A consideration of challenges to psychological assessment instruments used in forensic settings: Rorschach as exemplar. *Journal of Personality Assessment, 83*(2), 141–152.

Kane, A. W., & Dvoskin, J. A. (2011). *Evaluation for personal injury claims: Best practices in forensic mental health*. New York: Oxford University Press.

Lilienfeld, S. O., Wood, J. M., & Garb, H. N. (2000). The scientific status of projective techniques. *Psychological Science in the Public Interest, 1*, 27–66.

Mayhew, K. P., Flay, B. R., & Mott, J. A. (2000). Stages in the development of adolescent smoking. *Drug and Alcohol Dependence, 59*(1), 61–81.

Melton, G. B., Petrila, J., Poythress, N. G., Slobogin, C., Otto, R. K., Mossman, D., & Condie, L. O. (2018). *Psychological evaluations for the courts* (4th ed.). New York: Guilford.

Meyer, G. J., & Archer, R. P. (2001). The hard science of Rorschach research: What do we know and where do we go? *Psychological Assessment, 13*, 486–502.

Meyer, G. J. (2016). Neuropsychological factors and Rorschach performance in children. *Rorschachiana, 37*, 7–27.

Meyer, G. J., Viglione, D. J., Mihura, J. L, Erard, R. E., & Erdberg, P. (2011). *Rorschach performance assessment system: Administration, coding, interpretation, and technical manual*. Toledo, OH: Rorschach Performance Assessment System, LLP.

Mihura, J. L., Meyer, G. J., Bombel, G., & Dumitrascu, N. (2015). Standards, accuracy, and questions of bias in Rorschach meta-analyses: Reply to Wood, Garb, Nezworski, Lilienfeld, and Duke (2015). *Psychological Bulletin, 141*(1), 250–260.

Mihura, J. L., Meyer, G. J., Dumitrascu, N., & Bombel, G. (2013). The validity of individual Rorschach variables: Systematic reviews and meta-analyses of the comprehensive system. *Psychological Bulletin, 139*(3), 548–605.

Noll, J. G., Trickett, P. K., & Putnam, F. W. (2003). A prospective investigation of the impact of childhood sexual abuse on the development of sexuality. *Journal of Consulting and Clinical Psychology, 71*(3), 575–586.

Pollack, D. (2015). Understanding sexual grooming in child abuse cases. *American Bar Association, 34*(11), 165–168.

Sewell, K. W. (2008). Dissimulation on projective measures. In R. Rogers (Ed.), *Clinical assessment of malingering and deception* (3rd ed.). New York: Guilford Press.

Society for Personality Assessment. (2005). The status of the Rorschach in clinical and forensic practice: An official statement by the Board of Trustees of the Society for Personality Assessment. *Journal of Personality Assessment, 85*, 219–237.

Sugarman, S. D. (2000). A century of change in personal injury law. *California Law Review, 88*(6), 2403–2436.

Terr, L. (1990). *Too scared to cry: Psychic trauma in childhood.* New York: Harper & Row.

Van der Kolk, B. A., & Ducey, C. P. (1989). The psychological processing of traumatic experience: Rorschach patterns in PTSD. *Journal of Traumatic Stress, 2*(3), 259–274.

Viglione, D. J., Towns, B., & Lindshield, D. (2012). Understanding and using the Rorschach inkblot test to assess post-traumatic conditions. *Psychological Injury and Law, 5*(2), 135–144.

Wood, J. M., Garb, H. N, Nezworski, M. T., Lilienfeld, S. O., & Duke, M. C. (2015). A second look at the validity of widely used Rorschach indices: Comment on Mihura, Meyer, Dumitrascu, and Bombel (2013). *Psychological Bulletin, 141*(1), 236–249.

Wood, J. M., Lilienfeld, S. O., Garb, H. N., Nezworski, M. T. (2000). The Rorschach test in clinical diagnosis: A critical review, with a backward look at Garfield (1947). *Journal of Clinical Psychology, 56*, 395–430.

Wood, J. M., Nezworski, M. T., & Stejskal, W. J. (1996). The comprehensive system for the Rorschach: A critical examination. *Psychological Science, 7*, 3–10.

Wood, J. M., Nezworski, M. T., & Stejskal, W. J. (1997). The reliability of the comprehensive system for the Rorschach: A comment on Meyer. *Psychological Assessment, 9*(4), 490–494.

10   Interviewing Children about Sexual Abuse

Jacqueline Singer

It is difficult to determine the rate of sexual abuse. In 2002, the World Health Organization (WHO) estimated 73 million boys and 150 million girls under the age of 18 years had experienced some form of sexual violence. A meta-analysis conducted in 2009, which included 65 studies from 22 countries, estimated 7.9% of males and 19.7% of females were victims of sexual abuse prior to the age of 18 years (Singh et al., 2014). The National Child Abuse and Neglect Data Systems estimates 8.8% of children were sexually abused in the United States (Miller et al., 2007) whereas a report authored by Advocates for Youth estimated 1–3% annually (Conklin, 2000) and Freyd et al. (2005) estimated 20% of women and 5–10% of men have reported sexual abuse as a child. Direct experience of sexual victimization by children has been estimated to be 1 in 12 (Finkelhor et al., 2005; Finkelhor et al., 2013). Rates of false allegations also vary depending upon the way abuse is defined, the data source and the context. As O'Donohue, Cummings and Willis (2018) note,

> methodological problems such as unclear or invalid criteria used to judge truth or falsity of an allegation, unrepresentative samples, and ignoring important contextual variables such as the stage at which an allegation is made, currently all render the determination of actual rates of false child sexual abuse allegations to be unknown. (p. 459)

While they concluded the vast majority of allegations are true, false allegations range from 2% to 5%, with false reporting occurring at a much higher rate in child custody disputes.

Cases involving allegations of sexual abuse are complex just by their very secret nature. Not only is sexual abuse rarely witnessed but physical findings on medical exam are often nonexistent (Heger et al., 2002). As noted by Block and Williams (2019), less than 5% of sexual abuse cases have medical evidence available. It is not often that photos or videos of the abuse exist or that perpetrators confess. Typically, it is "soft psychosocial evidence," (Herman, 2009) that is gathered to prove abuse occurred. This includes the child's verbal statements, the quality of the child's narrative and his or her non-verbal behavior understood within the psychosocial context of the child's report, and the psychosocial history of the child and others who are involved in the case.

While false reports occur infrequently, they can be made by adults or children. False reports are more likely to be made in the context of divorce (see Faller, 2007b for review) but not all are conscious attempts to seek vengeance against an ex-spouse. False reports can be due to mental illness in a parent, a parent who has a genuine belief the abuse has occurred, misinterpretation of a child's normal sexual behavior, poor parental boundaries and enmeshment with the child, psychological disturbance in a child, misinterpretation of behavior by the child, exposure to sexual overstimulating but non-abusive situations, difficulty distinguishing reality from fantasy, social desirability in responding, poor interviewing techniques or wanting to punish a parent (Faller, 2007b). False positives, that is

DOI: 10.4324/9780429397806-11

when an allegation is found to be true when it is not (Herman & Freitas, 2010), can lead to the loss of a relationship between the child and the alleged abuser and loss of liberty for the accused, and in the cases of familial abuse allegations create significant psychological consequences for the child, the accused parent and even siblings.

However, false negatives can also occur. That is, an allegation is not found to be credible when in fact abuse did occur. Studies in which there was a confession (Sorenson & Snow, 1991), compelling medical evidence (Lyon, 2007; Sorenson & Snow, 1991), or audiovisual evidence of sexual abuse (Sjoberg & Lindblad, 2002) but no disclosure by a child suggest false negative rates are higher than false positive rates (Faller, 2007a). Non-disclosure rates have found to vary considerably, from 33 to 92% for women (Bagley & Ramsey, 1986; Finkelhor et al., 1990; London et al., 2005; Russell & Bolen, 2000) and 42 to 88% for men. (Finkelhor et al., 1990; Johnson & Shrier, 1985; London et al., 2005). In the case of false negatives, a child can be left unprotected from an abuser, and in addition to potential future abuse, the child can experience feelings of helplessness in a system that could not provide protection.

Challenges with memory and suggestibility, source monitoring, coaching, the child's level of cognitive development and language skills, and the complex dynamics of family systems can make these cases challenging for professionals. It is essential to consider multiple hypotheses in these investigations. This chapter will provide an overview of concepts that impact child abuse investigations and then provide case examples gathered from different venues which illustrate various aspects of understanding children's statements. No case presented in this chapter is meant to include all aspects of the investigation or analysis but will be used to illustrate some of the concepts important to interviewing children in sexual abuse cases and the factors that may influence their statements. Each case example is an amalgam of cases evaluated or reviewed by this author.

Standards of Proof

Allegations of sexual abuse can present themselves in several court venues. For cases that result in criminal charges in either adult or juvenile proceedings, it must be proven beyond a reasonable doubt that the allegations are true. In juvenile dependency cases, children can be removed from their parents' care if there is substantial risk of danger and no reasonable means to protect without removal and come under the jurisdiction of the juvenile court by a preponderance of the evidence. Clear and convincing evidence is the standard of proof for a juvenile petition to be sustained and parental rights to be terminated. In family law cases, child custody determinations are made by a preponderance of the evidence.

Regardless of the standard of proof[1] required in any of these jurisdictions, the child's statements are often the only "proof" of the allegation and those gathering this evidence by interview of the child must ensure that interviewing methods are sound and that factors which may affect the child's statement have been considered. This chapter is not meant to be a substitute for the excellent chapters on memory and suggestibility in this volume (see Chapters 3 and 4, this volume), nor will it be a thorough review of sound interviewing practices that can be found in a number of publications (Lamb et al., 2007; Lamb et al., 2008; Lamb et al., 2018). This chapter is not meant to be a guide to conducting interviews in a multidisciplinary team interview setting but rather will provide guidance on sound interviewing practices, and discuss how context, suggestibility, memory and source monitoring may impact a child's statements. Additionally, I will consider the complexity of the case dynamics and the development and testing of multiple hypotheses as a way of understanding how to evaluate the allegations presented and determine their likely veracity to ensure that innocent people are not wrongly punished and adequate protections are put in place for children who need them. This chapter will look at cases in adult and juvenile criminal court, juvenile dependency proceedings, and family court settings where allegations of sexual abuse have been made.

Interviewing Practices

While there are many interviewing protocols being used in sexual abuse cases (see APSAC Advisor, September 2020 for a review of protocols), the National Institute of Child Health and Human Development (Lamb et al., 2008; Orbach et al., 2000) developed an interviewing protocol[2] that has become the gold standard for interviewing children when there are allegations of sexual abuse in that its scripted approach allows for fewer interviewer errors. The protocol is used to elicit a narrative account of events from the child. There are 11 stages of the NICHD interview. The revised NICHD protocol[3] (RP) (Hershkowitz et al., 2013; Lamb et al., 2018), emphasizes rapport building, the identification of signs of reluctance, and the provision of nonsuggestive, supportive comments. Rapport building promotes the child's comfort, trust, and cooperation and precedes, rather than follows, an explanation of the ground rules. Interviewers express interest in the child early in the interview and offer supportive but nonsuggestive comments geared toward promoting rapport, reinforcing the child's efforts, offering emotional support and encouragement, and helping the child see the interviewer as trustworthy. The RP calls for rapport building and narrative practice to occur first. Narrative practice might include asking the child about events unrelated to the allegations, such as describing a holiday or birthday celebration, or activities done over the prior weekend or that day at school. This stage teaches the child to understand what is expected, to respond to open-ended questions and to provide details in his or her response. Next, the child is asked to promise to tell the truth, to correct the interviewer if something is misstated and to tell the interviewer if a question is not understood or the child does not know the answer. Additional rapport building and training of episodic memory (memory for specific events) precedes the substantive phase of the interview when the child is asked questions about the allegations, starting with open-ended questions (invitations) and using information provided by the child to ask follow-up prompts with close-ended or specific questions being asked only at the end of the interview after disclosures have been made. The use of anatomical dolls is not incorporated in the NICHD protocol because they have been demonstrated to create high rates of both false positives and false negatives for young children (Bruck et al., 2000; Lamb et al., 1996; Thierry et al., 2005). Anatomical (human figure) drawings may be used but only after verbal inquiry (Aldridge et al., 2004).

As a professional who is interviewing children, knowledge of proper interviewing protocols is essential. In most circumstances, interviewers do not know if a child has been abused, but pressure on a non-abused child can lead to false allegations (Ceci & Bruck, 2006) as can coercive interviewing techniques including stereotype induction (convincing the child the alleged abuser is bad), the use of authority (informing the child of the parent's statements) (Saywitz et al., 2018) and repetition of suggestive questions.

While many investigative interviews follow NICHD procedures, the questions of "first responders," that is teachers, parents, grandparents, friends or untrained social workers, therapists and police officers are unlikely to be guided by these principles. Further, prosecution or defense counsel can question children in a way that either makes prior credible testimony appear confusing or noncredible statements seem true. Children are susceptible to leading questions or suggestions that may come from an unskilled interviewer, an anxious parent or a biased questioner. The influence on children by unskilled interviewers creates challenges for understanding the child's statements. Tracking the disclosures a child has made and to whom they were made is an essential part of the investigation of sexual abuse allegations.

Interviews of children can be contaminated by first responders, including parents, friends or family members and professionals (therapists, doctors, social workers, teachers). This contamination can never be undone as questions, suggestions or statements can be incorporated into the child's memory of the experience (Hritz et al., 2015). If there is concern about sexual abuse, the child should be asked to state what happened and questions, if asked, should be open-ended (tell me what happened; tell me more), not leading, and only enough to determine if a report to child protective services should be made. Parents should listen but not ask questions until after forensic interviews have occurred, and even then should limit discussion of issues as cases may require additional forensic interviews or go to trial when the issue of influence, coaching or challenges with source monitoring are alleged.

Context

A child's disclosure of sexual abuse can be impacted by the child's age and personality characteristics, developmental and cognitive functioning and the cultural, familial and socioeconomic environments. The interpretation of statements or behaviors of a child by a care provider who may have heightened anxiety or concern regarding sexually inappropriate behavior of the alleged perpetrator can also influence disclosures. Sometimes, children's normal sexual curiosity, or even a child's normal reaction to stress, such as bedwetting, nightmares, sexualized, clingy or regressive behavior can be misinterpreted as a sign of sexual abuse (Kuehnle & Connell, 2009). Additionally, children can be influenced to recant an allegation by a non-protective care provider. Children's responses to sexual abuse are not predictable, nor do they present with a symptom picture that easily identifies them as a victim of sexual abuse. Children, depending upon their age, can be reliable reporters of events, but those who are younger or who have cognitive or developmental delays can show difficulty in recounting events and are more susceptible to suggestion or leading questions. Finally, without an understanding of developmentally normative sexual behavior in children (see Friedrich et al., 1998; Poole & Wolfe, 2009; Kenny & Wurtele, 2013), a parent can become concerned, especially if other factors exist, such as a parent's use of pornography, or a child custody dispute which can then result in leading questions and accusations which in turn impact the lives of both the child and the alleged perpetrator. For juvenile perpetrators, understanding the context of their behavior can also provide important information related to rehabilitation and treatment.

In addition to considering developmentally normative sexual behavior in children, cultural views regarding sexuality and acculturation must be considered (Meston & Ahrold, 2010). Not only can these views affect how certain behaviors are interpreted but cultural views can also affect how or whether reports of sexual abuse are made (Fontes, Cruz, & Tabachnick, 2001; Fontes, 2008). Finally, how a child reacts to the trauma of the alleged abuse must be examined when evaluating a child's ability to disclose or provide a coherent narrative about abuse. Trauma responses may affect a child's willingness to report (Ziegler, 2002) or the memory for events (Feiring & Taska, 2005; Fivush, Peterson, & Schwarzmueller, 2002).

Memory and Suggestibility

An excellent review of children's memory can be found in this volume (Baker-Ward, Ornstein & Thomas, Chapter 3). There are some important issues to highlight for this chapter on child interviews in sexual abuse cases. While infants can encode olfactory, visual and auditory memories, their ability to retrieve verbally these experiences is not supported by their level of cognitive development. That is, the ability to report events which occurred before a child is verbal are likely to be sparse and contain errors. Once children can speak, they can provide information about events or issues related to themselves. By the age of 3 or 4, children can recall both recent and distant events, provide information in response to open-ended questions and answer more focused queries. The amount of information children are able to provide increases with age. By early adolescence, narratives can include context, sequence and reflection.

While there is research to suggest children can provide accurate account of events, (Saywitz et al., 2018), the issue of suggestibility must be considered when evaluating children's statements. Ceci and Bruck (1993) define suggestibility as "the degree to which children's encoding, storage, retrieval, and reporting of events can be influenced by a range of social and psychological factors" (p. 404). Even one suggestive interview can have an impact on children's reporting and memory of events. While suggestibility decreases with age (Ceci et al., 2007) and younger children are more susceptible to misleading suggestions and false memories, there is variation within age groups (see Hritz et al., 2015 for review). Bruck and Melnyk (2004) synthesized the results of 69 studies which examined demographic, cognitive and psychosocial factors and children's suggestibility. There were no consistent findings related to race, socioeconomic status or gender, though children with limited cognitive ability were more susceptible to suggestion. At the same time, children age 5 to 8 who were highly creative were more likely to be suggestible, creating elaborate narratives for suggested events. Language ability may also affect suggestibility in younger children, with increased language ability being correlated with increased resistance to suggestion. When examining psychosocial factors, greater risk for suggestibility was found in children with poor self-concept, children who had unsupportive relationships with either parent, and children whose mothers had an insecure attachment in their romantic relationships. Finally, cultural factors should be considered as some children may be hesitant to disclose due to fear of the consequences of disclosure or may provide information they believe the interviewer wishes to hear in order to terminate an uncomfortable conversation (Fontes & Plummer, 2010; Hritz et al., 2015). Further, cultural issues can impact perceptions about locus of control, the experience of the basic social unit, time orientation, communication style, information sharing and view of authority figures (Fontes, 2008,), all of which may have an impact on a child's disclosures.

Source Monitoring

Johnson (2006) in her article *Memory and Reality* recounts a story from her childhood which, it turns out, was a mixture of her own experience and her imagination. Source monitoring refers to a cognitive process by which individuals attribute mental events to their origins, that is, from what source an experience is derived. As children are questioned about sexual abuse experiences, they must be able to differentiate between their own experience of the events and memories that come from other sources. Baker-Ward, Ornstein and Thomas (this volume, Chapter 3, pp. 22–26) discuss the influence that conversations with others including, for example, a parent, therapist, social worker, police officer or peer can have on the child's understanding, memory and recall of events. According to Lindsay (2008)

> "Source" is a multidimensional construct that includes (a) the environmental context in which a past event occurred (e.g., Did X happen at work or at home?), (b) an event's temporal context (e.g., Did X happen yesterday or last week? Before or after Y? In the morning, midday, or evening? Summer or fall?), (c) the agents involved in an event

(e.g., Who said X?), and (d) the sensory modalities and media through which the event was encountered (e.g., Did I read the book or see the film? Did I see a knife or only hear mention of a knife?). People quite often experience difficulty in remembering the sources of their recollections. Moreover, they sometimes misremember aspects of a source. (pp. 748–749)

The challenge when interviewing children regarding possible sexual abuse experiences, especially when they have been questioned by others who may have their own views of what occurred, is the child's memory of the events can be influenced by the questions they have been asked (Pezdek et al., 1997), by repeated recounting (Garry & Polaschek, 2000; Loftus & Kaufman, 1992) or by the way in which information provided to the child through suggestion can influence their recollections (Poole & Lindsay, 2001). The questions and the child's responses can then be incorporated into the child's now remembered experience.

Coaching is another factor to consider when examining children's statements about sexual abuse. Beginning in the preschool years, children's ability to lie develops rapidly with age (Lee, 2013) and they can keep secrets or maintain fabricated stories of abuse if coached to do so (Fogliati & Bussey, 2015). While fabricated reports can be detected more easily when children are asked to answer follow-up questions or provide longer narratives (Talwar & Lee, 2002), as coaching time increases, children are able to maintain their fabrication, even when directly questioned, and the longer coaching occurs, the more difficult it is to differentiate false reports from true ones (Talwar et al., 2018). This may be relevant especially in custody cases when false allegations against a parent may result in a loss of custody (Black et al., 2012; Engle & O'Donohue, 2012; Trocmé & Bala, 2005; and Bala et al., 2007).

Developing and Testing Multiple Hypotheses

Equally important is the consideration of multiple hypotheses to explain a child's statements when sexual abuse allegations are made. Kuehnle (1996, p. 4) outlines a series of hypotheses that should be considered in when sexual abuse of a child is alleged.

- The child is a victim of sexual abuse, and the allegation is credible and accurate.
- The child is a victim of sexual abuse, but due to age or cognitive deficits, does not have the verbal ability to provide a credible description of his or her abuse.
- The child is a victim of sexual abuse, but due to fear, will not disclose his or her abuse.
- The child is a victim of sexual abuse, but due to misguided loyalty, will not disclose his or her abuse.
- The child is not a victim of sexual abuse and is credible but has misperceived an innocent interaction.
- The child is not a victim of sexual abuse but has been unintentionally contaminated by a concerned and hypervigilant caregiver or authority figure.
- The child is not a victim of sexual abuse but has been intentionally manipulated by a caregiver or authority figure into believing that he or she has been abused.
- The child is not a victim of sexual abuse but knowingly falsely accuses someone of sexual abuse because of pressure by caretakers or authority figures who believe the child has been abused.
- The child is not a victim of sexual abuse but knowingly falsely accuses someone of sexual abuse for reasons of personal aggrandizement or revenge.

A systematic consideration of possible hypotheses generated based upon the specifics of a case can help evaluators sort through the data gathered during a sexual abuse investigation.

Criminal Case: Did I See It; Did We Play It or Did He Do It?

During a weekend at her father's house, Mia was invited to Kristen's for a sleepover. Kristen, who lives with her dad and little brother, lived next door to Mia's father. Six days later, Mia, a quiet, sweet and innocent 4-year-old who attended the local Waldorf school and had limited exposure to media, told her mom, Linda, she had seen a movie with "penises and butts and penises inside butts and rubbing vaginas." Further, Mia told Linda that Kristen's dad, Rob, asked, "Would you ever do this?" to which Mia responded, "No" and went to bed. Linda asked Mia some questions regarding the movie and determined it was animated pornography. Linda was concerned as she had never trusted her ex-husband to provide adequate supervision for their daughter. The following day, Linda contacted the police and reported she had questioned Mia further and had used puppets and "role played" to further determine what had occurred. Through this role play, Linda determined Rob was wearing pajamas and Mia saw his penis. Linda did not know if more had transpired. According to Linda, Rob went downstairs to take Mia to the bathroom because she was afraid of the dark and when they went back upstairs, he "took her back to the computer where the movie was still playing and told her, 'This is all for you.'" Mia continued to watch the movie and then went to sleep.

A week later, Mia was interviewed by a social worker at the local child advocacy center. A police summary of the interview and the interview itself were available for review. Oftentimes, the discrepant information in these two sources of data (Cauchi & Powell, 2009) can shed light on the way in which perspective or bias can influence how information obtained from children is interpreted and reported. The police report stated Mia "looked up from where she was lying on the floor in the same room and asked the suspect if she could watch what he was watching." She described this as "real and pretend people naked." The "real people were grown up men and women putting their private spots in other private spots." Mia reported she watched this for "a long time." "She first said she did not see any part of the suspect's body, but then admitted his pajama bottoms were 'partway down' and she could see his 'private part.'" She was asked what his private part looked like and she responded, "What he goes to the bathroom with." She also reported Rob asked her if she wanted to do what she was seeing on the computer, to which she replied, "No." Mia circled a penis on a (nude) drawing of a male, when asked what part of Rob she had seen. She could not describe his penis but stated that it was "pointing out." When it was determined that the child was "visibly tired and reluctant to talk," the interview was terminated. The investigative interview was video recorded as is best practice[4] (Kuehnle, 2003).

There is consensus regarding the importance of recording investigative interviews of children (APSAC Taskforce, 2012). Even when experienced interviewers are asked to recall information obtained during child interviews, they are unable to accurately reconstruct information verbatim. Additionally, untrained interviewers often do not rely on open-ended questions, and ask leading questions (Warren & Woodall, 1999). Further, when taking contemporaneous notes, interviewers can misrepresent the statements used to elicit information from children (Lamb et al., 2000). The degree of precision necessary for forensic purposes cannot be obtained without recording. In Mia's case, without recording the initial conversation and then subsequent questioning and role play between Mia and her mother, it is impossible to determine what Mia said or what her mother may have asked that led to Mia's alleged statements. Interviewer bias can also color what the child says. If Mia's mother believed Mia had been inadequately supervised and sexually abused, this could have influenced the questions asked. Secondly, when an interviewer moves beyond free recall into questioning a child directly, the interviewer risks suggesting to the child what the interviewer believes occurred (Saywitz, Goodman, & Lyon, 2002).

It is equally important that those interviewing children including police officers or investigators be trained in proper interviewing techniques. Not only do these techniques improve the quality and informativeness of investigative interviews with children, they also improve dramatically the reliability of the information obtained (Lamb et al., 2007; Lamb et al., 2018). Improperly trained interviewers, including parents, can ask suggestive and leading questions which produce responses that are inaccurate. This can also occur if the interviewer has a preconceived notion about what has occurred. Interviewer bias can affect the questions posed to the child and the responses obtained (Ceci et al., 2007). Statements made by Mia in the video recorded interview may be influenced by information she incorporated from the questions and role play which occurred with her mother creating challenges in determining the source of Mia's information.

A review of the social worker's video recorded interview of Mia tells a somewhat different story from what was reported in the police summary. When Mia was first asked if she ever saw any part of Rob's body she said "No." When asked a second time if Rob ever tried to show her any private part on his body, Mia said, "No." She then stated, "I was almost going to say yes, but said no." Since she had taken a long time to answer, the interviewer asked her what she was thinking about when she took so long to answer, to which Mia replied she was thinking about her brother, what he does to her and that he hit her and broke her doll leg. Near the end of the interview, Mia was asked, "Did Rob ever try to show you his private part" to which she responded, "No." She was then asked, "Did you talk with your mommy about Rob's pajama pants being down – like down around his legs or part way down?" To which Mia replied, "Part way down." When asked what she saw, she said "his private part." The interviewer asked four times "what did it look like" but did not get a response. When asked if there was anything Mia could tell her about Rob's private part she said, "No." The interviewer asked a number of questions related to Rob's pants being "part way down." To this series of questions, Mia's only response to "did you see his pants come part way down?" was "Yeah, just a second." When Mia was asked, "The whole time you were watching the computer, how were Rob's pants?" she replied, "Brown." She was then asked, "Were they part way down the whole time?" Mia replied, "No, yeah, I came over there. He said, 'Do you want to try that?' And I said no." Finally, Mia was asked if Rob touch his own private part, and she responded, "No."

Twelve days later, Mia was interviewed at the advocacy center a second time. Mia told the social worker her mom wanted her to come back and talk. She and her mom were at her grandparents' house where they talked about Rob. Mia told the social worker her mother wanted to have the meeting "so I could remember to say it to you." Mia told the interviewer she does not see Kristen anymore "because Rob did the bad thing." Mia then recounted the events which she and the interviewer previously discussed referring to them as "the real thing." In this description, Mia reported she went downstairs to use the bathroom and Rob pulled down his pants. Rob then went downstairs, pulled back up his pants and he said, "This is all for you" and then she fell asleep.

When asked, "Did you see Rob pull down his pants?" Mia nodded yes, then shook her head no, and then responded "no" when the question was asked again. When asked when Rob said, "This is all for you," Mia replied it was when she finished going to the bathroom. She was asked a series of questions to try and establish when and why Rob pulled up his pants including "Why was he going downstairs?" and "What was he doing when he went downstairs?" to which Mia replied it was "to clean up his milk." Information regarding the milk had not been shared during the first interview. After further questioning, Mia reported Kristen was spinning in a chair which made a glass break and the milk spill. Mia was not able to clarify if the glass broke before or after she saw things on the computer, stating "after, before" twice, though Mia reported she neither saw the glass break nor the milk spill. As a result of Mia's statements, Rob was charged with annoying and molesting a child under the age of 18.

This case provides examples of a) suggestibility in children, b) interviewer bias and its potential effect on children's recall, c) source monitoring; that is, the ability of children to determine the source of information they provide and how information from various sources can be incorporated into a child's narrative, d) the impact of repeated interviews on children's testimony, e) the ability of interviewers to recall their interviews with children, and f) the impact of maternal questioning on children's testimony.

There are several factors which must be considered in understanding these statements by Mia. First, Mia was 4 years old at the time of this event. As reported by Lamb et al. (2018) younger children typically recall less information about events than older children and they may require more prompts from interviewers which can then result in less accurate accounts. Preschool age children are also more likely to respond to suggestive questions with erroneous responses, though individual differences such as cognitive/intellectual ability, attachment and temperament, fantasy, knowledge, source monitoring, language skills and conversational ability can impact a child's report. Focusing only on fantasy for this analysis, the animated nature of the pornography coupled with the puppet role play Mia engaged in with her mother, create challenges in differentiating the real actions versus imagined components of Mia's report. Further, repeated questions could cause Mia to feel the answer she was giving was wrong and result in her changing her response. While this phenomenon has been studied in laboratory settings and found to be an influence on children's responding (Fivush & Schwarzmueller, 1995), there is also evidence to suggest the impact of repeated questions may be limited (Andrews & Lamb, 2014; La Rooy & Lamb, 2011).

Second, Mia was interviewed multiple times. She was questioned by her mother twice before Mia's first interview at the advocacy center. Mia's mother also used props including puppets and role play to gather further information. She was questioned again at her grandparents' house and interviewed a second time at the advocacy center. Children are susceptible to misleading and suggestive questions (Ceci & Bruck, 1993) and children can incorporate suggestions about salient events after a single interview (Garven et al., 2000). Further, false beliefs can be created even when interviews are only mildly suggestive (Poole and Lindsay, 2001). Repeated interviews can also have an impact on a child's memory and produce false reports (Quas et al., 2007). Repeated demands for retrieval may increase confabulation due to social pressure. While repeated interviews can benefit memory when a to-be-remembered event is true, they can also distort memory when the to-be-remembered event is false (Quas et al., 2007). Repeated questioning can also contribute to a child's suggestibility, and result in the child changing her answers in deference to the adult (Fivush & Schwarzmueller, 1995). Finally, during Mia's interview at the advocacy center, she was asked some questions multiple times and only changed her answer after she was reminded of the source of her response, her conversation with her mom. Source monitoring, that is determining the source of one's information, is also relevant. In this case, sources include Mia's experience, questions by Mia's mother and Mia's imagination which could have been created by the role play in which Mia and her mother engaged. Mia may have confused what happened with what was suggested to her or what she and her mom role played.

Third, Mia's conversations with her mother were not recorded and as such it is unknown what kind of questioning occurred, when the puppets were introduced, and the impact the questions and puppet role play had on Mia. Because Linda's conversations were not audio recorded, it is impossible to determine if questions posed to Mia were leading or repetitive, if the "role play" Mia engaged in with her mother or interviewer bias affected Mia's statements and in what ways this may have been incorporated into Mia's narrative. If Mia's mother believed that Rob was attempting to molest her daughter, the conversation/

questions asked of Mia by her mother could have influenced both Mia's interpretation *and* her experience of events (Poole and Lindsay, 2001). It is unknown how Mia's mother reacted to what she heard and how that might have affected not only her questioning of Mia but Mia's reaction, responses and experience of the events that occurred. Children are susceptible to misleading and suggestive questions (Ceci & Bruck, 1993) and can incorporate suggestions about salient events even after a single interview (Garven, Wood, & Malpass, 2000). A child can accept false information as true and then incorporate into her subsequent memory for an event. This danger is increased if a child cannot distinguish between her memory of the original event and her memory of the suggestive questions. As noted by Lamb, Brown, Hershkowitz, Orbach and Esplin (2018), younger children are more susceptible to providing false information in response to yes/no questions, misleading questions, or suggestions. "Risky questions are even riskier when addressed to children aged 6 and under ..." (Lamb et al., 2018, p. 125).

Information was also available from interviews of Rob and his children who were in the home at the time of these incidents. Rob acknowledged he was watching pornography on the computer at midnight when he thought the children were asleep. He was not sure when Mia awoke, but when she asked, "What is that?" Rob quickly closed the browser and said, "That is not for you." He was wearing pajamas when he took Mia downstairs to use the bathroom. He denies he pulled his pants down, or that he showed Mia his penis. In fact, Rob reported he was mortified when he heard Mia's voice. A glass of milk had spilled earlier in the evening and the glass broke when his daughter was spinning in a chair at the desk and knocked it over. He had gone downstairs to get a towel and cleaned it up. Neither Kirsten nor her older brother reported they were awake when their dad took Mia to the bathroom. The children both recounted the milk spilling and their dad being upset. Neither child had seen anything playing on their father's computer. The police interview suggested Rob showed poor judgment by watching pornography in the room in which the children slept but his behavior was not specifically directed at Mia in a sexual manner.

Finally, there are many confusing statements made by Mia regarding what happened when the milk was spilled, when she went to the bathroom relative to when Rob allegedly showed her his penis, when or whether his pants were down or when he pulled them up, and when she eventually went to sleep. At one point, Mia reported Rob pulled up his pants when he went to get his milk. Was this the same glass of milk that Rob and his children reported was spilled earlier in the evening? These kinds of challenges in temporal sequences are not unusual for a preschool age child (Lamb et al., 2018).

Entertaining alternative hypotheses can guard against selectively reinforcing information that is consistent with a preconceived notion of what has taken place. Rob may have been trying to seduce Mia by showing her pornography and exposing himself. He admits he was watching pornography on his computer when Mia awoke but he may not have intended for her to see it. He may have attempted to close the computer by "clicking" as Mia described in her interview. His robe or his pajama bottoms may have fallen open, but it was unrelated to the pornography or any sexual intent toward Mia, or he may have had an erection from viewing the pornography. The belief that he was trying to lure Mia into sexual activity and expose himself with the intent of seducing, grooming or molesting her can color the way that a parent or an interviewer questions a child.

Unfortunately, because it is impossible to obtain accurate information about conversations Mia had with her mother related to these allegations, it is impossible to determine which of her statements are an accurate recounting of the events of that evening and which are a result of poor or biased questioning leading to poor source monitoring. Mia gives no coherent sequence of events related to that evening. This could be due to developmental factors or because she had just woken and was groggy and confused or because information from her mother's questioning and their role play became part of Mia's story or because Mia blocked out part of what occurred because she experienced it as traumatic. Mia denied during the first three times she was asked in the videotaped interview seeing Rob's penis. It was not until Mia was reminded about her conversations with her mother that Mia said she saw it, though the information she gave about his penis was limited. Regardless, one must keep in mind that Mia's statements, even in the formal interview were subject to suggestion by Mia's mother and may not be accurately reported. In a case with this kind of fact pattern, it is impossible to know precisely which events occurred. Expert testimony in this case must focus on the factors that could have influenced the child's statements. Ultimately, these issues will affect the weight given to Mia's testimony.

Juvenile Criminal Proceedings: I Don't Remember

In juvenile criminal cases the focus is on rehabilitation and intervention for the perpetrator which must be balanced against community safety.[5] It is important to consider the totality of circumstances when determining the most appropriate interventions and placements. The following case provides examples of individual and cultural issues which can impact a juvenile's sexual behavior and how this information is used in making recommendations about treatment. For a further review of issues that impact immigrant children see Hass' chapter (8) in this volume.

Bastian was a 16-year-old refugee from El Salvador who was arrested after his parents contacted a local counseling center to express concern because they found Bastian lying on top of his 7-year-old sister who later reported that Bastian had touched her vagina. His parents were home during the incident and his mother saw Bastian getting off the bed and pulling up his pants when she walked into the bedroom. Bastian had suffered a significant head injury four years prior when he was run over by a motorcycle in El Salvador after he refused to be "jumped in" by a gang, a ritual whereby a number of members of the gang attack the new member and expect him to fight back (Taylor, 2013). He was comatose for 5 days, suffered severe traumatic brain injuries including impairment to the frontal lobe, and received treatment for two years while in El Salvador. His father described Bastian as "suspended in a different age, not 16, due to the accident."

Bastian was a tall, muscular handsome boy who presented much younger than his chronological age. He ran to hug his father after my interview with him and then lay his head on his father's shoulder. He was described as socially isolated and doing poorly in school. He was inattentive and distractible, could be impulsive according to his parents, and often had to be reminded to keep his hands to himself. During our interview, he would lose focus, often smiled despite the seriousness of the topics being discussed and flapped his hands. He had trouble following directions. Bastian's father had been asking for help since Bastian came to the United States approximately one year ago. He had been living in El Salvador with his maternal aunt and grandmother. His parents had come to the United States when Bastian was five years old. Bastian arrived in the United States after a perilous, two-month journey from El Salvador, having been transported by a coyote. Bastian struggles with short- and long-term memory, is not left alone by his parents and speaks little English. He had been evaluated by a neuropsychologist the year prior who documented his cognitive challenges.

Bastian was referred for a forensic evaluation as there were questions about his understanding of his actions and his Miranda Rights and whether he would be able to assist counsel. Bastian was interviewed with the assistance of a certified Spanish speaking translator. Despite the use of an interpreter in Bastian's native language, questions often had to be repeated and he did not always have a good understanding of what was being asked.

Bastian could not remember being interviewed by the police regarding the sexual assault of his sister and was unable to answer some basic questions. For example, when asked what school he attended, he incorrectly reported "Santa Clara," the city in which he lived. He could not state in what year he was born and his issues with verbal comprehension were evident. He would take only elements of a statement he understood and then confabulate an answer. He recalled some aspects of his time in El Salvador but other aspects he did not. His responses about what he should do clearly came from what he had been told. For instance, when asked at what age boys should have sex, Bastian stated, "I would say when you are over the legal age." When asked what age that was, he reported 18 or 20. When asked what age a girl should be, he said he imagined the same. While he acknowledged he was lying on top of his sister, he said he was giving her a "hug." He did not recall touching his sister's vagina or having his pants down but he did recall his parents told him he needed "psychology" and "help."

Bastian seemed to have some understanding that having sex with a 7-year-old would be wrong but it is unclear if he could apply this knowledge to a real-life situation. When asked if he thought having sex with a 7-year-old would be good or bad, right or wrong, at first he said he did not know and then he said, "I would imagine it would be a bad thing," stating he had been told so by his parents. While Bastian acknowledged he was forced to have sex with a prostitute in El Salvador, it was unclear if his behavior toward his sister was intentionally sexual or driven by poorly controlled impulses, secondary to his head trauma given his lack of recall of the events surrounding his actions, his cognitive impairment, his challenges with receptive speech, and his emotional immaturity.

Bastian's understanding of his Miranda Rights was evaluated using the Miranda Rights Comprehension Instrument (MRCI) (Goldstein et al., 2014). Bastian was unable to provide an explanation, in his own words, for any of the Miranda statements. He did not know what a "right" was. He stated, for example, "Anything you say can be used against you" meant "What I say can be bad or something like that." He claimed he did not have an attorney and did not know what "You have a right to talk to a lawyer before we ask you any questions" means. When asked what "If you cannot afford an attorney, one will be appointed for you" means, he responded, "The attorneys from here, I don't know if they really help anybody." When asked again, he said he did not know what it meant and repeated that he did not have an attorney. Additionally, when questioned by the police investigator about his Miranda Rights the word "court" was translated as "un tribunal," a word Bastian did not know. Out of 10 points for comprehension of Miranda Rights, Bastian received 1. He scored 0/32 for the Miranda Rights vocabulary. He could not correctly define any words and gave the following definitions to the words noted: consult (a consultation when you are sick and they take you to the hospital), questioning (it means you have to reply to them; when you don't know something and another person is asking questions to another person who is a specialist and they would know the answer), right (a person who uses their right hand), advice (an object), appoint (give a name to someone), represent (now). When examples were given to test his comprehension, Bastian used the example and then confabulated a response from the example.

When questioned by the police, Bastian was asked: (translated from Spanish), "Quickly in Spanish, I want to read this to you. You have the right to not say anything. Anything that you say can and will be used against you in court. You have the right to speak to an attorney and to have an attorney present before and during the questioning. If you cannot afford an attorney, one will be appointed for you, totally free, to represent you before and during questioning, if you wish. Do you understand each of these rights that I have just explained to you? Yes or no?" And Bastian responded "Yes." Despite his response, Bastian did not understand these rights, nor were they explained to him.

Regarding competence, Bastian was interviewed using the Juvenile Adjudicative Competence Interview (JACI) (Grisso, 2005). His responses suggest he had no recollection of the crime of which he was accused, did not understand the legal process, did not understand the roles of the different attorneys, the probation officer or the judge (he listens and tells you what to do), could not help his attorney and could not make decisions as they relate to his case. He stated, "They always tell me I did something but I have no idea what I did." He did not recall touching his sister and reported he did know what "private part" means. At the time, he would not have thought it was a serious offense but reports he was told by his father that it is. He believed using a gun in a crime or stealing gum from a store would both be more serious offenses than touching his sister. He understood in a very rudimentary way why he might go before a judge (to find out if I did something wrong, but I don't know why I am here). He believed it is more "dangerous" to be in court than to be in the principal's office at his school. He did not know what pleading guilty was or what happens if you do so, noting "I have not been to court before." He did not understand the difference between a not guilty plea and the act committed nor did he understand punishments for guilty pleas. When asked why he had been in juvenile hall, he reported that "They said I did something but I have no idea." He did not understand what a plea bargain was. For example, when asked why a prosecutor would offer a lighter sentence if you plead guilty (keep in mind, Bastian does not know what a prosecutor does or what pleading guilty means), he replied, "Somebody could do something they didn't know what they were doing." Regardless of the question, Bastian had no capacity to apply a concept beyond his own situation, and responded, if he understood at all, as if it were directly related to him. When explanations were given in order to teach the concept, he would weave these details into his own recounting. Even with a translator, Bastian would not be able to understand a legal proceeding.

Challenges in this case included Bastian's cognitive and memory challenges and cultural and language differences. Bastian's cognitive and memory challenges preexisted the current allegations and appear consistent with his difficulty remembering what occurred. Lamb et al. (2008) provide guidelines for interviewing youthful suspects (see Appendix 3, pp. 305–315). Further, Bastian's history of head injury which caused frontal lobe impairment may impact his impulse control. It is not uncommon for juvenile perpetrators to initially deny their actions (Barbaree & Cortoni, 1993) and though denial is not a risk factor for reoffence in juvenile sex offenses per se (Worling & Långström, 2006), all issues related to risk factors for recidivism, including impulsivity should be explored (Riser, Pegram, & Farley, 2013).

Additional challenges in this case were a product of language and cultural differences as well as the multiple traumas experienced by Bastian. Fontes (2008) provides guidelines for preparing the interpreter for the interview. Especially in forensic interviews, it is important for a verbatim interpretation of both the questions and the responses, without modifying the level of language skills or the words used. It is necessary to consider how culture affects all aspects of the interview including building rapport, non-verbal communication, language competency, bilingualism and its impact on language and memory, cultural issues which may affect communication style, word choice, self-disclosure, deference to authority or other factors. Bastian's trauma may also impact his episodic and emotional memory resulting in challenges in his ability to recall and report his actions.

While this case involved interviewing an adolescent in a juvenile criminal proceeding about allegations of sexual abuse, it is important to note that the goal of juvenile criminal court, unlike an adult criminal proceeding, is rehabilitation of the minor through appropriate intervention as warranted by the circumstance. In this case, determining if Bastian was a danger to his community and what interventions would be appropriate under the circumstance were some of the goals of this assessment. Consideration was given to whether Bastian's intent was sexual or whether his behavior was a function of poor impulse control due to his frontal lobe impairment. Treatment must focus on teaching Bastian the difference between appropriate and inappropriate behavior by repetitive instruction, enlisting the cooperation of Bastian's parents to supervise Bastian's contact with his sister, and providing education to her about her brother's condition and appropriate boundaries in order to ensure her safety. Due to Bastian's trauma, his lack of understanding of English and his cognitive delays, placement in a treatment program is unlikely to serve the purpose of rehabilitation as Bastian's ability to learn new information would be further hampered by his confusion and the potential trauma he would experience by being removed from his family and placed in a facility.

Juvenile Dependency Case: It's All a Lie

In juvenile dependency cases, children can be interviewed multiple times prior to formal interviews. Police or child protective services may be involved. The children may tell their story to teachers, grandparents, their appointed attorneys or their foster parents. Source monitoring can be a challenge. Additionally, the environment in which these children reside is often complicated by domestic violence, drug use and neglect, multiple contacts with child protective services or police over the course of their lives, and sometimes prior removals from their home making these children wary of authority figures and afraid if they make a disclosure, they will never be able to see their parents again.

Melissa, age 8, and her sister Karen, age 11 were removed from their parents' care as a result of neglect due to the unsanitary conditions in the home, and alcohol and cocaine abuse by both their mother and father. After their placement in foster care, both Melissa and Karen told another teen in the foster home that their father had given them white powder and made them drink vodka. They were also hit with sticks by their father and kicked in the stomach by their mother. Karen was told she was a "slut" and a "whore" who deserved to be beaten. Both girls were told if they said anything, they would be beaten "even harder."

The girls also reported their father exposed them to pornography. Both girls disclosed he would kiss them on their mouths, hold them down and make them watch. Karen reported her parents would "do nasty things" while watching the pornography. When her father caught her watching them, he made her watch more pornography and when she tried to cover her eyes, he peeled her hands away. Both girls also told the teen their father would hold them down and "stick his thing in" them. They would scream, "No" and told him it hurt, in hopes he would stop. They further reported he would videotape them doing these things, though he later threw the tape away.

A week after their disclosure to the teen, Karen and Melissa disclosed to the foster parent that their father used to kiss them on the mouth, hold them down and make them watch pornography. Karen said she was scared, embarrassed and ashamed and wrote in her journal: "My dad made us watch porn videos and had [sic] nasty stuff with me and my sister he raped us it was so scary[sic]." She reported he would hold them down one at a time and try to "put his thing" into them and they would cry and say it hurt. Their mother would watch and call them "sluts" and "whores." Melissa recounted similar behavior to her foster mother during a separate interview, stating she was in the room during the incident and that their mother was holding Karen down. Her parents threatened if Karen told anyone she would "get beat."

Karen and Melissa also had interviews with the social worker. Karen also told her social worker her father was watching porn and called Karen and her sister into the bedroom and made them take their clothes off. He then took all his clothes off and lay on top of her. He started kissing her on the lips and then rubbed his body against hers. He put his penis inside of her and it hurt "really bad." Later Karen told her social worker that everything she said was true, except she only had to watch pornography once as a punishment. Karen recalled the incident occurred around Easter time. Her father came to school the next day and brought her lunch.

When Melissa spoke to the social worker, she wanted to know if the social worker knew what happened to Melissa and her sister. She wanted to know if they had already spoken to her sister because Melissa did not want to talk about it and said it was embarrassing. When asked what was embarrassing, Melissa said she was referring to, "What my dad did to us" and when asked to elaborate she said, "He raped us." Melissa explained her father held Karen down and laid on top of her. Melissa was also on the bed and her mother was holding Karen down. Melissa thought her dad was wearing underwear. Melissa did not want to share more, stating she had already told her foster mom what happened.

Eleven weeks after their initial disclosure to the teen in the foster home, the children were interviewed at the local advocacy center. The interview was conducted using the NICHD protocol. A practice narrative and a promise to tell the truth were followed by open-ended questions and then follow-up questions asking when and where. The interviewer was not suggestive, did not repeat questions nor were forced choice or yes/no questions asked. Karen's disclosure was spontaneous. She reported she had been sexually abused by her father, providing details which were consistent with her prior reports. Karen was upset when describing what had happened to her and reported she did not wish to return home. Melissa's interview was conducted by the same interviewer using the NICHD protocol. Melissa was a reluctant participant. Her narrative in response to an open-ended question was followed by some forced choice questions, though no repeated questions were asked. Melissa told the interviewer she did not want her parents to go to jail and while she disclosed physical abuse, she said her sister made up the sexual abuse because Karen was mad and wanted her parents to get in trouble. Melissa was reluctant to answer questions, claimed the physical abuse only happened once and often said she did not remember or that she did not want to talk about it. Melissa appeared quite agitated during the interview and said she was scared.

A few additional incidents were noted that may be relevant to the relationships in this family and have an impact on assessing these sexual abuse allegations and recantation. Money and earrings were missing from another foster child in the home, and Melissa was watching pornography on someone's cell phone. Karen reported that she saw Melissa give a pair of earrings and $20 to their biological mom after a visit and then Melissa admitted she had stolen these items after previously denying she had done so. Melissa admitted she had been instructed by her mother to steal these items from foster parents' home and give them to her biological mom.

An analysis of this case will focus on Melissa's recantation. From a review of available material, the following issues appear relevant in determining the credibility of the allegations and the recantation. Melissa and Karen's first disclosures of sexual abuse were made to a teen foster child, then to the foster parent and later to the social worker. The foster teen reported Melissa and Karen told her of the abuse when they were all sharing why they had been removed from their birth families and placed in foster care. The teen reported Melissa shared first by reporting what she had witnessed. The foster teen had been removed from her parents' care because her 3-year-old brother suffered broken bones. She had no sexual abuse in her history. The details of the conversation among the girls were, however, unknown. Melissa and Karen could have been influenced by the teen or by each other in their disclosures. They may have been asked leading questions by the teen, or foster mother which could have been incorporated into their memory of events. All these elements would have an impact on the disclosure made during their formal interview. This may be because Melissa and Karen both experienced what was reported or it may be that one child influenced the other to make similar statements. This hypothesis was considered in the analysis of this case.

After the children were removed, both parents were jailed, though the mother was soon released. The mother and children had not had any visits prior to the initial disclosures to the teen and foster mother. By all reports, there was consistency in the children's statements to the teen, foster mother and social worker. No visits with the mother occurred during this time. The children had ten supervised visits with their mother prior to their formal interview. She had to be admonished twice not to speak about the reasons for removal or how unfair it was that the father remained in jail. She blamed both Karen and Melissa for "messing up" the family. She told the girls their father would be out of jail soon and they "better say sorry." She denied entirely any sexual abuse of the children and was hostile to any questions she was asked about the living arrangements in the home including the children's exposure to pornography or sex. Karen's story remained consistent during the advocacy center interview, whereas Melissa recanted. The incident with the earrings suggested the mother had influence over Melissa and her recantation could have been a function of this influence. Further, as research shows, a non-supportive caregiver and domestic violence in the home can also have an impact on recantation (Malloy et al., 2016).

This case is further complicated by neglect, drug and alcohol abuse, physical abuse, and exposure to pornography and adult sexual acts. There appears to be a high degree of chaos in the home. Children are at increased risk for victimization when they live in a home where parents' abilities to nurture and supervise are substantially compromised by violence, substance abuse, poverty, and single-parent status (Finkelhor, 2008; Sedlak & Broadhurst, 1996). Children in families of low socioeconomic status (SES) are twice as likely to be sexually abused than their counterparts in higher-SES homes and are at greater risk for other forms of abuse (Sedlak et al., 2010). Additionally, "parentally abused children with low levels of family support" will exhibit lower disclosure rates and higher recantation rates than other abuse victims (London et al., 2008, p. 38; Lippert et al., 2009; Malloy et al., 2007).

A child's age and how disclosures occur may impact whether a child discloses again during a formal interview. Studies suggest that children who have been questioned by someone about abuse prior to a formal interview are more likely to make a disclosure in the formal interview (Keary & Fitzpatrick, 1994). Additionally, older children who previously disclosed were more likely than younger children to disclose again during formal interview (Ghetti et al., 2002).

Recantation rates range from 23.1 to 27% with the highest rates found in studies where there was the least certainty of the allegations (Malloy et al., 2007; Malloy & Mugno, 2016; Malloy et al., 2016). Recantation may be the result of a child withdrawing a true statement of abuse or a child withdrawing a false statement of abuse (London et al., 2005). Recantation is more likely to occur for a young child abused by a parent figure who lacks support from the non-offending parent or feels the non-offending parent does not believe them (Malloy et al., 2007). Recantations can come from internal or external sources (Lyon & Ahern, 2011). Internal sources include embarrassment and shame, expectations that they would be blamed, or that they would not be believed or helped. External sources include not wanting to upset anyone or wanting to protect the abuser. While it is difficult to differentiate false allegations of abuse from true allegations that have been recanted (Faller, 2003), those children who fully recant tend to be younger, have a closer relationship with the perpetrator and lack maternal support (Faller, 2007b).

Where does this leave an investigation if a child recants? Investigating the issues surrounding the recantation is important (Sites & Southern Regional Children's Advocacy Center, 2017). How detailed was the original disclosure; to whom did the child disclose; and what were the child's demeanor and circumstances at the time of the disclosure? Who did the child recant to and what were the motivations to recant? Did other victims recant at the same time? What role may the family have played in the recantation? When a child recants, it can leave more questions than answers.

In the case of Melissa and Karen, the fact of both children initially reported to the teen in the foster home, the foster mother and the social worker, and Melissa changing her story only after being influenced by her biological mother suggests that this was a recantation of a true allegation of abuse. In order to make recommendations in this case, all case factors must be considered to ensure the children are protected from the abuse and neglect they experienced and reunified with their parents if or when appropriate interventions for remediation have been satisfactorily completed. If a successful criminal case is not brought against the parents, there will need to be a determination about whether reunification with one or both parents is the case plan goal. If it is, the Department of Social Services will start by determining the services required for each member of the family so that the children can reunify. This will include education about proper sexual boundaries and child sexual abuse, appropriate parenting practices including the development of empathy and understanding the impact that their behavior has had on their children, and treatment for other deficits including drug and alcohol abuse and anger management. All services will need to be completed within the statutory time frame which, for example, in California is 12 months for children over the age of 3 who have been removed from their parents.[6] For the children, treatment will need to focus on the trauma they have experienced due to physical and sexual abuse and neglect, in addition to their exposure to domestic violence and drug use by their parents. Both girls will need help to understand their own feelings of anger, guilt, embarrassment, and shame as it relates to their parents' behavior and gain the necessary skills and insight so the cycle of abuse is not repeated.

Child Custody Case: It's a Family Affair

When sexual abuse allegations arise within the context of child custody issues, alienation of a child from the alleged perpetrator, coaching, or misinterpretation of behavior should be explored. When there is a history of parental conflict, visitation refusal or lack of visitation support, all possible explanations for the difficulties in the parent-child relationship should be considered, including possible alienation, and multiple hypotheses should be developed. Additionally, allegations of abuse can give the parent make the allegation a legal advantage as the safety of children must take precedence over all other best interest factors (Brown, 2003).

The parameters of a comprehensive child custody evaluation which includes allegations of sexual abuse are often defined by statue. Among other things, including reviewing the criminal records of both parents, any medical exams of the child, all multidisciplinary interviews, police reports, and child protective service records, comprehensive interviewing of all parties, observation and psychological testing of parents and children are conducted. The facts presented below are only part of a comprehensive evaluation that was conducted on a family where sexual abuse allegations occurred within the context of a child custody dispute. Sally, a 12½-year-old, 7th grade student was reserved when she was seen in my office. Her medium length strawberry blonde hair covered part of her face, and her baggy sweatshirt, her body. She was petite for her age, and presented as a much younger child, reluctant to come into the office without her mother and carrying a teddy bear. She mumbled as she spoke and slouched in the chair as if she did not want to be seen. She answered questions about her relationship with her parents and the allegation she had made about her father as though she was talking about someone else. Her affect was flat, though her mother later reported Sally sequestered herself in her room for three days after our meeting, refusing to eat or speak and mostly sleeping.

Sally's demeanor changed little over the course of the 18 months from her formal interview to her participation in a custody evaluation. When discussing the allegations, she provided her narrative in a matter of fact fashion and without many prompts. She had refused to see her father, Nate, for three months prior to her accidental disclosure to her guitar teacher which ultimately led to a Child Protective Services referral and subsequent interview of Sally. Sally was having a hard time at a lesson and told her teacher she was uncomfortable with her dad who made sexual comments and came into her room when she was dressing which made her feel uncomfortable. When Sally's mother, Megan, was informed by the teacher of Sally's statement, Megan said was dumbfounded. Megan thought she and Sally had an open relationship and that Sally shared freely her feelings and experiences. Megan knew Nate to be insensitive to the children's needs as she had seen this firsthand when Nate and Megan were married. Megan believed little had changed in the five years since their separation. Sally had complained about Nate's treatment of her during visits for the year before her refusal to go, though according to Nate's new wife, they all got along and Sally seemed happy when she was at dad's home. Sally and Megan talked briefly after Sally's disclosure to her teacher, though according to Megan and confirmed by Sally, Sally revealed no more about her father's behavior. Megan called the police.

During Sally's contact with the police officer she told him her father said she had a nice figure and patted her bottom when she walked into the kitchen and this made her uncomfortable. Megan was told these behaviors did not rise to the level of a criminal act. Two months later, Megan called the police again reporting Sally had provided additional details in her journal about Nate's inappropriate behavior toward her. Sally was then referred to the multidisciplinary team for an interview. Megan reported she was still unaware of the extent of Sally's allegations.

During a multidisciplinary interview, Sally revealed the abuse by her father started when she was 5 years old and continued until she refused to go to his home any longer when she was almost 12. Sally recalled her father would let her watch cartoons on his computer. A couple of times, she saw pornography on this computer and she believed her father left it there for her to see. Her father would often take her shopping for clothes and Sally claimed he suggested inappropriate items for her to try. One time, he wanted her to buy a two-piece bathing suit and, on another occasion, he suggested she try on a lacy tank top which Sally found creepy. He told Sally she had a nice figure and she should show it off. She also reported there was a "no door locking" policy in the house and once her father walked into her bedroom when she was changing. Another time, he came in to use the bathroom while she was showering. She could hear him, though she could not see him as the shower curtain blocked her view. Sometimes, she had nightmares and her father would come into her bedroom at night and lie down next to her. There were other times she had dreams he was molesting her and she would go into his room seeking comfort and he would hold her. This also started to make Sally uncomfortable. Her father had been touching her bottom for as long as she could remember but this especially started to bother her when she turned 11. She asked him to stop but he just ignored her pleas. She also reported while she, her dad and her stepmom were watching television, he would touch Sally's thigh, and sometimes his finger touched her private area. This really made her uncomfortable and though she would push his hand away, he kept doing it. The social worker, who listened to the multidisciplinary interview, told Megan that Nate's behavior was a clear sign of grooming and she should file for sole custody and move out of the area. This frightened Megan. A temporary restraining order was issued and Sally began therapy with a therapist who specialized in treating victims of sexual abuse and trauma victims. Sally's therapist, when interviewed, said she believed Nate was a pedophile.

As an overlay to these challenges was the contentious and conflictual relationship between the parents, multiple live-in partners or dating relationships in each parent's home and Nate's remarriage after a brief courtship two years prior. For about six months, Sally complained she did not want to go to Nate's for his scheduled weekends as she was bored, or she said her dad would drag her along to do activities in which he was interested, such as fishing at nearby lakes. She learned to fish when she was 7 but she does not like fishing anymore. When they were home, he made her do art projects or tried to take photos of her and was constantly videotaping her. While Sally liked her stepmom when she and Sally's dad were dating as they would often bake cookies, do craft projects or go out to lunch, Sally now thought her stepmom should stop trying to be her mom by telling Sally what to do. This often led to arguments which ended when Sally retreated to her room.

Sally wanted to stay at her mom's house where she could read, was not forced to go out or do activities in which she was not interested. Sally loved her mom's new boyfriend who never tried to interfere or tell her what to do and did not seem to take up her mom's attention in the way that her stepmom did with her dad. While her mom told Sally she should talk to her dad, her mom also understood and empathized with Sally. After Sally's interview at the advocacy center, Megan told Sally about Megan's own history of abuse by her uncle which started when Megan was 6. Megan had loved her uncle and looked forward to seeing him at monthly family gatherings. He told Megan she was his favorite niece. She would sit on his lap and he would bring her little gifts. He then asked her into another room to play some games, showed her pornography and would grope her. She was told it was "their little secret." When she was 10, he tried to have sex with her but Megan was able to get away. She did not tell anyone about the abuse. Her uncle moved to another state and she saw him rarely. Megan also shared with Sally why she and Nate split up when Sally was 7. Nate was never around on weekends as he had an interest in fishing which led him to leave before dawn on weekend mornings and not return until after dark. He missed Sally's kindergarten graduation as he left on a Friday for a weekend fishing trip, her piano recital in the 1st grade which fell on opening day for the fishing season, and her 6th birthday because he was at a fly fishing tournament. He was so obsessed with fishing that he was rarely around. Megan also told Sally Nate watched pornography and this often resulted in arguments between Megan and Nate. Ultimately, the divorce occurred because Megan found out Nate was having an affair with Sally's teacher. Sally loved this teacher but did not know about the affair.

Nate was an emotionally fragile and highly sensitive man who cried when he talked about the allegations. He often got wrapped up in his feelings and at these times was more concerned about how events affected him than their impact on Sally. He longed for his relationship with his daughter to return to the way it was before her mother started to interfere with their visits. It was around the time Nate married his current wife that Megan often made it impossible for him to see Sally, claiming she did not want to come to his house or that she had other plans. Nate felt he was being replaced. Megan insisted Sally call Megan's new boyfriend "Dad" even though Nate did not ask Sally to call her stepmom "Mom." Nate knew about Megan's history of abuse and he wondered if she was making these allegations against him as another ploy to keep Sally from him. While he admits he watched some pornography during the marriage, he always closed the browser and did not allow Sally to have access to it. When Nate was questioned about Sally's allegations, he had an explanation for each of them. He denied he had ever intentionally showed pornography to Sally or left it open on his computer and said he could not remember the last time he even watched it as he was now, finally, in a sexually satisfying relationship. Sally sometimes had nightmares and Nate could hear her crying. If her door were locked, he could not go into her room to comfort her, so he asked she keep it unlocked. He once walked in on Sally while she was changing. He was embarrassed and apologized. They had one bathroom and, on occasion, Nate would have to use it while Sally was showering, though he does not recall this happening since she was 10. He admits he has touched Sally's bottom frequently, an affectionate pat when she walks into the room and knows she has said "STOP!" but he saw this as the "not so untypical tension" between a father and daughter as she got older and became more embarrassed about her body. While he does not remember specifically putting his hand on Sally's thigh, it would not surprise him if he did. She would often sit next to him, leaning her head on his shoulder, while they watched their favorite television show, Seinfeld.

In the beginning of the 7th grade, Sally cut her hair short and started wearing black. Her classmate started to call her "dyke" and suggested she was a lesbian. Sally did not tell her mom of this treatment by her peers but began to retreat further into reading, stopped going to school events and eventually asked to be home schooled. At the time, it was unclear if Sally was exploring her own sexual identity. After the disclosure to her teacher, Sally started to see a therapist who specialized in trauma and sexual abuse. Sally developed symptoms of anxiety and depression and was placed on medication. She was diagnosed with PTSD by her therapist who told Sally her symptoms were consistent with abuse and she should not have to see her father under any circumstance. Sally's anxiety increased whenever there was a court date, or when she thought about running into her dad. When he sought an evaluation in an attempt to resolve these issues, Sally felt suicidal.

Psychological testing showed Sally's need for external support and approval in order to maintain her self-esteem. She was exploring her sexual identity. She was sensitive to loss and rejection, and dependent on others for support and guidance, yet she was apt to misinterpret others' motives. As circumstances became more complex, Sally's reality testing suffered. She experienced considerable conflict within her relationships, and felt she needed to take sides to protect herself. Her fears created paralysis. Rather than using active coping strategies, she retreated but this only served to increase her anxiety. Sally was influenced by her mother, whom she found to be empathic, and her therapist who supported and believed Sally.

There were a number of factors that complicated Sally's disclosure. Sally reports her abuse spanned a period of seven years starting with exposure to pornography and culminating in being touched inappropriately by her father. It is impossible to determine if Sally's recollection of events has merged certain memories together and given them sexual meaning or if the source of her memories is her own experience, a dream, or something she has been told or was suggested. For example, Sally reports she saw pornography on a computer, then had dreams she was being molesting by her father and sought comfort from him which then made her uncomfortable. Sally does not provide descriptions of the pornography she viewed but her initial viewing seems to coincide with Megan's reports of Nate's watching pornography in the home. It is unclear if Sally's experiences were influenced by seeing the pornography, if her dreams became real for her, if she gave sexual meaning to her father's behavior when the behavior was not intended to be sexual, or if the behaviors she alleges did occur and were sexual in nature. There are things she remembers which have not been confirmed, such as her father insisting she purchase a two-piece bathing suit or a lacy top, or even if they are true, had no sexual intent, or his intentionally leaving pornography on his computer for her to see. Nate admits to almost all of behaviors alleged by Sally but provides a different context for and meaning to them.

There are other confounding factors that make it difficult to determine if Sally's reports are influenced by her mother's sharing details of her own abuse with Sally, the challenges in the marital relationship including father's viewing of pornography and having an extra-marital affair with Sally's teacher or Sally's experience of father's own intense neediness. Further, the dynamics in the family suggest Sally had readily accepted mother's new boyfriend as her father. Issues associated with alienation by Megan were also explored. Mother's knowledge of the sexual abuse perpetrators in father's family and father's own neediness may also have influenced how Megan or Sally viewed Nate. Finally, when a therapist's focus is only on abuse, the therapist has formed an opinion that the abuse has occurred, and determined without evaluating or even meeting the father that he is a pedo-phile, these conclusions could influence and solidify the child's feelings or perceptions about what happened to her.

False allegations of sexual abuse are more common in cases where there are also custody disputes. In Thoennes and Tjaden's study (1990), rates of false allegations varied by age of the child. For children aged 1 to 3 years, 38% of the allegations were false, whereas 44% of the claims were false in children aged 4 to 6 and 29% were false in children 7 years and older. Trocmé and Bala (2005) found 4% of allegations in custody cases to be intentionally fabricated and in more recent studies in which allegations of abuse in families involved in a child custody disputes were examined (Black et al., 2016; Saini et al., 2013), child sex-ual abuse allegations represented approximately 5% of reports to child protective services with the overall rate of malicious allegations ranging from 13 to 25%. However, research has also found that social workers lack training in investigating these challenging cases (Saini et al., 2012) and may believe parental anger fuels these allegations (Brown, 2003), resulting social workers feeling overwhelmed by these cases (Saini et al., 2019).

However, not all false allegations are the same. One must differentiate intentionally false allegations which may stem from a lie by a parent or a child, from suggestive influence by a parent or forensic interviewer, misinterpretation or confabulation of benign experiences, or adult or child psychopathology (O'Donohue et al., 2016). While there is some range of cases that are known to be false (see O'Donohue et al., 2018; and Saini, Laajasalo & Platt, 2020 for reviews), the true rate is unknown and not all reasons for false allegations have been studied. If false allegations in custody disputes include inaccurate memories and false statements which stem from suggestive questioning or socially desirable responding, the rate ranges from 23% to 35% (Ceci & Bruck, 1995), whereas if only calculated lying is considered, the rate of false allegations is around 4% (Trocmé & Bala, 2005).

In this case the following hypotheses were considered: 1) Sally is a victim of sexual abuse, and her allegation is credible and accurate; 2) Sally is not a victim of abuse and is credible but misperceived innocent interactions; 3) Sally is not a victim of abuse but her mother's concerns have contaminated Sally's perceptions; 4) Sally is not a victim of abuse but she has been intentionally manipulated by her mother to believe she was abused; 5) Sally is not a victim of abuse but has falsely accused her father of abuse due to being pres-sured by her mother for purposes of winning in the custody dispute or for revenge. When a clear conclusion cannot be reached, recommendations which address the issues raised in the investigation and offer treatment for the child, the alleged abuser and the family system must be considered. As the rate of the recidivism of sexual offending for incest offenders is low (4.4% to 8.4% for convicted sex offenders) (Hanson, 2002), reoffence is unlikely, especially since there is scrutiny on the family. Understanding the literature related to sex offenders, and incest perpetrators in particular, is also important (Seto, 2018).

Sally's disclosures were made with the backdrop of her exploration of her own identity, her father's remarriage, and the conflict between her parents. She appears extremely dis-tressed when describing Nate's actions and has been paralyzed by her experience of being abused. Her therapist believes she has been molested, though this belief may also be an influencer. There are events Sally has given sexual meaning while the intent of the behavior may not have been sexual in nature, such as her father asking her to keep doors unlocked, his suggesting a two-piece bathing suit, or his holding her when she climbed into his bed after a bad dream. Sally also describes some behaviors by Nate, such as touching her with sexual intent while her stepmom was in the room, which suggests Nate's boundaries are extremely poor or he is brazen, though there is scant evidence to support either of these explanations.

A thorough review of the timeline, disclosures and family system dynamics do not support the hypothesis that Sally was intentionally manipulated or coached by Megan. However, there were aspects of Megan's history which may be relevant and influenced Sally's experiences. Megan was molested by her uncle around the same age Sally alleges the abuse by Nate started and Megan was also shown pornography. After Megan's parents separated, her mother made it difficult for her to see her father. When Megan and Nate separated, Megan felt Sally should be able to decide if she wanted to spend the night at her father's house. There were other indications that Megan was not fully supporting Sally's relationship with her dad, though Megan tried to help Nate to be empathic to how Sally was feeling. In Nate's family, his father had molested his cousin and upon discovery of this, Nate's parents separated. Nate had limited contact with his father. Subsequently, Nate's father committed suicide though Nate did not learn of the reason for his father's death until he was 22 as it, like the sexual abuse, was kept a secret. Nate felt abandoned and experienced trauma as his mother spoke negatively about his father and though Nate understood his father's behavior as unacceptable, he still experienced a profound loss. Nate had a series of relationships after his separation from Megan, which would form quickly and end abruptly as Nate's high dependency needs seemed to overwhelm others. He had always been very affectionate with Sally and his behavior could have been misinterpreted or expressed too intensely and possibly inappropriately. While Megan was angry about the affair which ended the marriage, she now saw Nate as a child molester which could have resulted in her interpreting Nate's past behaviors as sexually inappropriate, thus influencing Sally's experience.

Unfortunately, as can be the case when there are complex dynamics and multiple factors that influence each member of a family and the relationship between the parents, it is sometimes impossible to know if a child has been abused given the multiple influences on the child's statements and ways in which data can be compromised over time (Deutsch, Drozd & Ajoku, 2020). Recommendations must balance the need for protection of Sally, taking into consideration that it is impossible to know if the allegations are in fact true, and the benefits of repairing the familial relationships. Treatment recommendation for Sally must also help her work through the trauma she is experiencing. Sally's treatment should focus on six core areas: 1) Safety, 2) Self-regulation, 3) Self-reflective information processing, 4) Traumatic experiences integration, 5) Relational engagement, and 6) Positive affect enhancement (Cook et al., 2005). A treatment plan may also include improving coparent communication, education around appropriate boundaries within the family, and the introduction of therapeutic visits for Sally and her father where reparation of their relationship can begin in a safe environment where Sally can be assured nothing inappropriate will happen.

Conclusions

Cases involving allegations of sexual abuse are often complex. The stakes are high as false allegations can lead to the disruption of relationships and false negatives can result in children remaining unprotected. Best evidence is frequently a child's statement regarding the abuse. However, these statements can be affected by a number of factors including a child's cognitive development, language skills, conversational ability, temperament, attachment style and personality characteristics, cultural, familial and socioeconomic environments, suggestibility, memory, source monitoring, coaching and pressures to recant. Clinicians and investigators working with these children should be familiar with the factors that impact a child's statements. Standardized interviewing protocols should be used to gather data from children and multiple hypotheses should be considered when evaluating children's statements. Finally, recommendations must be geared toward the specifics of the case and the venue in which they are being investigated.

Notes

1. https://www.hg.org/legal-articles/different-standards-of-proof-6363
2. http://nichdprotocol.com/
3. http://nichdprotocol.com/wp-content/uploads/2013/03/RevisedProtocolTMWH2final-1.pdf
4. 90% of child abuse interviews are video recorded at Child Advocacy Centers. See: Midwest Regional Children's Advocacy Center (MRCAC). 2014. *Key Survey Findings: National Multi-Site Survey of Children's Advocacy Centers*. St. Paul, MN: Author. Available online: www.mrcac.org/wp-content/uploads/2014/02/2013-Key-Survey- Findings.FINAL_.pdf
5. See Wilson, this volume Chapter 1, for further information about the development of the juvenile justice system and the balance between providing protection for society and rehabilitation for the juvenile.
6. See Welfare and Institutions Code: https://leginfo.legislature.ca.gov/faces/codes_displaySection.xhtml?sectionNum=361.5.&lawCode=WIC

References

Aldridge, J., Lamb, M. E., Sternberg, K. J., Orbach, Y., Esplin, P. W., & Bowler, L. (2004). Using a human figure drawing to elicit information from alleged victims of child sexual abuse. *Journal of Consulting and Clinical Psychology, 72*(2), 304–316. https://doi:10.1037/0022-006X.72.2.304

Andrews, S. J., & Lamb, M. E. (2014). The effects of age and delay on responses to repeated questions in forensic interviews with children alleging sexual abuse. *Law and Human Behavior, 38*(2), 171–180. https://doi:10.1037/lhb0000064

American Professional Society on the Abuse of Children (APSAC). (2020). *Forensic interviewing: Critical updates for professionals. APSAC Advisor, 32*(2), 4–91. Retrieved from: https://www.apsac.org/apsac-advisor

American Professional Society on the Abuse of Children (APSAC) Taskforce. (2012). *Forensic interviewing in cases of suspected abuse*. APSAC Practice Guidelines. Retrieved from: https://www.apsac.org/guidelines

Bagley, C., & Ramsey, R. (1986). Sexual abuse in childhood: Psychosocial outcomes and implications for social work practice. *Journal of Social Work and Human Sexuality, 4*, 33–47. https://doi:10.1300/J291v04n01_07

Bala, N., Mitnick, M., Trocmé, N., & Houston, C. (2007). Sexual abuse allegations and parental separation: Smokescreen or fire? *Journal of Family Studies, 13*, 26–56. https://doi:10.5172/jfs.327.13.1.26

Barbaree, H. E., & Cortoni, F. A. (1993). Treatment of the juvenile sex offender within the criminal justice and mental health systems. In H. E. Barbaree, W. L. Marshall, & S. M. Hudson (Eds.), *The juvenile sex offender* (pp. 243–263). New York: Guilford Press.

Black, F., Schweitzer, R., & Varghese, F. (2012). Allegations of child sexual abuse in family court cases: A qualitative analysis of psychiatric evidence. *Psychiatry, Psychology and Law, 19*, 482–496. https://doi:10.1080/13218719.2011.613905

Black, T., Saini, M., Fallon, B., Deljavan, S., Theoduloz, R., & Wall, M. (2016). The intersection of child custody disputes and child protection investigations: Secondary data analysis of the Canadian Incidence Study of Reported Child Abuse and Neglect (CIS2008). *International Journal of Child and Adolescent Resilience, 4*(1), 143–157.

Block, S. D., & Williams, L. M. (2019). The prosecution of child sexual abuse: A partnership to improve outcome. NCJRS. Retrieved from: https://www.ncjrs.gov/pdffiles1/nij/grants/252768.pdf

Brown, T. (2003). Fathers and child abuse allegations in the context of parental separation and divorce. *Family Court Review, 41*, 367–380. https://doi.org/10.1111/j.174-1617.2003.tb00898.x

Bruck, M., & Melnyk, L. (2004). Individual differences in children's suggestibility: A review and synthesis. *Applied Cognitive Psychology, 18*, 947–996. https://doi:10.1002/acp.1070

Bruck, M., Ceci, S. J., & Francoeur, E. (2000). Children's use of anatomically detailed dolls to report genital touching in a medical examination: Developmental and gender comparisons. *Journal of Experimental Psychology: Applied, 6*(1), 74–83. https://doi:10.1037/1076-898X.6.1.74

Cauchi, R., & Powell, M. B. (2009). An examination of police officers' notes of interviews with alleged child abuse victims. *International Journal of Police Science & Management, 11*(4), 505–515. https://doi:10.1350/ijps.2009.11.4.147

Ceci, S. J., & Bruck, M. (1993). Suggestibility of the child witness: A historical review and synthesis. *Psychological Bulletin, 113*(3), 403–439. https://doi:10.1037/0033-2909.113.3.403

Ceci, S. J., & Bruck, M. (1995). *Jeopardy in the courtroom: A scientific analysis of children's testimony.* Washington, DC: American Psychological Association. https://doi:10.1037/10180-000

Ceci, S. J., & Bruck, M. (2006). Children's suggestibility: Characteristics and mechanisms. In R. V. Kail (Ed.), *Advances in child development and behavior, vol. 34: Advances in child development and behavior* (pp. 247–281). Cambridge, MA: Elsevier Academic Press.

Ceci, S. J., Kulkofsky, S., Klemfuss, J. Z., Sweeney, C. D., & Bruck, M. (2007). Unwarranted assumptions about children's testimonial accuracy. *Annual Review of Clinical Psychology, 3*, 311–328. https://doi:10.1146/annurev.clinpsy.3.022806.091354

Conklin, K. Washington DC: Advocates for Youth; 2000. [Last cited on 2020 April 9]. Child sexual abuse. An overview of statistics, adverse effects and prevention strategies. Available from: www.advocatesforyouth.org/storage/advfy/documents/child-sexual-abuse-i.pdf

Cook, A., Spinazzola, J., Ford, J., Lanktree, C., Blaustein, M., Cloitre, M., DeRosa, R., Hubbard, R., Kagan, R., Liautaud, J., Mallah, K., Olafson, E., & van der Kolk, B. (2005).Complex trauma in children and adolescents. *Psychiatric Annals, 35*(5), 390–398.

Deutsch, R., Drozd, L., & Ajoku, C. (2020). Trauma-informed interventions in parent—child contact cases. *Family Court Review, 58*, 470–487. https://doi.org/10.1111/fcre.12483

Engle, J., & O'Donohue, W. (2012). Pathways to false allegations of sexual assault. *Journal of Forensic Psychology Practice, 12*, 97–123. https://doi:10.1080/15228932.2012.650071

Faller, K. C. (2003). *Understanding and assessing child sexual maltreatment.* Thousand Oaks, CA: Sage Publications.

Faller, K. C. (2007a). Coaching children about sexual abuse: A pilot study of professionals' perceptions. *Child Abuse and Neglect, 31*, 947–959. https://doi:10.1016/j.chiabu.2007.05.004

Faller, K. C. (2007b). *Interviewing children about sexual abuse: Controversies and best practices.* New York: Oxford University Press.

Feiring, C., and Taska, L. (2005). The persistence of shame following sexual abuse: A longitudinal look at risk and recovery. *Child Maltreatment, 10*(4), 337–349. https://doi:10.1177/1077559505276686

Finkelhor, D. (2008). *Interpersonal violence series. Childhood victimization: Violence, crime, and abuse in the lives of young people.* New York: Oxford University Press.

Finkelhor, D., Hotaling, G., Lewis, I. A., & Smith, C. (1990). Sexual abuse in a national survey of adult men and women: Prevalence, characteristics, and risk factors. *Child Abuse & Neglect, 14*(1), 19–28. https://doi:10.1016/0145-2134(90)90077-7

Finkelhor, D., Ormrod, R., Turner, H., & Hamby, S. L. (2005). The victimization of children and youth: A comprehensive, national survey. *Child Maltreatment, 10*(1), 5–25. https://doi:10.1177/1077559504271287

Finkelhor D., Turner, H. A., Shattuck, A., & Hamby, S. L. (2013). Violence, crime, and abuse exposure in a national sample of children and youth: An update. *JAMA Pediatrics, 167*(7), 614–621. https://doi:10.1001/jamapediatrics.2013.42

Fivush, R., & Schwarzmueller, A. (1995). Say it once again: Effects of repeated questions on children's event recall. *Journal of Traumatic Stress, 8*(4), 555–580. https://doi:10.1002/jts.2490080404

Fogliati, R., & Bussey, K. (2015). The effects of cross-examination on children's coached reports. *Psychology, Public Policy, and Law, 21*, 10–23. https://doi:10.1037/law0000036

Fivush, R., Peterson, C., & Schwarzmueller, A. (2002). Questions and answers: The credibility of child witnesses in the context of specific questioning techniques. In M. Eisen, J. Quas, & G. Goodman (Eds.), *Memory and suggestibility in the forensic interview* (pp. 331–354). Mahwah, NJ: Lawrence Erlbaum Associates.

Fontes, L. A. (2008). *Interviewing clients across cultures: A practitioner's guide.* New York: Guilford Press.

Fontes, L. A., & Plummer, C. (2010). Cultural issues in disclosures of child sexual abuse. *Journal of Child Sexual Abuse, 19*, 491–518. https://doi:10.1080/10538712.2010.512520

Fontes, L. A., Cruz, M., & Tabachnick, J. (2001). Views of child sexual abuse in two cultural communities: An exploratory study among African Americans and Latinos. *Child Maltreatment, 6*(2), 103–117. https://doi:10.1177/1077559501006002003

Friedrich, W. N., Fisher, J., Broughton, D., Houston, M., & Shafron, C. (1998). Normative sexual behavior in children: A contemporary sample. *Pediatrics, 101*(4), e9. https://doi:10.1542/peds.101.4.e9

Freyd, J. J., Putnam, F. W., Lyon, T. D., Becker-Blease, K. A., Cheit, R. E., Siegel, N. B., & Pezdek, K. (2005). The science of child sexual abuse. *Science, 308*, 501. https://doi:10.1126/science.1108066

Garry, M., & Polaschek, D. L. L. (2000). Imagination and memory. *Current Directions in Psychological Science, 9*(1), 6–10. https://doi:10.1111/1467-8721.00048

Garven, S., Wood, J. M., & Malpass, R. S. (2000). Allegations of wrongdoing: The effects of reinforcement on children's mundane and fantastic claims. *Journal of Applied Psychology, 85*(1), 38–49. https://doi:10.1037/0021-9010.85.1.38

Ghetti, S., Goodman, G. S., Eisen, M. L., Qin, J., & Davis, S. L. (2002). Consistency in children's reports of sexual and physical abuse. *Child Abuse & Neglect, 26*(9), 977–995. https://doi:10.1016/S0145-2134(02)00367-8

Goldstein, N. E. S., Zelle, H., & Grisso, T. (2014). *Miranda Rights Comprehension Instruments (MRCI) manual for juvenile and adult evaluations.* Sarasota, FL: Professional Resource Press. https://www.prpress.com/Miranda-Rights-Comprehension-Instruments-MRCI_p_157.html

Grisso, T. (2005). *Evaluating juveniles' adjudicative competence: A guide for clinical practice.* Sarasota, FL: Professional Resource Press.

Hanson, R. K. (2002). Recidivism and age: Follow-up data from 4,673 sexual offenders. *Journal of Interpersonal Violence, 17*, 1046–1062. https://doi:10.1177/088626002236659

Heger, A., Ticson, L., Velasquez, O., & Bernier R. (2002). Children referred for possible sexual abuse: Medical findings in 2384 children. *Child Abuse and Neglect, 26*, 645–659. https://doi:10.1016/S0145-2134(02)00339-3

Herman, S. (2009). Forensic child sexual abuse evaluations: Accuracy, ethics, and admissibility. In K. Kuehnle and M. Connell (Eds.), *The evaluation of child sexual abuse allegations: A comprehensive guide to assessment and treatment* (pp. 247–266). Hoboken, NJ: John Wiley & Sons.

Herman, S. & Freitas, T. (2010). Error rates in forensic child sexual abuse evaluations. *Psychological Injury and Law, 3*, 133–147. https://doi:10.1007/s12207-010-9073-0

Hershkowitz, I., Lamb, M. E., Katz, C., & Malloy, L. C. (2013). Does enhanced rapport-building alter the dynamics of investigative interviews with suspected victims of intra-familial abuse? *Journal of Police and Criminal Psychology, 30*, 6–14. http://dx.doi:10.1007/s11896-013-9136-8

Hritz, A. C., Royer, C. E., Helm, R. K., Burd, K. A., Ojeda, K., & Ceci, S. J. (2015). Children's suggestibility research: Things to know before interviewing. *Anuario de Psicología Jurídica, 25*(1), 3–12. https://doi:10.1016/j.apj.2014.09.002

Johnson, M. K. (2006). Memory and reality. *American Psychologist, 61*(8), 760–771. https://doi.org/10.1037/0003-066X.61.8.760

Johnson, R., & Shrier, D. (1985). Sexual victimization of boys: Experience at an adolescent medicine clinic. *Journal of Adolescent Medicine, 6*(5), 372–376.

Keary, K., & Fitzpatrick, C. (1994). Children's disclosure of sexual abuse during formal investigation. *Child Abuse & Neglect, 18*(7), 543–548. https://doi:10.1016/0145-2134(94)90080-9

Kenny, M., & Wurtele, S. K. (2013). Child sexual behavior inventory: A comparison between Latino and normative samples of preschoolers. *The Journal of Sex Research, 50*(5), 449–457. https://doi:10.1080/00224499.2011.652265

Kuehnle, K. (1996). *Assessing allegations of child sexual abuse.* Sarasota, FL: Professional Resource Press/Professional Resource Exchange.

Kuehnle, K. (2003). Child sexual abuse evaluations. In A. M. Goldstein (Ed.), *Handbook of psychology: Forensic psychology*, vol. 11 (pp. 437–460). Hoboken, NJ: John Wiley & Sons.

Kuehnle, K., & Connell, M. (2009). Evaluating child sexual abuse allegations. In R. Galatzer-Levy, L. Kraus, & J. Galatzer-Levy (Eds). *The scientific basis of child custody decisions.* Hoboken, NJ: Wiley & Sons.

La Rooy, D., & Lamb, M. E. (2011). What happens when interviewers ask repeated questions in forensic interviews with children alleging abuse? *Journal of Police and Criminal Psychology, 26*(1), 20–25. https://doi:10.1007/s11896-010-9069-4

Lamb, M. E., Brown, D. A., Hershkowitz, I., Orbach, Y., & Esplin, P. W. (2018). *Tell me what happened: Questioning children about abuse.* Hoboken, NJ: John Wiley & Sons.

Lamb, M. E., Hershkowitz, I., Orbach, Y., & Esplin, P. W. (2008). *Tell me what happened: Structured investigative interviews of child victims and witnesses.* Hoboken, NJ: John Wiley & Sons.

Lamb, M. E., Hershkowitz, I., Sternberg, K. J., Boat, B., & Everson, M. D. (1996). Investigative interviews of alleged sexual abuse victims with and without anatomical dolls. *Child Abuse & Neglect, 20*(12), 1251–1259. https://doi:10.1016/S0145-2134(96)00121-4

Lamb, M. E., Orbach, Y., Hershkowitz, I., Phillip W. Esplin, P. W., & Horowitz, D. (2007). Structured forensic interview protocols improve the quality and informativeness of investigative interviews with children: A review of research using the NICHD Investigative Interview Protocol. *Child Abuse & Neglect, 31*, 1201–1231. https://doi:10.1016/j.chiabu.2007.03.021

Lamb, M. E., Orbach, Y., Sternberg, K. J., Hershkowitz, I., & Horowitz, D. (2000). Accuracy of investigators' verbatim notes of their forensic interviews with alleged child abuse victims. *Law and Human Behavior, 24*(6), 699–708. https://doi:10.1023/A:1005556404636

Lee, K. (2013). Little liars: Development of verbal deception in children. *Child Development Perspectives, 7*, 91–96. https://doi:10.1111/cdep.12023

Lindsay, D. S. (2008). Source monitoring and eyewitness memory. In B. L. Cutler (Ed.), *Encyclopedia of psychology and law* (pp. 748–750). Thousand Oaks, CA: Sage.

Lippert, T., Cross, T. P., Jones, L., & Walsh, W. (2009). Telling interviewers about sexual abuse: Predictors of child disclosure at forensic interviews. *Child Maltreatment, 14*(1), 100–113. https://doi:10.1177/1077559508318398

Loftus, E. F., & Kaufman, L. (1992). Why do traumatic experiences sometimes produce good memory (flashbulbs) and sometimes no memory (repression)? In E. Winograd & U. Neisser (Eds.), *Emory symposia in cognition, 4. Affect and accuracy in recall: Studies of "flashbulb" memories* (pp. 212–223). Cambridge: Cambridge University Press.

London, K., Bruck, M., Ceci, S., & Shuman, D. (2005). Disclosure of child sexual abuse: What does the research tell us about how children tell? *Psychology, Public Policy, and the Law, 11*, 194–226. https://doi:10.1037/1076-8971.11.1.194

London, K., Bruck, M., Wright, D. B., & Ceci, S. J. (2008). Review of the contemporary literature on how children report sexual abuse to others: Findings, methodological issues, and implications for forensic interviewers. *Memory, 16*, 29–47. https://doi:10.1080/09658210701725732

Lyon, T. D. (2007). False denials: Overcoming methodological biases in abuse disclosure research. In M. E. Pipe, M. Lamb, Y. Orbach, & A. Cederborg (Eds.), *Disclosing abuse: Delays, denials, retractions, and incomplete accounts* (pp. 41–62). Mahwah, NJ: Lawrence Erlbaum Associates.

Lyon, T. D., & Ahern, E. C. (2011). Disclosure of child sexual abuse. In J. Myers (Ed.), *The APSAC handbook on child maltreatment* (3rd ed., pp. 233–252). Newbury Park, CA: Sage.

Malloy, L. C., & Lyon, T. D. (2006). Caregiver support and child sexual abuse: Why does it matter? *Journal of Child Sexual Abuse: Research, Treatment, & Program Innovations for Victims, Survivors, & Offenders, 15*(4), 97–103. https://doi:10.1300/J070v15n04_06

Malloy, L. C., Mugno, A. P. (2016). Children's recantation of adult wrongdoing: An experimental investigation. *Journal of Experimental Child Psychology, 14*, 11–21. https://doi:10.1016/j.jecp.2015.12.003

Malloy, L. C., Lyon, T. D., & Quas, J. A. (2007). Filial dependency and recantation of child sexual abuse allegations. *Journal of the Academy of Child and Adolescent Psychiatry, 46*(2), 162–170. https://doi:10.1097/01.chi.0000246067.77953.f7

Malloy, L. C., Mugno, A. P., Rivard, J. R., Lyon, T. D., & Quas, J. A. (2016). Familial influences on recantation in substantiated child sexual abuse cases. *Child Maltreatment, 21*(3), 256–261.

Meston, C. M., & Ahrold, T. (2010). Ethnic, gender, and acculturation influences on sexual behaviors. *Archive of Sexual Behavior, 39*(1), 179–189. https://doi:10.1007/s10508-008-9415-0

Miller K. L., Dove, M. K., & Miller, S. M. (2007, October). A counselor's guide to child sexual abuse: Prevention, reporting and treatment strategies. Available from: www.ncbi.nlm.nih.gov/pubmed/1186016

O'Donohue, W. T., Cirlugea, O., Bennett, N., & Benuto, L. T. (2016). Psychological and investigative pathways to untrue allegations of child sexual abuse. In W. T. O'Donohue & M. Fanetti (Eds.), *Forensic interviews regarding child sexual abuse: A guide to evidence-based practice* (pp. 257–273). New York: Springer Publishing. https://psycnet.apa.org/record/2016-01980-014

O'Donohue, W. T., Cummings, C., & Willis, B. (2018). The frequency of false allegations of child sexual abuse: A critical review, *Journal of Child Sexual Abuse, 27*(5), 459–475, https://doi:10.1080/10538712.2018.1477224

Orbach, Y., Hershkowitz, I., Lamb, M. E., Esplin, P. W., & Horowitz, D. (2000). Assessing the value of structured protocols for forensic interviews of alleged child abuse victims. *Child Abuse & Neglect, 24*(6), 733–752. https://doi:10.1016/S0145-2134(00)00137-X

Pezdek, K., Finger, K., & Hodge, D. (1997). Planting false childhood memories: The role of event plausibility. *Psychological Science, 8*(6), 437–441. Retrieved from: www.jstor.org/stable/40063230

Poole, D. A., & Lindsay, D. S. (2001). Children's eyewitness reports after exposure to misinformation from parents. *Journal of Experimental Psychology: Applied, 7*(1), 27–50. https://doi:10.1037/1076-898X.7.1.27

Poole, D. A. and Wolfe, A. W. (2009). Child development: Normative sexual and nonsexual behaviors that may be confused with symptoms of sexual abuse. In K. Kuehnle and M. Connell (Eds.), *The evaluation of child sexual abuse allegations: A comprehensive guide* (pp. 101–128). Hoboken, NJ: John Wiley & Sons.

Quas, J. A., Malloy, L. C., Melinder, A., Goodman, G. S., D'Mello, M., & Schaaf, J. (2007). Developmental differences in the effects of repeated interviews and interviewer bias on young children's event memory and false reports. *Developmental Psychology, 43*(4), 823–37. doi: 10.1037/0012-1649.43.4.823

Riser, D. K., Pegram, S. E., & Farley, J. P. (2013). Adolescent and young adult male sex offenders: Understanding the role of recidivism. *Journal of Child Sexual Abuse, 22*(1), 9–31. https://doi:10.1080/10538712.2013.735355

Russell, D. E. H., & Bolen, R. (2000). *The epidemic of rape and child sexual abuse in the United States.* Newbury Park, CA: Sage.

Saini, M., Black, T., Fallon, B., & Marshall, A. (2013). Child custody disputes within the context of child protection investigations: Secondary analysis of the Canadian incident study of reported child abuse and neglect. *Child Welfare, 92*(1), 115–137.

Saini, M., Black, T., Godbout, E., & Deljavan, S. (2019). Feeling the pressure to take sides: A survey of child protection workers' experiences about responding to allegations of child maltreatment within the context of child custody disputes. *Children and Youth Services Review, 96*, 127–133. https://doi:10.1016/j.childyouth.2018.11.044

Saini, M., Black, T., Lwin, K., Marshall, A., Fallon, B., & Goodman, D. (2012). Child protection workers' experiences of working with high conflict families. *Children and Youth Services Review, 34*, 1309–1316. https://doi:10.1016/j.childyouth.2012.03.005

Saini, M., Laajasalo, T., & Platt, S. (2020). Gatekeeping by allegations: An examination of verified, unfounded, and fabricated allegations of child maltreatment within the context of resist and refusal dynamics. *Family Court Review, 58*, 417–431. https://doi.org/10.1111/fcre.12480

Saywitz, K. J., Goodman, G. S., & Lyon, T. D. (2002). Interviewing children in and out of court: Current research and practice implications. In J. Myers, L. Berliner, J. Briere, C. T. Hendrix, C. Jenny, & T. Reid (Eds.), *The APSAC handbook on child maltreatment* (2nd ed., pp. 349–377). Thousand Oaks, CA: Sage.

Saywitz, K. J., Lyon, T. D., & Goodman, G. S. (2018). When interviewing children: A review and update. In J. B. Klika & J. R. Conte (Eds.), *APSAC handbook on child maltreatment* (4th ed., pp. 310–329). Newbury Park, CA: Sage.

Sedlak, A. J., & Broadhurst, D. D. (1996). *Third national incidence study of child abuse and neglect.* Washington DC: US Department of Health and Human Services.

Sedlak, A. J., Mettenburg, J., Basena, M., Petta, I., McPherson, K., Greene, A., & Li, S. (2010). *Fourth National Incidence Study of Child Abuse and Neglect (NIS–4): Report to Congress.* Washington, DC: U.S. Department of Health and Human Services, Administration for Children and Families.

Seto, M. C. (2018). *Pedophilia and sexual offending against children: Theory, assessment, and intervention* (2nd ed.). Washington, D.C.: American Psychological Association.

Singh, M. M., Parsekar, S. S., & Nair, S. N. (2014). An epidemiological overview of child sexual abuse. *Journal of family medicine and primary care, 3*(4), 430–435. https://doi:10.4103/2249-4863.148139 Retrieved from: https://www.ncbi.nlm.nih.gov/pmc/articles/PMC4311357/

Sites, J., & Southern Regional Children's Advocacy Center. (2017). *Considerations for the multidisciplinary team/children's advocacy center approach to recantation: A research-to-practice summary.* Huntsville, AL: Southern Regional Children's Advocacy Center.

Sjoberg, R., & Lindblad, F. (2002). Limited disclosure of sexual abuse in children whose experiences were documented by videotape. *American Journal of Psychiatry, 159*(2), 312–314. https://doi:10.1176/appi.ajp.159.2.312

Sorenson, T., & Snow, B. (1991). How children tell: The process of disclosure of sexual abuse. *Child Welfare, 70*(1), 3–15.

Talwar, V., & Lee, K. (2002). Development of lying to conceal a transgression: Children's control of expressive behaviour during verbal deception. *International Journal of Behavioral Development, 26*(5), 436–444. https://doi:10.1080/01650250143000373

Talwar, V., Hubbard, K., Saykaly, C., Lee, K., Lindsay, R. C. L., & Bala, N. (2018). Does parental coaching affect children's false reports? Comparing verbal markers of deception. *Behavioral sciences & the Law, 36*(1) 84–97. https://doi:10.1002/bsl.2331

Taylor, S. S. (2013). Why American boys join street gangs. *International Journal of Sociology and Anthropology, 5*(8), 339–349. https://doi:10.5897/IJSA12.073

Thierry, K. L., Lamb, M. E., Orbach, Y., & Pipe, M.-E. (2005). Developmental differences in the function and use of anatomical dolls during interviews with alleged sexual abuse victims. *Journal of Consulting and Clinical Psychology, 73*(6), 1125–1134. https://doi:10.1037/0022-006X.73.6.1125

Thoennes, N., & Tjaden, P. G. (1990). The extent, nature, and validity of sexual abuse allegations in custody/visitation disputes. *Child Abuse & Neglect, 14*, 151–163. https://doi:10.1016/0145-2134(90)90026-P

Trocmé, N., & Bala, N. (2005). False allegations of abuse and neglect when parents separate. *Child Abuse & Neglect, 29*, 1333–1345. https://doi:10.1016/j.chiabu.2004.06.016

U.S. Department of Health & Human Services, Administration for Children and Families, Administration on Children, Youth and Families, & Children's Bureau. (2020). *Child Maltreatment 2018*. Retrieved from: https://www.acf.hhs.gov/cb/resource/child-maltreatment-2018

Warren, A. R., & Woodall, C. E. (1999). The reliability of hearsay testimony: How well do interviewers recall their interviews with children? *Psychology, Public Policy, and Law, 5*(2), 355–371. https://doi:10.1037/1076-8971.5.2.355

Worling, J. R., & Långström, N. (2006). Risk of sexual recidivism in adolescents who offend sexually. In Barbaree, H. E. & Marshall, W. L. (Eds.). *The juvenile sexual offender* (2nd ed.). New York: Guilford.

Ziegler, D. (2002). *Traumatic experience and the brain: A handbook for understanding and treating those traumatized as children.* Phoenix, AZ: Acacia Press.

11 Interpersonal Violence and Children

Nancy W. Olesen

One setting very likely to involve children is Family Court, where the child is at the center of many of the disputes. (Property and custody are the main areas of conflict that end up in Family Court.) This chapter will concern the issues that arise when there are allegations of Intimate Partner Violence (IPV) in Family Court and the role of the children in the families in these situations. There are psychological and psycholegal parameters to the cases and if a mental health professional (MHP) is serving as evaluator or mediator or therapist for one of the parents, they need to have some knowledge in both the psychological and the psycholegal areas.

In this chapter, I will use "she" and "her" to describe the victims of IPV and "he" or "him" to refer to the perpetrators. This does not imply that there are no cases in which the female is violent and controlling and the male is victimized (Tjaden & Thoennes, 2000); indeed in same sex relationships, these same dynamics may occur. As will be described later in this chapter, depending on the type of IPV and depending on the population sample used in the research, there are some gender differences. However, the choice to use the stereotypical genders is for simplicity of writing and reading. Studies have consistently reported a high prevalence of IPV during the history of the relationship reported by divorcing-litigating partners (Newmark et al., 2004). Estimates vary greatly due to sampling and measurement differences, but a fair expectation is that over 50% of litigating, former intimates report IPV of some form and severity (see Kelly & Johnson, 2008 for a review). Bow and Boxer reported in 2003 that 51% cases with IPV had a male instigator, 11% had a female instigator, with the other groups consisting of bidirectional or mutual instigation.

How IPV Cases Get to the Mental Health Professional (MHP)

The ways that an MHP may become involved with the court in such IPV cases are actually quite varied. Some roles are known to be neutral with regard to the primary questions of whether the violence really happened, by whom, and what the level of future risk may be. An MHP could, for example, be named as a neutral court-ordered mediator or evaluator. As an evaluator in cases that involve allegations of IPV, the MHP can expect that their professional history will be deeply scrutinized for signs of bias. It is important to develop a protocol for evaluation that ensures that the inquiry is thorough, balanced and even-handed. Good note-taking skills and record-keeping skills are essential. One must know the outlines of the information that will be sought from the parties, from documents, from other witnesses and those should be disclosed in advance. Signed releases should be sought (and kept) before talking with others – doctors, schools, and the like. Often times the evaluator will need to request from the court, orders to obtain specific information such as police reports and CPS records. Additionally, should a parent not wish to sign a release,

DOI: 10.4324/9780429397806-12

the evaluator may try to seek a court order if that source of information is deemed critical to the psycholegal issue being assessed.

One can also work as therapist for the child in the family and probably be expected to maintain a neutral position in support of the child's relationship with both parents.

In a non-neutral role the MHP might work with the individual alleged victim as a therapist, for example, or as an advocate through an agency that works with IPV victims. In that case, the professional is not expected to be neutral, but instead to provide support to the victim or to provide the court with understanding of the underlying dynamics of family violence and such dynamics as the research based reasons that genuine victims may not have disclosed IPV earlier, or why they return to their abusers. One can also be retained by an attorney to assess the potential lethality of individual case situations to facilitate accurate and effective interventions that the attorney can request from the court.

Another non-neutral role may be as therapist to the alleged perpetrator, either to provide support during the investigations or to provide guidance and psycho-education about ways to improve his interpersonal functioning in whatever ways have been identified as leading to danger to his family members. These might be likely to include anger management, improving emotional regulation and information about child development among other things.

Legal Issues to be Considered by Evaluators

There are legal facts and factors one needs to know when entering into an evaluation that may involve Intimate Partner Violence in Family Court. The first is that there may be different definitions of Domestic Violence under the Family Code, Criminal Code and Civil Code in a particular state. Presumptions for the implications for child custody associated with findings of IPV may vary from state to state. The evaluator must know the relevant definitions for the jurisdiction in which he is practicing.

There can be serious potential effects of prior judicial findings in the case that the evaluator needs to know. For example, California law (FC3044) states that there is a rebuttable presumption that it is not in the child's best interests for the alleged perpetrator of family violence to have sole or joint custody. Therefore if, for example, there has been a judicial finding of IPV in a state like California with a rebuttable presumption that governs future custody, it is not proper for the evaluating psychologist to state a conclusion contrary to the judicial finding. (The evaluator may choose to describe the facts that could lead to a contrary conclusion, yet may not explicitly describe the court's findings as wrong.) Note that the issuance of a temporary restraining order or emergency protective order does not ordinarily constitute a judicial finding of domestic violence.

In addition, it is important for the clinician to learn whether there has been a civil or criminal restraining order and whether the case is also involved in another court (criminal, for example). This may impact the protocol for interviewing the parents. It is not the job of the mental health professional to sort out differences between the demands of different courts but rather to be aware of the potential conflicts in the demands of these courts. For example, interviewing the alleged perpetrator may be blocked by his criminal defense attorney in the interests of preserving his constitutional rights to not incriminate himself. Occasionally, the Family Court will choose to wait for a final ruling from criminal court before proceeding with the custody hearings but that will be the decision of the court, not the evaluator.

The law in California describes various behaviors or factors that would serve to rebut the presumption described above. Such a legal conclusion in the case requires the evaluator to gather information related to factors that might rebut the presumption. These may include actions such as completion of a 52-week Batterers Intervention Program (BIP), therapy focused on behavior such as anger management, or evidence that the child has had a deep and meaningful relationship with the offending parent such that the loss of that relationship would be detrimental. The evaluator should be knowledgeable about the factors that are relevant in the jurisdiction in which they practice and describe their relevance in their reports.

In family matters the legal standard is Best Interests of the Child (BIC). This is a term that can be seen through different lenses and sometimes there is disagreement on the meaning. Fortunately, many states have listed the factors that make up BIC determinations. Michigan, for example, has a list of 12 factors that is often used in other states as a model, as it is considered thoughtful and comprehensive. The eleventh factor in the Michigan BIC list (after elements such as love and affections, stability, parental capacity and mental and physical health) is "Domestic violence, regardless of whether the violence was directed at or witnessed by the child." (Michigan Best Interest Standards, FINDLAW) This statement hints at the different kinds of exposure to violence and those different kinds of exposure to IPV will be discussed later in this chapter. In California and some other states allowing a child to be exposed to IPV is considered child abuse. (It should be noted that these laws may secondarily victimize the victims of IPV. Women in violent relationships may find themselves caught between making the decisions they feel they must make to keep their children safe and the risk of being accused of child endangerment on the one hand or interfering with the parental rights of their partner on the other.)

In summary, because there are legal factors that have a bearing on IPV determinations, it is important for the clinician/evaluator to get information about the state laws defining IPV and the legal case history which may have characterized the case in certain ways that make some referral questions moot in terms of the psychological assessment of the parties or the child. It is not the job of the mental health professional to sort out differences between the demands of different court systems but rather to be aware of the potential conflicts in the demands of the courts. For example, the alleged perpetrator may be instructed by his criminal defense attorney not to cooperate with the custody evaluation, in the interests of preserving his constitutional rights to not incriminate himself while being expected to cooperate honestly with the Family Court.

Psychological Issues to be Considered

Over the past two decades or more there has been movement in family psychology and family violence thinking, leading to more nuanced and specific knowledge about IPV. The recent developments in the IPV field include more information and agreement about the types of IPV, the impact of IPV on children in the family, and the best practices for evaluation, intervention and custodial arrangements. Following an interdisciplinary conference in 2008 at the Wingspread Conference Center, the Association of Family and Conciliation Courts (AFCC) published a series of papers outlining the areas of agreement on a list of types of IPV (referred to as the Wingspread Report). This group of specialists argued that differentiation of the various types allows for focused and appropriate court orders and interventions to keep families safe and ensure the well-being of children in these families, including guidance for developing parenting plans in families where there has been IPV.

One issue of great importance in the effort to differentiate types of family violence is the question of how likely it is that the violence, or the controlling dynamics, will continue after separation. Another issue is the need to make appropriate arrangements for safety and for services according to the specific family's needs. When courts saw family violence that did not fit old models of "battering" and therefore decided that the behavior in question represented simple conflict, the orders often provided little protection for the victims and children. Similarly, when courts saw all family violence as "battering," they often made orders that led to the loss of the child's relationship with an otherwise "good enough" parent and the loss of opportunities for services such as mediation and family therapy. Narrow thinking can lead to increased risk of future harm of the one hand and potential loss of relationships and resources on the other. In addition to the Wingspread papers, AFCC recently published best practice Guidelines for Child Custody Evaluations in Cases with IPV (2016).

The types of IPV identified in a preliminary way by the Wingspread conference are considered to depend on the context in which the violence occurs, the history of and direction of the violence, the forms of abuse (financial, sexual) other than physical aggression and more (Ver Steegh & Dalton, 2008). While theirs was not considered a definitive or final list, there was clearly an advantage in going beyond the one-size-fits-all simple definitions of IPV that had been used previously. (Many of these definitions remain gender-based in their descriptions and to some extent the ways that we understand them. Genuinely neutral understanding of the issue of interpersonal family violence will need to wait for further analysis. Until that time, we will deal with the definitions we presently have.)

Coercive Control

Violence used by a perpetrator in the exercise of control over the victim, in which physical violence is used "as one tactic in a larger escalating pattern aimed at intimidating and controlling the victim" (*op cit.*, p. 458). This type is the closest fit with classic "battering" and has been shown to have damaging effects on the parent victim and the children. The goal oftentimes is to break down the self-esteem and identity of the victim. Among other things, attachment relationships are often disrupted by the child's experience that the attachment figures to whom they need to turn for safety are the ones who either threaten their safety directly or indirectly or the ones who demonstrate an inability to protect the child or themselves. For a further discussion of attachment, see Chapter 7 of this volume by Attorney Jurney. This pattern is associated with a continuing risk of violence, when the perpetrator may feel the need to maintain control of the now ex-partner. Litigation can be used in this regard as another form of Coercive Control and threat. Earlier research suggesting that the period immediately after separation was the time of greatest danger of physical harm or death to the victim parent and/or child fits with this observation (Hardesty, Haselschwerdt, & Johnson, 2012).

Children often feel divided loyalties in these situations, fearing the violent parent and also looking to him for security and safety, as the child may experience the victim parent as too weak to provide safety.

Coercive Control will almost always involve fear in the victim and controlling behavior in the perpetrator. The violence is in the service of maintaining control over the other. There may be control over finances, with the victim lacking independent access to money or facing demands to account for all household money spent. There may be strict control over where the victim may go and with whom she can interact. The victim may need permission from her spouse to visit her friends or family or to spend any money on their children.

Coercive Control also involves continuing efforts to denigrate and humiliate the victim to lead her to lose self-confidence and self-esteem. Negative statements about her appearance, competence, parenting ability and history of failure are frequent and become increasingly effective in breaking down the confidence of the victim with repetition over time. It is common that there is violence to enforce the coercion, sometimes wildly out of control and overtly violent, but sometimes also subtle and hidden and very controlled. These are situations in which the violence may be deliberately inflicted on her body in places where the bruises or marks will not be seen. There may be threats to take the children away, to publish embarrassing things about her to workmates or family. There is always the repeated threat that no one will ever believe her or trust her word against his, because they will see how "useless and bad" she is. The most common paradigm for coercive control is with a male perpetrator and a female victim.

One frequent outcome of these coercive control dynamics is trauma in the victims. Such trauma may interfere with effectively seeking help, with effective parenting, and create a negative feedback loop reinforcing her negative identity presented by the abuser. Often the abusive party appears to professionals as more functional than the victim.

The mere fact of the parents not living together or not needing to interact directly does not lessen the risk of future violence from a coercively controlling parent. They may follow or stalk their former partner, may repeatedly call or send hundreds of daily text messages. They may even come unbidden and illegally into her home or place of work and into her social media. These acts sometimes function as a way to convey that he refuses to be controlled by her, sometimes as desperate attempts to rekindle the relationship or as ways to punish her for leaving or to check on whether she may be dating.

When a woman has been the victim of Coercive Control, often she does not recognize it as such. If asked directly whether she has experienced IPV, many women in these relationship will say "no, of course not." Sometimes, they think it has not been IPV if they have not had a broken bone or been hospitalized; sometimes, they are embarrassed to think of themselves as one of the victims they have held in pity and contempt in the past. So, it is important to ask many questions, both general and specific about how conflict was managed in the relationship, how money was handled, who made decisions about the children, what happened when one of the parents was upset etc. A very thorough list of screener questions (created by Leslie Drozd, Ph.D.) can be found in Appendix 2 at the end of this volume.

The effects of coercive control are pernicious, both on the victim and the children. The fear generated may be truly traumatic in itself, leading to interference with effective functioning as a parent. Some victims are afraid of their own very young children; when the child is angry or has a tantrum, the mother may react to the child as though he is the aggressive ex-partner.

"Helpless caregiving" creates destructive issues in the attachment process especially for young children (Solomon & George, 2011). The loss of self-respect may make it difficult to face the many things that need doing after any separation, including finding an attorney, moving to a new home, arranging school enrollment or child care, organizing paperwork and finances, etc. For further discussion of trauma see Chapter 4.

Violence Driven by Conflict

This is violence that arises out of an argument or fight that escalates through loss of emotional control but without a pattern of unidirectional coercive control. It may involve one or both people and neither fears the other nor tries to exert control. Instead there is an explosive loss of control of anger without any plan to control the other with the anger. The effects on children can be serious, as they may be terrified and experience their parents as dangerous, unable to maintain their control and emotional regulation. Dysregulation is a common problem in children from these families. In evaluating the parents, psychological testing may provide insight into the parents' capacity for emotional regulation and future self-control. For a further discussion of psychological testing, see Part Two of this volume.

In families that show this pattern, future violence is less likely when there is a defined plan for the exchange of information, exchange of belongings, and for the transfer of the child from one to the other. These can be specified to be in a public place, during daylight hours, with a third party available – all factors that minimize the intimacy of the encounter and the opportunity for provocations that lead to angry outbursts. Such plans can serve to prevent the parents from having inflammatory interactions, while maintaining close contact with both parents for the child.

A subset of conflict-based violence is that which is caused by or accelerated by **substance abuse.** The evaluator is responsible for addressing the presence of, levels of and future risks of substance abuse in one or both parents. The evaluation should describe the effects on the child of exposure to the substance abuse, the likely risks of the parent relapsing and recommendations for treatment and ways to monitor abstinence for child safety. At a minimum, the parenting plan must specify no ingestion of substances 8 hours before the visit, as well as during the visit. Regular testing, for example by Soberlink (www.soberlink. com), may be instituted.

Separation-Instigated Violence

This occurs when the violence occurs for the first time at the time of separation in response to the trauma of separation and loss where there has been no prior history of violence. This type of violence may have both male and female perpetrators. Both the victim and the perpetrator may be surprised by the outbreak of violent behavior and usually this does not continue after separation. While this can be dangerous or disruptive to the child, there is a different context and meaning in this violent outburst. Often it is easier for both parents to reassure the child that there was no intention to harm the parent or child, that the parent "just got too upset and lost it" and that he or she is now getting help to make sure it doesn't happen again." Such explanations, of course, require agreement between the parents about what happened and the violent parent's commitment to getting help. This type of violence is less likely to occur in the future, and therefore need not be a major factor in developing a post-separation parenting plan, beyond the obvious need to recommend appropriate treatment for all in the family who are in need of treatment.

Violence Stemming from Severe Mental Illness

In this case, the IPV arises from the compromised emotional and cognitive functioning of one of the parents, who has a serious mental or emotional disorder. The presence of Bipolar Disorder, psychosis or a major personality disorder makes it essential for there to be clearly defined parameters for safe contact and behavior, including demonstrated compliance with treatment. Again, in this situation, psychological testing can be helpful in determining the nature and severity of the mental health problems and suggesting possible interventions such as medication, or specific treatment such as Dialectical Behavior Therapy (DBT). General recommendations for unspecified and generic "therapy" are rarely helpful. Recommendations should state the focus of the treatment, identify named professionals who are known to be skilled in this type of treatment, define goals of the treatment, and ways to measure cooperation and progress. Often there are "Step-up" plans for increasing contact between parent and child as progress is demonstrated (Pruett et al., 2016).

Defensive or Reactive Violence

In these cases the victim may take violent action to protect herself and her children and in so doing she may be accused of being herself the instigator of violence. The evaluator will need to be very clear in their assessment of this accusation, relying on police reports, medical reports, and witness statements (including from the children).

Children in the Middle of the Conflict

When children are involved in situations that involve Intimate Partner Violence (IPV), they may be in any one or more of the roles outlined elsewhere in this volume. They may be witnesses, providing information about what happened during the violent event. In that case all the considerations of developmental level, language competence, reliability and memory are relevant as described in Chapters 3 and 4 of this volume. They may be direct victims of violence by the same perpetrator who is accused of harming their parent. In that case considerations of the corroborating evidence, such as physical injury, medical records, recorded interviews, witnesses, and the like are relevant. These types of records are described in Chapters 9, 10, 13, 14 and 15 of this volume. They may be secondary victims, harmed by exposure to witnessing IPV on a loved parent. They may be accused of lying about what happened in an "unholy alliance" with the alleged victim to gain an advantage in Family Court.

Often the person who describes what the child was exposed to is the victim parent, who then faces the double burden of convincing the authorities of their own victimization and that of their child. The child thus may be suspected of conspiring with the parent with whom they are aligned to blame the other parent for violence not actually committed. On the other hand, in some cases the child actually may be providing false information to police or other authorities, either based on loyalty to the alleged victim, fear of the alleged aggressor (but not fear of IPV), or based on immature or faulty understanding of the events. It can be difficult for children to respond to all the pressures on them and they may be seen as lying, or as victims themselves. Children in these emotional binds feature prominently in discussions of "Resist-Refuse" dynamics, as will be discussed in Chapter 14 of this volume

When the child refuses to have contact with one of the parents, insisting on maintaining their relationship solely with the preferred parent, there is a knotty problem for the court to resolve. The issue of Resist-Refuse dynamics and Alienation in separating families requires extensive knowledge and experience in an evaluator, presented in a recent special series of a leading journal (*Family Court Review*, 58[2]). Before accepting an evaluation with such issues, the evaluator should ensure they are knowledgeable about the best current thinking on the subject.

The child may also be invisible to the court, without anyone considering them at all as affected by the events. We see court decisions about parenting roles, in families where there has been IPV, where no consideration has been given about the effects on the children or the plan for future contact with both parents. It is incumbent on the MHP to consider the elements of the child's role in the IPV and help the court see the child as a separate person with their own experiences and needs. In one widely publicized case, O.J. Simpson's custody litigation with the family of his late wife, the court ruled that it was not relevant how the children's mother died, only that they had a living parent who was available and "good enough." The judgment was reversed on appeal. It is clear that all elements of the family dynamics are "relevant."

Case Examples

"Sheila" was an 8-year-old child whose family was referred to me for a comprehensive child custody evaluation. It is a case that illustrates Coercive Control IPV. I conducted a standard evaluation, including interviews, parent-child observations in the office, home visits in both homes, psychological testing plus interviews with collateral informants. Her father frequently railed against her mother, criticizing her appearance, parenting, her housekeeping, her education, her intelligence and all aspects of her person. Occasionally, he threatened violence, and broke objects and struck holes in walls and doors. The mother was overweight and timid, rarely "talking back" to her husband and trying to follow his requirements for her behavior, which included how much time she spent with her friends, how much money she spent, what she and her daughter ate, and other aspects of daily life for which he attempted control. Post-separation, he had her followed and, on one occasion, disabled her car so she could not drive to work. He took his ex-wife to court to demand half of the firewood left at the family home. He also controlled the child post-separation, to the extent of demanding that she bring her clothes (even underwear), after a dance recital, to him because they "belonged" to him (i.e. he had purchased them) rather than being allowed to wear them to the mother's home at transition time after the recital. Initially the child presented herself as perfect, a good student, an exemplary obedient child. On psychological testing, she showed an awareness of intense danger around her. One Rorschach response was of a small helpless animal being ripped apart by two predators. (See Part Two of this volume for a discussion of psychological testing and Chapter 8 for more detail about the Rorschach Inkblot Method.)

Sheila explained to the evaluator how she helped her little sister when their father was raging. She said she brought the younger child into the cubbyhole under the desk in her bedroom and played music so that the younger girl would not hear the screaming in the house. She admitted that this effort was not always successful but seemed pleased and proud to be able to help her younger sister stay calm and feel safe. Nevertheless, she initially had said she wanted to spend equal time with each of her parents.

As the post-separation phase stretched into the evaluation, the child began to express her wish to see her father less than the half-time the parents has agreed at the direction of the court mediator. She complained that her father was always critical and angry and constantly said negative things about her and her mother. Father denied ever saying anything the slightest bit negative about the child or the mother and insisted that the mother was campaigning to turn the child against him. Interestingly, during the home visit, he talked at some length with me and his daughter about how poor the mother's cooking was and how superior he was as a cook. In a later interview, when asked about the conflict between his assertion of always making positive statements and the statements the evaluator and the child heard, he extended his conversation about the mother's failings her weight problems and said he was simply telling the truth about her to his child.

Based in part on the evidence of repeated efforts to control his ex-wife, it was the recommendation of the evaluator and the order of the court that the time-share should not be 50–50, that the father immediately should attend treatment to reduce his level of anger and increase his awareness of the effects of his behavior on his child. The court ordered that the child should be in psychotherapy.

"George" was 4 years old when his parents separated. They had avoided arguments in front of him and as far as George knew, they presented a calm and harmonious picture of the family. At the point when father discovered that mother was having an affair with a family friend, he became enraged, got drunk and took an axe to the dining room table, screaming that they would not be needing a family dining area any longer. Both parents agreed that this violent outburst was completely out of character for him and was deeply distressing to their son.

Father left the home, began therapy the next day with an MHP with experience in substance abuse, and got the therapist's help in crafting an apology for his son. Mother was concerned about the level of rage displayed but agreed it was not characteristic of his prior behavior. They agreed in mediation to a stipulation that he would not drink for 8 hours before or any time during his parenting time with George. They arranged for an experienced child therapist to see George in therapy. In this case, what was needed in the assessment was different than it was in the case of Sheila. In Sheila's family case, the primary emphasis was on understanding and describing what happened, the effects on the child and her sister and the safeguards that would be needed for safe contact between parent and child, and parent and parent. In George's family, there was no disagreement about the events; everyone agreed on what happened and needed deeper understanding of the meaning of the events and the best ways to move forward.

Where there has been violence arising from the mental illness of a parent, the child has almost always been aware that something was wrong with that parent. The MHP needs to carefully look into the history of the mental illness (if it has been documented previously), and the current symptoms. Even more importantly, the MHP must look carefully at the impact of the mental illness on parenting itself. The parent may need specific treatment for the mental illness and ongoing visitation with the impaired parent may need to be contingent on reliable information that the parent is compliant with treatment, such as medication compliance. The child may need sensitive and age-appropriate information about that parent and their behavior. A therapist may be able to help the child understand the mental illness in the parent, including the fact that the child did not cause it and is not responsible to heal the parent. The non-impaired parent may need coaching about appropriate ways to talk with the child about the parent's mental illness. Supervised visitation can help the child and parent continue their relationship, while minimizing emotional damage to the child during the period when there remains uncertainty about the parent's functioning. The evaluator may get useful information from the visitation supervisors as well.

Exposure vs Victimization

It should be noted that children suffer from "exposure" to IPV, even when they were not in the room when it occurred – even when they were not in the home when it happened. The effects of an episode of IPV can be intense and far-reaching. When children are in another room or upstairs in bed during an episode of IPV, the MHP should operate from the assumption that the child did hear the fight. Children frequently try to shield their parents from knowing that they were heard, perhaps because they want to pretend it did not happen, but even more because they will try to protect the parent from the parent's distress about having upset the children. When the children have been out of the house, they return to a home in which a parent may be crying, or show evidence of having been crying, a home in which things may be broken or damaged, or a home in which both parents are "walking on eggshells" or otherwise behaving strangely. The expectation is almost always that the children will not acknowledge that they see that something has happened. But those children are burdened by their knowledge; knowledge that they will not be able to discuss with any trusted person.

Summary and Conclusions

In evaluations, MHP need to carefully describe the events of the alleged IPV; this includes creating a time-line of events, laying out the source of each piece of information and noting the reliability of each source, cross-checking pieces of data when possible. When the evaluator reaches an understanding of the dynamics, he must articulate that understanding and the basis for it. The evaluator needs to fit the facts of the case against the types of IPV articulated in the literature (Austin & Drozd, 2013).

Then the evaluator needs to provide a description of ways for the family to move forward into the future – structures, schedules, treatments and future potential changes in all the structures and schedules, etc. as progress is made or set-backs occur.

There is extensive information about how to organize parenting plans in families with concerns about IPV. For example, Johnston, Roseby, and Kuehnle (2009), and Jaffe, Johnston, Crooks, and Bala (2008) provide comprehensive, thorough analyses of specific family dynamics and how best to address promoting the child's best interests post-separation and divorce in these families.

In addition to describing the violence that did occur, the partner dynamics, and the factors suggesting risk for future violence, the evaluator must be knowledgeable about and describe the specific effects on the child or children (Osofsky, 1999).

There is a strong correlation noted in the research literature between the existence of IPV and child abuse (Bancroft et al., 2012). Child abuse should be considered first as a separate issue in IPV families, even when it has not been raised by either parent and subsequently, it should be integrated into the overall description of the dynamics in the family.

In IPV cases, more than most, evaluators face problems with maintaining their neutrality, working within a systematic approach, using valid assessment tools (see Rossi et al., 2013 for a thorough discussion). The evaluator must consistently review all the data available, including police reports, hospital or medical records, witness statements, and any other relevant documents. If there are, as there should be, video-recorded forensic interviews with the children done soon after the events in question, the evaluator must watch them. Those can be compared with the child's interviews with the evaluator.

It will be important to know the research literature on the effects of family violence on children and propose interventions to lessen the potential impact (Jaffe et al., 2008). There will be considerable demands on the evaluator's sense of empathy, usually from the victim mother, but also sometimes from the alleged aggressor father. The evaluator may feel threatened by the prospect of lawsuits by the parents or public exposure in the local media.

It is incumbent on the evaluator to attend conferences and trainings on IPV, to work with a group of experienced professionals with whom they can discuss these difficult families (disguised as to identity, of course). Knowledgeable colleagues can help provide additional clarity on the issues and emotional support in the storms that may come in such cases.

References

Association of Family and Conciliation Courts. (2016). *Guidelines for Examining Intimate Partner Violence: A Supplement to the AFCC Model Standards of Practice for Child Custody Evaluation.* Madison WI: Association of Family and Conciliation Courts.

Austin, W. G., & Drozd, L. M. (2013). Judge's bench book for application of the integrated framework for the assessment of intimate partner violence in child custody disputes. *Journal of Child Custody: Research, Issues, and Practices, 10*(2), 99–119.

Bancroft, L., Silverman, J., & Ritchie, D. (2012). *The batterer as parent: Addressing the impact of domestic violence on family dynamics* (2nd ed.). Los Angeles, CA: Sage Publications.

Bow, J. N., & Boxer, P. (2003). Assessing allegations of domestic violence in child custody evaluations. *Journal of Interpersonal Violence, 18*(12), 1394–1410.

Hardesty, J. L., Haselschwerdt, M. L., & Johnson, M. P. (2012). Domestic violence and child custody. In K. Kuehnle & L. Drozd (Eds.), *Parenting plan evaluations: Applied research for the family court.* (pp. 442–475). New York: Oxford University Press.

Jaffe, P. G., Johnston, J. R., Crooks, C. V., & Bala, N. (2008). Custody disputes involving allegations of domestic violence: Toward a differentiated approach to parenting plans. *Family Court Review, 46*(3), 500–522.

Johnston, J. R., Roseby, V., & Kuehnle, K. (2009). In the name of the child: A developmental approach to understanding and helping children of conflicted and violent divorce (2nd ed.). New York: Springer Publishing.

Kelly, J. B., & Johnson, M. P. (2008). Differentiation among types of intimate partner violence: Research update and implications for interventions. *Family Court Review, 46*(3), 476–499.

Osofsky, J. D. (1999). The impact of violence on children. *The Future of Children, 9*(3), 33–49.

Newmark, L., Rempel, M., Diffily, K., & Kane, K. M. (2004). Specialized felony domestic violence courts: Lessons on implementation and impacts from the Kings County experience. In B. S. Fisher (Ed.), *Violence against women and family violence: Developments in research, practice, and policy* (p. III–8–1). National Counsel of Juvenile and Family Court Judges. https://www.ojp.gov/pdffiles1/nij/199701.pdf

Pruett, M. K., Deutsch, R., & Drozd, L. M. (2016). Considerations for step-up planning: When and how to determine the "right" time. In L. M. Drozd, M. A. Saini, & N. W. Olesen (Eds.), *Parenting plan evaluations: Applied research for the family court* (2nd ed., pp. 535–554). New York: Oxford University Press.

Rossi, F. S., Holtzworth-Munroe, A., & Rudd, B. N. (2016). Intimate partner violence and child custody. In L. M. Drozd, M. A. Saini, & N. W. Olesen (Eds.), *Parenting plan evaluations: Applied research for the family court* (2nd ed., pp. 346–373). New York: Oxford University Press.

Rossi, F. S., Holtzworth-Munroe, A., Applegate, A. G., Beck, C. J. A., Adams, J. M., & Hale, D. F. (2013). Detection of intimate partner violence and recommendation for joint family mediation: A randomized controlled trial of two screening measures. *Psychology, Public Policy, and Law, 21*(3), 239–251. https://doi.org/10.1037/law0000043

Solomon, J., and George, C. (Eds.). (2011). *Disorganized attachment and caregiving: Research and clinical advances*. New York: Guilford Press.

Tjaden, P. and Thoennes, N. (2000). Prevalence and consequences of male-to-female and female-to-male intimate partner violence as measured by the national violence against women survey. *Violence Against Women, 6:142*. Los Angeles: Sage Publications.

Ver Steegh, N., & Dalton, C. (2008). Report from the Wingspread Conference on domestic violence and family courts. *Family Court Review, 46*(3), 454–475.

12 Giving Voice to Children in Non-Traditional Families

Deborah Wald and S. Margaret Lee

Children come before our family courts in many ways, and as culture and technology have changed, families' forms, structures and roles have become increasingly diverse. As historically depicted in the literature, families have had one mother and one father, most typically a biological mother and a presumed biological father, her husband. This has long been treated as the norm. Laws in family court established what should happen when this normative family underwent a divorce, with the specific laws being based on cultural beliefs and social science literature as they evolved over time. Thus, children as the father's property moved to the tender years doctrine and eventually laws allowing for shared custody following divorce. However, many of these laws continued to be based on an assumption that all children were raised by one mother and one father who preferably were married when the children were born.

Since the 1970s, issues related to families in general – and to parenting in particular – have only become more complex. Two predominant areas of familial evolution have impacted a push towards revision of the laws that affect families: (1) the emergence into the open of same-sex parents has led to debates regarding what we mean when we refer to "parents," e.g., how to manage non-biological parentage, who is legally a parent, who is a psychological parent and how many "parents" a child can have; (2) the increasingly open use of assisted reproductive technology has created a new range of biological relationships and psychological relationships, as we differentiate between "donors," "surrogates" and "parents." From sperm and egg donation to surrogacy, conflicts arising in the definition and resolution of who is a parent, and what relationships should be protected/promoted legally, have become critical issues for the courts to address.

This chapter is primarily written by a family law attorney, who will review the history of legal questions that have arisen in response to these identified societal changes. Since many of the conflicts seen in court arise within the context of the child's interest in maintaining attachment relationships, the editors have summarized the area of parent–child attachment and will comment (frequently in footnotes) on the psychological issues that arise in the legal processes occurring within the courts. Our goal is to assist readers in addressing multi-parent families, non-biological parents and, generally, how to keep apace with rapidly changing cultural and technological changes in how families are formed and defined.

As will be discussed in this chapter, the laws needed to accommodate both the issues raised by attachment relationships and the expanded recognition of a wide variety of families, are slowly leading to an evolution in the law.

Historical Perspective

The definitions of who are parents, what should happen following a separation and what should happen to the children, has changed significantly over the past 100 years in the

DOI: 10.4324/9780429397806-13

United States. In part this has been due to changing cultural norms and in part due to advances in the research of the social sciences. During the time frame when this chapter and book was being written, there has been societal upheaval that has highlighted the systemic aspects affecting so many areas of the United States and its organizing principles, including the law and its historical development. Thus, prior to elaborating on where we currently are in terms of the legal system and the issue of "who is a parent," it is important to articulate the foundations and possibly, systematic problems, in the family law arena.

When America was founded we based our legal system on the English system, which was adversarial, patriarchal and all judges and attorneys (barristers) were male. As a young country only landed, Anglo males had rights. As will be described, societal changes and research has resulted in shifting beliefs and has empowered women and resulted in an increasing focus on the importance of children's needs and interests. However, these changes have historically been driven by patriarchal, Anglo, middle-class segments of the society. Twin or competing issues about who should raise children and who should be financially responsible for children run through this narrative. Cost and access to the court (and attorneys) lead most families to resolve their differences without court involvement. The high-profile cases that set legal precedents depend on legal representation and involvement of the courts. Cases involving disadvantaged minorities are less likely to reach the high courts where precedents are established.

For some years, there has been professional discussion regarding whether "family issues" should even be assessed within an adversarial system. Might it not be better that a system be developed that focuses not on who was right and wrong but how children's needs can best be addressed and what tools are needed by parents to resolve differences? Expanding legal definitions of who might be a "parent" and what constitutes a "family" highlight the need to seriously consider which adults children rely on, what it means to lose important adults and whether there might be a better system to address these issues holding the children's best interests as paramount.

Historical Views and Social Science Research

Up until the 20th century, children were essentially seen as property of their fathers. Children's emotional needs for attachment figures were not taken into consideration when families separated.

This began to change during the 20th century, as the emotional ties between mothers and their children (at least in the dominant paradigm) began to be valued. The "tender years doctrine" emphasized the needs of infants and young children to be in the primary care of their mothers. These changes reflected societal and cultural shifts as well as changes in societal values, and impacted the status and value given to children and women. Additionally, with Freud and his focus on the critical nature of a child's experiences during development informing later adult functioning, the child as an individual with a unique psychology was emphasized.

Another factor that contributed to a shift of focus to the individual child's development was the lowering of childhood mortality rates, allowing for more emotional investment by parents likely to result in an ongoing relationship with their child. During World War II, in part prompted by voluntary parent–child separations due to bombing in London and the U.K., John Bowlby (1969/1982) explored the idea that the parent–child attachment relationships during the early years represented the major line of development; that attachment relationships significantly impact various areas of development; and that separations and losses of these attachment relationships can result in potentially permanent impairments to development. Bowlby theorized that attachment relationships not only serve to facilitate the child's safety, it is within these relationships that the child develops a view of the self, a view of the world and a view of others, which facilitates a "theory of mind." Furthermore, within these relationships a child learns to label, understand and manage emotions; and, finally, these relationships become an avenue for developing internal templates for developing future intimate relationships and eventual caregiving relationships.

Also during this historical period, Anna Freud was expanding the idea of children needing a "psychological parent" in order to ensure the child's psychological development and health (Goldstein, Freud & Solnit, 1973). In mid century it was assumed in the social science literature that the mother's care was unique; that there was a hierarchy of attachment relationships and that mothers, unless significantly impaired or damaged, were more important to children than fathers. When there was divorce, young children would typically be raised by their mothers, both because mothering was seen as unique and mothers tended to be the "primary caregiver." The cultural stereotype of the stay-at-home mom and the working father reflected the dominant culture's reality and a certain level of economic stability. Needless to say, these stereotypes were based largely on a white, patriarchal, financially comfortable norm; racial, ethnic, sub-cultural and class differences, among other variations, bring with them myriad other family structures based on different cultural values in addition to different economic realities.

In the latter part of the 20th century there was a shift in the dominant culture, with more white Anglo women joining the workforce and there being a move, in the dominant culture, for fathers to become more involved with their children; there was also the development of effective birth control so that couples could plan their families to balance work and parenting. These factors prompted the expansion of research involving fathers and other, non-biological, parenting figures (Kelly & Lamb, 2000). The research began to demonstrate (not without controversy) (Lamb, 2016) that children could have multiple attachment relationships, that attachment relationships were not determined by biology, and that the maintenance of these important relationships significantly informed the child's development of a sense of security about self, others and the world (Smith, Coffino, Van Horn & Lieberman, 2012). Secure attachments have been shown to be associated with other psychological benefits such as social competence, academic advantage and even physical health (Sroufe, Egeland, Carlson & Collins, 2005). Furthermore, the disruption or loss of an attachment relationship can result in decreased or impaired functioning, depression, anxiety and loss of security and can have lifelong implications (Bowlby, 1969/1982). This more nuanced understanding of attachment relationships coincided with cultural changes that resulted in substantial shifts in thinking that are explored hereafter in this chapter.

It should be noted that research indicates that attachment relationships have been found to be similar across cultures and classes (Van Ijzendoorn and Sagi-Schwartz, 2008); however, when families and children experience cumulative stresses, traumas and losses, the child's experience of security can be eroded. Thus, separations from attachment figures, exposure to conflict and violence, the stress of income instability, and myriad other factors can erode a child's sense of security and the security in their parent–child relationships (Kelly & Lamb, 2000).

Legal Outgrowths from Cultural Shifts

Cultural concepts of what constitutes a family began to shift in the late 1960s and early 1970s, starting with a reexamination of the concept of "illegitimate" children. Legally, the issue of the treatment of "illegitimate" children reached the United States Supreme Court in 1972, causing them to state that:

The status of illegitimacy has expressed through the ages society's condemnation of irresponsible liaisons beyond the bonds of marriage. But visiting this condemnation on the head of an infant is illogical and unjust. Moreover, imposing disabilities on the illegitimate child is contrary to the basic concept of our system that legal burdens should bear some relationship to individual responsibility or wrongdoing. Obviously, no child is responsible for his birth and penalizing the illegitimate child is an ineffectual – as well as an unjust – way of deterring the parent. Courts are powerless to prevent the social opprobrium suffered by these hapless children, but the Equal Protection Clause does enable us to strike down discriminatory laws relating to status of birth where – as in this case – the classification is justified by no legitimate state interest, compelling or otherwise. (*Weber v. Aetna Casualty & Surety Company*, 92 S.Ct. 1400, 1406–07 (1972))

This decision was a catalyst for the drafting of the first Uniform Parentage Act (UPA) in 1973, the explicit purpose of which was to provide equal protection to children regardless of whether they were born into or out of wedlock.

In addition to largely eliminating the concept of "illegitimacy," the 1973 UPA, which was adopted in some form by all 50 states, set the stage for recognition of legal parentage based on behavior rather than biology or marriage. It included a provision that a man is presumed to be a child's legal father if "while the child is under the age of majority, [the man] receives the child into his home and openly holds out the child as his natural child" (See 1973 UPA §4(a)(4)). This, in turn, led to the emergence in the 1980s of cases that put a legal focus on the role of non-biological parents; that is, people who had raised children as their own despite the lack of a biological or adoptive connection. Many of these cases pitted biology against the child's attachment relationships. Prominent examples include the United States Supreme Court's decision in *Michael H. v. Gerald D.*, 109 S.Ct. 2333 (1989), in which a child brought a court action asking that her relationship with the man who had raised her – with whom her married mother had had an extended adulterous relationship – be recognized as her legal father, rather than her mother's husband (who also was her genetic father). That is, the child was trying to have the court override the marital presumption of paternity and allow her attachment to her non-biological father to prevail. A plurality of the Supreme Court upheld the state's application of the marital presumption, and its favoring of the mother's husband over the man the child looked to for fathering. However, the Supreme Court did not *require* this result; it simply found this result constitutional when mandated by state law. This case led to a gradual reexamining of biology versus attachment in family law. Expansion of the definitions of what constitutes a parent, and the subsequent need to create new and broader laws that protect parent–child relationships, has been informed by the concept of attachment relationships between children and their parents or other adults and the resulting social science research from this area of investigation.

In addition to uncertainty about the continuing role of biology in determining legal parentage, when we redefine and broaden what we mean by the term "parent" – presumably with the goal of taking the child's perspectives and "best interest" into consideration – more and more situations arise where more than two people fit our expanded definitions. As we increasingly consider intentions and attachment and experience – and not just biology or marriage – in determining whom to recognize as "parents" under a broad variety of circumstances, it becomes clear that there are many children being raised by more than two "parents."

As we look at broadening understandings of parenting and parentage, a final issue that needs to be addressed is the area of gender identification, both when parents are transgendered and when children identify as transgendered. How the legal system manages these issues often strikes at the heart of cultural stereotypes and can pit societal confusion about gender and children's best interests against each other.

The focus of this chapter is on how our court system can (or should) adjust its laws to accommodate these new definitions of parents and the biological and social science research that is currently available.

Given some of the underlying biases associated with same-sex relationships, as well as concerns in the assisted reproduction area (such as "am I really a parent if I am not biologically related to my "child"?), commentary will be made about the need for cultural sensitivity on the part of mental health professionals and suggestions will be provided for professionals working with these families.

We start the chapter with some cases that have come before the courts, to assist the reader in understanding the context in which the questions we are addressing are being raised. Following these brief vignettes, there will be a review of how these complex cases have been resolved historically and in the current law.

A wife has a brief affair, but soon ends it without ever telling her husband. When they find out they are expecting a baby, they are overjoyed. They assume the baby is the husband's, until blood tests taken at the baby's birth exclude the husband as a possible biological father. At this point the wife admits that she had a brief affair with a close family friend. After some counseling, husband and wife are able to resolve their marital conflict and they remain living together, raising the baby as their child. However, they also allow the baby's biological father and his wife to spend time with the baby, including weekly overnights starting when the baby is three months old; and when the biological mother has to go back to work, the biological father's wife assumes childcare responsibilities for the baby.

When the baby is 3 years old and getting ready to start preschool, the biological mother and her husband decide that it is too awkward and embarrassing to have to explain their family to the public, and that it is not in the child's best interests for her biological father and his wife to be involved with their family any longer. They cut off contact between them and the toddler.

From a legal and psychological perspective, how many parents does this child have?[i]

A lesbian couple has a child together, using an old friend as their sperm donor. The child is raised by the women, but spends time with the donor each week including occasional overnights and vacations. The child calls the donor "dad" and knows the donor's parents as a third set of grandparents. When the women decide to move across country, the donor tries to stop the move. Who are this child's legal parents? What is the significance of the child's relationship with the donor if he does not qualify legally as a parent?

A woman gives birth to a baby boy. Within a few months, her 16-year-old daughter – who lives with her – also gives birth to a baby. Mother and daughter raise the two babies together, and the daughter cares for – and breast feeds – both babies while her mother is at work.

When her mother is killed in a car accident, the daughter continues to raise both babies as her own. She also has one more baby, and the three children are raised as siblings and consider the young woman their mother.

When this young woman gets arrested for peripheral involvement in a drug case, all three children are temporarily taken from her and put into foster care. As a mother, she is

---

i   The development of attachment relationships predominantly occurs over the first four years of life. By 3 years old a child will have established specific attachment relationships with their caregivers, which are further consolidated and internalized during the fourth year of life. The loss of important caregivers when 3 years old would represent a significant risk to psychological development.

entitled to reunification services with her two biological children, but the third child – her biological brother – is in danger of being separated from the other two children and placed for adoption.

What is the legal and psychological relationship of this young woman and this child?

A child is adopted as an infant by a single mother. After the adoption is final, the woman enters into a committed relationship with another woman who co-parents with her for the next eight years. By the time they break up, the child is 10 years old and cannot remember a time when the two women were not both in his life as his parents. However, the women never went to court to address the partner's relationship with the child – nor did they marry – so the woman who did not participate in the original adoption does not have an established legal relationship with either the other woman or the child.

Does her failure to adopt the child mean that she is not a parent? What is the relevance of the child's experience of whom his parents are?[ii]

A young man and woman get together when they are in their late teens. The young woman has an infant. She is estranged from her own family and moves in with the young man and his parents. Together, they raise the baby for the next several years, but their relationship doesn't last and eventually the young woman – now in her 20s – moves on; however, recognizing that by now the baby is firmly settled into the home and family of the young man, the young woman leaves the baby where he is and visits him on weekends as she is able given her own lack of a stable job or residence. The baby's biological father has no involvement in the baby's life, and the baby is raised to believe the young man is his father.

When the baby is 10 years old, the mother marries a man with a stable job and home and decides it is time to bring her family back together. She tells her ex-boyfriend that she wants the child back. The ex-boyfriend refuses to return the child to her, arguing that he has raised the child as his own since infancy and that the child deserves the stability of remaining where he is in the home he knows and with the family he loves. They end up in a court battle over custody.

Who is this child's legal family? Where should he live? What is everyone's appropriate role going forward?

A husband and wife have a young son. When the son is 5 years old, the father comes out as transgender and fully transitions to female. The marriage does not survive the transition. The couple share a 50/50 parenting plan, whereby the child is in the care of each parent on alternating weeks. Six months into this arrangement, it becomes apparent that on the original mother's custodial weeks the child is frequently late to school and arrives with homework left uncompleted; whereas on the original father's custodial weeks the child consistently arrives at school on time and fully prepared. The original father therefore goes to court to request that the child be in her care on all school nights. The case is referred to Family Court Services for assessment, and the assessment comes back determining that the child should be in the original mother's care except for alternating weekends to protect the child from gender confusion about his father's transition.

Is this an appropriate basis for a change in custody? If so, under what criteria should the child's adjustment to his parent's gender transition be assessed?[iii]

ii   It is cases such as these that were so difficult when the law precluded or there failed to be legal status. Given the fact pattern it would be reasonable to assume that the child experienced both of her mothers as parents/ as attachment figure, and that contact with both should be assured regardless of the relationship status.

iii   Without an established protocol for determining "best interest" factors, cases like this are very vulnerable to societal biases and individual prejudice that assumes that a transgendered parent would cause gender confusion and this would necessarily be detrimental to a child.

A husband and wife are divorced. Their son and daughter live primarily with their mother, with monthly weekends with their father and his new wife and baby. When the daughter is 10 years old, she starts expressing that her authentic identity is male; she asks to be called by a male name, prefers traditionally male clothing, and is attracted to things generally identified as "masculine." The mother accepts these changes and supports her child; but when the child goes to their father's house, the father is upset and hostile to the child's efforts at gender expression and blames the masculine behaviors on the mother. The father refuses to have the child for weekends any more unless the child dresses as and "acts like" a girl, allegedly out of fear the child will influence the father's new baby.

How should the courts, and any mental health professionals working with the family, assess the child's gender issues in the context of what is now a custody dispute between the parents? How should they differentiate between cause and effect (i.e., is the parental conflict caused by the child's gender non-conforming behavior or is the child's gender non-conforming behavior a reaction to parental conflict)?[iv]

Children Being Raised by Non-Biological Parents

What is meant by the word "parent" is evolving due to a combination of factors including the increased acceptance of adoption and assisted reproduction, as well as social science research on the importance to children's healthy development of maintaining stable attachments. The visibility of same-sex families – where by definition there is likely to be at least one parent not genetically related to the child – also is having an influence on this change.

Historically, a child's "mother" was the woman who gave birth and the child's "father" was that woman's husband. The children of unmarried women were "illegitimate" and had no legal fathers. In this sense, "father" always has been a social construct – primarily, a way to assign financial responsibility for children to an individual man, rather than to society at large. It only is relatively recently that we have had a way to easily determine who a child's genetic parents are, which scientific advancement has led some to defer to genetics as the sole factor determining whom a child's "real" parents are. Exclusive reliance on genetics to determine "real" parentage is ahistorical and does not take into account the many other factors that make someone a parent.

Family courts around the country are wrestling with what makes someone a legal parent in the current era. As our courts and legislatures grapple with solving this puzzle, the primary factors they have looked to are procreative intentions, genetics, marital presumptions, and parental conduct. In the model "traditional" heterosexual family, all these factors point in the same direction: i.e., that the husband and wife are the parents of the child. In other words, in a model "traditional" family, the genetic parents have intentionally conceived their children within the context of their marriage, and will be acting in the role of parents with regard to those same children. However, both interesting and challenging legal and social policy issues arise when all of these factors *don't* point to the same people.

Further, as we redefine and broaden what we mean by the term "parent," more and more situations arise where more than two people fit our expanded definitions. When we look to intentions and conduct – and not just biology or marriage – it quickly becomes clear that there may be more than two people in a child's life who are candidates for the legal title "parent."

iv   The probable need for a child custody evaluation performed by a Forensic Mental Health Professional with education and experience with gender issues would likely be helpful in aiding the court and determining the dynamics underlying the conflict.

While most states remain reluctant to find more than two parents for any given child, due to some combination of distaste for "non-traditional" families and concern about putting children in the middle of increasingly complex custody disputes, there are starting to be some exceptions. For example, in 2013 the California Legislature passed a law by which a child could have more than two legal parents under certain specific circumstances, by adding a section (c) to California Family Code section 7612, providing that:

> In an appropriate action, a court may find that more than two persons with a claim to parentage ... are parents if the court finds that recognizing only two parents would be detrimental to the child. In determining detriment to the child, the court shall consider all relevant factors, including, but not limited to, the harm of removing the child from a stable placement with a parent who has fulfilled the child's physical needs and the child's psychological needs for care and affection, and who has assumed that role for a substantial period of time. A finding of detriment to the child does not require a finding of unfitness of any of the parents or persons with a claim to parentage.

Examples of families where children have more than two parents include polyamorous families, where the children are intentionally conceived with the intention of more than two people parenting; families where there was a break-up while the child was young, and then a regrouping, so children are raised from a young age by a mother, a father, and the newer stable partners of one or both original parents; and families where the children were conceived with the assistance of known egg or sperm donors who have gone on to play a meaningful and consistent role in the children's lives.

Same-Sex Couples

Lesbian and gay couples have long parented children; however, up until fairly recently the majority of children being raised by same-sex couple were born into heterosexual relationships which later dissolved. It still is true that many children being raised by same-sex couples were conceived through heterosexual sex; but increasingly, same-sex couples are choosing to become parents through adoption or assisted reproduction without other known individuals involved.

Children adopted or conceived into stable same-sex relationships tend to do well by all measures. A study published in 2018 by the Williams Institute of the UCLA School of Law found that 25-year-olds raised by lesbian parents do as well on multiple measures of psychological health as their peers. The researchers compared relationships, educational/job performance, and behavioral, emotional and mental health problems in the two samples and found no significant differences.[1]

> "When I began this study in 1986, there was considerable speculation about the future mental health of children conceived through donor insemination and raised by sexual minority parents," says the study's lead author, Dr. Nanette Gartrell. "We have followed these families since the mothers were inseminating or pregnant and now find that their 25-year-old daughters and sons score as well on mental health as other adults of the same age."

The results of the Williams Institute study are consistent with results of another study published in the *Journal of Developmental & Behavioral Pediatrics* which followed three groups of families in Italy: 70 gay fathers who had children through surrogacy, 125 lesbian mothers who had children through donor insemination, and 195 heterosexual couples who had children through spontaneous conception. "Our findings suggested that children with same-sex parents fare well, both in terms of psychological adjustment and prosocial behavior," said Prof. Roberto Baiocco, PhD, of Sapienza University of Rome. The scores for psychological adjustment for the children in all three groups were within the normal range, with no major differences.[2]

Despite the consistency of the research on same-sex couples raising children, these families continue to experience biases within the court system. It is common for mental health professionals interacting with these families to focus on which parent is the "real" (meaning genetic) parent and to assume that the child's attachment to this parent will be stronger. This is not necessarily true. For example, in a case that gained some notoriety due to its tragic ending, a lesbian couple had two kids together, first a girl and then a boy. The biological mother was the primary breadwinner for the family, while her partner took primary child-rearing responsibility. This was contrary to all stereotypes, especially because the partner was quite "butch" in appearance.

When the couple broke up, they initially agreed that the daughter would stay with the non-biological mother while the son – who was four years younger – would stay with the biological mother. This lasted approximately three years, until the biological mother wanted to change the custody arrangement. When the non-biological mother resisted, the biological mother took her to court and obtained a judgment that she was the children's only legal parent because the non-biological mother had never adopted the children (although they both bore her last name and she had co-parented them for their entire lives). The non-biological mother was found to be a legal stranger to the kids, with no right to even visitation. The daughter was forced to move back with the biological mother, and remained there until her pediatrician intervened after she became clinically depressed and the biological mother reluctantly allowed her to return to her non-biological mother's care.

Shortly after the daughter returned to live with her non-biological mother, the biological mother and the son moved to a very conservative state to live with the biological mother's new girlfriend. On the Fourth of July they were in a tragic car accident in which the biological mother was killed. The son woke up in a hospital bed and, once fully conscious, was asked who his father was. Unable to identify his father (having been conceived through sperm donation), and with the state he was in not then recognizing same-sex families as having any legal rights, the child was on his way into foster care when the biological mother's parents intervened to take custody of him and deliver him safely back into the care of his non-biological mother and his sister, where he remained for the rest of his childhood. Needless to say, both of these children wouldn't have suffered such substantial trauma had the legal systems with which they interfaced been willing to acknowledge their experiences of whom their parents were.

Gay men parenting children tend to encounter even greater bias. The myth that gay men are more likely to molest children still casts a shadow over these families, and they are likely to be particularly (and justifiably) sensitive to any hints of prejudice. Further, the assumption that young children need mothers can lead to significant negativity about gay men raising kids. Finally, nurturing babies and young children is so counter to what our society considers "masculine" that being a devoted, hands-on father often creates gender insecurity even for heterosexual dads; and for a gay man – whose masculinity already is subject to societal skepticism – this insecurity can evidence itself in a variety of ways that can prove challenging in the context of a custody dispute. It is essential that mental health professionals interacting with gay parents be sensitive to all these dynamics and more.

Finally, it is important to note that many people are not exclusively hetero- or homosexual, and this leads to some complex parenting situations. Based on the collective experience of members of the National LGBT Bar Association's Family Law Institute – a national body of attorneys practicing LGBT-oriented family law – it seems safe to conclude that polyamorous[3] families with children are far more common throughout the country than is publicly acknowledged. Further, lesbians and gay men continue to conceive children as a result of extra-marital affairs with people of the opposite sex, whether intentionally or accidentally. People interacting with same-sex couples and their children should make no assumptions about how the children were conceived or whom they rely on for parenting. Instead, as with heterosexual couples, there is no replacement for an unbiased inquiry into the actual history and dynamics of each specific family.

Assisted Reproduction

The significance of cases involving assisted reproductive technologies (ART) in the evolution of parentage law is threefold. First, these cases have called into question the value we place on genetics in assigning parental rights, since many ART cases involve children who are intentionally conceived on behalf of "parents" to whom they are not genetically related. Second, many of these cases have attempted to apply contract principles to parentage determinations, undermining the longstanding rule that contract principles do not apply in family law. Third, these cases have highlighted the issue of procreative intentions as a basis for establishing legal parentage. By doing so, ART cases have paved the way for many of the cutting-edge developments in family law, and they therefore are critical to a modern examination of the legal issues involved in determining parentage.

Sperm Donation Cases

One of the critical functions of family law is to determine which adults will be responsible legally and financially for children. Historically, there was no issue with determining which woman was a child's mother – the mother was the woman who gave birth to the child. But determining the father was far more complicated – at least until the 1960s, when HLA typing created the first accurate method for determining genetic paternity. Up until then, determining paternity was almost entirely a matter of public policy, and many of the rules developed prior to accurate paternity testing continue to exist in our Family Codes to this date (e.g., the "marital presumption").

Because there is an historical assumption in family law that men may be reluctant to take financial responsibility for their offspring, we make it hard – if not impossible – to "opt out" of legal fatherhood. Generally speaking, we hold biological fathers legally and financially responsible for their offspring regardless of whether the men intended to become parents – and even regardless of whether the men knew of the children's existence. As stated by one California judge: "If you have sexual intercourse with a woman of child-bearing years ... you have good cause to believe that you may have just created a human being ..." (*In re Zacharia D.* (1993) 6 Cal.4th 435, footnote 8). "Polyamorous" in this context refers to families where ongoing intimate relationships are maintained between more than two adults – typically either one man with two women or two men with one woman. Often these triads live together and share financial and household as well as child-rearing responsibilities.

Sperm donation attempts to carve out an exception to this well-established rule. It provides a way for men to knowingly help women conceive children without the men becoming legally or financially responsible for those children. It also provides a way for single women, lesbian couples, and heterosexual couples struggling with male factor infertility to conceive children without the legal and social complications of having the sperm donors obtain rights to – or bear responsibilities for – the children. However, because the legal recognition of certain men as "sperm donors" rather than "fathers" allows some men to avoid legal and financial responsibility for their genetic offspring, the category of "sperm donors" tends to be strictly defined and narrowly construed.

States have adopted different requirements for differentiating a sperm donor from a father; and different states have taken more or less rigid stances on maintaining these distinctions. California and Virginia have contrasting statutes, and each have recent – and controversial – appellate decisions that illustrate the issues raised, and thereby are instructive on the range of possible approaches.

Up until 2016, when a new expanded sperm donation statute went into effect, California was one of many states where, in order to qualify as a "sperm donor," the sperm had to be donated to a licensed physician rather than directly to the intended recipient(s). Effective January 1, 2016, the California sperm donation statute now reads: "(1) The donor of semen provided to a licensed physician and surgeon or to a licensed sperm bank for use in assisted reproduction by a woman other than the donor's spouse is treated in law as if he were not the natural parent of a child thereby conceived, unless otherwise agreed to in a writing signed by the donor and the woman prior to the conception of the child. (2) If the semen is not provided to a licensed physician and surgeon or a licensed sperm bank as specified in paragraph (1), the donor of semen for use in assisted reproduction by a woman other than the donor's spouse is treated in law as if he were not the natural parent of a child thereby conceived if either of the following are met: (A) The donor and the woman agreed in a writing signed prior to conception that the donor would not be a parent. (B) A court finds by clear and convincing evidence that the child was conceived through assisted reproduction and that, prior to the conception of the child, the woman and the donor had an oral agreement that the donor would not be a parent." As stated by one California Court of Appeal:

> the California Legislature has afforded unmarried as well as married women a statutory vehicle for obtaining semen for artificial insemination without fear that the donor may claim paternity, and has likewise provided men with a statutory vehicle for donating semen to married and unmarried women alike without fear of liability for child support. Subdivision (b) [of California Family Code § 7613] states only one limitation on its application: *the semen must be 'provided to a licensed physician.'* Otherwise, whether impregnation occurs through artificial insemination or sexual intercourse, there can be a determination of paternity with the rights, duties and obligations such a determination entails. (*Jhordan C. v. Mary K.* (1986) 179 Cal.App.3d 386, 392, emphasis added)

By way of contrast, Virginia adopted a broader definition of "sperm donor" in their "assisted conception" statute. The statute defines a "donor" as "an individual, other than a surrogate, who contributes the sperm or egg used in assisted conception" (Virginia Code § 20–156). Virginia Code § 20–156 defines "assisted conception" as

> a pregnancy resulting from any intervening medical technology, whether in vivo or in vitro, which completely or partially replaces sexual intercourse as the means of conception. Such intervening medical technology includes, but is not limited to, conventional medical and surgical treatment as well as noncoital reproductive technology such as artificial insemination by donor, cryopreservation of gametes and embryos, in vitro fertilization, uterine embryo lavage, embryo transfer, gamete intrafallopian tube transfer, and low tubal ovum transfer.

Both California and Virginia have recent appellate cases that test the limits of their respective sperm donor statutes. In both cases, men attempted to establish paternity, custody and visitation with regard to their genetic offspring and the mothers of those offspring countered by arguing the men were sperm donors and not fathers. Both states' courts of appeal ultimately determined that the men were fathers rather than sperm donors, albeit for very different reasons. These two decisions graphically illustrate how narrowly sperm donation statutes continue to be construed, and how strongly inclined courts still are to find that men are legal fathers when provided with an opportunity to do so.

In the California case, *Jason P. v. Danielle S.*, the man and woman had cohabited for many years, but never married. They had tried to conceive a child together through intercourse but had been unable to do so. In 2009, they underwent an *in vitro* fertilization and embryo transfer procedure by which a child, G., was conceived. The parties gave conflicting testimony as to whether or not they were together as a couple at the time of the IVF procedure, and they also gave conflicting testimony about whether at the time of the IVF procedure it was their intention that Jason would be a sperm donor or a father. However, there was uncontroverted evidence that G. knew Jason and called him "dada," and that the three had lived together for some period of time after G. was born.

The trial court dismissed Jason's paternity action, finding that he was a sperm donor rather than a father as a matter of law because he had provided his sperm to a physician for purposes of assisted reproduction by a woman who was not his wife. The Court of Appeal reversed and remanded, *not* because they disagreed that Jason met the statutory definition of a sperm donor, but because they agreed with Jason's argument that even a statutory sperm donor can become a legal father if he subsequently receives the child into his home and openly holds the child out as his own child. As stated by the Court of Appeal: "we hold that [California Family Code] section 7613(b) should be interpreted only to preclude a sperm donor from establishing paternity based on his biological connection to the child, and does not preclude him from establishing that he is a presumed parent ... based on post-birth conduct." Thus, G. ended up with a legal father based on the California appellate court's insistence on taking a holistic approach to viewing G.'s situation, rather than a formulaic approach whereby they simply applied the strict language of California's sperm donation statute and stopped there.

In the Virginia case, *Bruce v. Boardwine*, a single woman (Bruce) approached a longtime friend (Boardwine) and asked him to be a sperm donor. The two never had been sexually intimate and never had lived together. After some hesitation, Boardwine agreed. Without a physician's involvement and without a written contract, Boardwine went to Bruce's home on multiple occasions and provided her with sperm samples. Bruce used these samples to inseminate herself using "an ordinary turkey baster," and ultimately conceived a child. With apparently conflicting expectations about the degree of involvement Boardwine would have in the child's life, the two quickly ended up in court.

The court in *Bruce v. Boardwine* determined that Boardwine was a father and not a sperm donor because Bruce inseminated herself using a turkey baster whereas the assisted conception statute defines assisted conception as "a pregnancy resulting from *any intervening medical technology*" (California Fam. Code § 7613, subd. (b)). As stated by the Court of Appeals:

> The word "medical," in its ordinary use, means "of, relating to, or concerned with physicians or with the practice of medicine" and "requiring or devoted to medical treatment." ... The statute does not encompass all technology. Instead, its language is limited to "medical technology." *The plain meaning of the term "medical technology" does not encompass a kitchen implement such as a turkey baster.* (*Bruce v. Boardwine* (Va. Ct. App. 2015) 64 Va.App. 623, 630, emphasis added)

The court in *Bruce v. Boardwine* did exactly the opposite of what the California court did in *Jason P. v. Danielle S.* – instead of taking a holistic look at the situation, they very strictly applied the language of Virginia's assisted conception statute and stopped there. And the child J.E., like little G., ended up with a legal father.

The flip side of the sperm donation issue is what the legal status is of a husband whose wife gives birth as a result of an artificial insemination procedure involving the sperm of another man. The Uniform Parentage Act (UPA) has long addressed this issue, providing that where a husband consents to his wife's insemination with donor sperm, the husband will be treated for all purposes as the natural father of the child. California has modernized its sperm donation statute to make it both gender neutral and marital status neutral. The California sperm donation statute now provides, in relevant part: "If a woman conceives through assisted reproduction with semen or ova or both donated by a donor not her spouse, with the consent of another intended parent, that intended parent is treated in law as if he or she were the natural parent of a child thereby conceived. The other intended parent's consent shall be in writing and signed by the other intended parent and the woman conceiving through assisted reproduction" (California Fam. Code § 7613, subd. (a)). As noted by the Maryland Court of Special Appeals in a recent case, this provision is consistent with the more general "presumption of 'legitimacy' for children born to a married mother," aka, the marital presumption (*Sieglein v. Schmidt* (2015) 224 Md.App. 222, 239). The decision of the Maryland Court of Special Appeals subsequently was affirmed by the Maryland Court of Appeals in *Sieglein v. Schmidt* (2016) 447 Md. 647.

The *Sieglein* case raised the issue of whether the artificial insemination statute should be interpreted to apply to an IVF procedure by which a married woman had an embryo transferred into her uterus, which embryo had been created from anonymously donated eggs and sperm. When the marriage fell apart just weeks after the baby was born, the wife petitioned the court for child support and the husband took the position that he was not legally responsible for the baby because he was not the genetic father and there had been no "artificial insemination" procedure as described in the statute. The Court of Special Appeals rejected the husband's argument, noting:

> Artificial insemination and IVF are two of many procedures used today that change or substitute for human reproduction by sexual intercourse, and we are not called upon here to explore or explain any scientific, practical or ethical distinctions. By enacting ET § 1–206(b), the General Assembly evinced its intention to acknowledge the role of medically assisted, non-traditional conception of a child in establishing a parent's rights and obligations. Under Maryland law, within the context of marriage, the precise physical procedure has no necessary impact on the relationships of the parties involved—mother, father, and child. Therefore, we interpret ET § 1–206(b) as also encompassing IVF, and hold that a child conceived via artificial insemination or IVF with the consent of the parties and born during a marriage is the legitimate child of the marriage and legal parentage is established as to both spouses. In the matter before us, where Mother and Father were married at the time of conception and birth, and willingly and voluntarily agreed to conceive a child through assisted reproductive services using anonymously donated genetic material, we hold that ET § 1–206(b) applies to establish the legal parentage of both Mother and Father. (*Sieglein v. Schmidt, supra*, 224 Md.App. at 242–243; accord, *Okoli v. Okoli* (2012) 81 Mass.App. Ct. 371, 963 N.E.2d 730)

The lesson to be learned from these very different cases – and from the different approaches of California, Maryland and Virginia – seems clear: courts will embrace opportunities to find that a child has a legal father if given an opportunity to do so. And while both the California and Virginia cases involved single women attempting to be recognized as single mothers, rather than lesbian or gay couples seeking joint parental rights, in many states a courts' interest in assuring that children are connected to both a mother and a father may cause similar outcomes in cases involving same-sex couples. Professionals interacting with children born through artificial insemination would be well-advised to have some familiarity with state law in order to help them determine the legal status of a child's genetic parents, in order to assure that they are engaging in the appropriate inquiries when discussing the various involved adults with the children. It is worth noting that with the advent of genetic tracing services such as 23andMe and Genealogy.com, an increasing number of donor-conceived young adults are identifying and locating their donors as well as "donor siblings" and forming new extended "families" based on these previously anonymous relationships.

Surrogacy Cases

There are two types of surrogacy: "traditional surrogacy" and "gestational surrogacy." With gestational surrogacy, the surrogate is impregnated by way of an embryo transfer using eggs from someone else – either the "intended mother" or an egg donor – so the surrogate is not genetically related to the child. In a "traditional" surrogacy, the surrogate is impregnated via artificial insemination – often with sperm of the "intended father" – pursuant to an agreement that, even though she is the genetic mother, she is bearing the child for someone else. The laws for these two types of surrogacy tend to differ. Whereas gestational surrogacy has attained fairly broad acceptance, traditional surrogacy remains far more controversial because it involves a woman giving up a baby that is genetically her own.

Gestational Surrogacy

When a heterosexual, married couple conceives a child using the wife's egg, fertilized *in vitro* with the husband's sperm, but the baby is carried to term by a "gestational surrogate," there are two possible mothers: the genetic mother and the gestational mother. Most states that have ruled on this type of surrogacy arrangement have found that the husband and wife are the legal parents of the child, and that the woman who carried the child is not a parent, based on consideration of some combination of intentionality and genetics.

The lead case in this area comes from California. In *Johnson v. Calvert* (1993) 5 Cal.4th 84, the California Supreme Court resolved a dispute between a child's genetic/intended mother and the gestational surrogate by placing dispositive weight on the parties' pre-birth intentions. The Court found that "although the [Uniform Parentage] Act recognizes both genetic consanguinity and giving birth as a means of establishing a mother and child relationship, when the two means do not coincide in one woman, she who intended to procreate the child – that is, she who intended to bring about the birth of a child that she intended to raise as her own – is the natural mother under California law" (*Id.* at 94).

Johnson v. Calvert was followed by a far more complex California case, *In re Marriage of Buzzanca* (1998) 61 Cal.App.4th 1410. The *Buzzanca* case involved a married couple, John and Luanne Buzzanca, who – like the couple in *Sieglein* – wanted to have a child but both were infertile. They obtained the eggs of an anonymous egg donor, which they had fertilized *in vitro* with the sperm of an anonymous sperm donor, and the resulting embryos were implanted into the womb of a married surrogate. This child had at least six adults involved in her procreation: an egg donor/genetic mother, a sperm donor/genetic father, the

Buzzancas as "intended parents," the surrogate and the surrogate's husband (who would be presumed to be the child's father, based on a traditional application of the marital presumption, since his wife was the one giving birth). Then, while the surrogate still was pregnant, the Buzzancas filed for divorce. In the dissolution papers, Luanne indicated that the baby was a child of the marriage; John responded that there were no children of the marriage, maintaining that he should not be held legally responsible for a child that was not genetically his, was not genetically his wife's, and was not even being gestated by his wife.

The trial court agreed with Mr. Buzzanca, finding that the baby had *no legal parents.* The Court of Appeal that heard the case disagreed, finding that when a married couple – unable to procreate without medical assistance – causes the conception of a child by use of reproductive technology and with the intent to parent the child, they must be held to the status of legal parents regardless of genetics.

Ohio has taken a completely different philosophical approach to determining parentage in the surrogacy context – albeit one that often will result in the same outcome. Explicitly rejecting California's intent-based analysis as too confusing and prone to uncertainty, Ohio has chosen to rely exclusively on genetics, finding that: "The test to identify the natural parents should be, 'Who are the genetic parents?'" According to Ohio law,

> when a child is delivered by a gestational surrogate who has been impregnated through the process of in vitro fertilization, the natural parents of the child shall be identified by a determination as to which individuals have provided the genetic imprint for that child. If the individuals who have been identified as the genetic parents have not relinquished or waived their rights to assume the legal status of natural parents, they shall be considered the natural and legal parents of that child. (*Belsito v. Clark* (1994) 67 Ohio Misc.2d 54, 66)

Whether relying on genetics or intentions or some combination of the two to determine legal parentage, the majority of states now are recognizing gestational surrogacy as a valid way for infertile or same-sex couples to become parents. The same cannot be said for traditional surrogacy.

Traditional Surrogacy

While the *Buzzanca* case elevated intentions over genetics and other more traditional family law factors, California appellate courts so far have drawn a line at recognizing "traditional surrogacy" arrangements. In *In re Marriage of Moschetta* (1994) 25 Cal.App.4th 1218, Robert and Cynthia Moschetta wanted to have a child, but Cynthia was sterile. Elvira Jordan agreed to be inseminated with Robert's sperm, and to carry the baby to term for the Moschettas and then give it to them to raise. Pursuant to their written agreement, Elvira was to allow Robert sole custody, and was to consent to adoption of the child by Cynthia. However, when the Moschettas broke up during her pregnancy, Elvira decided to keep the baby; although when the couple reconciled she relented and allowed the baby to go home with them. Seven months later, the Moschettas broke up for good. Cynthia petitioned the court for parental rights, arguing that she was the baby's legal mother, not Elvira, based on the terms of the written surrogacy contract and the fact that the baby had lived with Cynthia for most of its short life. The courts disagreed, holding that *Johnson v. Calvert* did not apply since Elvira was both the genetic and the gestational mother. According to the court, enforcing a pre-birth contract to give up one's baby would go against broader public policies relating to parentage and adoption. Legally, based on their genetic relationships to the baby, Elvira was the mother and Robert was the father.

Much more recently, and after careful and detailed analysis, the Supreme Court of Tennessee reached a similar conclusion. In *In re Baby* (2014) 447 S.W.3d 807, an unmarried man and woman from Italy, who were unable to have children together without reproductive assistance, engaged the services of a surrogacy program in the United States to help them find a surrogate. They were matched with a married surrogate in Tennessee. The parties entered into a written surrogacy agreement, and the Surrogate subsequently was inseminated with the Intended Father's sperm. According to the decision, the Intended Parents paid the Surrogate approximately $42,000 to cover her medical and legal fees, plus some $31,000 as compensation for pain, suffering and other expenses related to the pregnancy and birth.

Approximately a month before the due date, the two couples petitioned the court and obtained a pre-birth order terminating whatever parental rights the Surrogate and her husband otherwise would have and finding that the Intended Father was the legal father of the child and that the Intended Parents should have full custody immediately upon birth. The Intended Parents were present at the birth; however, medical personnel advised them that they should have the Surrogate breast feed the baby for the first week "in the interest of ensuring the best possible nutrition for the Child." By the end of that week, the Surrogate had obtained new counsel and filed a motion requesting custody of the child and a determination that she was the child's legal mother.

After careful consideration of the case, including a review of both Tennessee law and the decisions of other states that have addressed the complex family law issues raised by traditional surrogacy, the Tennessee Supreme Court concluded that, pursuant to Tennessee statutory law, a woman who gives birth to her own genetic child is a mother. Because a mother's rights to her child cannot be terminated before the child's birth, nor can she consent to an adoption before the child's birth, the trial court's order was invalid. As explained by the Court:

> Our adoption code provides that a woman may qualify as the "[l]egal parent" of a child in two ways: (1) by being "[t]he biological mother of a child," ... or (2) by being "[a]n adoptive parent of a child," ... Once a woman attains the status of a legal parent, her parental rights may only be terminated in three ways." Those ways include an involuntary termination by a court in the best interests of the child, consent by the mother to an adoption as part of an adoption proceeding, or relinquishment of the child to an adoption agency. (*In re Baby, supra*, 447 S.W.3d at 829–830, internal citations omitted)

The Court went on to note:

> Other state courts considering traditional surrogacy agreements have declined to allow parties to circumvent statutory procedures in regard to the termination of a surrogate's parental rights. When considering the validity of a traditional surrogacy agreement, a California appellate court found that absent compliance with statutory procedure, the surrogacy contract was insufficient "to deprive the 'surrogate' of the legal parental tie she would otherwise possess." [Citing *In re Marriage of Moschetta, supra*.] ... Like these courts, we conclude that the enforcement of a traditional surrogacy contract must occur within the confines of the statutes governing who qualifies as a legal parent and how parental rights may be terminated ... Just as parents may not use a private agreement to deprive courts of their designated role in determining the best interests of a child in a custody determination ... a parent may not avoid judicial oversight of the termination of parental rights by the terms of a contract. Hence, a

traditional surrogate, as the biological mother of the child, is a legal parent until her parental rights are terminated through one of our statutory procedures ... In a traditional surrogacy, an intended mother — who, by definition, is not genetically related to the child — may only attain the status of a legal parent through adoption. (*In re Baby, supra,* 447 S.W.3d at 830–831, internal citations omitted)

The Court went on to clarify that:

the public policy of our state does not preclude the enforcement of traditional surrogacy contracts. Their enforceability, however, is not without bounds. Compensation may not be contingent on the surrender of the child or the termination of parental rights ... Moreover, the terms of a surrogacy contract may not dispense with a judicial determination of the best interests of a child. Likewise, the terms of a surrogacy contract may not circumvent the statutes governing a person's status as a legal parent or the statutory procedures for terminating parental rights. Finally, termination of parental rights in an involuntary proceeding may not occur absent a finding that the parent is unfit or that substantial harm to the child will result if parental rights are not terminated. (*Id.* at 833)

Having fully analyzed the proposed traditional surrogacy from a traditional family law perspective, and consistent with the relevant statutes, the Court concluded:

Because the Surrogate is the biological mother of the Child ... she qualifies as a legal parent ... Our statutes provide no mechanism by which a biological birth mother – including a traditional surrogate – may use a contract to avoid attaining the status of a legal parent or to negate parental status prior to the birth of a child ... Our statutory procedures unequivocally prohibit the voluntary relinquishment of a biological birth mother's parental rights prior to birth through either surrender or parental consent to adoption ... Thus, the provisions of the contract at issue that attempt to circumvent statutory procedure by terminating or negating the parental rights of the Surrogate prior to birth contravene the public policy of our state. Those provisions are therefore unenforceable and without legal effect ... In summary, the statutory procedures for terminating the parental rights of a traditional surrogate are limited to involuntary termination [based on a court's finding of unfitness], parental consent to adoption, and surrender. Because neither the parties nor the juvenile court complied with any of these procedures in this instance, the juvenile court's order terminating the parental rights of the Surrogate must be set aside ... Our ruling does not preclude the termination of the parental rights of the Surrogate in a future proceeding. Absent a basis for involuntary termination, however, the termination may only occur if the Surrogate executes a surrender or consent to a petition for adoption. (In re Baby, supra, 447 S.W.3d 834–836, internal citations omitted, emphasis added)

The case therefore was remanded to the juvenile court for a determination of visitation and child support.

Starting with Cultural Competence

It still is common for psychologists and social workers within the family law world to use outmoded language on their intake forms. If the form provides pre-printed spaces for information about the "mother" and the "father," a same-sex couple already will have concerns about whether the mental health professional interviewing them will be biased against them or their family before the interview even begins. If there are two spaces in which to identify a child's parents, single parents – or families where the children are being raised by more than two parents – may immediately feel marginalized.

The same is even more true where there may be issues of gender identity with one or both parents, or with the child. Transgender parents are subject to enormous bias in our court system, and gender non-conforming children and youth are at particular risk. Mental health professionals should be sensitive to the vulnerabilities of these populations and make sure that sensitivity is reflected in their initial presentations, whether through websites or intake forms or releases that must be signed in order for the work to begin. An intake form that offers three options for gender – "male," "female" or "other" – immediately will alert a vulnerable client that the practitioner is aware that not everyone fits into a binary model of gender and will greatly increase the opportunity for an open and honest clinical or forensic interaction.

Families created through assisted reproduction or adoption may be comparably sensitive to questions that assume a biological connection between parent and child. Many parents whose families are the result of either gamete donation or adoption have very little information about their children's genetic histories. Questionnaires asking for detailed information about genetic parents without a clear way to indicate that this information is unavailable may unintentionally alienate these families.

If mental health professionals who interface with the family law system want to get a clear and honest picture of a family, the documents they rely on to gather information must leave room for family members to define their own roles in terms of gender identity, position in the family, etc. By being open in initial paperwork and presentation, the professional will indicate to family members that it is safe to be honest about who they are; an indication that is essential if the goal is to get an accurate picture of the family system and the dynamics that may be causing stress to that system and to the children being raised in it.

Children of Transgender Parents

Transgender parents interfacing with our family courts are subject to a great deal of bias. There are many cases, from around the country, where a transgender parent has lost custody of his or her child for no reason other than the court's discomfort with the parent's gender identity or expression. Take the following true example:

When his child is 4 years old, a husband finally admits that he is transgender and decides to transition from male to female. His wife is deeply distressed and decides to end the marriage. It is important to note here that, contrary to common assumptions, approximately half of marriages survive the gender transition of one of the spouses. Although in this particular example, the husband's gender transition led to the end of the marriage, no conclusions should be drawn about the general impact on marriages of one spouse transitioning genders. Once the husband is through his transition, and as they settle into their new lives, the couple shares custody of the child on an alternating 2–2–5–2 schedule whereby the child is with the original mother on Monday and Tuesday nights, with the transitioned mother on Wednesday and Thursday nights, and alternates weekends between the two homes.

The transitioned mother is an excellent parent, attentive to the child's social and emotional needs and involved with the child's school and community. The original mother is far less focused on the child's needs. After several years of co-parenting, the transitioned mother becomes aware that the original mother is consistently getting the child to school late without his homework completed, and that the child is in danger of being expelled from school due to his chronic tardiness on the mornings he is in his original mother's care. There is no problem with attendance on the days the child is in his transitioned mother's custody.

Based on her concern about her son's education, the transitioned mother goes to court to request a change in the parenting plan to grant her physical custody on all school days. The court refers the couple to Family Court Services to meet with a "Child Custody Recommending Counselor." The counselor meets with both parents and the child, and rather than focusing on the child's educational needs the counselor becomes fixated on the fact that the child calls the transitioned mother "dad" in private (as he did prior to the transition) while referring to her as "mom" in public (to avoid embarrassment or confusion). The counselor concludes that this demonstrates that the child is under significant psychological stress and makes this the focus of her report to the court, in which she recommends full custody for the original mother despite the original mother's documented neglect of the child's education and despite the child's strong attachment to the transitioned mother.

In this case, it took the pro bono efforts of multiple attorneys and a complaint to the licensing board in order to get the court evaluation back on track and focused on the child's educational needs. In a community less rich in resources than the San Francisco Bay Area – where the case occurred – the court almost certainly would have followed the recommendations of the counselor and the transitioned parent almost certainly would have lost custody of her child.

Gender Non-Conforming Children

If the experience of transgender parents in the court system is bad, the experience of gender non-conforming children often is worse. This is an issue of increasing importance as more and more children are expressing gender non-conformity at younger and younger ages.

While many children experiment with gender identity during their childhoods without being transgender, there are children who *consistently*, *persistently* and *insistently* identify with a gender other than the one assigned at birth – whether the "opposite" gender or something in between the two genders. For these children, affirmation of their authentic sense of gender is likely to be critical to their emotional and psychological well-being.

According to a 2018 study by the American Academy of Pediatrics of adolescents aged 11–19:

> Nearly 14% of adolescents reported a previous suicide attempt; disparities by gender identity in suicide attempts were found. Female to male [transgender] adolescents reported the highest rate of attempted suicide (50.8%), followed by adolescents who identified as not exclusively male or female (41.8%), male to female [transgender] adolescents (29.9%), questioning adolescents (27.9%), female adolescents (17.6%), and male adolescents (9.8%). Identifying as nonheterosexual exacerbated the risk for all adolescents except for those who did not exclusively identify as male or female (ie, nonbinary). For transgender adolescents, no other sociodemographic characteristic was associated with suicide attempts.[4]

The incidence of suicidality in transgender youth should be enough to convince any mental health professional that taking a young person's gender identity and expression seriously is critical to their health.

There are few published cases of custody disputes centered on the gender identity of a child, but those that exist should be shocking to anyone sensitive to the psychological needs of children. The most commonly cited one is *Smith v. Smith*, a 2007 Ohio case involving the custody of two children (both born boys) whose parents divorced when they were 6 and 2 years old. The mother was designated as the primary residential parent for both children and the father had very little ongoing contact with the children.

When the kids were approximately 9 and 5, the mother moved with them to a new county and enrolled the older child in school as a girl. She took the child to a transgender support group and indicated a willingness to allow the child to transition genders when the child got older. On this basis, the father petitioned for a change in custody and the court issued temporary orders removing both children from their mother's care and placing them in the home of their father. To the extent the mother was allowed to continue exercising custody, she was ordered "to stop any treatment or counseling for gender disorder; to stop the child from attending transgender support groups; to stop addressing the boy as Christine or any other female name; and to stop allowing or encouraging him to wear girl's clothing ... The court absolutely prohibited the parties from treating or counseling the boy for gender identity disorder (hereinafter "GID") throughout the pendency of the dispute."

The court acknowledged that the child had "displayed some female tendencies, including an attraction to female clothing, as early as age two." Among the evidence produced at trial was a video the child sent the father when the child was approximately 9 years old. As described in the decision:

> The videotape recorded the child sitting in a chair and talking about his gender, trying to explain the situation to his father. The boy stated numerous times on the tape that he is a girl, wants to be a girl, and that he would like to live a normal life as a girl. He stated that he looked forward to the time when he could wear girl's clothes all the time. He stated that he is a girl even if he does not have all the body parts of a girl. He expressed a desire to either go to school as a girl or be home-schooled. He also stated a number of times that he hoped his father would understand the situation, but that no matter what, he intended to become a girl.

Following a trial at which multiple experts testified, the court issued a final judgment granting the father primary physical custody with the mother only having the children on weekends. The court also issued the following orders:

> The boy was not to be encouraged or permitted to wear girl's clothes. He was not permitted to go by a girl's name or be referred to as "she" or "her." ... The child was not permitted to attend transgender support groups and was to become "disassociated with that lifestyle," absent agreement of both parties or further order of the court.

Following further proceedings – during which a psychologist who had conducted an evaluation of both parents and the child testified that both parents were well-meaning and attempting to act in their child's best interests, and that the child was effeminate but not necessarily transgender and was depressed and possibly suicidal – the court issued final orders granting sole custody of both children to the father.

When last heard from by one of the attorneys who consulted on this matter, the child – now in his 20s – was still alive but struggling with severe depression as well as substance abuse issues. Neither he nor his mother had recovered in any way from the traumas they suffered through the court proceedings. One can hope that this young man will find a way to make sense of his experiences and find peace with his gender identity, whatever it may be. One also can hope that the court system has become more sensitive to gender issues in the 20 years since this case was adjudicated. Sadly, more recent experiences suggest this may not be true.

In a fairly recent case that occurred in the San Francisco Bay Area – an area far more socially progressive than rural Ohio – a family found themselves in a similar situation to the one that occurred in *Smith*. The child – born male – lived primarily with his mother. His father had little contact with the child. The child began expressing his identity as a girl when he was a toddler, and by the time he was 5 or 6 he consistently was choosing girls' clothing and preferred to be called by a girl's name. His mother did research and sought out experts and committed to affirming her child's gender identity. When the father became aware of the situation, he took the mother to court. The father's position was that the mother was turning their son into a little girl, and he set about trying to counteract her influence. The Bay Area court, in an attempt not to pick sides, granted the parents joint custody and allowed each of them to parent their child as they saw fit during the time the child was in their care. What this meant, for the child, was that during the time he was with his mother he wore girls' clothing, went by a girl's name, and saw a gender-affirming therapist. When he was with his father he only was allowed to wear boys' clothing, was required to go by a boy's name, and was taken to a therapist affiliated with the father's church who counseled the child about his "god-given" sex. If one wanted to design an experiment to see if a psychologically healthy child can be led by parental conflict about the child's fundamental identity to engage in a confused, if not distorted, thought process, it would be hard to come up with a better one than this.

Conclusion

Children are being raised in so many different types of families, professionals make assumptions at their own peril. For our court system to be responsive to the needs of all the children who rely on it – whether in the context of custody or dependency proceedings or otherwise – it must have an expansive view of what constitutes a parent. The professionals who interact directly with the children play a critical role in making sure the decision-makers (typically the judges) have an accurate picture of the children's needs. Keeping an open mind, setting aside biases, and asking curious questions without presupposing the answers all are critical tools for people interviewing children being raised in non-traditional families. Without these tools, these children are at particular risk.

Some examples: intake forms can be edited to allow space for more than two parents and to eliminate gendered assumptions about who those parents are (e.g., prompts can be "Parent" and "Parent" and "Are there any additional parents I should know about?" rather than "Mother" and "Father"). Allowing families to feel seen at the intake stage is more likely to produce accurate results regarding family configurations and alignments. Rather than asking children about their "mom and dad," even very young children can be asked open-ended non-leading questions like "who is in your family?" This will allow children to identify a beloved donor, or stepparent, or whomever that child is attached to without assumptions that can cause some of the child's most significant relationships to be overlooked. A child's expression that they have more than two parents can be treated with compassion rather than skepticism. Children can be encouraged to choose toys to play with from a broad array of objects, not pre-selected based on any assumptions about gender preference. Practitioners can have books in their bookcases and posters on their walls that demonstrate openness to lots of kinds of families. Coming to a family with curiosity and an open mind will allow that family – and that family's children – to present themselves with authenticity without feeling the need to defend against the interviewer. This will, in turn, lead to a much more accurate interview and much more reliable results.

Notes

1. See "Mental Health of Adult Offspring of Lesbian Parents"; National Longitudinal Lesbian Family Study, July 2018; Authors: Nanette Gartrell, Henny Bos, Audrey S. Koh. (https://williamsinstitute.law.ucla.edu/publications/nllfs-mental-health-offspring/)
2. See "Same-Sex and Different-Sex Parent Families in Italy: Is Parents' Sexual Orientation Associated with Child Health Outcomes and Parental Dimensions?" by Baiocco, Roberto PhD; Carone, Nicola PhD; Ioverno, Salvatore PhD; Lingiardi, Vittorio MD; Journal of Developmental & Behavioral Pediatrics: September 2018, Volume 39, Issue 7, pp. 555–563.
3. "Polyamorous" in this context refers to families where ongoing intimate relationships are maintained between more than two adults – typically either one man with two women or two men with one woman. Often these triads live together and share financial and household as well as child-rearing responsibilities.
4. © 2018 American Academy of Pediatrics, *Pediatrics*, October 2018, volume 142 / issue 4.

References

Bowlby, J. (1969/1982). *Attachment and loss, vol. 1: Attachment*. New York: Basic Books.

Goldstein, J., Freud, A., & Solnit, A. J. (1973). *Beyond the best interest of the child*. New York: Free Press.

Kelly, J. B., & Lamb, M. E. (2000). Using child development research to make appropriate custody and access decisions for young children. *Family and Conciliation Review, 38*(3), 297–311. doi:10.1111/j.174–1617.2000. tb00577.x

Lamb, M. E. (2016). Critical analysis of research on parenting plans. In L. Drozd, M. Saini, & N. Olesen (Eds.), *Parenting plan evaluations: Applied research for the family court* (2nd ed., pp. 170–202). New York: Oxford University Press.

Smith, G., Coffino, B., Van Horn, P., & Lieberman, A. (2012). Attachment and child custody: The importance of available parents. In K. Kuehnle, and L. Drozd (Eds.), *Parenting plan evaluations: Applied research for the family court* (pp. 5–24). New York: Oxford University Press.

Sroufe, L. A., Egeland, B., Carlson, E., & Collins, A. (2005). *Development of the person*. New York: Guilford Press.

Van Ijzendoorn, M. H., & Sagi-Schwartz, A. (2008). Cross-cultural patterns of attachment: Universal and contextual dimensions. In J. Cassidy & P. R. Shaver (Eds.), *Handbook of attachment: Theory, research, and clinical applications* (pp. 880–905). New York: Guilford Press.

13 Hague Convention Cases

S. Margaret Lee and Brent D. Seymour

Hague Convention Cases

This chapter is written by an attorney and a psychologist and focuses on cases involving the Hague Convention where a child has allegedly been wrongfully retained or wrongfully removed from his or her country of habitual residence and a Petition for return of the child has been filed. After placing these cases within the context of other international cases involving children, the Hague Convention will be explained, including the exceptions to the Hague which allow for the child to remain in the country where he or she has been retained. Although many Hague cases are resolved solely through legal argument, some cases lend themselves to the involvement of mental health professionals. Specifically, cases where the issue of the "grave risk of harm" exception is raised, the issue of "sufficient age and maturity" for a child to object to their return is raised and/or the issue of "habituation"/"acclimatization" is raised, lend themselves to expert evaluation and opinions by mental health professionals. In this chapter the authors will focus on the last three issues. The "grave risk of harm" exception is beyond the scope of this chapter and is currently being rethought. Those interested in that literature could begin with "assessing Grave Risk of Harm Under the Hague Convention (Melcher, 2013).

There are several court systems within which children may be involved in international cases. Children are referred to immigration courts when they have entered the United States seeking asylum, refugee status or have accompanied their parents, who lack legal status. This court venue and associated cases is described in Chapter 8 of this volume, written by Giselle Hass. In the literature, there has been some discussion when "abduction cases" may involve both immigration courts assessing asylum and a Hague Convention action (Garbolino, 2019).

The other groups of cases involving international matters and the question of where children will reside involve families engaged in custody disputes. International child custody disputes are not uncommon as nearly one in four U.S. children have at least one foreign-born parent (Shear & Drozd, 2013). In our increasingly global world, with international dating sites and relatively easy and affordable ways to maintain long distance relationships, this is not surprising.

In cases where the United States is the country of habitual residence and one parent wishes to relocate with the children to another country, typically to return to his or her native country, that parent will request, in Family Court, permission to move with the children. In these cases the legal standard applied is the issue of the "best interests of the child" (BIC). There is a large body of literature discussing relevant factors that should be considered when analyzing BIC, given general relocations disputes within the U.S. If the reader is interested in that body of literature, the following authors and articles are recommended as a basis for review (Parkinson, Taylor, Cashmore, & Austin, 2016; Austin,

DOI: 10.4324/9780429397806-14

2008; Kelly & Lamb, 2003) Additionally some states, such as California, have specified factors that must be considered when determining whether a move is in the child's best interest (La Musga).[1] There is a far more limited body of literature that describes the complexities involved in determining BIC in international relocations, particularly in terms of how to assess and prioritize factors (Warshak, 2013; Shear & Drozd, 2013, Morley, 2013). Evaluators and judges need to understand that in allowing the move to a foreign country there is a risk that future jurisdiction regarding custody and access will be changed from the U.S. to the other country. In addition to this jurisdictional issue, questions regarding language fluency, educational issues, cultural influences arise. Finally, practical issues such as different time zones, cost of transportation and the family's resources become critical in assessing whether children will be able to maintain relationships with both of their parents. A primary source of information describing how to evaluate international relocations can be found in a special issue of the Journal of Child Custody (2013).[2]

Unfortunately, many evaluators hold a misconception regarding the jurisdictional issues in international relocation cases. There is an erroneous belief that if a country is a "Hague" country, that country will insure that children will be returned to the United States for visitation with the left behind parent and/or that U.S. orders will be enforced by foreign courts (Morley, 2013; Shear & Drozd, 2013).

There are some protections that may optimize continued access between the left behind parent and children, including mirror orders, posting a bond and assessing whether the parent who is allowed to move with the children has sufficient ties to the U.S. that they would be unlikely to abduct the child permanently as they would not want to give up the possibility of coming to the U.S. (Morley, 2013).

Unlike the cases described above, where the court determines which country the children in a family dispute will primarily reside, other cases arise when a parent wrongful removes or retains a child from the U.S. without the other parent's or the court's permission. Or, wrongfully removes a child from another country and retains the child in the U.S. without parental permission or court approval. When a child is abducted from the U.S. and wrongfully retained in a non-Hague country, there is very little that can be legally done to return the child. According to data from the Department of State, "approximately forty percent of abduction cases involve children taken from the United States to countries with which the United States does not have reciprocal obligations under the HCAC" (Pahrand, 2017). At times parents hire "recovery agents" to abduct children and return them to the left behind parent (Yaffe-Bellany, 2020). On the other hand, if the child is wrongfully removed or retained in a country that is a signatory to the Hague Convention, return is possible as the Hague Convention was established to protect the jurisdiction of the country of habitual residence. However, different countries have differing records for acting in a prompt manner to returning children (Messitte, 2020).

There are some important similarities and differences between the two types of international family disputes. As noted above increasing numbers of families are multi-national and multi-cultural. The increases in international travel and Americans working abroad lead to an increased number of both intentional and unintentional situations where children have parents from different countries (Lesh, 2011; Moskowitz, 2003). This has been accompanied by an increase in international child abduction (Pahrand, 2017).

There are important similarities and differences between these two different types of international cases. Thus, both types of cases involve resolving disputes about where children will primarily reside, what culture will likely be their primary culture and what social capital will be most readily available to them.

Both these types of cases also involve the question of when and how the child's voice should be considered and the weight that their opinion should carry (Fernando, 2014).

The U.N., in Article 12 of the United Nations Convention on the Rights of Children ("UNCRC"), states that children's voices should be heard in any legal proceeding affecting them. Their voices are typically heard through an expert, through an attorney or through their direct testimony (Fernando, 2014). In international relocation cases heard in Family Court, the child's voice and the weight of that opinion is typically brought in through a mental health professional performing a child custody evaluation. In Hague cases, the child's voice is most critical if the child objects to being returned to its home country. In both domestic cases and Hague cases, there is a need to determine whether the child's opinion has been independently formed, and is not based on undue influence, typically by one parent's behavior.

The major differences between domestic cases and Hague cases involve the legal stand-ard applied and the scope of cases before the court. Thus, potentially any family where one parent requests an international relocation can do so and the case will be analyzed using the BIC standard. In such a situation the child's preference for a parent may be a relevant factor, also preference for a country may be considered. In Hague cases, there are very limited conditions defining which families may apply for relief. The psycho-legal question is whether one of the exceptions to the Hague's general policy of returning children to their country of habitual residence is applicable and therefore it is, essentially, a jurisdictional question. The goal of the Hague Convention is to "restore abducted children promptly to their pre-abduction circumstances" (Reynolds, 2006). The children's preference for a parent plays no role in determining the outcome, nor does a preference for one country over the other country, and the merits of the case are not at issue. Once it is determined as to whether the child will be returned to its home country or remain in the U.S., the child's best interests will be decided within that jurisdiction in Family Court.

The Hague – Legal Issues

The Hague Convention of October 25, 1980 on the Civil Aspects of International Child Abduction ("the Convention") is an international treaty focused on child abduction of children across international borders by one of the child's parents. The United States is a Contracting State to the Convention, along with approximately 100 other countries. The International Child Abduction Remedies Act (ICARA) 22 U.S.C. §§9001 et seq. implements the Convention in the United States.

The objects of the Convention are:

1 To secure the prompt return of children wrongfully removed to or retained in any Contracting State (Article 1(a)); and
2 To ensure that rights of custody and of access under the law of one Contracting State are effectively respected in the other Contracting States (Article 1(b)).

The Convention does not apply a "best interests" standard" and may not be used to litigate child custody and visitation. Furthermore "[a] decision under [the] Convention concerning the return of the child shall not be taken to be a determination on the merits of any cus-tody issue." (Article 19) Rather, the focus is on which Contracting State has jurisdiction to determine custody and visitation issues (i.e., the child's habitual residence).

The State Department's Office of Children's Issues acts as the Central Authority for the United States. When an application is received from another country, the State Department will help the applicant to discover the whereabouts of the child and refer the applicant to local counsel, if requested. If the applicant does not have counsel, the State Department will forward the application to the District Attorney of the county in which the child is located. The District Attorney will then file the Hague Petition, but will not represent the applicant. The applicant must either retain counsel or represent him or herself. In other countries, the Central Authority may take a more pro-active role in resolving the dispute.

The Petitioner may instead file a petition under the Convention in State or Federal Court, without going through the Central Authority. (Article 29) The State courts and the Federal Courts have concurrent jurisdiction over matters brought under the Convention. If the Petitioner files in State Court, the Respondent may remove the proceedings to Federal Court at his or her option. The Convention requires that the adjudicating court "act expeditiously." Six weeks is the suggested time for return of the child. (Article 11)

The Convention requires that a child be returned promptly to its habitual residence if the Petitioner establishes the following:

1   The child was removed or retained from a Contracting State.
2   The child was habitually resident in the Contracting State at the time of removal or retention (Article 4).
3   The child is under the age of 16 (Article 4).
4   The removal or retention was in breach of petitioner's rights of custody under the laws of the country in which the child was habitually resident at the time of removal or retention (Articles 3 and 5(a)).
5   At the time of removal or retention, those rights of custody were actually exercised (Article 3(b)).

Additionally, the Hague Convention must be in effect between the United States and the country of the child's habitual residence at the time of removal or retention (Article 35) and the child must be located within the jurisdiction of the Court in which the petition is filed.

The Court is not bound to order the return of the child if the Respondent establishes any of the following defenses:

1   Petitioner was *not actually exercising his or her rights of custody* at the time of removal or retention (Article 13(a)).
2   Petitioner *consented* to removal or retention of the child (Article 13(a)).
3   Petitioner subsequently *acquiesced* in the removal or retention of the child (Article 13(a)).
4   There is a *grave risk* that return would expose the child to physical or psychological harm or place the child in an intolerable situation (Article 13(b)).
5   The child *objects* to being returned and has attained an *age and degree of maturity* at which it is appropriate for the Court to take account of the child's views (Article 13).
6   The judicial proceedings have been commenced *more than one year* from the date of removal or retention and the child is *well settled* in the new environment (Article 12).
7   The the return of the child would not be permitted by the fundamental principles of the requested State relating to the protection of human rights and fundamental freedoms (Article 20).

If the Respondent has commenced any custody proceedings in the State Court, all custody proceedings shall be stayed pending resolution of the Hague Petition.

> After receiving notice of a wrongful removal or retention of a child, the judicial or administrative authorities of the Contracting State to which the child has been removed or in which it is being retained shall not decide on the merits of rights of custody until it is be determined that the child is not to be returned under this Convention

or unless an application under this convention is not lodged within a reasonable time following receipt of the notice. (Article 16)

Habitual Residence

The Convention requires that the judicial authority determine the child's habitual residence. Habitual residence was purposely left undefined by the drafters of the Convention in order to leave room for judicial interpretation and flexibility and in order to prevent mechanical application of the term.

The U.S. Supreme Court recently decided the case of *Monasky v. Taglieri,* 140 S.Ct. 719 (2020) and, for the first time, addressed the determination of habitual residence under the Hague Convention. The Supreme Court held, "[A] child's habitual residence depends on the totality of the circumstances specific to the case. An actual agreement between the parents is not necessary to establish an infant's habitual residence" (*Monasky v. Taglieri,* at 722). This opinion was intended to resolve the differences among the circuits in determining habitual residence, noting the Sixth Circuit's holding in *Taglieri v. Monasky,* 908 F.3d 404 (6th Cir. 2018) (acclimatization as the "primary approach"), the Ninth Circuit's approach in *Mozes v. Mozes,* 239 F.3d 1067 (9th Cir. 2001) (shared parental intent), and the Seventh Circuit's approach in *Redmond v. Redmond,* 724 F.3d 729 (7th Cir. 2013) (rejecting "rigid rules, formulas, or presumptions").

Writing for the Court, Justice Ginsburg stated a child's residence in a particular country can be deemed "habitual," however, only when her residence there is more than transitory. "Habitual" implies "[c]ustomary, usual, of the nature of a habit ... The place where a child is at home, at the time of removal or retention, ranks as the child's habitual residence" (*Monasky v. Taglieri,* 140 S. Ct. at 726).

Determination of habitual residence requires "a fact-sensitive inquiry, not a categorical one." It is important to note that the habitual residence is determined at the time of the removal or retention – not at some future time, such as time of trial or even when the petition is filed.

No single factor is dispositive of all cases. For example, the ages of the children involved may require a different focus of the habitual residence inquiry: facts indicating the child's acclimatization may be "highly" relevant for older children who are capable of acclimating to their surroundings, while the "intentions and circumstances" of the parents are relevant in cases involving children who are unable to acclimatize due to their youth or other reasons. Likewise, a child that has been abducted to another country, will have had little or no time to acclimatize, so absent prior history in the new country, acclimatization will be of little relevance.

While *Monasky v. Taglieri* shifts the focus of the habitual residence inquiry from any one particular factor such as shared parental intent or acclimatization to a totality of the circumstances, both factors are still important factors and must be addressed. See, e.g., *Grano v. Martin,* 2020 WL 1164800 (S.D.N.Y., 2020), citing *Monasky v. Taglieri* ("the parents' last shared intent is a relevant consideration, but it is by no means dispositive of the habitual residence inquiry").

Mozes v. Mozes, 239 F.3d 1067 (9th Cir. 2001) is useful for determining whether there was a shared intent. *Mozes* instructs that before a child may acquire a new habitual residence, the court must determine "whether there is a settled intention to abandon a prior habitual residence." The parent's intent must be mutual; the unilateral action of one parent to move a child to another country does not alter the child's habitual residence. *Gitter v. Gitter,* 396 F.3d 124, 135 (2d. Cir. 2005).

Monasky also requires that the Court consider whether or not the child has acclimated to the new home. And importantly, acclimatization must be determined at the time of the unlawful retention – facts relating to the child's subsequent acclimatization and activities in the new residence after the date of abduction or retention are not relevant to the inquiry.

To determine whether a child has acclimatized, the court should consider the length of time the child has spent in the new country, as well as how integrated the child has become into the new society. The court will consider such factors as the child's schooling, activities, language ability, and adaptation to the new culture.

Exercising Parental Rights

To establish a wrongful removal or retention, the Petitioner must establish that he or she had rights of custody under the laws of the child's habitual residence and that he or she was actually exercising those rights. *Abbott v. Abbott*, 560 U.S. 1, 8–9 (2001). Rights of custody include rights relating to the care for the child and, in particular, the right to determine his or her residence (Article 5(a)). The Convention distinguishes rights of custody from rights of access, which include the right to take a child for a limited time to a place other than the child's habitual residence (Article 5(b)). Breach of rights of access, alone, will not sustain an action for return of the child under the Convention.

The proof of exercise of rights of custody has a low threshold. A court should "liberally find exercise [of custody rights] whenever a parent with de jure custody rights keeps, or seeks to keep, any sort of regular contact with his or her child." *Friedrich v. Friedrich*, 78 F.3rd 1060, 1065 (6th Cir. 1996).

> If a person has valid custody rights … that person cannot fail to "exercise" those rights under the [Convention] short of acts that constitute clear and unequivocal abandonment of the child. Once it determines that the parent exercised custody rights in any manner, the court should stop – completely avoiding the question whether the parent exercised the custody rights well or badly. These matters go to the merits of the custody dispute and are, therefore, beyond the subject matter jurisdiction of the federal courts. (*Id.* at 1066)

Consent and Acquiescence

Consenting to, or subsequently acquiescing in, the removal or retention is a defense under the Convention. Consent and acquiescence are two separate and "analytically distinct" affirmative defenses. *Padilla v. Troxell*, 850 F.3d 168, 175 (4th Cir. 2017), 850 F.3d at 175. The defense of consent "concerns the petitioner's conduct before the contested removal or retention" and acquiescence "concerns whether the petitioner … agreed to or accepted the removal or retention [after it had already occurred.]" *Id.* "For both the consent and acquiescence defenses, the inquiry turns on the petitioner's subjective intent." *Padilla*, 850 F.3d at 176).

The defense of consent requires less formality than the defense of acquiescence … "[A] petitioner's statement or conduct – formal or informal – can manifest consent." *Padilla,* 850 F.3d at 176; to establish consent, courts "focus on the parties' conduct *prior* to the removal or retention." *Id.* However, "conduct after removal can be useful in determining whether consent was present at the time of removal." *Gonzalez-Caballero v. Mena*, 251 F.3d 789, 794 (9th Cir. 2001). To establish the defense, the respondent must prove by a preponderance of the evidence, that the petitioner subjectively intended to allow the respondent to remove the child permanently from its habitual residence. A parent's consent to the children going to another country with the other parent for a limited period of time will not sustain the defense. Thus, the fact that a petitioner initially allows children to travel, and knows their location and how to contact them, does not necessarily constitute consent to removal or retention under the Convention. *Baxter v. Baxter*, 423 F.3d 363, 371 (3d Cir. 2005). It is important to note that consent may be withdrawn before the removal. *Khalip v. Khalip*, 2011 WL 1882514 (E.D. Mich. May 17, 2011) (same). In *Khalip*, the petitioner signed a notarized application consenting to the respondent permanently moving with the children. However, before the respondent actually removed the children, the petitioner signed another notarized application, revoking his consent. Because the petitioner revoked his consent before removal, the court found that the respondent failed to demonstrate consent. *Id.*, 2011 WL 1882514 at *6.

The defense of acquiescence concerns a petitioner's subjective intent *after* the removal or retention. *Padilla*, 850 F.3d at 176. Additionally, "the defense of acquiescence has been held to require 'an act or statement with the requisite formality, such as testimony in a judicial proceeding; a convincing written renunciation of rights; or a consistent attitude of acquiescence over a significant period of time.'" *Baxter*, 423 F.3d at 371 (quoting *Friedrich v. Friedrich*, 78 F.3d 1060, 1070 (6th Cir. 1996)).

Sufficient Age and Maturity

The defense of sufficient age and maturity requires that the Court find: (1) the child objects to being returned and (2) has attained an age and degree of maturity at which it is appropriate to take account of its views. The defense is discretionary and even if the Court makes those findings, it may choose to return the child.

A child's desire to remain in the new country is not sufficient: the child must object to being returned to its habitual residence. "The court must distinguish between a child's objections as defined by the Hague Convention and the child's wishes as in a typical child custody case. A child's "generalized desire" to remain in the United States is not necessarily sufficient to invoke the exception. The child must "include particularized objections to returning to" the former country of residence. Where the particularized objection is "born of rational comparison" between a child's life in the new country and the country of habitual residence, the court may consider the child's objections to be a mature objection worthy of consideration." *Alcala v. Hernandez*, No. 4:14-CV-04176-RBH, 2015 WL 4429425, at *14 (D.S.C. July 20, 2015), aff'd in part, appeal dismissed in part, 826 F.3d 161 (4th Cir. 2016) (citations omitted).

Determining the age and level of maturity issue, requires more analysis and is dependent on the particular child. The Pérez-Vera Report on the Convention notes that "'all efforts to agree on a minimum age at which the views of the child could be taken into account failed, since all the ages suggested seemed artificial, even arbitrary. It seemed best to leave the application of this clause to the discretion of the competent authorities.'" *De Silva v. Pitts,* 481 F.3d 1279, 1286 (10th Cir.2007). The courts that have addressed the issue have found children as young as 8 years old sufficiently mature (see *Blondin v. Dubois*, 238 F.3d 153 (2d Cir. 2001)) while others have found a 13-year-old insufficiently mature (see *England v. England*, 234 F.3d 268 (5th Cir. 2000)).

The court must also consider the extent to which the child's views have been influenced by the abducting parent, or if the objection is simply that the child wishes to remain with the abductor. When a child says that he or she prefers to stay with the taking parent or uses age-inappropriate language to explain that preference, further investigation is advised.

Grave Risk of Harm

The court is not required to return the children if the Respondent proves by clear and convincing evidence that returning the children will expose them to a grave risk of physical or psychological harm or otherwise place the children in an intolerable situation. (Article 13(b)) The exception is to be interpreted narrowly. Courts are not to engage in a custody determination. Nor is Article 13(b) to be used to litigate the best interests of the parents or the relative qualities of the respective parents. See *Walsh v. Walsh*, 221 F. 3d. 204, 218–219 (1st Cir. 2000).

Even if a grave risk of harm is found, a Court will usually order the child returned if "reasonable accommodations" can be made in the other country to protect the parent and child pending a court hearing in that country.

One Year and Settled

If the petition is filed more than one year from the date of the removal or retention and that the child is now settled in the new environment, the Court is not required to order the return of the child. (Article 12).

Determination of a child being settled in the new environment typically requires evidence of integration into the new family, and the new community.

The one-year period will not be extended. In *Lozano v. Alvarez,*134 S. Ct., 1224 (2014), the left behind parent delayed filing the Hague application and petition until after a year after the abduction because he could not locate the child. The US Supreme Court held that the one-year period was not tolled even where the abducting parent had concealed the location of the child.

Article 18 provides that the provisions of this chapter do not limit the power of a judicial or administrative authority to order the return of the child at any time. Thus the court may order the child's return in the exercise of its discretion even where a defense has been established. In *Lozano*, in his concurring opinion, Justice Alito stated that even after a year has elapsed and the child has become settled in the new environment a variety of factors may outweigh the child's interest in remaining in the new country such as a child's interest in returning to his her original country of residence with which he or she may still have close ties despite having become settled new country; the child's need for contact with the non-abducting parent; the non-abducting parent's interest in exercising the custody to which he or she is legally entitled; the need to discourage inequitable conduct such as concealment by adopting parents; and the need to deter international abductions generally.

Mental Health Involvement and Case Illustrations

Mental health professionals may be brought in to render expert opinions in Hague cases involving sufficient age and maturity when a child has voiced an objection to returning to its home country and/or to assess whether the child has become habituated in the U.S. As noted earlier there is very little literature regarding the assessment of these issues. Some articles mention the psychological damage to children of abduction in general terms (Reynolds, 2006), but a review of the literature revealed no articles regarding the assessment of these Hague exceptions.

Despite this apparent lack of specific guidance, the issues of children's opinions, the weight to place on these opinions and whether a child's opinion is independent from parental pressure are common concerns in child custody evaluations performed in many conflicted, divorcing families.

In the following sampling of cases a combination of procedures were used to assess the psycho-legal questions. Access to data and what data was available was quite variable for a number of reasons. In these cases the evaluator was hired by one parent's attorney and therefore did not necessarily have access to the other parent. In one case there was an agreement between the attorneys that the evaluator would have full access to both parents and the children and thus, the evaluation was conducted similarly to a neutral evaluation as is typically done in Family Court (however with a different psycho-legal question). When only one parent is available, and that parent has access to the children, an evaluator must be vigilant regarding "retention bias" (Murrie et al., 2013) and "confirmatory bias," since one is getting "one side" of the story.

The evaluations consisted of interviewing the adults, interviewing the children, individually and as a sibling group and performing some cognitive testing to assess abstract thinking and general cognitive abilities. When possible, the evaluation can include the interviewing of collaterals, primarily teachers as they have the opportunity to observe, overtime, the child's cognitive functioning, peer relationships, adjustment and may have awareness of a child's opinion. Interviewing collaterals and reviewing documents can be difficult (or impossible) given language barriers or problems obtaining documents from overseas. It is possible to make use of interpreters to facilitate interviews or translate documents.

When interviewing children a focus is on determining whether they actually have an objection to returning to their country of habitual residence and, if they do, what are the reasons for that objection. Interviewing also provides the opportunity to obtain an understanding of the child's view of both countries and their experiences in each country. By in-depth interviewing of these topics, the complexity of the child's thinking and their understanding of the implications of various outcomes can be assessed. Finally, in questioning children regarding how they formed their opinions, what conversations they have had with their parents and clinical observations as to the manner in which they recite their narrative, allow for the assessment of the independence of their opinion.

As noted, the main limitations in doing these Hague assessments include access to only one parent, potential lack of access to collateral informants, language barriers and cultural barriers, in addition to a lack of standard guidelines for these evaluations.

Rachel

The evaluator was hired by mother's attorney, after father filed a Hague motion alleging that Rachel had been wrongfully retained in the U.S. and that she should be returned to Israel. Rachel's mother objected to Rachel's return to Israel stating that Rachel objected to returning to Israel, was of sufficient age and maturity that her opinion should be afforded significant weight and further, that Rachel had become settled in her life in the United States.

Rachel was evaluated when she was 13 years old. She had spent her first 11 years living in Israel, first in an intact family and then in a shared custody situation following her parents' divorce when she was eight years old. She had an Israeli father and an American mother. As a child she had limited English skills, and Hebrew was considered her mother tongue; however, there were limits to her fluency as her mother was her primary caregiver and a non-native Hebrew speaker with limited fluency.

When Rachel was 11 years old, her mother requested of her ex-husband that she be allowed to bring the child to the United States for a year. Rachel was enrolled in a local, private Jewish school and provided with extra tutoring in English. After the initial year, Rachel's father agreed to extend their stay in the U.S. on the condition that Rachel have a visit with him in Israel. Mother was concerned that Rachel would not be returned so only allowed contact between Rachel and her father in the United States. Father then filed a Hague petition to have Rachel returned to Israel. At the time of the assessment, Rachel had been in the United States for two years.

To assess this child's maturity, the independence of her opinion and the degree to which she was settled in the new environment where she had lived for two years, the evaluator interviewed her mother for background information, interviewed Rachel, reviewed school records from both Israel and the United States, including a past psychological assessment performed in Israel, and administered selected subtests from the Wechsler Intelligence Scale for Children – Fourth Edition (WISC-IV). The evaluator was unable to obtain information from father.

In providing the family history, mother explained that following the divorce Rachel lived primarily with her but had frequent and regular contact with her father. This pattern was similar to the caregiving prior to the divorce. Once in the United States, it became apparent that Rachel was quite behind academically both because she was not fluent in either English or Hebrew, and the curriculum had been more limited in the Israeli school system so she lacked a broad fund of general knowledge. Within a year her English had vastly improved and she had caught up academically.

In Israel, Rachel had been a shy child and had relied on her peers to talk for her. Given her lack of fluency in Hebrew, she had performed poorly in preschool and elementary school. Her teachers had not considered the potential language deficits but rather saw Rachel as a below-average student. In later elementary school, Rachel was increasingly targeted by her peers, and was the brunt of significant rejection. Regarding these peer problems she did not get a lot of support from the school staff whose attitude was that she should "toughen up."

Rachel was eager to come to the United States, threw herself into learning English, getting caught up in all her academic areas, and worked on peer relationships, learning how to stand up for herself. By the beginning of her second year in the United States, she had largely adjusted.

In clinical interviews, Rachel was engaging and cooperative. She appeared fluent in English, at least on a conversational level. She appeared to be an accurate historian, providing information about her family and her school experiences. She had nuanced views of her parents, aware of each parent's strengths and limitations. She also freely described missing her father. She did not appear polarized as can be seen when children have been strongly influenced by one parent. Rachel was able to describe the difficulties she had had in Israel both academically and socially and the lack of support or help provided by the school.

Rachel described her experience in the United States in a detailed manner. She talked about her initial fear and the need for significant help. She noted that the move had been hard but worth it. She described her commitment to hours of extra tutoring and homework on a daily basis for a year in order to master English. She stated that she had learned a lot more in U.S. schools and had developed a strong peer group that she "loves." She was also engaged in numerous extracurricular activities that balanced out her studies.

Asked if she had an opinion about staying in the United States or returning to Israel, Rachel was clear that she wanted to remain here. She cited the school and social difficulties in Israel, her good adaptation here and the fact that her Hebrew had further deteriorated so she felt that she would be unable to function at a high school level should she return. Finally, she expressed an interest in attending a US college. Rachel's articulation of her thinking and the reasons she objected to being returned were logical, thoughtful, and appeared to be independent. She stated that her mother had not talked negatively about her father and that her mother values her opinions, which she feels free to voice.

To further assess Rachel's cognitive abilities, particularly her ability to think abstractly, the evaluator reviewed the school records and administered selected subtests of the WISC-IV. Given the question of true language fluency, those subtests that are not verbally based were administered. This allowed a measure of her processing speed and of her perceptual reasoning. One language-based subtest, comprehension, was administered in order to obtain an estimate of how well she has picked up an understanding of social mores and appropriate response to everyday, social, problems and her fund of general information.

Rachel demonstrated a talent for making sense of abstract, nonverbally mediated, spatial problems. One subtest score was in the very superior range (Matrix Reasoning), suggesting a capacity to recognize complex interrelationships and the ability to solve novel problems. She was able to solve spatial, constructional problems at the superior level. On another subtest, also requiring her to generalize regarding common features between objects, Rachel obtained a score in the average range. These findings suggest that Rachel is a very bright child and in particular, has excellent abstract reasoning abilities.

Tasks measuring Rachel's processing speed suggested that when the task required Rachel to write a response she did so carefully and somewhat slowly, resulting in an average score. However, when there was not this requirement, she worked at the very superior level. Thus, she processes nonverbal information very quickly although she may be slowed down depending on what output is required.

The evaluator's opinion given the psycho-legal question was that: Rachel is a teenager who is voicing a strong objection to returning to Israel and can provide cohesive reasons that support her objection. Rachel's experience in Israel was quite painful as she struggled with Hebrew, had difficulties in school, and had significant peer problems. She was, apparently, also seen at her school as not particularly bright.

Rachel has thrown herself into learning English, becoming a more organized and effective student and has blossomed socially. The school she has attended in the United States is small, and she experiences it as very accepting and the faculty as very helpful in terms of her initial adjustment and acceptance. She describes having two very close friends (a new experience for her) and is well integrated with the other students. She now feels comfortable and confident in English.

Although Rachel has been aware of some of the difficulties and disputes between her parents, she has not taken a polarized position. She misses her father and is very empathic to his distress. She maintains a balanced view of him, recalling fun times but also expressing her frustration that he won't understand her position. In her most recent visit with her father, she experienced pressure from him to change her stated desire to stay in the U.S. and stated that, in fact, he became angry during one discussion. Thus, her father's consistent mentioning of returning to Israel and his inability to accept Rachel's feelings appears to be making it more difficult for Rachel to enjoy her time with her father.

Finally, Rachel appears to be very "settled" in the United States and her community, and has been since the end of her first year in the U.S. She has progressed well in school, has improved her English significantly, has formed a satisfying social network, and feels supported by her family. She is involved in extracurricular activities such as sports and music. She presents as a capable, confident teen, who is thinking about how to make important decisions such as where to attend high school and what is involved in attending a good college. The idea of returning to Israel brings up concerns about whether she would be able to function well academically and socially which, given her past experiences, appear to be reasonable concerns. It also seems clear that when in Israel, the school system was not responsive to Rachel's language deficits or her social difficulties that were affecting her self-esteem, whereas they have been successfully addressed in her current school.

This case was litigated in the Federal District Court, which has a comprehensive alternative dispute resolution (ADR) program. The parties elected to try to resolve their issue with the help of a magistrate judge appointed as a settlement judge. After several sessions, the parties came to a settlement that allowed Rachel to remain in the United States, but required summer and other holiday visits with her father in Israel.

Maria and Clara

In another case with the same psycho-legal questions posed, the focus of the evaluation shifted to issues of cognitive abilities versus maturity of thinking processes and the factor of parental influence. In this case, the children had lived in the United States during their early years but four years prior to the evaluation had returned to Spain, where their parents had met and married and lived prior to having children. Both father and mother were Spanish citizens and both parents had also obtained citizenship in the United States. After several years in Spain, mother decided to return to the United States. There was a dispute as to whether the parents had agreed that in the event that Mother established a viable life that the children would join her and primarily reside with Mother. This speaks to the issues of intent and consent as discussed above in the section concerning legal issues.

In the summer of 2016, the parents did agree that the children, two girls aged 9 and 11, would spend a month with their mother and then return to Spain to be with their father and resume their schooling in the fall. The day prior to the scheduled return to Spain, mother informed father that the girls would not be returned and had been enrolled in school in the United States. Father immediately filed a Hague motion requesting the return of his daughters. In response, mother alleged that there had been an agreement that the children could relocate with her, that the children objected to returning to Spain and that they had become acclimatized to their lives in the United States, which had been their birth country. Mother further alleged they had not previously become acclimatized to their lives in Spain during the four prior years. By the time the girls were evaluated they had lived in the United States for 11 months.

The evaluator was hired by father's attorney; however, mother's attorney agreed that mother would be involved in the evaluation process and would cooperate by bringing the girls, Maria and Clara, to appointments. As was done in the previous case example, the girls were interviewed and their cognitive functioning was assessed using the WISC-V. Both parents were interviewed on several occasions. The evaluator was able to interview both girls' teachers and counselors in Spain and in the U.S. Interviewing the Spanish teachers and counselor was accomplished by using an interpreter. Additionally, in this case both sides had submitted documents to the court that outlined the legal issues and each parent's perspective and significant family history.

The parents were interviewed initially to obtain a history of their marriage and of both girls in order to have a context for the current evaluation. In these interviews both parents made serious allegations against the other parent; such as allegations of domestic violence, mental illness and incompetent parenting. Given that the focus of this evaluation was not to determine the children's best interests, the truth of these allegations was not evaluated as one would in a child custody evaluation. The information obtained was included in the evaluation as it was pertinent to understanding the children's feelings and could possibly play a part in opinions that they are currently voicing. It seemed at the very least, these girls were likely somewhat traumatized, that they were exposed to their parents' conflict and to a very dysfunctional household for several years. The fact of such serious allegations did indicate that this was a "high conflict" family and that it was likely that the children had been pulled into the middle of parental disputes.

Relevant history regarding the girls included that they were bilingual in Spanish and English and that they were physically healthy. Maria, the older daughter, had experienced some anxiety, distractibility and behavioral acting out at various points in her history, primarily associated with times when there were major changes in her life, such as starting school, moving to Spain and moving back to the U.S. It was also reported that both parents were expecting to divorce and had been living semi-separated for some time.

Other important information obtained in the interviews with the parents included how they portrayed the other parent and their willingness to acknowledge their own contributions to difficulties. Whereas father did describe his concerns about mother, he was also able to describe positive times during their marriage and her positive attributes. Father was also able to acknowledge some of the children's statements that reflected negatively on him, in a non-defensive manner. He described in detail his efforts to keep the children out of the middle of his disputes with mother, a fact confirmed by the children. Although mother was very cooperative and charming during the interviews, she had a consistently demeaning attitude regarding father and took credit for all of the positive experiences in the children's lives. Throughout the interviewing there was a strong emphasis on her need/wish to be in the United States, and that that is where she feels comfortable. There was little analysis of what this might mean for the children. This focus suggested a sense of entitlement that her needs should be determinative. It was also noted that on one occasion, in the evaluator's office, with the children present, mother made demeaning comments about the father.

Mother also described that she had made the decision to stay in the U.S. in collaboration with the children, that they had had conversations and decided together that they would not return to Spain.

Maria, the older daughter, was immediately engaging with the examiner. She was told that nothing she said would be confidential and that the information provided would be included in a report that her parents would read and that the evaluator's job is to get to know children and their thoughts and feelings to help the judge make a decision, in this case the decision as to whether they would stay in the U.S. or return to Spain. During the interviews, Maria described, in a rather superficial manner, aspects of her life, things that she didn't like in Spain and what she liked in the U.S. She mostly focused on playing video games. Periodically, during the interviews, when asked about positive and negative attributes of her parents, she would stop and state that she shouldn't say negative things about her mother as that might "hurt their case." Likewise, when she said positive things about her father, she would stop herself and then add something negative. Although Maria stated that she wanted to stay in the U.S., some ambivalence was expressed when her guard was let down. When asked how it would feel if the court said that she had to return to Spain, she talked about how great it would be to see her friends. Thus, although Maria stated a preference to remain in the US, she did not really voice a strong, well-articulated objection to returning to Spain. Also concerning was the fact that incidents that she cited underlying her wish to stay in the US, were superficial and similar to complaints of both her sister and her mother.

The clinical impression following this initial interview of Maria was of a somewhat scattered, fidgety child who chattered easily with the examiner but had difficulty engaging in deeper, more thoughtful discussion. In the second appointment with Maria, the WISC-V was administered during which she was amazingly focused and concentrated. Given the observations from the first interview, her focus on video games, her rather simplistic reasoning about forming opinions and her, at times, antsy behavior and loss of focus, her excellent focus and extremely high level of performance on the cognitive testing (as will be analyzed below) was quite surprising. It seemed clear that she liked the intellectual challenge.

Maria's "sign off" in the evaluation was to state that if her father stopped the case, they would be able to move into a bigger house.

The question of whether a child is of sufficient age and maturity to have an opinion that should be considered, in part, depends on their cognitive abilities. Cognitive functioning informs one's ability to solve problems, understand multiple perspectives and consider future implications. These abilities develop with age. This baseline data can then be used to assess a child's real-life application of their abilities. In this situation, I reviewed Maria's current report card, commentary by her teachers, both in Spain and in the United States and administered selected subtests from the WISC-V (the Wechsler Intelligence Scale of Children, Fifth Edition). I administered the primary subtests that measure Verbal Comprehension, Visual Spatial functioning, and Fluid Reasoning. These subtests were chosen as they are most related to understanding a child's overall cognitive capacity, including abstract reasoning. Based on other data collected in this evaluation, I had no reason to question Maria's fluency in English.

The test results indicated that Maria functions in the Very High to Extremely High ranges of cognitive functioning. Her greatest strength is in the area of Visual Spatial Reasoning, her performance being the age equivalent of a 16-year-old, another way to describe this is that her score was in the 99th percentile. This means that she can easily and quickly make sense of her visual world, seeing complex patterns, deconstructing and constructing designs and patterns and is attentive to visual details and nuance. Strengths in this arena can be associated with right brain functioning and novel problem solving. Maria scored very high on tasks involving verbal comprehension and fluid reasoning. Her vocabulary is the equivalent of a 13-year-old and her ability to solve more abstract, linguistically based problems is similar to a 16-year-old. Overall Verbal Comprehension was at the 92%. Fluid reasoning, which looks at abstract thinking capacity, was at the 92%. Taken together, these scores would suggest that her General Ability is Very High, at the 97% and she is likely a gifted child.

The first issue to address was Maria's objections and preferences. Maria expressed a preference to staying in the U.S., and was not highly ambivalent about that preference. Maria's discussion of the various issues suggested, that for her, it was more of a preference than a true objection to returning to Spain. Thus when asked how she might feel about being returned to Spain, her response suggested that she would actually like being with her friends there. Thus, although her preference was to stay here for reasons articulated below, the idea of returning to Spain was not hugely disconcerting to her.

In looking at the "mature child's objection," there are various factors that are useful to explore. Maria is extremely bright and can think in ways well beyond her age peers. As is true with very bright children, the question often becomes their ability to utilize that brainpower for understanding their internal worlds, applying their thinking to solving everyday problems in the world and their ability to use their good reasoning to bear on life problems. As is also true with very bright children, they may rely on these strengths for coping and avoid strengthening other lines of development. This appears to be the case with Maria

Maria is a child who has struggled to engage fully in the world, to manage her emotions and to learn appropriate defenses in the face of her emotional sensitivity. One thing that seems to have helped Maria is that she appears to have pretty well-developed social skills and has made friends in both countries. It should be noted that Maria has been dealing with an emotionally charged family environment, which at times has likely been somewhat traumatic. Exposure to conflict and violence can interfere with a child's emotional development and maturity unless there are direct efforts to resolve the trauma and change the environment. Thus, it is not surprising that although Maria is very bright and creative she is underdeveloped emotionally and seems quite immature. This was noteworthy in the way she explained her preference to remain in this country. Her reasons are quite superficial and disjointed. It is clear that she has not made a rational comparison between the two countries nor has she thought about the bigger implications that growing up in one country versus the other might have in her life. This is not surprising, just as most 11-year-olds are more focused on the here and now and don't engage in more complex, abstract reasoning, Maria is similar to her age peers. Maria has not provided a more complex, cohesive explanation of her preference with collateral informants, who also saw Maria as bright but immature emotionally. In part this seems due to Maria's tendency towards avoidance, i.e., she did not appear to sort through issues on a deeper level, remained more on the surface and put her energy into her creative cognitive endeavors.

Maria's younger sister, Clara, presented as a very poised, chatty child. She easily launched in to all the ways that life in the U.S. was better than life in Spain. Although there were various differences Clara cited regarding the schools, friends and the environment, her strongest sentiment was that Spain was awful because her mother was not there. Clara could not think of anything good to say about her father. During the questioning about her father, Clara became silly, tangential and generally managed to avoid much discussion. Clara's polarized view of her family and her very negative views about both her father and sister, were concerning. The polarization and black and white thinking was reminiscent of the dynamics seen in "refuse/resist" families (see Chapter 14 in this volume).

Much like her sister, her intense ability to focus during the cognitive testing was impressive and somewhat surprising, given her simplistic thinking about the family situation. She was also highly competitive, several times noting that her sister was "dumb" and that she was "smart." In fact the results of the cognitive testing were very similar to those of her sister, indicating that she is also a gifted child. The test results were consistent with her teacher's descriptions of her academic work.

In considering the data collected to apply to the question of whether Clara has an objection to being returned to Spain, whether she demonstrates sufficient maturity for that objection to be given significant weight and whether hers is an independent opinion, the following conclusions were rendered. Like her sister, although extremely bright, Clara did not present as having a mature and integrated opinion and by far the biggest concern with Clara was the independence of her opinion. She presented as a child who was in charge and quite sure of herself. At times it does seem that she derives some of her confidence through putting her sister down. However, Clara appears to have a polarized view of the world that is rather black and white and lacks nuance – Spain is boring, dirty and the school has many problematic features, most of which are quite superficial. The U.S. is good. This polarized view of the world extends to her parents where Mom is pretty much all good, except for the yelling and there is little that she likes about her father. Thus, her stated reasons for her objections lack depth, are not well integrated nor well-reasoned. Furthermore, they seem driven by her connection/alliance to her mother. It is very worrisome that she doesn't allow herself to miss her father. Her counselor confirmed her being a "mommy's girl" and that in their work together, Clara does not articulate a more comprehensive, integrated objection to returning to Spain.

Thus, from the data collected, neither child appeared to have the maturity to render an opinion that should carry much weight in this matter, nor have they formed a maturely articulated objection.

Regarding the possibility of mother influencing the girls and therefore there being a lack of independence, Maria indicated that mother was exposing the children to way too much information that would likely influence them – the information about the case and about their father. Both children were well aware of how finances were playing out in this "case" and that their father could stop the case. If the case was dropped they would then not need to worry about being homeless, they would also be able to get a townhouse and take trips to New York City. Maria directly talked about instructions from her mother that she should not say anything bad about the United States and should not say that she misses anything about Spain. This has contributed to a breach in the relationship with her father, as she feels very constrained in her contact with her Dad. Finally mother's very negative view of father, is likely picked up by the children as it seems unlikely that she screens it – as noted by her comments about her distrust of him to me in front of the children. It should be noted that in the incidental observations of her interactions with the children she is warm, light hearted and engaged, this positive aspect of her parenting may make her negative actions have more effect.

Thus, is addition to my concerns about these children's ability to form mature opinions, I am very concerned about the independence of the opinions that they have voiced.

Outcome

Settlement was not possible in this case, so it proceeded to trial, Father offered testimony from his mental health expert and himself. Mother offered only her own testimony. Mother did not follow up on her "sufficient age and maturity" defense and did not request that the Court hear from the children.

At the end of the trial, the judge ordered the parties to submit written closing arguments. In her closing argument, Mother conceded that the children's habitual residence was Spain. She did not address the children's alleged objections. Her sole defense was that father had consented to the children moving to the United States.

In its written opinion, the Court found that Father had not consented, or that if he ever had, that consent had been withdrawn before the children left for their visit with Mother. The Court also found that Mother was aware that Father did not consent to the children remaining in the United States.

Finding for Father, the Court ordered Mother to return the children to Spain. Mother did not cooperate, so Father came to the United States to take the children back to Spain, where they are now living and going to school.

Nikos and Melina

A third case will be briefly described as the outcome of the case demonstrated how once jurisdiction has been determined, the best interests of the children are then determined in the Family Court of the country with jurisdiction and, that these processes are entirely separate.

In this family, both parents are from Greece and the children, a son aged 11 years and a daughter, aged 6 years, had been born and raised in Greece. Mother had been offered a job in the U.S. and initially the children remained in Greece with their father. After several months, both parents agreed that the children would live with their mother in the U.S. for a year. At the time that the children joined their mother, this was an intact family. The children arrived in the U.S. knowing no English. The children were enrolled in school and provided with extra help in English. After several months, mother filed for divorce in the U.S. and father then filed a custody motion for divorce in the Greek courts. Mother did not receive notice of the hearing in Greece as papers were sent to her address there, not her address in the U.S. As mother did not attend the hearing in Greece, the courts there granted the father's request for sole legal custody, two days of parenting time per month for mother to be with the children, with no overnight visitation. The father then filed a Hague petition to compel the return of his children to Greece. Mother responded indicating that the children objected to their return to Greece and that they were of sufficient maturity that their opinion should be considered. As in the previously detailed cases, the mother was interviewed, as were the children. The older child, Nikos, was administered cognitive testing utilizing the WISC-IV. The material provided to the Greek courts was reviewed. There was no access to the father in this case.

Mother provided the following family history: she had been the main source of economic stability for the family. Her husband had long periods of unemployment but not wanting to accept the extra work of caring for the children or running the household. Both children had periods of psychological difficulties when they were younger Nikos had eating difficulties and Melina had difficulties with emotional expression. Both children had been provided with psychological services. It should be noted that prior to mother moving to the U.S., there had been talk between the parents regarding divorce.

When the children arrived in the U.S., mother noted that they had lice, they were both thin and they talked about having missed their mother.

Despite the children knowing no English, by the end of the academic year the children were adapting well. The children were caught in discussions with their parents about what might happen in the future. Mother had been advised to be honest with her children and talk about the separation whereas father had stated that he didn't want a divorce and his wife was lying to the children. Nikos stated that his father was often very negative about his mother and this was very difficult for him.

Mother stated that she provided father with information and facilitated calls between the children and their father. However, Nikos became involved in court issues during these calls. His father described the court's findings that the children should return to Greece and that they would live with him however, he also stated that they could see their mother anytime. In response, mother showed Nikos the decree which described the limited access to mother. This situation resulted in Nikos being increasingly negative about returning to Greece.

The evaluation of Melina indicated that she was very immature, was not fluent in English although she was cooperative and engaging. She had an interesting approach to being asked questions. It was noted that in response to some questions she did what younger children do when they don't really understand, they engage in "mental surfing." For example when asked what she liked about living here, she mentioned the beautiful houses, couches, chairs and offices, while looking around my office and naming things she saw. Regarding her life here she listed a number of friends, including her teacher and her brother. She explained that she has learned a lot since being here, especially learning English. She described having play dates with a number of friends and being involved in activities such as going to the park, reading books and playing outside. Her interests in TV reflected age appropriate ones such as princess movies, Dora the Explorer and mermaids. When asked about her brother, she explained that they both played together and sometimes fought, noting that sharing is hard.

She did talk about missing her father and relatives in Greece. She noted that she loved both countries. The following is the conclusion of the evaluation.

Based on contact with Melina and review of her school work, one could not determine whether Melina had a real opinion about staying in the United States or being in Greece and even if she did, she did not appear to have sufficient maturity for any opinion to be given determinative weight. Her thinking was very much in the here and now and these was no evidence of particular sophistication in her thinking. However, given her more limited English skills, it is certainly possible that if interviewed in her mother tongue her thinking could reflect greater sophistication. It was noted, that Melina's love for her father, holding on to positive feelings about him, being able to express that she misses him, all indicate that mother supports her daughter's emotions and is not trying to influence her. Mother also freely acknowledged that Melina enjoyed talking with her father and missed him.

Nikos, as an 11-year-old, had a clearer and more sophisticated understanding of the situation. Nikos immediately informed me that he liked being in the U.S. better than being in Greece. He proceeded to explain that school was better because it was easier and the teachers didn't yell all the time. He also described that when in Greece he had to take an hour-long bus ride to school, had to eat breakfast at school and that on weekends they had a lot of homework. He liked his friends here better and played with them more. He noted that he hadn't had a best friend in Greece. He noted that he liked the parks here, it was safer here and there were special lanes for riding bikes. He also noted that the street dogs don't bite and there were more policemen, lending to the feeling of safety. In my final interview with Nikos, shortly after school started, he was very excited about his new teacher, feeling good about having better friends than last year and excited about being able to ride his bike to school (with his sister and a friend). This fall, he is involved in karate, piano and soccer.

Nikos had many complaints about his father. He stated that when in Greece his father didn't help him with homework and even when he didn't have a job he wouldn't want to go out and play. He noted that after his mother left when his father did help on one school project, he did it wrong and he got yelled at by the teacher. During his time in Greece with his father it appears that the nanny was the one who cooked for the children and was with them on weekends. Nikos noted that the nanny yelled a lot. Furthermore, Nikos described his father's inability to accept anything positive in his life in the U.S. Despite these complaints about his father, Nikos understood that his father's actions came from a place of missing his children. Nikos did not have a black and white perspective about the U.S. versus Greece and could describe the difficulties he had had in both countries.

Nikos had a relatively reasoned view of his situation. Both of his parents apparently involved him in too many discussions regarding the divorce and the other parents' actions. On cognitive testing, Nikos performed solidly in the average range. He did hold the opinion that he would prefer to stay with his mother in the U.S. There did not appear to be evidence of mother coaching him although she did expose him to more court information than is ideal, but so did his father. Nikos did appear more affiliated with his mother, who seemed more sensitive to his developmental needs and more attuned to who he is.

This case ended up as a case where one child did not have an opinion whereas the older child had an opinion that appeared reasonably well thought out. However, the court determined that the children should be returned to Greece and that their best interests should be determined by the Family Court there. Although the father had obtained an order giving him sole legal and physical custody of the children, upon rehearing the case, with mother's involvement, the court reversed their finding, giving mother sole legal and physical custody of the children, in recognition of father's significant limitations as a parent.

Conclusion

Again, in this case, a settlement was reached. Mother agreed to return to Greece with the children. Over Mother's objections, the District Court ordered custody of the children to Father upon return, pending proceedings in the Greek court. Mother and the children were met at the airport in Athens by Father and his attorney, who immediately took custody of the crying and resistant children. For the next several weeks, Father would not permit Mother to see the children. At the first hearing in the Greek court, temporary custody was reversed with Mother having primary custody. The end result, after additional hearings, was that Mother was given sole custody of the children. Ironically, under the local law, that gave her the absolute right to relocate with the children wherever in the world she desired, without obtaining Father's consent. She chose not to return to the United States.

Summary

In our increasingly global world, disputes as to where children should reside and be raised are becoming more common. The ultimate decision as to which culture, which language, which parent will have the dominant influence is huge and likely to have immense impact on the children experience and development. In the best of all possible worlds, parents are mutually committed to maintaining deep relationships between the child and both parents, both cultures, optimizing the social capital that can come from this diversity and range of options. As noted by Drozd and Shear (2013), it may come down to – do you trust the other parent to support the relationships despite the distance?

The Hague Convention is an attempt to stop "jurisdiction shopping" and develop a reasonable system for how to determine the best interest of children in a global world. Given the enormous potential impact of where a child's fate will be determined and who/which country will determine what that child's life and contact with both parents will look like, it is critical that attorneys and mental health professionals understand the issues involved in our increasingly global world.

Readers will hopefully understand the difference between determining the issue of which country has jurisdiction to make parenting determinations and what those countries determine as the BIC, has been made clear.

Perhaps one of the more important aspects of the Hague Convention is the further articulation of how we should understand children's "voices" and their opinions and how they can weigh in on situations that affect their lives. In the early 1900s children's opinions had no weight, as they were owned by their parents, in the 1980s, in divorce proceedings their voice was silenced so that they were not brought into the marital conflict and currently there is a discussion as to their rights to have a voice in legal proceeding that affect their future – the Hague Convention and the Elkins Committee in California (2010) are good examples of this changing viewpoint.

Given that children can be manipulated, especially in family matters, it is our responsibility to insure that children's opinions have been independently formed. It is also important that children feel respected when voicing their opinion even if their opinion is not determinative.

Notes

1. In re Marriage of Lamusga 32 Cal. 4th 1072
2. Journal of Child Custody, Vol. 10, Numbers 3–4, 2013

References

Austin, William G. (2008). Relocation, research, and forensic evaluation: Part II: Research in support of the relocation risk assessment model. *Family Court Review*, Vol. 46 No. 2, April 2008 347–365.

Elkins Family Law Task Force Final Report and Recommendations (2010). Available at www.courts.ca.gov.

Fernando, Michelle (2014). Family law proceedings and the child's right to be heard in Australia, the United Kingdom, New Zealand, and Canada. *Family Court Review*, Vol. 52 No. 1, January 2014 46–59.

Garbolino, James D. (2019). Intersecting issues involving asylum in the United States and cases arising under the 1980 Hague Convention on the civic aspects of international abduction. *Family Court Review*, Vol 57 No. April 2, 2019 159–174.

Kelly, Joan B. & Lamb, M. E. (2003). Developmental issues in relocation cases involving young children: When, whether, and how? *Journal of Family Psychology* Vol. 17 No. 2, 193–205.

Lesh, Eric (2011). Jurisdiction friction and the frustration of the Hague Convention: Why international child abduction cases should be heard exclusively by Federal Courts. *Family Court Review*, Vol. 49 No. 1, January 2011 170–189.

Melcher, Christopher C. (2013). The role of the mental health professional in assessing grave risk of harm under the Hague Convention on the Civil Aspects of Child Abduction. *Journal of Child Custody*, Vol. 10 No. 3–4, 2013.

Messitte, Peter J. (2020). Getting tough on international child abduction. *Family Court Review*, Vol. 58 No. 1, January 2020 195–210.

Morley, Jeremy D. (2013). The impact of foreign law on child custody determinations. *Journal of Child Custody* Vol. 10 No. 3–4, 2013.

Moskowitz, Galit (2003). The Hague Convention on international child abduction and the grave risk of harm exception: Recent decisions and their implications on children from nations in political turmoil. *Family Court Review*, Vol. 41 No. 4, October 2003 580–596.

Murrie, D. C., Boccaccini, M. T., Guamera, L. A., & Rufino, K. A. (2013). Are forensic experts biased by the side that retained them? *Psychological Science*, 24(10), 1889–1897.

Pahrand, Mishal (2017). Not without my children: the need for the modification of international child abduction law. *Family Court Review*, Vol. 55 No. January 1, 2017 139–151.

Parkinson, Patrick, Taylor, Nicola, Cashmore, Judith & Austin, William G. (2016). Relocation, research, and child custody disputes. In Drozd, Leslie, Saini, Michael & Olesen, Nancy (Eds) *Parenting Plan Evaluations: Applied research for the family court*, New York, NY: Oxford University Press, 2016, pp. 431–463.

Reynolds, Sara E. (2006). International parental abduction: Why we need to expand custody rights protected under the child abduction convention. *Family Court Review*, Vol. 44 No. 3, July 2006 464–483.

Shear, Leslie E. and Drozd, Leslie M. (2013). To speak of all kinds of things: Child custody evaluations and the unique characteristics of relocations to foreign countries. *Journal of Child Custody* Vol. 10 No. 3–4, 2013.

Yaffe-Bellany, David (2020). The three abductions of N. In the New York Times Sunday, August 16, 2020, Business Section.

Warshak, Richard A. (2013). In a land far, far away: Assessing children's best interests in international relocation cases. *Journal of Child Custody* Vol. 10 No. 3–4, 2013.

Cases

Abbott v. Abbott, 560 U.S. 1 (2001)

Alcala v. Hernandez, 2015 WL 4429425 (D.S.C. 2015), aff'd in part, appeal dismissed in part, 826 F.3d 161 (4th Cir. 2016), cert. denied, 137 S. Ct. 393 (2016)

Baxter v. Baxter, 423 F.3d 363 (3d Cir. 2005)

Blondin v. Dubois, 238 F.3d 153 (2d Cir. 2001)

De Silva v. Pitts, 481 F.3d 1279 (10th Cir.2007)

England v. England, 234 F.3d 268 (5th Cir. 2000)

Friedrich v. Friedrich, 78 F.3rd 1060 (6th Cir. 1996)

Gitter v. Gitter, 396 F.3d 124 (2d. Cir. 2005)

Gonzalez-Caballero v. Mena, 251 F.3d 789 (9th Cir. 2001).

Grano v. Martin, 2020 WL 1164800 (S.D.N.Y., 2020)

Khalip v. Khalip, 2011 WL 1882514 (E.D. Mich. May 17, 2011)

La Musga, In re Marriage of La Musga (2004) 32 Cal 4ᵗʰ 1072

*Lozano v. Alvarez,*134 S. Ct., 1224 (2014)

Monasky v. Taglieri, 140 S.Ct. 719 (2020)

Mozes v. Mozes, 239 F.3d 1067 (9th Cir. 2001)

Padilla v. Troxell, 850 F.3d 168 (4th Cir. 2017)

Redmond v. Redmond, 724 F.3d 729 (7th Cir. 2013)

Taglieri v. Monasky, 907 F.3d 404 (6th Cir. 2018)

Walsh v. Walsh, 221 F. 3d. 204 (1st Cir. 2000)

14 Resist Refuse Dynamics in Family Law with a Young Child

Ginger C. Calloway and S. Margaret Lee

Introduction

One court system devoted to child issues and the participation of children is Family Court (see Chapters by Olesen, Singer and Wald in this volume). Divorce is relatively common in the United States and, although most child custody disputes are resolved through parents negotiating their own arrangements, parents using alternative dispute resolution (ADR) mechanisms, such as mediation, parents' attorneys negotiating settlements, a small percentage of cases require court intervention for resolution of disputes regarding post-divorce parenting plans. The small percentage of families unable to resolve disputes in a less adversarial manner are considered "high conflict"[i] and the children in these families are at greater risk of difficulties adjusting to their parents' divorce. These families also demand the lion's share of the court's time and attention, as they tend to return to court repeatedly. One group of families that has been concerning and has ignited significant attention in the family law community are those families where a divorce leads to the loss, or potential loss, for the child, of his/her relationship with one parent. Early research in divorce demonstrated that children in high conflict divorces have poorer adaptation to their parent's divorce and tend to have more psychological scars. There is a tendency in these families for the children to be pulled into the middle of their parents' conflict and are under pressure to "choose" a side or, alternatively, to find a way to maintain alliances with "opposing camps." The latter is often at the expense of their own optimal psychological development as their energy is devoted to managing these alliances, figuring out what can be said to what parent and how not to get further caught in the complex family dynamics.[ii] In these families, children often have too much power, they have the power to get one parent "in trouble" with the other parent, the power to get police called and sometimes to have courts change the structure of their lives.

A subgroup of these "high conflict" families include a phenomena that was originally named "parental alienation syndrome" by Richard Gardner.[iii] The original idea of a "syndrome" connoted that there was a known cause and a predictable course and outcome to the phenomena. The phenomena itself was well known to professionals in family law; a child refuses to have contact with one parent following divorce, often accompanied by allegations of abuse, evidence of fear and a wish to completely cut off the relationship. Gardner proposed this was caused by one parent engaging in "alienating" behaviors, essentially brain washing a child into having a false belief about the other parent as being dangerous, unloving, untrustworthy and the cause of fear, even terror.[iv] As the concept of alienation was highlighted, families started presenting for evaluation where the essential referral question was "is this alienation or is this abuse," or "is this alienation or is this domestic violence.[v]" Evaluators are encouraged to hold alternative hypotheses such as these and then collect data to confirm and/or disconfirm the hypotheses, to then,

DOI: 10.4324/9780429397806-15

hopefully provide understanding of a family's dynamics and provide recommendations regarding how to help the family find resolution, define what safety measures are needed if there has been DV or child abuse and recommend interventions that will support the best interests of the children.

In the past 20 years, there has been an expansion in the understanding of this phenomena and the development of various models of intervention to reunify alienated children and to develop safeguards for them. In addition, interventions aim to teach parents to understand the implications of their actions and to educate them as to the need to develop a co-parenting relationship that does not damage their children. The latter is accomplished either through learning to actively co-parent or, at a minimum, learning how to parallel parent.

One of the major shifts in our understanding regarding "alienation" is that there is not one cause, not one dynamic. It is vastly more complex than our earlier question of "is it abuse or is it alienation?" These families are on a continuum and there are usually multiple factors that have contributed to the family dynamic. For example, "realistic estrangement" refers to situations where a child does not want contact with a parent because, in fact, that parent had been abusive or was the perpetrator of domestic violence. This is seen as different from an "alienated child"[vi] who previously had a good enough relationship with a parent, who had not been traumatized but had come to believe that one parent was dangerous and abusive. In this situation, the child has rewritten history. There are also situations where a child just gets along better with one parent and has a preference for that parent. The latter is not a pathological situation. A major change in our understanding of these families has been an understanding that we rarely see what might be considered a pure case of "alienation," instead we see multiple factors[vii] that have contributed to the development of what is now referred to as "refuse/resist" dynamics. Some of the factors that are common include alienating behaviors on the part of one or both parents, less than ideal parenting on the part of the rejected parent and vulnerabilities within a particular child.

This more nuanced understanding of "alienation" has led to a range of interventions thought to be helpful that include removing the child from the parental conflict and re-establishing normalized relationship with both parents. This facilitates more optimal development in children of divorce as long as both parents provide a safe environment.

"Alienating behaviors" include "bad mouthing" the other parent, bringing the children into the conflict and attempting to influence them, rewriting the narrative about an incident that occurred in the other home. An example of the latter is when a parent disciplines a child and the other parent describes it as unfair/mean/abusive, thus encouraging the child to hold onto negative feelings or thoughts about the other parent. Another tactic frequently seen in parents who engage in alienating behaviors includes "restrictive gatekeeping"[viii] which basically involves interfering with the other parents' access to the child. This can be seen when a parent interferes with or sabotages visits and/or restricts or regulates distant contact. This is often done in the name of protecting the child.

In these high-stake cases that may involve active attempts to alienate a child from one parent, may involve abuse or domestic violence and may involve vulnerable children, having a comprehensive child custody evaluation ordered by the court can be crucial for determining what interventions may help the family attain optimal functioning – questions such as legal decision making, parenting scheduling, therapeutic interventions and case management are central to the purpose of the comprehensive child custody evaluation.

Context of the Comprehensive Child Custody Evaluation

Comprehensive child custody evaluations (CCE) are highly risky evaluations for evaluators, in that parents are typically very angry, have sufficient finances to litigate their desires and wishes, and are often skilled at persuasiveness. Angry litigants unwilling to settle their litigation after the findings from a CCE are issued frequently use consultants to review the evaluator's work and appear at Hearings on Permanent Custody. In some jurisdictions, where mean incomes are higher than other places in the United States, it is not uncommon for multiple consultants to be hired by both parents, through their attorneys, following the completion of a CCE. For evaluators who are psychologists, it is recommended by risk managers for malpractice companies to purchase an additional rider to a policy to cover anticipated costs should a parent, parents or others file a complaint against the evaluator with oversight bodies. This rider pays for legal fees and associated costs, such as copying substantial amounts of paperwork provided to evaluators, in representing the psychologist to an oversight body.

Suggested guidelines by several organizations for the conduct of a CCE resulted in part from the litigious nature of these evaluations. Evaluators are not only encouraged, they are generally expected to follow these guidelines by oversight bodies, such as licensing boards, and by colleagues conducting these evaluations who might review their work. In some jurisdictions, like California, evaluators are mandated to have annual training updates in topics related to performing child custody evaluations, in addition to separate updates in the area of Domestic Violence, this is in addition to an initial required training in these areas. Furthermore, in California, there are guidelines for performing evaluations that must be followed, California Rules of Court 5.225. In addition to guidelines, many texts exist for the proper and just conduct of a CCE,[ix] continuing education is offered by a variety of organizations,[x] and training programs are available for evaluators wishing to conduct these types of evaluations. Supervision is recommended for new evaluators, due to the litigious and complex nature of these evaluations, and collegial consults for more advanced evaluators can be extremely helpful in checking potential biases and in analyzing complex matters.

CCE's are civil matters and thus are heard through the mechanism of hearings by judges, not trials with juries, with the exception of one state, Texas, which does allow for some, limited trials by jury. In civil matters, depositions, statements taken under oath and conducted by an attorney, are allowed and it is not unusual for attorneys to depose any number of individuals prior to a CCE beginning or subsequent to the findings of a CCE being issued, when litigants are unhappy with the findings. The standard of proof in these matters is generally "clear and convincing", although in some states such as California, preponderance of the evidence may apply, and the prevailing legal standard generally adhered to is "best interests of the child."[xi] Hearings are typically conducted in Family Court, where the Family Court is a part of District Court, although in some jurisdictions, may be part of the state Superior Court. As with many matters in forensic practice, practitioners should learn the applicable standards of proof, legal questions, and particular courts in which their work takes place.

It is recommended that evaluators seek appointment as the Court's expert in a Consent Order. This allows the evaluator to assume a neutral, objective role as the Court's expert, rather than as an expert for either side. As the Court's expert, the data gathered during a CCE remains under the control of the Court and cannot be released without the Court's direction. Typically, a CCE is handled by a sole judge throughout the course of the CCE and for any associated hearings following the CCE. The notion of one judge one family is one that has arisen over the past decades as family courts have moved from being more adversarial to a more judicial management format that recognizes the value of understanding a family over time for repeat or "revolving door" families, is more effective. Before beginning a CCE, evaluators often use a set of stipulations they have parents/caregivers and attorneys sign and collect a deposit in advance of appointment as the expert for the CCE. The set of stipulations used by one author for this chapter were vetted by a Family Law specialist. It is wise to hold a joint meeting or telephone conference with both attorneys or alternatively, have both attorneys submit separate letters to the custody evaluator with copy to opposing counsel with referral questions outlined during the conference or in the letter.

Historically, parents engaging in custody trials were represented in court by attorneys. The affordability of representation, especially for families who engage in ongoing disputes can be prohibitive. Currently, in some jurisdictions, the number of parents who represent themselves in Family Court, outnumbers the parents with representation, sometimes by large numbers. Performing an evaluation having one or both parents unrepresented by counsel is particularly challenging for evaluators and therefore some evaluators only accept cases where both parents have representation. Maintaining a transparent process, avoiding the need to have calls with "attorneys" (who are actually parents serving pro se as their own attorney) and deciding whether the court's assistance is required in distributing the report are some possible solutions.

A joint meeting with the parents/caregivers can be useful to obtain all consent forms that will go to various providers and agencies, to explain Informed Consent to parents/caregivers, and to have parents/caregivers sign Informed Consent forms. In situations where domestic violence is substantiated and a protective order preventing contact is in place, the evaluator may have to meet with parents separately or make arrangements for the joint meeting to be held in ways that protect the victim of the domestic violence. See the chapter by Olesen in this volume for more on domestic violence. The collection of data, in the context of evaluating and interviewing multiple individuals in a CCE, can be immense and adds another level of complexity to these types of evaluations. Oftentimes, there is more than one legal question to address. Maintaining a primary focus on the child's needs and best interests can be challenging in the midst of dramatic, emotional parent dynamics that can include multiple allegations.

Process of the Evaluation in This Case

Background and Referral

The attorneys contacted the custody evaluator jointly in a three-way phone conversation with the following information about Sarah and her parents. This phone call occurred after receipt of the Order naming the evaluator as the Court's expert and after the evaluator received a deposit. Sarah, a 6-year old girl was the only child of David and Jane, both in their early 40s. Sarah's parents separated abruptly when her mother surreptitiously left the family home and moved to an undisclosed location when Sarah was 5 years old. Sarah's mother, Jane, alleged that her husband, David, was abusive to her and to Sarah, was mentally ill and drank heavily. She further alleged that both she and Sarah were frightened of David. This fear was Jane's stated reason for moving out abruptly without informing David. He did not know their whereabouts for several months when Jane, on the advice of her family law attorney, contacted David to discuss divorce and supervised visits between him and Sarah. The custody evaluation, sought by attorneys for both parents and arranged by an agreement memorialized through a court order, started when Sarah was 6 years old. The evaluation began roughly a year after the separation, at which point in time, David had exercised no overnight visitation with Sarah. Initially, any visits he had with Sarah were limited in time and number and were supervised by Jane and/or her parents, who moved to where David and Jane lived. Subsequently, the attorneys negotiated a schedule for visitation that had Sarah making frequent exchanges between these two "warring" parents. Throughout the custody evaluation, Jane refused to give David her new address and insisted they meet in various parks or child centered locales for his visitation. Initially, she did not want to provide her address to the custody evaluator and was adamant that the address should not be provided to David. She further insisted that the exchange of Sarah between her and David, orchestrated by their separate attorneys' joint agreement before the custody evaluation started, occur some distance away from her new home and in parking lots or at police stations. Jane would not leave her car to escort Sarah to her father's car and would not agree to David approaching her car to retrieve or deliver Sarah.

Sarah's parents were each in their 30s when Sarah was born and she was their only child. Sarah's parents lived with Sarah's maternal grandparents for a brief period of time until they moved out on their own and into a different city. Jane, who was very close to her family of origin, wanted to return to where they lived and spoke often of "going home," whereas David wanted to stay where they had moved, as he had secured well-paying, satisfactory employment, following his training as a physical therapist. Jane was a homemaker from the time of Sarah's birth and for the duration of the custody evaluation. The couple engaged in some couples' therapy with two different therapists, one of whom convinced David to stop drinking altogether. When he relapsed, it was shortly thereafter that Jane left the home, to the surprise of the couples' therapist, who was not informed and who thought the couple could have negotiated a separation with the therapist's help. One therapist they contacted for co-parenting work terminated the intervention with them, due to their high level of hostility and inability to compromise and to negotiate.

At some point, Sarah started having frequent tantrums, was "bossy" and "mean" to other children in her first-grade class, was more aggressive at home, had some "toileting" accidents, cried easily and could not be easily soothed. This seemed to coincide with increased visitation with David and with a "campaign" by Jane. This campaign was pursued relentlessly to convince the custody evaluator, neighbors of the father, Jane's friends who were mothers to Sarah's playmates in school, Sarah's pediatrician, and Sarah's psychotherapist, chosen by the attorneys from names given by both parents that David was "crazy," volatile and unstable. Some collateral sources described Jane as "desperate" to convince them that David was abusive, was a "drunk," and that Sarah was highly fearful of him.

Referral questions from the attorneys were sent to the evaluator after the initial, joint phone call with them and each copied the other on their letter sent to the evaluator. The attorney for Jane had many, detailed questions about "appropriate parenting" she wanted addressed. She laid out a very detailed set of parenting styles and options she considered ideal and sought rigid rules for parenting to be employed by Sarah's parents. This attorney also stated that she and Jane wanted David's visits with Sarah indefinitely supervised and infrequent in number and advocated for Sarah's wishes for a parenting schedule to be enacted. This attorney's referral questions did not address the issue of re-location which was frequently raised by Jane throughout the course of the custody evaluation.

David's attorney remarked on David pursuing his advanced degree after Sarah's birth, working while he pursued the degree, and allowing Jane to work as a homemaker during Sarah's early years. This attorney expressed concern for and asked the evaluator to address what David perceived as Jane's "alienating" behaviors. These included, according to the attorney, restriction of Sarah's time with David both during and after the marriage, Jane's abrupt and secretive manner of leaving the marriage, Jane's denigrating of and stereotyping David as an abuser and a "drunk" to multiple individuals and her comments made in front of Sarah, overheard by David and others, that Jane had "no choice" about Sarah's visitation with David and "had to make" her go with him for visits. David's attorney said David wanted sole custody of Sarah, due to his worries about Jane's alienating behaviors, and asked the evaluator for recommendations about a parenting plan of visitation following the custody evaluation.

Initial Interview with the Parents

The initial, joint interview with the parents occurred after they were mailed a packet of forms, including a Parenting History Survey[xii] each was to complete separately. Although Jane alleged domestic violence (DV) by David, there were no police reports of domestic disputes, no emergency hearings for protective order and therefore no protective orders, and no reports to psychotherapists, women's shelters or agencies that work with victims of DV. To accommodate Jane's concerns, David was told he needed to arrive a half hour prior to Jane arriving and would need to leave a half hour after her departure. He waited in the evaluator's waiting room, within sight of the evaluator and her assistant, until Jane arrived. Jane texted the evaluator when she arrived in the parking lot, David was escorted into the evaluator's private office, and the evaluator went to the door of the building to let Jane in. A similar, reverse procedure was followed at the conclusion of the four and a half hours with the parents. The evaluator used the time to explain the procedures to be used in the evaluation, to have parents provide all names of any medical or mental health provider and other sources of information to be contacted, to sign all necessary release of information forms to be mailed to agencies, companies and individuals and finally, to discuss both how they started their relationship and marriage and how the marriage ended. In addition, dates were established for the evaluator to make home visits, to observe transition of Sarah from Jane to David and from David to Jane, and to set times for the videotaped interactions of each parent with Sarah in a structured procedure. These videotaped observations occurred at a setting outside the examiner's office where one-way mirrors were available and a colleague was available to play the part of a stranger in a variant of the Strange Situation.[xiii] See the Jurney chapter in this volume for more information on attachment relationships and for a diagram of the Circle of Security.[xiv]

Procedures Employed

The evaluator used multiple data sources, multiple types of data, and multi-method psychological measures. Multiple sources of information are preferable in any forensic evaluation, to allow evaluators varying viewpoints and perspectives, to allow for the formation of multiple hypotheses in arriving at conclusions and recommendations, and to assess congruence and lack of congruence in the entire set of data. See the Singer chapter in this volume for more on multiple hypotheses in sexual abuse matters, the Levy chapter for the Specialty Guidelines for Forensic Psychologists, and the Calloway chapter on teen homicide. Document review is a major source of information or data for any CCE, is often voluminous in nature, and can include pediatrician reports, school and educational records, reports from agencies like Child Protective Services when abuse and neglect are substantiated or alleged (see the Mercer chapter for more on dependency issues), psychotherapist records, and documentation of training or degrees, for some examples. Due to the allegations of David's alcohol abuse from Jane, he was asked to submit grocery and loyalty card receipts for a period of time specified by Jane and he was asked to submit copies of debit and credit card statements from the same time period. Jane provided an extensive number of audio recordings taken by her that she said were examples of David's abusive behavior and his behavior while drinking alcohol. Unsure of the legality of these recordings, a request to the attorneys to provide an Order to review was made. Although not typically relying on recordings in data collection, the evaluator agreed to review a limited sample of 4 hours, selected by the two attorneys.

Multiple types of measures were given to the parents and differing types of measures were used in obtaining information from and about the parents. For example, they each completed a Developmental History Form for Sarah, completed a Parenting History Survey, and were observed multiple times in varying ways by observation of transitions, observations within each home, structured observations that were videotaped, and structured and unstructured interviews. Each parent submitted emails they received from the other parent and these were reviewed. Interviews with collateral sources included phone conversations with various psychotherapists, Sarah's pediatrician, teachers, and neighbors, friends and family members, whose names were submitted by Jane and David. Informed consent and lack of confidentiality were obtained from and explained to all collateral sources.

Multi-method psychological testing was used with Jane, David and Sarah in order to analyze whether congruence existed or not from the different types of psychological measures used. For example, interviews were obtained in meeting face to face and from interview forms such as the Parenting History Survey. In addition to interviews, specific psychological measures like a checklist called The Child Behavior Checklist (CBCL),[xv] was given to each parent to complete about Sarah and the Parenting Stress Index (PSI)[xvi] was completed by each parent about their parenting of Sarah. These measures where the parents complete the form and interviews with them are *self-report* measures where the subject provides an evaluator with information that subject chooses to provide. These parents were also individually administered the Personality Assessment Inventory (PAI) and the Conflict Tactics Scale, both self-report measures. These self-report measures can be influenced by response style.[xvii] (See the Levy chapter in this volume for more on the PAI and response style).

To achieve multi-method assessment, the evaluator administered the Rorschach Inkblot Method (see the Levy chapter for more on this measure) and the Wechsler Abbreviated Scale of Intelligence (WASI). There are few *performance* measures available for use by evaluators in a CCE and both the WASI and the Rorschach are performance measures. Performance measures allow an evaluator to sample behavior of interest and to score that behavior by particular and specific rules and guidelines contained in scoring manuals. Hence, an evaluator can examine the behavior of a subject, or what that subject does, that results from performance measures, and compare to a normative sample of subjects (see the Lee chapter on assessment in this volume) and can compare the subject's self-report of the same behaviors of interest that result from self-report measures. This allows for a fine-grained examination of behaviors of interest and allows for determining congruence and lack of congruence in the entire data set.

In CCE's parents generally wish to present their case for why they should have sole custody or a major proportion of time with the child. There are self-interest reasons for this wish, as well as financial and self-esteem ones. For this reason and others, response style can be a critical component of a CCE. While a review of this area or research is beyond the scope of this chapter, the interested reader is referred to *The Art and Science of Child Custody Evaluations* by Gould and Martindale.[xviii] The variable of response style can be useful if not critical in some cases for an evaluator in a CCE to determine and sort out convergence and lack of convergence in the data.

Analysis of This Case

The evaluator's preferred method of writing a report on findings from a CCE is to provide: (1) a brief summary of the critical family events, often in a tabular form, (2) a summary of the attorney's referral questions and their summary of their client and that client's former spouse or partner, (3) a statement of the referral process, (4) a list of all documents reviewed and from where or whom they originated, (5) a list of all dates of service, including time and event, (6) a list of all collateral sources attempted and contacted and (7) the process of the evaluation. Following the setting of the context for the evaluation in this manner, this evaluator preferred to present findings about the child before presenting findings about the individual parent/caregiver. This is for several reasons. One, the CCE is about a child or children and their future caretaking relationship, in this case, Sarah's relationship with Jane and with David. By presenting findings about the child(ren) first, the reader is directed to a complete understanding of who this child(ren) is(are). CCE's are detailed and take considerable time for completion. The information about the child(ren) comes from multiple sources, both within and outside the family. A nuanced understanding of the child then becomes a part of the reader's thinking as they approach findings about each parent/partner. In the case of 6-year-old Sarah, it was important for the reader to have a good understanding of her experiences with each parent and importantly in this case, her ability to resist "alienating" behaviors from either parent given her age. Sarah reportedly exhibited some resistance to visits with David, according to Jane and disputed by David, and this was examined in the Discussion part of the report in terms of "resist and refuse" dynamics. Her relatively high intelligence level was another factor in addition to her age in affecting her ability to resist alienating behaviors.

Secondly, findings about parents/caregivers are typically complex and fraught with layers of issues such as response style, motivation, self-interest, and personality styles. The parental conflict can easily overwhelm the reader, especially when salacious details about parental behavior are part of the narrative and when the level of conflict and frequent pathology exceed the imagination of an average reader of a CCE. By placing findings about the child in the forefront, an evaluator can orient the reader to a specific child's interests, needs, developmental age and level of sophistication due to age, loyalties, suggestibility, and language, memory, and cognitive development in the context of data collected about the parents and their particular parenting styles, strengths and limitations, and personality and behavioral idiosyncrasies.

Sarah, an Adored Child

Sarah was the only child of her parents who were not likely to bear other children, primarily due to their age, and was adored by both parents. Some collaterals remarked on her overly mischievous ways before the separation of her parents and expressed astonishment that neither Jane nor David disciplined her for misbehaving in clearly socially and age inappropriate ways. Sarah could be alternately charming, playful and fun while at other times was controlling, volatile in her anger, and needy and whiny in appearance. She angrily directed the evaluator and other adults, including her mother, her father, a colleague who assisted during the videotaping sessions, and her psychotherapist to complete activities in the way she wanted them to be conducted or completed. This controlling and sometimes aggressive or angry behavior was also noted by several collateral sources of information. She was a physically attractive child, did very well in her school subjects, was considered "bright" by her teachers, was competitive and often "cheated" on games in the evaluator's office. She was observed during the structured observation with each parent to "lie" or "fib" about different matters, an observation offered by some playmates' mothers. Some fibs were obvious and puzzling, such as ones she told in the structured observations where videotaping took place. It was explained to Sarah prior to videotaping that she would be videotaped and therefore, she was aware of this. Generally, Sarah behaved more appropriately when no demands were placed on her and when she was allowed complete control over the sessions, games, or play.

Several collateral sources described Sarah as less well emotionally regulated following the abrupt separation of her parents that included a year of no overnights with David. Jane attributed the decline in Sarah's behaviors to the fact that she was "made" to visit

David, did not like these visits and did not want to go. David seemed clueless and lacking in awareness about the decline in Sarah's emotional regulation and typically reported she was "fine" at his home and during visits with him. When prodded or pushed with specific examples of her aggressiveness, however, David agreed she "didn't seem like herself" at those times. An interesting finding from the interview with Jane included a report by Jane that Sarah was not an easy baby, experienced considerable difficulty settling and falling asleep at night, and was often inconsolable. This finding suggested that Sarah might have a difficult temperament generally speaking, one that the separation and divorce did not "cause" as much as it exacerbated her natural tendencies and ultimately her various behaviors. During the evaluation, Jane was worried about Sarah's aggressiveness toward other children when she seemed to "go at them," as Jane noted. She was reported by Jane and David to intentionally hit family members with objects and on occasion to bite them. During observations of transitions, Sarah ran back and forth between her parents' separate cars multiple times and could be heard begging them to talk with one another. Roughly mid-way through the CCE, Sarah grew increasingly dysregulated, reportedly experienced greater difficulty separating from Jane, was reported by her psychotherapist and extended family members to have more "meltdowns," and was reported by her pediatrician to have more frequent urination than normal.

Sarah's psychotherapist reported Sarah talked about a "monster who ate part of her tongue," a comment the psychotherapist interpreted to mean Sarah thinks adults were not listening to her and that she had "no voice." Jane and the psychotherapist reported that Sarah screamed more frequently, jumped around on different pieces of furniture more often and did not respond to efforts to calm or soothe her. These variable, aggressive and anxious behaviors were diagnosed by Sarah's psychotherapist as anxiety due to high conflict separation and divorce. Some of these same behaviors were seen during the videotaped interactions of Sarah with each of her parents. She did not want David to leave the room, which is a part of the structured observation, and was highly resistant to the evaluator explaining he would return shortly. Once in the room alone, she tore at the blinds, nearly crashing them to the floor and threw toys and herself about the couch and room. When David returned, she told him a "fib" about completing the more difficult task the two worked on before he left, with which she had grown frustrated and said it was "stupid." She wanted David to leave immediately when he returned to the room and reluctantly engaged in clean up only after the evaluator intervened to have her and David clean up. During the videotaped observation of Sarah and Jane, Sarah complained loudly about the "baby toys" in the room, wanted to play with the toys in the cupboard to which Jane responded multiple times they would once the procedure was completed and complained about not being the one "to decide." She did not want Jane to leave, attempted to leave with her and complied with staying only after two instructions to do so. Once Jane returned, however, Sarah did not want to leave and persisted repeatedly in exchange with Jane that she did not want to leave. On the post video ratings, Jane said Sarah was, "frequently disobedient, bossy, anxious, and out of control in connection with caretaking activities, bedtimes, and on weekend evenings." Although no conclusion was offered from these observations about a specific pattern of attachment relationship for Sarah with each of her parents, the evaluator had concerns about Sarah's emotional dysregulation in multiple situations and her anxious style exhibited during the videotaped observations. There are some limits to using structured, standard procedures assessing attachment in the context of a child custody evaluation (Lee, Borelli and West, 2011.) but there is support for viewing behaviors through an attachment lens. In this case, the possibility of a disorganized attachment arose based on her behaviors in the taped observations with her parents, both the contradictory behaviors with her father and the bossy behaviors with her mother. Ultimately, no specific attachment pattern was diagnosed. For greater detail about attachment relationships, see the chapter by Jurney in this volume.

Completion of psychological testing with Sarah was exceedingly difficult in that Sarah broke pencils and threw them in the trash, impatiently asked the evaluator why she was wearing **that dress again**, and generally resisted anything other than playing games or directing the evaluator in ways she wanted her to behave. Some measures were not completed at all, due to her oppositional manner that included throwing test materials at the evaluator. When shown projective cards, Sarah repetitively stated, "I don't know. The parents are separating, everyone is sad." Most information about Sarah came from the numerous behavioral observations that occurred during separate home visits to each parent's home, observation of two transitions of Sarah from one parent to the other, the structured, videotaped observation of Sarah with each parent, interviews with her parents separately, multiple interviews with her psychotherapist, extended phone calls with her pediatrician, a phone call with her school teacher, observations gleaned from mothers of her school mates and play date friends, and information gleaned from her parents where they separately completed a Developmental History Form detailing her growth and development, a CBCL and the PSI-4.

Jane's scores rating Sarah's behaviors on the CBCL and PSI-4 were routinely in a clinical or significant range. This was true for interviews with Jane, too, where she typically described Sarah as "demanding, moody, aggressive and frustrating." She described Sarah through the CBCL in ways to suggest clinically significant emotional reactivity, sleep problems that included "extreme" difficulty falling asleep and going to bed, difficulties with soothing or being calmed, being a "picky" eater, and cruelty to animals. Findings from the PSI-4 suggested considerable stress for Jane in parenting Sarah and suggested Sarah's characteristics should be the focus of psychotherapeutic intervention, rather than other aspects of the parent–child relationship. Jane listed her concerns for Sarah as "Deterioration over the last two years from being a bright child developing well to an anxious, fearful child with self-regulation problems." Jane reported during interview that Sarah's diagnosis from her psychotherapist was Generalized Anxiety Disorder due to experienced trauma. Jane explained the trauma was from David's abusive treatment of her and Sarah and the ongoing stress to Sarah from the required visitations with David. Sarah's psychotherapist reported a diagnosis of Adjustment Disorder with anxious features due to high conflict separation and divorce.

On the CBCL that David completed, he endorsed problems for Sarah with sleeping, being a "picky" eater, having unfounded fears about various matters, talks in "baby talk" and "wants a lot of attention." He said, "Her environment is not stable due to her parents' previous dynamic." Clinically speaking, David rated Sarah as average in externalizing problems, as minimally significant in internalizing problems, and as significant in total problems. He perceived Sarah as less problematic, on the whole, than did Jane and had less to say about her problem areas during interviews. He said on one occasion that he thought much of Sarah's problems had to do with being "too dependent on her mother. Her mom needs to be more disciplined and structured with her." David had no clinical elevations on the PSI-4, suggesting that he was not experiencing stress in the parent–child system, perhaps due in part to his limited time with Sarah, relative to Jane's time with her, and perhaps due to an insensitivity, naiveté or lack of awareness regarding problematic behaviors. An additional hypothesis about David is that he was not included in medical or dental visits, teacher-parent conferences at school or in extracurricular activities for Sarah and thus was less aware of growing concerns about her behavior. Initially, he was not included in referral to Sarah's psychotherapist who declined to treat Sarah until David was notified. Jane usually notified David after the fact about these various conferences and visits with a summary of what transpired. When asked why he did not attend these various appointments and the like, he replied he did not know he could attend.

In summary, Sarah presented behaviorally as a child with many difficulties. She was more greatly unhappy, more needy or "clingy" with her mother as compared to her father, more dependent, less individuated, more moody and more irritable than other children her age. She also experienced greater needs to control and was oppositional much of the time. She was quite "bossy" with other children and was aggressive and careless with materials and in interpersonal relating. These behaviors were noted by multiple collateral sources, with differing reasons or explanations for the origin of the behaviors, and were noted by her parents, grandparents, psychotherapist and others. In addition, she was recently evaluated for frequent daytime urination that concerned her pediatrician for the fact this only seemed to occur at Jane's home. The pediatrician never met David, who reported to the evaluator that Sarah had no urination problems at his home. Jane reported night terrors and recorded an episode of this. She also reported nightmares and endorsed many of the behaviors noted here in this paragraph. She petitioned Sarah's pediatrician to place Sarah on medications for her anxiety and for her urination problems, against the advice of Sarah's psychotherapist and a psychiatrist included in a consult. David is concerned with Sarah's development, although he tends to rate her more like other children her age, perhaps due to his limited time with her that typically occurred on weekends only and perhaps due to his limited experience with her for almost a year. He also had less detailed information about her due to being excluded from appointments, conferences and referrals.

Sarah's Parents, David and Jane

Jane was the parent who produced the greatest amount of documentation during the CCE. On a Developmental History Form, for example, of roughly 15 pages, she submitted over 100 pages of notes. This massive elaboration characterized all forms she completed during the CCE. She produced many hours of audio recordings of David meant to illustrate his abusive behavior and "rages" while drinking. She also recorded Sarah at various times throughout the course of the CCE. Jane was attractive, pleasant, likeable, organized, thorough, and prompt for appointments. She also appeared vulnerable at times and slightly fearful, features of her presentation that elicited empathy from her psychotherapist, Sarah's psychotherapist and the evaluator. Both Sarah's psychotherapist and the evaluator agreed to listen to a limited number of recordings Jane produced documenting what Jane called David's nefarious and abusive behaviors, in part due to her appeal and vulnerability that elicited empathy and in part due to her persuasiveness that seemed genuine. She was highly articulate, very persuasive, and had her narrative of David as abusive, mentally ill, and abusing alcohol well organized and extremely documented. She was typically "low key" with regard to emotions, the only exception being toward the end of the CCE when various, possible parenting plans were discussed with regard to her willingness to accept or understand variants on her ideal parenting plan. At this point, she burst into tears and "couldn't imagine" a situation where anyone, including a judge, could possibly give David more time than he had at the time with Sarah.

During testing with Jane, she exhibited a consistent pattern of responding. Where measures were self-report, she responded with a response style suggesting she was not completely forthright, was reluctant to recognize or acknowledge even minor faults, and portrayed herself in an overly positive manner. Her responses suggested she attended well and was not careless in responding. Her presentation regarding response style also suggested she was presenting an overly positive picture of herself, such that it could be difficult to know exactly what she is like. The way in which she responded indicates she truly believed this presentation of herself to be accurate. Therefore, she had no clinical elevations on self-report measures and instead presented as stable, meek, mild mannered, unassuming, prefers to avoid leadership roles, and is confident and optimistic. Of note, there was nothing to suggest she was experiencing trauma or had trauma reactions from the way in which she responded to these various measures. Her psychotherapist stated during interview that Jane seemed like a "typical domestic violence victim" who dissociated when discussing difficult topics like her marriage to David. Results from the various self-report measures did not support an interpretation of her behavior as trauma based. Her reported dissociation had sources other than trauma, as revealed in reports from prior counselors and psychotherapists, from behavioral observations, from various behaviors exhibited during the CCE, from actions during the CCE like immediately informing even recent acquaintances about the "dangerousness" of David and his abusive treatment of her and Sarah, and from findings on the Rorschach Inkblot Method. All these data sources converged on similar conclusions. Additional findings about Jane from self-report measures that were consistent with findings from collateral sources' reports of her included a "lack of insight, looks for simplistic, concrete solutions that do not require self-examination, engages in blame and has substantial needs for acceptance and affection."

On more ambiguous measures, like the Rorschach and certain parts of the WASI, Jane's tangential thinking and overly elaborative response style were in evidence, just as they were during various observations, interviews, responses to forms she completed as a part of the CCE, her insistence on audio recording Sarah in multiple ways and various situations, and reports from collateral sources. Findings from the Rorschach suggested she had considerable internal resources for problem-solving and coping, yet due to a chronic, long-standing psychological overload or stress, she could not access her internal resources. Findings suggested she is a complex person who interprets the external world from her internal perspective that was not reality based. This made her quite vulnerable because she has only her internal world in which to anchor her perceptions and interpretations of the external world and needed a psychotherapist to anchor her perceptions in external realities, something the psychotherapist she had during the CCE was not providing and rather was reinforcing Jane's sense of self as a victim. Prior counselors described Jane as rigid, concrete, immutable and highly vulnerable. Her vulnerability and likeability caused others, including the evaluator, to respond to her with empathy. Vaguely uncomfortable with some test results, the evaluator sought consultation with a senior colleague who had national and international recognition as an assessment psychologist. This consultation resulted in a re-scoring, for example, of the Rorschach and a re-examination of all test results compared to other data points collected regarding Jane. This was a good example of the need to check one's potential biases and personal predilections as an evaluator, the value of consultation even as a seasoned evaluator, and the imperative to examine a data set from all angles.

What psychological testing contributed to this evaluation as regards Jane was a nuanced understanding of how Jane organized herself with self-report measures and structured interview and how she organized her thinking around themes, such as David's dangerousness, with this kind of framework. With more ambiguous measures or when probed to think beyond her preconceived notions, particularly when emotion was involved, Jane's thinking was highly tangential. At these times, she grew overly elaborative and grew more obsessive regarding her belief system, which she elaborated in a long winded and imprecise manner. She had no insight to her behaviors that others considered odd or unusual, such as writing her telephone number on Sarah's arm when she went for visits with David, securing a passport for Sarah in the event Jane wanted to leave the county, or contacting virtual strangers with reports of David's dangerousness. Jane had no understanding of an event where Sarah delayed leaving for visitation which Jane interpreted as resistance to the visitation. In this situation and as a consequence of Jane's frustration and her disturbed interpretation of reality, she assumed Sarah was fearful, grew fearful herself in response to Sarah and the two ended up in hours of crying to the point of exhaustion.

David appeared variously as lost, forlorn, often close to tears, clueless, hapless and slightly stilted. He was pleasant and cooperative and appeared intellectualized, detached and remote at times. He appeared naïve when he talked about the personal growth classes in which he participated as he spoke in glowing terms about his self-actualization. Collateral sources who attended these classes with him and who were contacted during the course of the CCE described David as wholesome, dedicated, hard-working and honest. Some of these individuals also socialized with David and denied ever seeing him drinking alcohol at all. One collateral source, whose name was submitted by Jane, adamantly stated she had "never" seen David inebriated or drinking to excess, which she declared would not happen at her parties. Although he often appeared stiff in posture, David cried openly in recounting a time he and Sarah were at a visitation and she cuddled up next to him saying, "Daddy I love you!"

It was puzzling how calm and passive David appeared when discussing the demise of his marriage, the allegations made by Jane about him, the absence of time with Sarah due to restricted visitation, and other conditions placed by Jane on conditions of visitation, once it started. He appeared impassive about all of this and did not aggressively pursue more time with Sarah nor did he challenge any of these conditions placed on his time with Sarah by Jane. This presentation was the same as in the first, joint interview with Jane who was verbally disdainful toward him. He did not react with anger or irritation to her tone or to her allegations about him. When asked about this absence of anger and his deference toward Jane during a subsequent, individual interview, David reported he had been reading books on non-violent communication as a part of his personal growth classes. His childhood friends, current friends, and family members all described him as "laid back," naïve and passive for the whole of his life.

A surprising piece of information came to light toward the end of the CCE. Jane insisted throughout the course of the CCE that David should not have her address because he would come uninvited to her new home, feared he would be threatening and abusive, and feared he would seek reprisals against Sarah and her for ending the marriage. A family member mentioned to the evaluator that David had known for almost a year where Jane had moved with Sarah, something he discovered in an accidental way. When asked why he did not share this information with the evaluator, he replied he was fearful of Jane finding out through the evaluator that he knew her address. He was fearful she would abruptly leave with Sarah again to an unknown destination and said he did not want Sarah to have that experience again of being isolated,. He also felt intimidated by some of Jane's family members, especially Jane's father, and by Jane's assertion that David's "abuse" toward her and Sarah was damaging to Sarah's brain. He added he felt threatened by Jane's recordings of all transition exchanges, of Sarah in Jane's home, and by Jane's family members who, when they were supervising visits between David and Sarah prior to the attorneys' involvement, asked him insulting questions he felt were intended for recordings.

Testing with David produced the following findings. He did not produce a discernible response style on self-report measures, which is to say findings about him suggested he was open, honest, forthcoming and not overly positive or overly negative about himself. He was somewhat defensive on one validity scale suggesting that he considered himself more virtuous than the average person and was not admitting to minor faults. He did not produce elevations on clinical scales although the pattern of his responses suggested he was hypervigilant and dependent. When his therapist was asked if she considered him hypervigilant, i.e., perhaps paranoid, she responded that of course he was, due to being intensely scrutinized and "maligned." The kind of dependency on others, or an intense desire to be liked and appreciated by others, was a characteristic finding about him from the self-report measures and the performance measures. When asked about David's possible dependency, Jane said, "Oh yes, he's very needy. It's all about him. His needs have to be met first. If he wanted something and I didn't respond, he thought I was cold, aloof and unemotional." David was forthcoming about his alcohol use on self-report measures and responded to these measures in ways that suggest he avoids confrontations, has a strong need for affection from others and is optimistic and trusting.

Across the Rorschach and PAI, as well as data collected from collateral sources and observations, David did not appear depressed, did not endorse suicidal ideation, and displayed thinking that was like that of other adults. In interviews, he acknowledged feelings of depression and suicidal thinking on occasion during his marriage. Jane and her family members thought David was mentally ill, depressed and suicidal, a finding not substantiated by other sources of information gathered during the CCE. Jane described his "rages" as due to a frontal lobe problem that she researched online, she reported. On the various measures administered to David, there was little evidence for aggressive thoughts or propensities toward aggressive actions. This was a finding supported by collateral sources, wherein collateral sources uniformly described David as passive, "laid back," and not prone to confrontation or angry displays.

On the Conflict Tactics Scale, David acknowledged areas of psychological aggression (swearing, insulting), consistent with what Jane reported on this measure during their marriage. Each parent acknowledged participating in this form of aggression toward each other. Both Jane and David denied major physical assaults, injuries or sexual coercion as routine, substantial areas of conflict on this measure. Including areas identified in the Spousal Assault Risk Assessment Guide (SARA) there were no areas of criminal assault that could be identified for David, few areas of psychosocial adjustment that were problematic for him, no identified areas of spousal assault history that could be identified, and no recent substantiated criminal offenses.

An area of concern for David that arose in interpretation of Rorschach findings was his immaturity, relative to other adults. He exhibited fewer resources for coping and therefore was more easily overwhelmed than other adults, even with minor stresses. This made him more impulsive at times than he might be otherwise. Two occasions happened just before and then during the CCE that demonstrated his impulsivity. He was exercising visitation with Sarah at a playground and left to go elsewhere, without notifying Jane of the change. On a second occasion, he grew frustrated with the absence of overnights and kept Sarah overnight without Jane's agreement. Both occasions were ones that Jane repeatedly referenced as evidence of his "dangerousness." The evaluator opined in the report on the CCE that it might be this behavior that alarmed Jane and her family members, who mislabeled this behavior as to origin, motivation and diagnosis.

Conclusions

This was a family system characterized by allegations of domestic violence, alcohol abuse, trauma, child abuse and mental illness. There were no domestic violence protective orders (DVPO), no ex parte filings for DVPO, no reports to Child Protective Services (CPS), no investigations by or findings from any CPS agency, no report of physical injuries to doctors or medical facilities sustained during incidents of domestic violence, no assault charges, and one police report documenting a call from a neighbor due to loud noise from intense argument. The police report documented no property destruction in the home, no sign of a struggle was mentioned, Sarah did not awaken during the argument, and police described hearing "yelling" from both parents when they approached the apartment. Jane elected to remain in the home that night after police asked her if she felt safe. Further, no report from police was made to Child Protective Services, as is usually the case for domestic violence cases when a child is present, in this jurisdiction where the police report originated.

After her parents' marriage dissolved, Sarah deteriorated in ways documented and described by numerous individuals. Mothers of her playmates who knew her before the marital breakup described her previously (prior to the breakup and when her parents lived together as a married couple) as confident and perhaps even bold. No one described her as fearful of David during the marriage. Since the breakup, Sarah was described as whiny, crying frequently, clinging unnaturally for extended periods of time to her mother, bossy, withdrawn, needy, aggressive, given to "meltdowns" at the slightest stress, avoidant and controlling. Since the breakup of her parents' marriage, Sarah looked disorganized, unregulated regarding her emotions and behaviors, experienced extreme difficulties in the parent–child relationship with her mother and was diagnosed with frequent daytime urination by her pediatrician, who recommended psychotropic medication in the absence of David's input to this pediatrician.

The timing of Sarah's deterioration seemed clearly connected to the marital breakup and the abrupt manner by which her relationship with David was severed. The "drumbeat"[xix] of how dangerous David was and how much he was to be feared was reinforced by Jane's imposition of supervised visitation overseen by her or family members, Jane's prevention of David's participation in teacher conferences, school related events, medical and dental appointments, and an attempt to thwart David's participation in Sarah's psychotherapy. David contributed to this family dynamic with his passivity and unwillingness to learn appropriate confrontation and/or directness, lack of assertiveness, self-absorption in being perceived as the angelic parent and insensitivity to and/or lack of attunement to Sarah's needs for him to be a more forceful and equal partner in co-parenting with Jane. Jane's father, a wealthy and aggressive C.E.O. of a large international conglomerate, added to the family conflict with an imposing manner generally and by wholeheartedly siding with his only daughter. He and his wife stoked and fanned the flames of Sarah's dissatisfaction with visitations and exchanges by joining with their daughter in continually placing blame on David for all problems, small and large, and by labeling David as mentally ill, ragefully angry and a "drunk."

Every visitation and especially the frequent exchanges between her "warring" parents was another occasion for Sarah to be subjected to the dual reality she experienced where she had fun, was playful with and was nurtured by David versus the reality of her beloved mother and grandparents, to whom she felt close and of whom she spoke warmly and who daily communicated in big and small ways, the danger and threat of David. In addition to her split experiences, she was a 6-year-old child who could not cognitively merge these highly discrepant perceptions and experiences alone. Sarah's security with her psychotherapist was undermined by Jane and her father, who lobbied for the psychotherapist's removal when she did not agree with the pediatrician's recommendation for psychotropic medication. This was despite the fact that the psychotherapist consulted with a psychiatrist regarding this medication, as the pediatrician recommended. In addition, Sarah's every word and move were scrutinized by Jane, either by daily and nightly video and audio recording, by sudden, unexplained trips to the bathroom with Jane to write Sarah's words down quickly, by sudden dashes of Jane to the computer to write down Sarah's words and/ or actions, and by Jane's random jotting down of Sarah's thoughts and words when Jane a drove and could make notes on grocery store receipts at stop signs or lights. Her mother's compromised hold on reality wherein her fight to "protect" Sarah became an organizing principle for her, the reinforcement of Jane's distortions by well-meaning and misguided professionals and family members, and the daily confusion for Sarah in figuring out reality was stunning and pervasive.

Sarah's complex set of behaviors and moods, the multiple discrepant ways her parents acted and of which she was aware, the fact that Sarah made multiple transitions in the midst of this high conflict family, the complexity of the family organization contributed to by Jane's father and mother, and Sarah's age are some of the sources of her resistance to visitations. Other contributors to her anger, aggression and confusion were the mixed messages she received from her parents and other caregivers, the damaging and inaccurate messages she received about David, and the inability of her psychotherapist, through no fault of the psychotherapist, to provide a safe haven[xx] (see Chapter 7 in this volume) for her while her parents struggled over control for her. Sarah's situation and the lack of flexibility in adjusting the family organization and dynamics to meet her needs was damaging to her and contributed to her maladaptive behaviors.

Recommendations

Control of the Family System by a Parenting Coordinator

There were many recommendations for containing the conflict in the family system, in order to provide protection to Sarah from this conflict and congruent with general principles about "resist and refuse" dynamics.[xxi] This included making recommendations that would address the individual contributions to this toxic dynamic in addition a structure that could monitor interventions, help prevent professionals from "splitting," (i.e., buying into their client's perspective) and losing sight of the overall family dynamic and move towards a goal of allowing Sarah to develop and maintain stronger, healthier relationships with both of her parents. A Parent Coordinator (PC),[xxii] to serve as referee and judge and with mental health qualifications and considerable forensic experience, was recommended to provide control of all decisions within the family system. Due to the fact that Jane's parents entered this fray as *intervenors* meant they had legal standing in the case and thus could be compelled in certain ways to comply with some orders from the PC. It was recommended that Jane seek part-time employment and that monitoring of David's alcohol consumption be managed by the PC. Exchanges of Sarah from one parent to the other were advised against for direct contact and were recommended to be handled by a supervisor of exchanges or at neutral locations such as school and gym.

Treatment Interventions

It was also recommended that the PC form a treatment team with a treatment team supervisor who coordinated input from all treatment providers, medical and therapeutic, for all family members. Recommendation was made for the grandparents to engage in an educational course of study, selected by the PC, of the growth, development and special vulnerabilities of children Sarah's age and of alienating dynamics in family systems. David was referred to a specialized program designed to enhance parenting skills and conducted by a seasoned child psychotherapist. Jane was referred to an educational "coach," someone other than her psychotherapist, to assist her in understanding "resist and refuse" dynamics, in understanding the damage to Sarah from demonizing David, and to provide readings as homework. It was recommended that all family members continue in the treatment interventions with which they were engaged. An increase from weekly to twice or three times weekly visits with Sarah's psychotherapist was recommended for the short term to give Sarah more of a "safe haven" and neutral ground. It was also recommended that neither parent could "fire" Sarah's psychotherapist without consultation with the PC In addition, it was recommended that Sarah have day care after school at a local gym, to increase socialization with other children and from which each parent have the opportunity to retrieve her. Other extracurricular activities were recommended to approval by the PC with input and participation by both parents.

Parenting Plans and Plan of Contact for the Parents

Recommendation was made for parental contact to occur through the PC, through monitoring of emails and software management systems. Eventually, direct contact was recommended (1) first, through brief, schedule management issues on a platform like Zoom or Google Meet Up, scaffolding later to brief conversations about matters deemed neutral and (2) second, to co-parenting intervention when deemed feasible by the PC.

A short period of roughly six months was planned for an alternating schedule of three days on and three days off with overnights for Sarah with each parent. Following this period of time, at which point Sarah was nearly 7 years old, a schedule of 2–2–5 was recommended. It was recommended that this schedule be monitored by the PC for any necessary changes, based on Sarah's needs as determined by input from her therapist. If any complaints or allegations arose such as occurred during the CCE, it was recommended that the PC meet with Sarah prior to and after transition to the other parent. Recommendation was made for the report detailing findings from the CCE to be shared with treatment providers and others at the discretion of the PC.

Notes

i   Johnston, J. (1994). High Conflict Divorce. *The Future of Children, 4(1),* 165–182. doi:10.2307/1602483.
Garrity, C.B. and M.A. Baris (1994). *Caught in the Middle: Protecting the Children of High Conflict Divorce.* New York: Lexington Books.
Ayoub, C.C., R. Deutsch and A. Maraganore (1999). Emotional Distress in Children of High Conflict Divorce: The Impact of Marital Conflict and Violence. *Family Court Review, 37(3),* 297–315. https://doi.org/10.1111/j.174-1617.1999.tb01307.x.
Doolittle, D.B. and R. Deutsch (1999). Children and High Conflict Divorce: Theory, Research and Intervention. In R. M. Galatzer-Levy and L. Kraus (Eds.), *The Scientific Basis of Child Custody Decisions* (pp. 425–440). New York: John Wiley and Sons.
ii Johnston, J. and V. Roseby (1997). *In the Name of the Child: A Developmental Approach to Understanding and Helping Children of Conflicted and Violent Divorce.* New York: The Free Press.
iii Gardner, R. A. (1998). The Parental Alienation Syndrome: What Is It and What Data Support It? *Child Maltreatment, 3(4),* 309–312. https://doi.org/10/1177/1077559598003004001.
iv Clawar, S.S. and B.V. Rivlin (1991). *Children Held Hostage: Dealing with Programmed and Brainwashed Children.* Chicago, IL: American Bar Association.
v   Lee, S.M. and N. W. Olesen (2001). Assessing for Alienation in Child Custody and Access Evaluations. *Family Court Review, 39(3),* 282–298. doi:10.1111/j.174-1617.2001.tb00611.x.
vi Kelly, J.B. and J.R. Johnston (2005). Commentary on Tippins and Williams "Empirical and Ethical Problems with Custody Recommendations: A Call for Clinical Humility and Judicial Vigilance." *Family Court Review, 43(2),* 233–241. https://doi.org/10.1111/j.1744-1617.2005.00022.x.
vii Friedlander, S. and M.G. Walters (2010). Finding a Tenable Middle Space: Understanding the Role of Clinical Interventions When a Child Refuses Contact with a Parent. *Journal of Child Custody: Research, Issues and Practices, 7(4),* 287–328. https://doi.org/10.1080/15379418.2010.521027.

viii Austin, W.G., L. Fieldstone and M.K. Pruett (2013). Bench Book for Assessing Parental Gatekeeping in Parenting Disputes: Understanding the Dynamics of Gate Closing and Opening for the Best Interests of Children. *Journal of Child Custody: Research, Issues and Practices, 10(1),* 1–16. https://doi.org/10.1080/15379418.2013.778693.

ix Stahl, P. (2003). *Complex Issues in Child Custody Evaluations.* Thousand Oaks, CA: Sage Publications.

x Association of Family and Conciliation Courts. https://www.afccnet.org/Resource-Center. American Psychological Association. https://www.apa.org.

xi Melton, G.B., J. Petrila, N.G. Poythress, C. Slobogin, R.K. Otto, D. Mossman and L.O. Condie (2018). *Psychological Evaluations for the Courts: A Handbook for Mental Health Professionals and Lawyers,* 4th Edition. Chapter 16: Child Custody in Divorce and page 706 (Glossary). New York: The Guilford Press.

xii Greenberg, Stuart and Humphreys. Contact chapter author at gcallowayphd@gmail.com.

xiii Cassidy, J. and P.R. Shaver (2016). *Handbook of Attachment: Theory, Research and Clinical Applications.* New York: Guilford Publications, p. 4.

xiv Cooper, G., K. Hoffman, R. Marvin and B. Powell (1999) in C. Zeanah (2009). *Handbook of Infant Mental Health,* 3rd Edition. New York: Guilford Press.
Lee, S. M., Borelli, J. L. and West, J. L. (2011). Children's Attachment Relationships: Can Attachment Data be Used in Child Custody Evaluations. *Journal of Child Custody, 8(3),* 212–242. https://doi.org/10.1080/15379418.2011.594736.

xv Achenbach, T.M. (1999). The Child Behavior Checklist and related instruments. In M.E. Maruish (Ed.). *The Use of Psychological Testing for Treatment Planning and Outcomes Assessment* (pp. 429–466). Mahwah, NJ: Lawrence Erlbaum Associates Publishers.

xvi Abidin, R.R. (2012). *Parenting Stress Index* (currently in 4th Edition). Lutz, FL: PAR.

xvii Rogers, R. and S.D. Bender (2018). *Clinical Assessment of Malingering and Deception,* 4th Edition. New York: The Guilford Press.

xviii Gould, J.W. and D.A. Martindale (2007). *The Art and Science of Child Custody Evaluations.* New York: Guilford Press.

xix Lee, Borelli and West (2011).

xx Cooper et al. (1999).

xxi *Fam Court Review* (2020).

xxii American Psychological Association. (2012). Guidelines for the Practice of Parenting Coordination. *American Psychologist, 67(1),* 63–71. doi:10.1037/a0024646.
Association of Family and Conciliation Courts. Guidelines for Parenting Coordination (2019). *Available at* https://www.afccnet.org/Resource-Center/Practice-Guidelines-and-Standards.

15 A Case of Juvenile Homicide with Complex Issues of Mental Illness and Developmental Disorder

Ginger C. Calloway

Introduction and Critical Elements to the Case

This young man, Andrew, was not an individual for whom sympathy naturally arises, due to his aggressive and angry behaviors that landed him in trouble with school authorities from an early age. The school system was vigilant in providing exceptional children's (EC) services to him and adjusting these to his ongoing needs and changing, unpredictable, and often volatile behaviors. As he progressed through school, accommodations to his Individual Education Plan (IEP) included more restrictive settings, limited contact with other children on school buses, home bound services at times, and occasional suspensions from school. His well-intended and highly involved parents were frequently confused by him and by a variety of professionals who offered differing diagnoses. Often, his aggressive behaviors were interpreted as intentional and deliberate, which led some professionals to question the diagnosis of intellectual disability (ID), despite consistent findings from measures of intelligence administered to Andrew over a multitude of years.

In efforts seemingly directed to assure his parents he would "grow out of" his aggressive behaviors and the inconsistent logic of his thoughts, or perhaps due to practitioner desire to appease exceedingly worried parents, some practitioners diagnosed Andrew with disorders like attention deficit/hyperactivity disorder (ADHD), autism spectrum disorder and oppositional defiant disorder (ODD). More often than not, Andrew carried diagnoses of bipolar disorder with and without psychosis and major depressive disorder (MDD), with and without psychosis.

Some reasons practitioners are reluctant to diagnose ID include the stigma and negative connotations attached to being labeled intellectually disabled, the common lay assumption that individuals with ID are incapable of any accomplishments, and the commonly held assumption that ID individuals can be identified by external appearance.[i] When children misbehave and fail to control their behaviors, it would not be uncommon for some teachers, parents and others to assume intention and willful disobedience, which may also be interpreted as having sufficient intelligence to commit the dysregulated and/or aggressive behaviors. This was the case for Andrew on occasion.

The interaction of a developmental disorder (e.g., ID), a mental illness (e.g., the diagnoses of bipolar disorder and MDD), his age as an adolescent and all that adolescence signifies regarding immaturity, dependence, and other descriptive factors, and his rigid adherence to a self-defense argument for the instant offense made for a complicated set of factors for his attorney's understanding of him and for the court's disposition of him. This chapter will examine the interaction of Andrew's diagnoses, the psycholegal question of competency to proceed posed by his attorney, the fact of his adolescence and key judicial decisions that apply because he was an adolescent, and the methodology by which the evaluation was conducted.

DOI: 10.4324/9780429397806-16

The Framework for the Instant Offense

Andrew was immediately arrested and incarcerated when he acknowledged to law enforcement that he shot the victim of the instant offense so that the victim could not harm him or his friend. His attorney was well respected and knowledgeable. He readily acknowledged to the evaluator, however, that he was unfamiliar with and had not represented many adolescents. Andrew was not yet 18 years old, which meant that the state could not pursue the matter as a capital crime and thus could not request the death penalty as a consequence or punishment.

In Chapter 1 of this book, Ms. Wilson covered the history of juvenile justice for delinquents and covered the various decisions by the Supreme Court of the United States (SCOTUS) that affect adolescents directly and that span the years roughly from 2005 to the present. The reader is directed to these decisions in the Wilson chapter, is encouraged to read these decisions and is encouraged to read the amicus briefs, called *amici curiae*, in support or disagreement with the request for SCOTUS to review the specific cases. The information available in these briefs and decisions is highly informative as to adolescent brain science and characteristics of adolescents that are widely accepted in the juvenile court system as a result of these varying SCOTUS decisions. In addition to the Wilson chapter, our bibliography contains multiple works by academic psychologists who address juvenile justice, SCOTUS decisions about juveniles, and adolescent brain science, and it also includes reference to a seminal textbook by Melton et al. to provide the reader with myriad ways in which to access the most extant literature in this area.[ii]

Andrew's adolescent age not only prohibited the state from pursuing the death penalty, his age also prevented an automatic sentence of life without parole, due to these SCOTUS decisions covered in the Stansell chapter and elsewhere.[iii] Although he was 16 years old at the time of the instant offense, he functioned much lower than an average 16-year-old, due to the presence of ID, and was classified functionally illiterate in some school records, by family and self-reports, and in some penal institution records. At age 6 years, he was identified as ID and carried multiple diagnoses that variously captured his problems with thinking, mood variations, and unpredictable behaviors. The legal issue of competency was immediately a question due to the presence of ID and mental illness, the two most prevalent diagnoses associated with competency to proceed[iv]. Once competency was determined, the state could pursue life without parole if the state could establish that Andrew was truly an "incorrigible"[v] adolescent. Other options for disposition could have included a plea offer from the state for life with parole, a Motion for hospitalization of Andrew indefinitely due to his being a danger to society, or other offers reached by negotiation between the state and the defense attorney.

The Referral

With no psychotropic medication to address his underlying thought disorder and no supportive community, Andrew mentally deteriorated in a matter of months. At the time of the instant offense, he reported he was using heroin and alcohol, additional factors that may have played a role in the symptoms of his deterioration. He was a very tall, not overweight though solidly built adolescent who wore antiquated eyeglasses and who frequently stared intently while remaining mute and non-communicative. His language difficulties and muteness were challenges to assessment. His physical appearance alone frightened some correctional officers in the county jail. Andrew started making odd noises, such as barking like a dog, grew increasingly more agitated, and precipitately called out the names of the victim (whom he previously knew and with whom he socially interacted) as well as his dead parent. He hid under his bed and in common areas of the jail such that correctional officers could not return him to his cell. Andrew experienced auditory and visual hallucinations, insomnia, irritability, labile mood, anxiety described as brief periods of syncope, agitation that included head banging, and odd behaviors. The local jail personnel referred him to a maximum security prison with facilities for inpatient hospitalization, medication compliance and treatment. There, he was placed on several psychotropic medications, including those used for psychosis, agitation and depression. Discharge diagnosis was MDD with psychotic features.

It was at this point, following transfer to an inpatient unit, that Andrew's attorney sought consultation from the forensic evaluator. The attorney initially asked for a "mental status exam." After further discussion, it was determined that Andrew's attorney did not understand Andrew's psychotic behaviors, wanted to understand his various diagnoses, and questioned Andrew's competency to proceed. The attorney understood that Andrew was a complicated individual with multiple diagnoses. In addition to questioning Andrew's competency to proceed, he also understood he needed assistance in evaluating Andrew as a cognitively limited individual who would likely experience considerable difficulty navigating legal procedures and decisions related to his disposition, should he be found competent to proceed. In discussion, the attorney and expert arrived at the following referral questions: (1) Is this youth intellectually disabled and/or does he have a mental illness? (2) Is this young man competent to proceed to trial? (3) What recommendations could the examiner provide regarding assistance to him in a trial, if he is found to be intellectually disabled and/or mentally ill, yet is deemed competent to proceed?

In Part Two of this book, Dr. Lee has outlined general assessment procedures, ethical obligations, need for Informed Consent that is particular to children and adolescents, and broadly defined scope for forensic evaluators who evaluate children and adolescents. Central to this assessment chapter is the notion of clearly identifying the referral question(s). It is not uncommon for attorneys to seek consultation from mental health experts without a specific or detailed understanding of what it is they seek to know and how it is that the expert can assist the attorney's defense. Such was the case with Andrew's attorney, who fortunately knew what he did not know, which is to say that he did not understand adolescents, did not understand the specific diagnoses that Andrew received from various practitioners, and had a vague notion that his client seemed incapable to proceed. How best to defend Andrew should he be deemed competent to proceed also concerned this attorney.

With regard to Informed Consent, Andrew's severe cognitive limitations rendered questionable whether or not he truly understood the notions of confidentiality and non-confidentiality given to him by the evaluator. After several repetitions of the parameters of Informed Consent, Andrew said, "You can talk to other people about it." As noted subsequently as an expert for the state who examined him, Andrew struggled with this notion of Informed Consent, even after repeated explanations at each evaluation session by the expert for the defense and by repetitions and prompting provided by the state's expert. A subject's limited understanding of Informed Consent is a thorny problem for practitioners who work with children and adolescents, due to limited cognitive abilities, lack of development of abstract thinking and undeveloped language skills, relative to adults. Both experts for the state and the defense, as required by professional ethical and code of conduct guidelines,[vi] reported separately in their reports, for differing reasons, that Andrew did not grasp all elements about the nature of the evaluations and the limits of confidentiality. The expert hired by defense struggled with whether defense counsel could consent to Informed Consent or if a guardian was required to do so. In discussions with defense counsel, Andrew's mother, and Andrew, it was decided that Andrew's understanding of Informed Consent was sufficient to proceed. The state's expert was required only to obtain "assent," because evaluation by the state was ordered by the Court.[vii] There are available specific forms for obtaining Informed Consent such as found in Melton et al.[viii]

The Assessment Process

Behavioral Observations

The examiner first met with Andrew while he was incarcerated in the prison unit for inpatient hospitalization. Andrew appeared highly vulnerable, sad, confused, frightened and dazed with regard to affect or emotion. He generally avoided eye contact or if eye contact was made, it was fleeting. He was soft spoken, mumbled and rarely made spontaneous comments. He replied "I don't remember" to many questions and he appeared lethargic, sluggish, worried and dull. He did not understand where he was located, even when a crude map was drawn for him showing him the location of the unit and the location of his hometown. When asked where he was located, for example, he replied, "Locked up." In the initial evaluation with him that spanned 15 hours over a number of days and months, he fleetingly smiled once and appeared irritable and suspicious during the last interview. He was routinely shackled at his wrists, ankles and waist. Correctional officers agreed to unshackle him for psychological assessment. In the records from this first unit, Andrew typically stood at the door to his cell, looked out and rarely said a word to anyone. He was generally described in the inpatient hospital records as "cooperative and passive."

After the initial contact that consisted of an interview only, Andrew was evaluated in a second penal institution where he continued to receive psychotropic medications and psychiatric and psychological treatment. This contact took place several months after the initial contact and roughly a year and a half after the instant offense. Andrew was more alert than on initial contact, although he continued to appear sad and frightened and verbalized that he felt sad and scared. He frequently voiced a wish to "go home." He was perpetually a limited historian and his unequivocal cognitive deficits became more obvious and evident as psychotic symptoms abated. He expressed himself in a simplistic manner and frequently said, "I don't know nuthin' about that – I can't read that good." When asked about his feelings, he usually repeated being sad and scared and once reported, "It's like it ain't real."

Andrew also reported that he frequently refused his medications because another inmate told him they were "poison." He expressed remorse for the instant offense and emphatically, continuously asserted the need for him to protect himself and his friend from the decedent. He reported recurring experiences of seeing and hearing dead people, most notably the victim of the instant offense and his father who died when he was a young teen. He said that these individuals told him to take his own life and "come to the other side." During incarceration at this site, Andrew attempted to hang himself with a sheet in his cell, fashioned a crude weapon with which to slash his wrists and used his wrist shackles in an attempt to strangle himself. He reported having "crazy dreams" in which he saw "people dying, blood and people coming for" him. In prison records, he was described as eating paper, barking like a dog, and standing at his cell door for hours on end, staring out without talking. The presence of hallucinations and delusions was repeatedly recorded by multiple practitioners with differing professional affiliations, although these abated over time and were less frequently experienced by Andrew, according to records reviewed.

Data Collection: Adhering to Standards in Forensic Psychology for Multiple Sources and Types of Data, for Transparency in Presenting Findings and for Considering Multiple Hypotheses in Interpretation of Findings[ix]

Voluminous records existed for the examiner's review, in part due to Andrew's age. There were extensive school records, due to the fact that he was identified as needing exceptional children's services in first grade and remained in special education until he quit and left school. Little time had passed since Andrew left school and the date of the instant offense. His parents had him evaluated by a number of mental health practitioners and those extensive records were available for review for some of the same reasons as the school records. His pediatric records remained available, with letters and reports back and forth from pediatricians to school personnel.

Interviews by law enforcement were made available, both visual and audio reproduction, as well as witness statement interviews. Because Andrew was taken into custody by law enforcement quickly, his mother and grandmother were able to secure his school records in full, before destruction of these records. These records were reviewed prior to choice of assessment instruments for this evaluation.

In addition to the ample records for review, the examiner administered a structured interview that required multiple sessions for completion, the Wechsler Adult Intelligence Scale, Fourth Edition (WAIS-4), the Wide Range Achievement Test, Fourth Edition (WRAT-4), and the Grisso Instruments for Evaluating Juveniles' Adjudicative Competence. The Grisso instruments included the Juvenile Adjudicative Competence Interview (JACI) that is administered directly to the juvenile, a Developmental History Form that was administered to Andrew's mother and grandfather, the Caretaker's Perception of Youth's Adjudication administered to Andrew's mother and grandfather, and the Forensic Evaluation Outline Form that was provided to Andrew's attorney.

Due to Andrew's striking cognitive limitations, his simplistic manner of speaking, his general lack of knowledge and the need to simplify questions asked of him, the examiner chose to audio tape the administration of the JACI. This choice was made because Andrew's cognitive limitations were clearly evident when listening to him and audio taping made it possible for another examiner to review his responses in their complete form and reach an independent conclusion. As matters progressed in the disposition of Andrew's case, this was a fortuitous decision, as it allowed for comparison of Andrew at different time periods by varying experts. It was expected that the state would vigorously defend a punitive consequence for the alleged crime and would employ any number of mental health experts to pursue its goal. Therefore, in the interests of transparency, required by psychological experts who perform forensic evaluations and who testify in forensic matters,[x] the examiner decided to preserve the interview regarding competency with Andrew in an audio recorded form to allow for completely independent review of Andrew's actual words, rather than a summary or interpretation by the examiner who was hired by defense attorney for Andrew.

The choice regarding various instruments selected for use with Andrew was based in part on the psycholegal questions provided on page six. The intelligence test, the screening measure for achievement (WRAT-4), the Diagnostic Assessment of Post Traumatic Stress (DAPS) and the Grisso instruments for assessment of juvenile adjudicative competency were all chosen to address the question of competency to proceed. Although Andrew was administered a number of intelligence tests from age 6 to age 14 by psychologists working for the school system, he was showing psychotic symptoms soon after arrest and incarceration. Further, he was diagnosed with MDD with psychosis after his deterioration. This led to a question of whether or not the decompensation resulted in cognitive decline. The intelligence test and the screening measure of achievement also allowed the examiner to know whether or not Andrew could read and reliably respond to measures of self-report.

The choice of the DAPS came about because of Andrew's inability to specifically describe his internal states and thoughts, due to his frequent repetitions when asked open-ended questions, and due to routine muteness. The DAPS was read to Andrew, due to his limited reading abilities. This situation of Andrew's difficulties with language comprehension and expression was frustrating and therefore, the evaluator elected to use this instrument, although it could not be scored and relied upon for conclusions. What was gained with the DAPS questions was an opportunity for Andrew to answer specific rather than open-ended questions and to provide a richer narrative to the behavioral observations of him through using his words and descriptions of his internal experiences. This administration, too, was audio-taped.

Malingering[xi] is of concern in any forensic evaluation because such a finding can play a decisive role in legal outcomes as it brings into question the credibility and veracity of the subject being evaluated.[xii] Malingering is a somewhat controversial concept,[xiii] in that defining intent to lie or deceive, a central aspect of the definition of malingering in the Diagnostic and Statistical Manual of Mental Disorders, Fifth Edition (DSM-5) is difficult to establish. Malingering is a diagnosis and is concluded by collateral data and measures of response style such as feigning and deception. For a more through treatment of the subjects of malingering, deception and response styles, the reader is referred to the several editions of *Clinical Assessment of Malingering and Deception*[xiv] in print. For coverage of validity indicators within some specific assessment instruments that allow for interpretation of response style, see Levy's chapter in this book.

For those with Intellectual Disability, there are no current standardized measures that are appropriate for this population with regard to feigning or malingering ID.[xv] For someone with a diagnosis of ID, the congruence of information or data about the individual's intellectual disability is a more reliable method for an opinion as to feigning cognitive deficit.[xvi] Therefore, no standardized measure of feigning for cognitive impairment was administered to Andrew. As regards feigning of his mental illness, reliance on record review, multiple opinions provided by differing practitioners beginning at age six through adulthood for Andrew, and congruence of all data was considered the most accurate way to assess his potential feigning of mental illness for him.

Additional Assessment

During the course of his incarceration, Andrew spent more than a year in a penal institution where he received court ordered competency restoration training. Two examiners had opined that Andrew was likely incompetent to proceed. Because determination about competency is a legal one, the presiding judge ruled Andrew incompetent to proceed at the time. Historically, findings of incompetency arose out of English Common Law and arose from concerns about defendants' mental state of mind, referred to by Blackstone as "unsane" and "becoming mad."[xvii] In the United States, the case of *Dusky versus the United States*[xviii] established the modern day standard for competency to stand trial,[xix] with additional cases and statutes refining and adding to the *Dusky* standard. Training to competency is intended to restore a defendant to sufficient present ability to allow for trials, hearings and legal disposition of a case to proceed. Where an individual is deemed "mentally ill," is ordered to training for competency, and is "restored" to a functional level by correct administration of medications or other treatment and educational interventions, restoration to competency accurately captures the outcome. In cases where a defendant is diagnosed with ID, however, "restoration" to competency is a misleading notion. ID is a developmental disorder and thus one cannot be "restored" to a condition where one no longer has that intellectual disability. More accurate description of training to competency for ID individuals is the notion of "attainment" to competency.[xx] Following this training where he was declared by staff at the penal institution as "unrestorable," Andrew was once more assessed by the two experts involved for the state and for the defense.

Assessment Findings

Relevant Background Information

The following is an account of his background and history that was provided by Andrew during multiple interviews, corroborated by third-party information sources, and by an interview with his mother and grandmother jointly, followed by two interviews with his mother by phone.

His birth history was uneventful, with the exception that he was born two weeks early and that his mother suffered from diabetes. His family history included first degree relatives with histories of psychiatric hospitalization, some developmental disorders, and psychiatric disorders including diagnosis of bipolar disorder. His father died in an automobile accident when Andrew was 13 years old. During his childhood years, Andrew had a period of time where he gained 50 pounds, the origin for which was uncertain.

As he was only 16 at the time of the instant offense, Andrew had never married and had never applied for or secured a full-time employment position. He did "odd jobs" here and there for neighbors or family friends. His mother and grandmother carefully monitored him in these various "odd jobs," for fear he would be taken advantage of, due to his naiveté and immaturity. He had no children or significant romantic relationships, although he may have had some romantic feelings toward the girlfriend of the victim of the homicide. He reported and family members concurred he "experimented" with marijuana and alcohol, meaning he tried marijuana and alcohol on occasion. Andrew reported to prison practitioners in the inpatient unit that he had tried heroin and told them he was using heroin and alcohol on the date of the instant offense. He never received treatment for substance abuse.

His educational and psychiatric history were documented in great detail and were the most noteworthy aspects of Andrew's developmental years. He was initially identified as learning disabled in school and placed in EC classes at age 6. When asked if he ever received special education, Andrew remarked he was in "crazy classes." Although he scored in a range consistent with identification as intellectually disabled, he was initially classified specific learning disability (SLD). Andrew continued to consistently score in a range of I.Q. congruent with ID throughout his years in school and also scored similarly on measures of adaptive functioning. His achievement in school was congruent with sub-average, general intellectual functioning, significant deficits in adaptive functioning and evidence of both these deficits prior to the age of 18.[xxi] Thus, it was evident from multiple, extensive sources that Andrew could be diagnosed intellectually disabled, congruent with definitions for ID found in various authoritative sources.[xxii]

In a similar vein to the progression of his ID, Andrew's psychiatric history started with behavioral problems at age six and was marked by various diagnoses from multiple providers or practitioners. For many years, it was unclear to educators, his parents, and the several providers with whom his parents consulted whether his aggressive behaviors were solely fueled by his learning handicap or whether they were distinct and indicative of other diagnoses. His emotional and behavioral problems were sometimes amenable to treatment and sometimes highly resistant to treatment. He experienced periods of stability and some progress in treatment and at other times, he declined dramatically and abruptly. He alternately felt threatened by other children and was threatening to them. There was no record of or reference to hallucinations or delusions until shortly after his incarceration. His mother and grandmother denied he experienced these as a child. He was administered a number of different medications, including antipsychotic medications and stimulant medications to address varying diagnoses of ADHD, bipolar disorder, autism and Tourette's syndrome. At times, he was diagnosed with oppositional defiant disorder (ODD), although interestingly, he never received a diagnosis of conduct disorder. His parents were dutiful and consistent in securing consultations and treatment and in adhering to recommenda-tions from various providers, although they did not follow through with lengthy treat-ment interventions. They faithfully attended school conferences and assisted him in ways recommended by teachers, physical and occupational therapists in the schools and other educational professionals. At some point around 10 to 12 years of age, Andrew was placed in self-contained classes for ID and emotionally handicapped students. He was provided detailed Individual Education Plans (IEP) with a host of varying, differentiated interven-tions that ranged from least to most restrictive. By recommendation of a mental health practitioner, he took a brief respite from school entirely. When he dropped out of school at age 16, he had attained only a first to second grade level of academic functioning. Records from agencies with which he came in contact afterward listed him as "functionally illit-erate." He frequently said of himself that he did not understand many questions posed during interview and often made statements like, "I can't read that good."

Findings from Specific Assessment Instruments

Intelligence and Achievement Measures, Current and Historic

Andrew was administered an intelligence test, on which he obtained a full-scale I.Q. of 60, well within limits of ID. This score was reported as an adjusted score of 57.6, an adjustment made for norm obsolescence.[xxiii] Norm obsolescence refers to a finding, attributed to James Flynn, that the mean I.Q., generally set at a score of 100 for most measures of intelligence, rises over time making the mean point of 100 a less accurate point of comparison.[xxiv] Extensive research over many years has shown that I.Q. scores increase slightly over time[xxv], which is why test publishers re-norm their tests approximately every 10–12 years. Colloquially, norm obsolescence is referred to as "the Flynn effect." In Andrew's case, this adjustment for norm obsolescence was less important than in other situations, such as when the death penalty can be pursued. However, the point is made in this chapter because there will be some I.Q. scores obtained by evaluators that are closer to the "borderline" range of intelligence, sometimes considered out of range for diagnosis and identification of ID. A more complete discussion of norm obsolescence and applying adjustment for norm obsolescence can be found in the references contained in endnote xxiv and in the source material within these references. In those situations where an I.Q. score falls within "borderline" limits, evaluators should also be knowledgeable about standard error of measurement (SEM) and how this phenomenon affects interpretation of scores. In addition, evaluators should be aware of the increasing reliance on identification of adaptive deficits in arriving at a diagnosis of ID,[xxvi] as compared to a period of time when greater reliance was placed on I.Q. scores.

The WRAT-4 was given to Andrew to obtain an approximation of his level of achieve-ment. The WRAT is a screening measure only and not as valid as more comprehensive measures of achievement such as the Woodcock-Johnson Tests of Achievement or other similar comprehensive measures. However, Andrew was administered a number of more comprehensive measures of achievement, received yearly end-of-grade testing in school, and received multiple administrations of standardized group measures of achievement yearly while in school. These were available for review from his extensive, lengthy school record and could be compared to his present level of functioning. Andrew's performance on all achievement measures, as well as his school grades in individual subject areas, was consistent and was congruent with his performance on measures of intelligence.

Andrew's teachers and parents were routinely administered measures of adaptive func-tioning, rating his adaptive behaviors, while Andrew was in school, with results congruent with intelligence and achievement testing. Therefore, no measures of adaptive functioning were administered to family or others who knew him, given the congruence of these various measures during the developmental period or prior to the age of 18. There was ample data to substantiate the diagnosis of ID, obviating the need for further investigation of this diagnosis. The current measure of intelligence and the screening measure of achievement were consistent with prior findings about his intelligence and achievement and suggested there was no further deterioration as a result of Andrew's psychotic experience and symptoms.

Behavioral and Social/Emotional Measures

Throughout his school years, Andrew's parents and various teachers rated his behavior on measures like the Preschool and Kindergarten Behavior Scales and the Behavior Assessment System for Children (BASC), with findings indicating severe difficulties in both internalizing and externalizing behaviors. He received several diagnoses related to behavioral and/or social/emotional functioning, as mentioned previously in this chapter. His behavior shortly after incarceration led to inpatient hospitalization. At the time of the current evaluation, Andrew received an initial diagnosis of schizophrenia and a discharge diagnosis of MDD with psychosis from the inpatient unit where he was transported shortly after incarceration for the instant offense.

Consistent with Andrew's self-report, he appeared very bothered, worried and severely affected by the events connected with the instant offense. He reported that he relieved the events of the instant offense in disturbing and distressing way and heard the victim "talking" to him in various ways. Consistent with the behavioral descriptions provided earlier in this report, Andrew seemed confused, dazed, highly distressed, and vulnerable. He appeared traumatized by the events of the instant offense and had a limited understanding of and no insight into the frightening images, emotions and thoughts he experienced since incarceration. During the various interviews with him, he repeatedly expressed a wish to harm himself and/or to die to the evaluator, to hospital staff at the inpatient unit, and to mental health professionals in the second penal institution where he was housed. As mentioned previously in this chapter, he attempted to harm himself on several occasions after incarceration.

Measures of Competency to Stand Trial or Competency to Proceed

Due to Andrew's impaired level of functioning, there were few choices[xxvii] for assessing his competency to stand trial (CST), also known as competency to proceed. In his case, selection of a multitude of psychological instruments was not necessary due to issues of co-morbidity, the existence of multiple clinical diagnoses, Andrew's adolescence and the issues of a developmental perspective on mental disorder for adolescents.[xxviii] For a number of reasons, Andrew was immediately transferred from juvenile court to adult court for disposition of his case. The only assessment method that was suitable for him was the collection of interviews contained in Evaluating Juvenile's Adjudicative Competence.[xxix] The Grisso interviews (I will refer to the collection of interviews in Evaluating Juvenile's Adjudicative Competence as the Grisso interviews) about competency assume the juvenile is adjudicated in juvenile court. This was not the case for Andrew, such that questions from the Juvenile Adjudicative Competency Interview (JACI), a part of this collection of interviews, were altered or omitted that referred to juvenile court, juvenile court judge and juvenile court counselor. In part due to this alteration and other reasons that include need for transparency and Andrew's simplistic language, the interview with the JACI was audio recorded and preserved. When the state requested the evaluator's files, the evaluator recommended to the defense attorney that he seek a protective order for the audio recordings, due to the copyright attached to the materials as well as need for compliance with the

American Psychological Association (APA) Ethical Principles of Psychologists and Code of Conduct. The presiding judge signed this order for protection.

One part of the Grisso interviews includes two interviews for family members: (1) the Caretaker's Perception of Youth's Adjudication and (2) Developmental and Clinical History. There are other forms within this set of interviews that can be used for preparation of youth and family or caretakers that were not applicable to Andrew's situation.

Interviews with Andrew's Mother and Grandmother

Andrew's mother and grandmother were first interviewed jointly and subsequently, Andrew's mother was interviewed alone. These family members described Andrew as child-like, immature and unsophisticated. They said he was very frustrated with school and did not learn much there. They described him as "easily led." After his transfer to the inpatient unit, it was roughly six to seven months before they saw him again in the second unit. They described him as tearful, sad and "bawling" and added, "He didn't talk much." They reported further that Andrew "always" experienced difficulty with memory and typically appeared "pitiful." His mother said Andrew experienced depression throughout his school years, particularly in the spring and fall, a phenomenon that his pediatrician classified as bipolar disorder. His mother reported that Andrew was also thought to be autistic.

His mother and grandmother denied that Andrew ever experienced hallucinations and reported he had not been hospitalized for psychiatric difficulties during his developmental years. They remarked that his older brother "heard things" and would run through the house as if someone was chasing him. When shaken, "he'd be all right. He was also bad to sleepwalk." They denied that Andrew engaged in any similar behaviors of that nature. Subsequently, however, when discussing Andrew's depression, they noted he went through a period of time where he refused to remove his clothing to sleep at night, "in case he had to get up and run." They reported a family history of Andrew's paternal grandmother being hospitalized three to four times for bipolar disorder and stated that several of Andrew's aunts were diagnosed with bipolar disorder. They also reported a family history of schizophrenia and ADHD (attention deficit/hyperactivity disorder). They were sure Andrew experienced depression when his father died and when his maternal grandmother moved away for a few years. They remarked on the substantial weight gains he had both times.

Since his incarceration, his mother and grandmother report that Andrew lost weight, is irritable, claims others are "picking" on him, reported seeing a dead person in the jail bathroom and reported seeing men behind him watching him all night. They emphatically denied he behaved in these ways as a child or young teen. They also denied he previously engaged in self-injurious behaviors or attempted suicide. They reported that Andrew typically used "poor judgement" that included bouts of volatility toward other children in school, being easily manipulated by others and requiring their oversight when completing "odd jobs" in the neighborhood. Andrew's mother remarked that he routinely relied on her for problem-solving and decision making.

Of note is that while Andrew did not have an extensive juvenile record of offenses, he did have contact with the juvenile justice system as a 12 year old, when a school resource officer (SRO) intervened during one of Andrew's aggressive periods that involved destruction of school property. Due to the school's "zero tolerance" policy, he was referred to the juvenile system.

Interview with Andrew: the JACI

Andrew exhibited severe limitations in his knowledge of the legal system and legal concepts, the nature and object of the proceedings against him, his ability to assist his defense in a rational and reasonable way, application of an understanding of the legal system and legal concepts to novel situations and his own case. For example, he did not know what a prosecutor, jury, judge or trial were and did not know the role or purpose of any of these individuals. When asked what a prosecutor is and what a prosecutor does, he replied, "I couldn't tell you." In an attempt to test his appreciation of what a prosecutor does, Andrew confused the role of defense counsel with prosecutor and stated the prosecutor would "tell my story, I guess. That's his job, ain't it?" The JACI allows for teaching or instruction about these roles. Following a brief explanation, he was again asked the role of the prosecutor and said, "It sounds like he's trying to get me in trouble." With regard to defense counsel, Andrew reported, "He's supposed to help me." He was unable to elaborate specific ways in which defense counsel might assist him.

When asked what crime he was charged with, he initially said, "Killing someone." When asked what that is called, he replied he did not know. When asked the same question later, he replied, "Murder." He was unable to elaborate what kind of murder charge, i.e., first or second degree, and was unable to detail or elaborate what kind of consequences could result if he was found guilty of charges against him. He did state that "they" told him it "was a pretty bad thing." On further inquiry, he stated "they" was a reference to police or law enforcement. After several questions during the first interview with him about these matters, he stated after several questions, "A lawyer told me I could get a life sentence." On further questioning, he stated when asked what that meant, "They can lock me up for the rest of my life."

Andrew was asked about pleas. He continually shook his head "no" when asked about pleas and when asked what does "pleading guilty" mean. When asked what would happen if he pled "guilty," he stated, "Guess you get to go home." In answer to what would happen if you pled "not guilty," he shrugged his shoulders and shook his head back and forth, indicating he did not know an answer. Additional questions about pleas resulted in Andrew stating, "I don't know nothing about the law." He was asked what could happen to him if he was found guilty during a trial. He replied, "I really don't know. Might get to go home, don't know." He was asked what could happen to him if he did not go home and he replied, "Guess you get locked up." He did not know how long he would be "locked up" and replied to this question, "A long time." He had difficulty defining "a long time." An effort was made through questioning to reference "a long time" to his current incarceration length. Ultimately with regard to "a long time" as it relates to the length of his current incarceration, Andrew stated, "I think my Mama said about 2 years." Additional questions to him about plea agreements resulted in his repeatedly stating, "I don't know" or "don't know." On the JACI where instruction is allowed, the concept of plea agreement was explained to him. When asked to explain this in his own words, he stated, "Trying to get me to say something that ain't true. I didn't do wrong, I didn't do nothing wrong." Additional questions about possible choices he might make or that the prosecutor might offer resulted in Andrew growing more adamant and insistent that he "couldn't lie" about what happened.

Summary and Conclusions about Competency/Incompetency to Proceed

Andrew had an inadequate knowledge base about the legal system and legal concepts, lacked a rational appreciation of how he might be impacted by pleas or by a decision of guilty with regard to his charges, and lacked an understanding of how to assist his attorney. He also lacked the capacity to retain anything he learned about the legal system. He was confused regarding the roles of defense counsel and prosecutor. In addition, Andrew has been diagnosed with two of the major diagnoses most likely to negatively affect competency to stand trial, i.e., ID and psychotic features.

Diagnostically, he was intellectually disabled throughout the developmental period or prior to the age of 18 years and remained intellectually disabled at the time of the evaluation. While housed in an inpatient unit during incarceration, he received a diagnosis of MDD, with psychotic features. The evaluator concurred with that diagnosis on the basis of his behavioral presentation during the evaluation and by multiple reports of differing practitioners during his stay on the inpatient unit and the unit to which he was referred for continued observation. Additionally, he was diagnosed in the inpatient unit with substance abuse disorder, polysubstance abuse, in remission due to incarceration. The evaluator concurred with this diagnosis. It was also suggested in notes about him from that same unit that bipolar disorder was a "rule out" diagnosis. His diagnoses, medications and recorded behaviors provided subsequently were consistent with these diagnoses and notes.

The question of Andrew's various diagnoses were complicated by his young age and family history, such that the question of schizophrenia, for example, still remains. The finding that he reported to inpatient staff he had used heroin and alcohol at the time of the instant offense also raised the question of whether his various symptoms could be explained by withdrawal and/or continued impact from this combination of drugs. His hallucinations were unusual for MDD and as a child, he had many odd behaviors and thoughts. Diagnosis for children is complex in part due to the fact that children are growing and developing and in part because thought disorder and depression can and do result in different symptoms for children than for adults.

Legal Proceedings

The Attorney's First Question

The attorney's first question: is this young man ID and/or mentally ill was answered yes for both disorders. The findings for this question quite obviously had a significant impact on the additional question of competency to proceed. In Andrew's case, there was substantial data to support both diagnoses and both diagnoses had tremendous impact on his subsequent performance in the program designed to provide sufficient competency to proceed. Andrew did not gain competency as a result of participating in this restoration program for more than a year.

"Research on the characteristics of defendants evaluated for competency to proceed shows that incompetent defendants are more likely to have lower I.Q.s and psychiatric disorders."[xxx] When defendants participate in programs to enhance competency, the time for this training can typically take upwards of two years for the ID.[xxxi] Oftentimes, the ID defendant can repetitiously provide answers to the roles of courtroom players like a judge, prosecutor or defense attorney. They may also be able to recite from memory what they learn about pleas and possible outcomes from a trial or as a consequence as their alleged crime(s). Where ID individuals experience greatest difficulty, however, is with active and meaningful participation in the trial process due to difficulties with abstract reasoning, a rational ability to cooperate with their attorney and to understand proceedings, gullibility and suggestibility, dependence on others, and language difficulties.[xxxii]

The Attorney's Second Question

The attorney's second referral question was: Is this youth competent to proceed? The evaluator answered that as an opinion, he was not and added that the determination of competence is a legal one.

The Attorney's Third Question: What do I do if the judge says he's competent?

Andrew's attorney who had some familiarity with ID individuals requested consultation on and recommendations for how to proceed with hearings, pleas or trial should the court rule that Andrew could proceed. Presenting these recommendations to the attorney in the evalua-tion report provided an answer to the attorney's third question. These included the following:

1   Andrew lacks the capacity to understand the proceedings against him, to comprehend plea discussions and agreements, and is incapable of assisting his attorney in his own defense.
2   Andrew should be held in custody in a suitable hospital facility for treatment pend-ing determination, by the court, of his fitness to proceed. He appears to have settled into an appropriate medication regime and treatment protocol where he is currently housed and might experience a deterioration in his mental status should he be trans-ferred to a facility where oversight and treatment interventions are not provided.
3   The stress of a trial or a hearing could exacerbate Andrew's symptoms and care should be taken to provide a supportive environment for him as he moves through the various legal proceedings. Therefore, it is recommended that an advocate/assistant be appointed by the court to help him with understanding plea offers, to assist in his ability to communicate with counsel and to help him understand generally the process of litigation. An advocate for the disabled, congruent with standards for the disabled, is recommended, although it is unlikely to be successful. Support for this option can be found in recent case law within this state and with reference to Accommodations Under the American Disabilities Act.
4   With his developmental disorder (ID) and long-standing behavioral problems, a "res-toration" to total competency is not likely. He could perhaps "attain" a level of com-petence that might result in greater knowledge of legal concepts and terms. He might profit from attending a program of attainment at a regional hospital with an established competency "restoration" program, as regards improvement of knowledge for him regarding legal concepts and terms. Application, however, of short-term gains from this training to his specific situation is likely to remain an insurmountable problem for him in the long run, when a trial or hearing might occur long after completion of "res-toration" training. Therefore, due to his age as an adolescent, his lack of mental matu-rity as a consequence of his ID, his oft cited dependence upon others regarding multiple areas of decision making, and his current confused, dazed state of mind, an advocate for the disabled is recommended as above. In addition, re-evaluation of his competency to proceed is recommended at each juncture just prior to a legal proceeding.

Adolescent Developmental Characteristics Not Central to This Case

Although Andrew's case was well documented and offered an obvious congruence of data as regards his dual diagnoses of ID and thought disorder, other adolescents may have more complex and less easily discerned situations. In Andrew's case, developmental considerations were overshadowed by his severe intellectual deficits, thought disorder and mood dysregu-lation. Developmental considerations take precedence in other adolescents whose situations are less stark than for Andrew. These developmental factors may play a part where ID, sub-stance abuse and mental disorders co-exist, although in different ways than for Andrew. In this evaluation, the evaluator was greatly assisted to evaluate the continuity, consistency and congruence of the data set regarding Andrew, due to the extensive amount of records over a period of 10–12 years. That data set may not always be available in other cases.

Those working with adolescents in the juvenile justice system who commit criminal offenses should be familiar with the progress in adolescent brain development that has occurred since the Supreme Court decision in *Roper vs Simmons*[xxxiii] in 2005.[xxxiv] "This landmark case was the first to use empirical evidence in place of common sense to draw legal bounda-ries between adolescents and adults."[xxxv] The *Roper* decision held that it is unconstitutional to impose capital punishment (e.g., sentence someone to death) for those younger than 18 years. The *Roper* decision was remarkable for the Court's consideration of scientific findings about adolescents and how they are different from adults. In several cases that followed, [xxxvi] the court more explicitly referenced adolescent brain development presented in the various amicus briefs[xxxvii] submitted by organizations like the American Medical Association, the American Psychological Association and the National Association of Social Workers. In the chapter in this book by Stansell, this progression of cases and their import is presented.

The reader is also referred to an excellent chapter in *The Handbook of Psychology and Juvenile Justice*[xxxviii] written by Nagel and colleagues on Adolescent Development, Mental Disorder and Decision Making in Delinquent Youths. Particularly noteworthy in this chapter is the author's note that "Historically, juvenile psychopathology was either ignored or considered merely a downward extension of adult psychopathology.[xxxix] Before the 20th century, adolescent mental disorder did not exist as a psychiatric specialty,[xl] and it was not until the 1980s that adolescent psychopathology was considered in the context of the unique changes and vulnerabilities of the developmental period.[xli] In contrast to prior theories that saw childhood mental health problems as either irrelevant to or entirely continuous with adult functioning, the new field of developmental psychopathology expected juvenile mental disorder to show both continuity and discontinuity in behavioral variation and developmental course.[xlii] The American Psychiatric Association's 2013 *Diagnostic and Statistical Manual of Mental Disorders* (5th edition; *DSM-5*), which is the most widely used classification system for mental disorders in the United States, generally fits adult psychopathology better than adolescent psychopathology because its system of diagnoses does not recognize these continuities and discontinuities inherent in the developmental experience."[xliii] These authors examine a developmental perspective on mental disorder in adolescents, distinctions between normal development and mental disorder, and continuity and discontinuity across the developmental period.[xliv]

Informative for practitioners who read this chapter referenced above, Table 6.1 on page 121 is especially significant. Table 6.1 presents prevalence of mental disorders among samples of detained and community adolescents. What is striking about the numbers in this table is: "Clearly a huge number of youths in the juvenile justice system have some form of mental problem, both in an absolute sense and in proportion to the number of mentally disordered youths in the community."[xlv] The implications of this finding are contextualized for whether or not treatment recommendations should be a part of an evaluator's report, the connection between delinquency and mental disorder, the experience of adolescents with mental disorders in the juvenile justice system and the responsibility and capacity to respond to this considerable mental health problem. Discussion of historical and legal explanations for the high prevalence of mental disorders, explanations for high prevalence and best practices for youths with mental disorders follows.

Practical Points

- Forensic evaluations require evaluators to be thorough in request for documents and in examination of all data.
- Clearly state one's referral questions and make sure you understand clearly what information the attorney is seeking.
- Examine all data sources for consistency, continuity and convergence of findings. Understand that examining a data set from one or two data points only can mislead an evaluator to inappropriate and/or ineffective conclusions.
- Adolescents are complex and evaluations of them require specialized knowledge, training, and experience. Understand child and adolescent development.
- Understanding and clinically working with/treating adolescents does not equal specific expertise required for particular types of forensic evaluations that have psycholegal questions.

- Assess honestly whether your skills and expertise are sufficient to address the specific psycholegal questions posed by the offense and offense disposition. Understand possible dispositions and sentencing.
- Stay up-to-date or current with relevant literature and how it applies to your case.

Notes

i   Blume, J.H. & K.L. Salekin (2015). "Analysis of Atkins Cases." In E.A. Polloway, Ed. *Intellectual Disability and the Death Penalty*. Washington, D.C.: The American Association on Intellectual and Developmental Disorders.

ii   Melton, G.B., J. Petrila, N.G. Poythress, C. Slobogin, R.K. Otto, D. Mossman and L.O. Condie (2018). *Psychological Evaluations for the Courts: A Handbook for Mental Health Professionals and Lawyers: Fourth Edition*. New York: The Guilford Press.

iii *Miller vs. Alabama*, 567 U.S. 460 (2012), *Graham v. Florida*, 560 U.S. 48 (2010), and *Montgomery v Louisiana*, 577 U.S., No. 14-280 (2016).

iv   Zapf, P.A. and R. Roesch (2009). *Evaluation of Competence to Stand Trial: Best Practices in Forensic Mental Health Assessment*. New York: Oxford University Press.

v   *Miller vs. Alabama*, 567 U.S. 460 (2012).
     Fairfax-Columbo, J., S. Fishel and D. DeMatteo (2019). Distinguishing "Incorrigibility" from "Transient Immaturity": Risk Assessment in the Context of Sentencing/Resentencing Evaluations for Juvenile Homicide Offenders. *Translational Issues in Psychological Science, Vol. 5 (12)*, 132–142. http://dx.doi.org/10.1037/tps0000194.

vi   American Psychological Association (2017). *Ethical Principles of Psychologists and Code of Conduct*. Washington, D.C.: APA. www.apa.org.
     Specialty Guidelines for Forensic Psychology (2013). *American Psychologist, Vol. 68 (1)*, 7–19. Washington, D.C.: APA. doi:10.1037/a0029889.

vii Melton et al. (2018), p. 153

viii Ibid, p. 97.

ix   Specialty Guidelines for Forensic Psychology (2013).
     Melton et al. (2018).
     Otto, R.K. & I. B. Weiner (2014). *The Handbook of Forensic Psychology: Fourth Edition*. Hoboken, NJ: John Wiley and Sons.

x   Specialty Guidelines for Forensic Psychology (2013).

xi   Rogers, R. and S.D. Bender (2018). *Clinical Assessment of Malingering and Deception: Fourth Edition*. New York: The Guilford Press.

xii Ibid.

xiii Otto, R.K. in Rogers, R., Ed. (2008). *Clinical Assessment of Malingering and Deception: Third Edition*. New York: The Guilford Press.

xiv Rogers, R. and S.D. Bender (2018).

xv   Salekin, K.L. and B. M. Doane (2009). Malingering Intellectual Disability: The Value of Available Measures and Methods. *Applied Neuropsychology, Vol. 16*, 105–113. doi:10.1080/09084280902864485.
     Ellis, J.W., C. Everington, and A.M. Delpha (2018). Evaluating Intellectual Disability: Clinical Assessment in Atkins' Cases. *Hofstra Law Review, Vol. 46, (4)*, Article 8. https://scholarlycommons.law.hofstra.edu/hlr/vol46/iss4/8.
     Keyes, D.W. and D. Freedman (2015). "Retrospective Diagnosis and Malingering." In E.A. Polloway, Ed., *Intellectual Disability and the Death Penalty*. Washington, D.C.: The American Association on Intellectual and Developmental Disorders.

xvi Everington, C. and J.G. Olley (2008). Implications of Atkins v. Virginia: Issues in Defining and Diagnosing Mental Retardation. *Journal of Forensic Psychology Practice, Vol. 8(1)*, 1–23. doi:10.1080/15228930801947278.
     Salekin, K.L. and B. M. Doane (2009).

xvii Zapf, P. A. and R. Roesch (2009).

xviii *Dusky versus United States*, 362 U.S. 402 (1960).

xix Zapf, P. A. and R. Roesch (2009).

xx   Ibid.

xxi American Association on Intellectual and Developmental Disabilities (2010). *Intellectual Disability: Definition, Classification, and Systems of Support: The 11th Edition of the AAIDD Definition Manual*. Washington, D.C.: AAIDD.

American Psychiatric Association (2013). *Diagnostic and Statistical Manual of Mental Disorders: Fifth Edition*. Washington, D.C.: American Psychiatric Publishing.

xxii   Ibid.

xxiii   Flynn, J.F. (1984). The Mean I.Q. of Americans: Massive Gains 1932 to 1978. *Psychological Bulletin, Vol. 95(1)*, 29–51. https://doi.org/10.1037/0033-2909.95.1.29.

xxiv   DeMatteo, D., M. Kessler, M. Murphy & H. Strohmaier (2015). "Capital Case Considerations." In B. Cutler and P. Zapf, Eds., *Handbook of Forensic Psychology*, Vol. I. Washington, D.C.: American Psychological Association.
American Association of Intellectual and Developmental Disabilities (AAIDD). (2010).
McGrew, K. (2015). "Norm Obsolescence: The Flynn Effect," pages 155–169. In E. Polloway, Ed., *The Death Penalty and Intellectual Disability*. Washington, D.C.: AAIDD.
Cunningham, M.D. and M. Tasse (2010). Looking to Science Rather than Convention in Adjusting I.Q. Scores When Death Is at Issue. *Professional Psychology, Research and Practice, Vol. 41*, 413–419. doi:10.137/a0020226.

xxv   Flynn, J.F. (1987). Massive I.Q. Gains in 14 Nations: What I.Q. Tests Really Measure. *Psychological Bulletin, Vol. 101(3)*, 427. https://doi.org/10.1037/h0090408.
Trahan, L.H., K.K. Stubing, J.M.Fletcher and M. Hiscock (2014). The Flynn Effect: A Meta-analysis. *Psychological Bulletin, Vol. 140(5)*, 1332–1360. https://doi.org/10.1037/a0037173.
Pietschnig, J. and M. Vorachek (2015). One Century of Global I.Q. Gains: A Formal Meta-Analysis of the Flynn Effect (1909-2013). *Perspectives on Psychological Science, Vol. 10(3)*, 282–306. doi:10/1177/1745691615577701.

xxvi   Polloway, E.A. (2015).

xxvii   Melton et al. (2018)
Heilbrun, K., D. DeMatteo & N.E.S. Goldstein, Eds. (2016). *APA Handbook of Psychology and Juvenile Justice*. Washington, D.C.: American Psychological Association. https://doi.org/10.1037/14643-000.
Zapf, P.A. & R. Roesch (2009).
Grisso, T. (2013). *Forensic Evaluation of Juveniles: Second edition*. Sarasota, FL: Professional Resource Press.

xxviii Nagel, A.G., L.A.Guarnera and N.D. Reppucci (2016) "Adolescent Development, Mental Disorder and Decision Making in Delinquent Youth." In Heilbrun et al., *APA Handbook of Psychology and Juvenile Justice*.

xxix   Grisso, T. (2013)

xxx   Everington, C. & K.L. Salekin (2015). "Criteria for Competence to Stand Trial." In E.A. Polloway, *Intellectual Disability and the Death Penalty*, p. 253.

xxxi   Zapf, P.A. and R. Roesch (2009).

xxxii   Everington, C. & K.L. Salekin (2015).

xxxiii *Roper versus Simmons*, 543 U.S. 551 (2005).

xxxiv   Galvan, Adriana (2017). *The Neuroscience of Adolescence*. New York, NY: Cambridge University Press.
Steinberg, L. (2017). Adolescent brain science and juvenile justice policymaking. *Psychology, Public Policy & Law, Vol. 23 (1)*, 410–420.
Grisso, T. and A. Kavanaugh (2016). Prospects for Developmental Evidence in Juvenile Sentencing Based on *Miller v. Alabama*. *Psychology, Public Policy and Law, Vol. 22 (3)*, 235–249.

xxxv   Luna, B. and C. Wright in Heilbrun et al. (2016), p. 94.

xxxvi   *Graham v. Florida (2010), Miller v. Alabama (2012)*.

xxxvii Brief for the American Psychological Association, American Psychiatric Association, and National Association of Social Workers as *Amici Curiae* in Support of Petitioners, *Miller v. Alabama* and *Jackson v. Hobbs*, 132 S. Ct. 2455 (2012), Nos. 10-9646, 10-9647; and *Graham v. Florida* and *Sullivan v. Florida*, 130 S. Ct. 2011 (2010), Nos. 08-7412, 08-7621.

xxxviii Heilbrun et al. (2016).

xxxix   Rutter, 2010 in Nagel et al., in Heilbrun et al. (2016).

xl   Rutter, 2010 in Nagel et al., in Heilbrun et al. (2016).

xli   Cicchetti, 1984 in Nagel et al. in Heilbrun et al. (2016).

xlii   Rutter, 2013 in Nagel et al., in Heilbrun et al. (2016).

xliii   Nagel et al. in Heilbrun et al. (2016).

xliv   Ibid.

xlv   Ibid, p. 121.

16 The Role of Advocates for Children in Dependency Court

Sally Wilson Erny

Introduction

Essay Excerpts from Akerman Academic Excellence Scholarship Winner – The Importance of a CASA/GAL Volunteer

Growing up I lived with my Great Grandparents until I was thirteen and I lost them both within 6 months of one another due to strokes. This happened when I was at the end of middle school. My mother struggled with a drug and alcohol problem and my father was in and out of prison and this is how I ended up in foster care. Being in foster care I changed group homes and foster homes a few times. When I was a sophomore, I lost my mom to drug addiction and found out my dad was being sent to prison for life without parole. Towards the end of high school my two older sisters got into trouble and both are serving state sentences. With everything that happened I always knew I wanted to go to college and I'm thankful to be here and receiving a college education.

I would say my biggest obstacle was grieving. Not only did I grieve the loss of my mother and Great Grandparents as well, but I had to move out of the house I knew as home for thirteen years. While all of this was going on, I had to grieve and I did so while moving homes and changing schools and friends. Consistency was the second. It was hard to build relationships because my counselors and caseworkers kept changing. There came a point where I got tired of telling my story, so I gave up on counseling. *That is where having a CASA is beneficial to me. I couldn't imagine my life without her. She is one of the biggest reasons on why I am in college today. Her impact on me motivates me to impact youth as she did.* Everything I encountered growing up has made me grow as a person and opened my eyes to so many things. I believe that regardless of what everyone goes through you gain a new perspective on things and become grateful for many things.

Idelia Robinson-Confer
2020 Akerman Academic Excellence Scholarship Winner
Sophomore, California University of Pennsylvania

National CASA/GAL Association for Children – The Origins of the Movement

Idelia's heartfelt story is one that is very familiar to court-appointed special advocate (CASA)/guardian ad litem (GAL) volunteers as a reflection of the long-lasting impact they have on a child's life. The positive impact that the CASA volunteer had on Idelia's life, is exactly the result the founder of the movement anticipated.

The inspiration for the CASA/GAL network came to Seattle juvenile court judge, David W. Soukup, in 1976 when he conceived the idea of using carefully screened and

DOI: 10.4324/9780429397806-17

trained community volunteers to speak for the best interests of children in court. He was concerned about making decisions relating to the lives of children who experienced abuse or neglect without enough information, after realizing he had insufficient information to make a life-changing decision for a 3-year-old who had suffered from abuse and was appearing before him in court.

In January 1977 the King County, Washington GAL Program was established and similar programs began developing around the country.

At a 1978 meeting of the Concern for Children in Placement Project (CIP) of the National Council of Juvenile and Family Court Judges (NCJFCJ), Committee Member Judge John F. Mendoza, Clark County District Court, Nevada, suggested the term court-appointed special advocate (CASA) to designate the lay court-appointed volunteers.

Judge Soukup recognized that the children, who had experienced abuse or neglect, needed trained volunteers speaking up in the courtroom for their best interests. Because of his awareness at that moment, more than 2.5 million[1] children have been served by a CASA/GAL volunteer during the past 40 years, with over 275,000[2] children served in the most recent year. Judge Soukup's visionary leadership created a single program based in Washington State that has grown to a national movement with nearly 1,000 member programs that span 49 states and the District of Columbia.

Over the decades, NCJFCJ's network of judges, along with other judges nationwide and National CASA/GAL and the national network of CASA/GAL programs, have collaborated to expand the programs to serve more children and families in need. As with the first program started in 1977 and with the nearly 1,000 programs started since, judges have always been essential to the success of CASA/GAL programs. Not only can there be no program without judicial support, a program cannot achieve the full benefit for the children served without strong judicial support. CASA and volunteer GAL programs have benefited tremendously from the support of countless judicial leaders across the country who have replicated the model conceived by Judge Soukup. The biggest winners have been the children.

On any given day, there are more than 440,000[3] children who are in foster care, and spend more than a year there. Together with state and local member programs, National CASA/GAL supports and promotes court-appointed volunteer advocacy so every child who has experienced abuse or neglect can be safe, have a permanent home, and the opportunity to thrive.

At the heart of the organization's work are CASA/GAL volunteers who are appointed by judges to advocate for children's best interests. They continue their advocacy for each child until the case is closed and the child is in a safe, permanent home. Volunteers work with legal and child welfare professionals, educators and other service providers to ensure that judges have all the information they need to make the most well-informed decisions for each child.

CASA/GAL volunteers form a one-on-one relationship with a child and get a full picture of the situation. With the information the volunteer collects, they report it to the judge. Judges depend on CASA/GAL volunteers for critical information to help them make the most well-informed decisions.

The CASA/GAL Model – Best-interest Advocacy

> CASA volunteers play a unique role on behalf of some of our most vulnerable children. Their commitment, vigilance and persistence offer hope where there has been little.
>
> – Marian Wright Edelman, Founder of the
> Children's Defense Fund

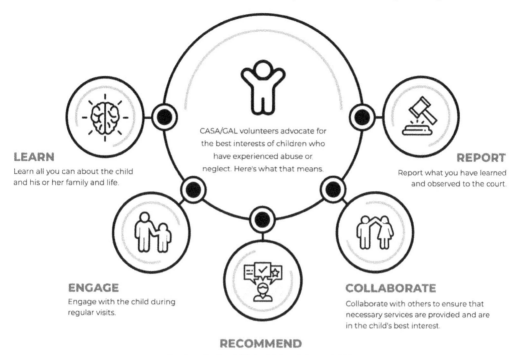

Figure 16.1 A diagram explaining how CASA/GAL volunteers advocate for the best interests of children who have experiences abuse or neglect. 5 bubbles come off the main diagram to highlight the five different methods volunteers use. In order they are Learn, Engage, Recommend, Collaborate, Report. Descriptions of what each of the below mean for CASA/GAL volunteers are below.

Best-interest advocacy is driven by the guiding principle that children grow and develop best with their family of origin, if that can be safely achieved. While most of the children CASA/GAL volunteers work with are in foster care, some are with their family of origin and, most children who leave foster care do so to return to their family.

The best-interest advocacy model comprises five components for volunteers to follow which include learn, engage, recommend, collaborate, and report in their work on behalf of the child, as illustrated in Figure 16.1.

- **Learn:** Learn all they can about the child, his or her family, and life.
- **Engage:** Engage with the child during regular visits.
- **Recommend:** Speak up for the child's best interest in court. Make recommendations regarding the child's placement and needed services, and monitor the child's situation until the case is released by the court.
- **Collaborate:** Collaborate with others to ensure that necessary services are provided and are in the child's best interest.
- **Report:** Report what they have learned and observed to the court.

Who are CASA/GAL Volunteers?

CASA/GAL volunteers, numbering nearly 100,000 in the most recent year, are ordinary people who come from all walks of life with a common interest in supporting and seeing children in need thrive. Volunteers are thoroughly screened and trained and receive ongoing support to help them advocate effectively on a child's behalf.

CASA/GAL volunteers, who donate over 5 million[4] hours of their time annually, receive extensive training through their local program. Each volunteer receives more than 30 hours of training before they begin working with a child, complemented by an additional 12 hours of continued education that is required annually.

CASA/GAL volunteers are assigned to only one or two children or sibling groups at a time so they have the necessary time to dedicate and stay involved from the time of appointment until the child achieves permanency. In addition, CASA/GAL volunteers are specially trained to consider issues relevant to the best interests of the child, which may be different than the interests of other parties.

Often, children in foster care have experienced abuse or neglect and other forms of trauma that can impact physical and mental health, academic achievement, and other vital elements of development. The support of a CASA/GAL volunteer can help children build resilience to counter those impacts. Abuse, neglect, and other trauma can mark a child for life but they need not define a life.

In 2017, 9 out of every 1,000[5] U.S. children were determined to be victims of abuse or neglect. Physical abuse and neglect are two of a number of highly stressful, potentially traumatic experiences known as "adverse childhood experiences," or ACEs. Children who have experienced abuse or neglect are far more likely than others to have experienced a large number of ACEs.

Research shows that having a stable relationship with a supportive adult can help children do well, even when they have faced significant hardships. CASA/GAL volunteers are trained to understand the impact of trauma on children and be a significant support.

They encourage services that strengthen parents' relationships with their children. Because they spend time with children and the people in their lives by talking to service providers, teachers, and social workers to gather information that will help them make informed recommendations to the court, volunteers also advocate for services that promote healing, that help children develop resilience.

Impact of CASA/GAL Volunteers on the Lives of Children

> It is our goal that every child in the dependency system has a trained CASA or GAL volunteer … We have seen first-hand that these volunteer advocates make a positive difference in children's lives.
>
> > 15 past presidents of the NCJFCJ expressing their view
> > of the importance of the role of CASA/GAL volunteers

The work of CASA/GAL volunteers is strongly supported by judges, seen as effective in its impact, and has evidence of long-lasting results.

CASA/GAL volunteers are highly effective in getting their recommendations accepted in court. In four out of five cases, all or almost all CASA/GAL volunteer recommendations are accepted. Children with a CASA/GAL volunteer, and their families, receive more services.

Judges support the work of CASA/GAL volunteers and see the benefit to having a volunteer on a case. A recent study by Chapin Hall at the University of Chicago, surveyed judges' perspective of the value of CASA/GAL advocacy. The study showed that 93%[6] of judges report positive to very positive overall experience with the CASA/GAL program, and 78%[7] of them say they would appoint more volunteers to cases if there were more of them available in their jurisdiction.

In addition, judges report the impact of CASA/GAL volunteers is most pronounced in promoting children's long-term well-being (92%),[8] encouraging appropriate services for children and families (83%), and promoting children's psychological well-being (80%).[9]

A child with a CASA/GAL volunteer is more likely to have better outcomes: children tended to perform better academically and behaviorally in school as measured by whether or not they passed all of their courses, whether or not they were expelled, and their conduct performance.

While CASA/GAL volunteers are typically assigned to the most complex cases, the outcomes for children with CASA/GAL volunteers are seen as effective. Children with a CASA/GAL volunteer are more likely to achieve permanency, and are as likely to be reunified with their birth parent as a child without a CASA/GAL volunteer. In addition, they are less likely to reenter the child welfare system, and those that do are consistently reduced by half.

A Call to Action

National CASA/GAL has grown to lead a significant national movement and offers training and technical assistance to state and local affiliates. The organization has standards to which state organizations and local programs adhere, engages in national public policy efforts, promotes volunteer advocacy through public awareness efforts, offers consultation and resources to help develop CASA/GAL programs and provides vital assistance to build the capacity of established programs.

National CASA/GAL Association is proud that, through its member programs, it serves over 300,000 children a year but there are thousands more who need our help. The organization's vision is to provide a CASA/GAL volunteer for every child that needs one. In order to accomplish this, the organization needs more volunteers.

You can learn more about volunteering or ways to contribute by visiting the organization's website: nationalcasagal.org.

Notes

1. National CASA/GAL Association For Children Internal Data.
2. National CASA/GAL Association For Children Internal Data.
3. Numbers and Trends May 2020, Foster Care Statistics 2018, Childwelfare.gov. https://www.childwelfare.gov/pubPDFs/foster.pdf.
4. National CASA/GAL Association for Children Annual Survey of Local Programs 2019.
5. Health and Human Services Administration for Children and Families, Administration on Children, Youth and Families Children's Bureau, 2002–2019, Child Maltreatment 2000–2017.
6. National CASA/GAL Association for Children's Judges Perspective Study, Chapin Hall, University of Chicago 2019.
7. National CASA/GAL Association for Children's Judges Perspective Study, Chapin Hall, University of Chicago 2019.
8. National CASA/GAL Association for Children's Judges Perspective Study, Chapin Hall, University of Chicago 2019.
9. National CASA/GAL Association for Children's Judges Perspective Study, Chapin Hall, University of Chicago 2019.

Appendix A

Specialty Guidelines for Forensic Psychology

Adopted by APA Council of Representatives, August 3, 2011 (Unofficial version-official version is in press, *American Psychologist*)

INTRODUCTION

In the past 50 years forensic psychological practice had expanded dramatically. The American Psychological Association has a division devoted to matters of law and psychology (APA Division 41, the American Psychology-Law Society), a number of scientific journals devoted to interactions between psychology and the law exist (e.g., *Law and Human Behavior, Psychology, Public Policy and Law, Behavioral Sciences and the Law*), and a number of key texts have been published and undergone multiple revisions (e.g., Grisso, 1986, 2003; Melton, Petrila, Poythress, & Slobogin, 1987, 1997; Melton, Petrila, Poythress, Slobogin, Lyons, & Otto, 2007; Rogers, 1988, 1997, 2008). In addition, training in forensic psychology is available in pre-doctoral, internship and post-doctoral settings, and the American Psychological Association recognized forensic psychology as a specialty in 2001, with subsequent re-certification in 2008.

Because the practice of forensic psychology differs in important ways from more traditional practice areas (Monahan, 1980) the Specialty Guidelines for Forensic Psychologists were developed and published in 1991 (Committee on Specialty Guidelines for Forensic Psychologists, 1991). Because

of continued developments in the field in the ensuing 20 years, forensic practitioners' ongoing need for guidance, and policy requirements of the American Psychological Association, the 1991 Specialty Guidelines for Forensic Psychologists were revised, with the intent of benefitting forensic practitioners and recipients of their services alike.

The goals of these *Guidelines* are to improve the quality of forensic psychological services; enhance the practice and facilitate the systematic development of forensic psychology; encourage a high level of quality in professional practice; and encourage forensic practitioners to acknowledge and respect the rights of those they serve. These *Guidelines* are intended for use by psychologists when engaged in the practice of forensic psychology as described below, and may also provide guidance on professional conduct to the legal system, and other organizations and professions.

For the purposes of these *Guidelines*, forensic psychology refers to professional practice by any psychologist working within any sub-discipline of psychology (e.g., clinical, developmental, social, cognitive) when applying the scientific, technical, or specialized knowledge of psychology to the law to assist in addressing legal, contractual, and administrative matters. Application of the *Guidelines* does not depend on the practitioner's typical areas of practice or expertise, but rather on the service provided in the case at hand. These *Guidelines* apply in all matters in which psychologists provide expertise to judicial, administrative, and educational systems including, but not limited to, examining or treating persons in anticipation of or subsequent to legal, contractual, administrative, proceedings; offering expert opinion about psychological issues in the form of *amicus* briefs or testimony to judicial, legislative or administrative bodies; acting in an adjudicative capacity; serving as a trial consultant or otherwise offering expertise to attorneys, the courts, or others; conducting research in connection with, or in the anticipation of, litigation; or involvement in educational activities of a forensic nature.

Psychological practice is not considered forensic solely because the conduct takes place in, or the product is presented in, a tribunal or other judicial, legislative, or administrative forum. For example, when a party (such as a civilly or criminally detained individual) or another individual (such as a child whose parents are involved in divorce proceedings) is ordered into treatment with a practitioner, that treatment is not necessarily the practice of forensic psychology. In addition, psychological testimony that is solely based on the provision of psychotherapy and does not include psycholegal opinions is not ordinarily considered forensic practice.

For the purposes of these *Guidelines*, "forensic practitioner" refers to a psychologist when engaged in the practice of forensic psychology as described above. Such professional conduct is considered forensic from the time the practitioner reasonably expects to, agrees to, or is legally mandated to, provide expertise on an explicitly psycholegal issue.

The provision of forensic services may include a wide variety of psycholegal roles and functions. For example, as researchers, forensic practitioners may participate in the collection and dissemination of data that are relevant to various legal issues. As advisors, forensic practitioners may provide an attorney with an informed understanding of the role that psychology can play in the case at hand. As consultants, forensic practitioners may explain the practical implications of relevant research, examination findings, and the opinions of other psycholegal experts. As examiners, forensic practitioners may assess an individual's functioning and report findings and opinions to the attorney, a legal tribunal, an employer, an insurer, or others (American

Psychological Association, 2010; American Psychological Association, 2011a). As treatment providers, forensic practitioners may provide therapeutic services tailored to the issues and context of a legal proceeding. As mediators or negotiators, forensic practitioners may serve in a third-party neutral role and assist parties in resolving disputes. As arbiters, special masters, or case managers with decision-making authority, forensic practitioners may serve parties, attorneys, and the courts (American Psychological Association, 2011b).

These guidelines are informed by the American Psychological Association's (APA's) Ethical Principles of Psychologists and Code of Conduct (hereinafter referred to as the EPPCC; APA, 2002). The term guidelines refers to statements that suggest or recommend specific professional behavior, endeavors, or conduct for psychologists. Guidelines differ from standards in that standards are mandatory and may be accompanied by an enforcement mechanism. Guidelines are aspirational in intent. They are intended to facilitate the continued systematic development of the profession and facilitate a high level of practice by psychologists. Guidelines are not intended to be mandatory or exhaustive and may not be applicable to every professional situation. They are not definitive, and they are not intended to take precedence over the judgment of psychologists.

As such, the *Guidelines* are advisory in areas in which the forensic practitioner has discretion to exercise professional judgment that is not prohibited or mandated by the EPPCC or applicable law, rules, or regulations. The *Guidelines* neither add obligations to nor eliminate obligations from the EPPCC, but provide additional guidance for psychologists. The modifiers used in the *Guidelines* (e.g., reasonably, appropriate, potentially) are included in recognition of the need for professional judgment on the part of forensic practitioners; ensure applicability across the broad range of activities conducted by forensic practitioners; and reduce the likelihood of enacting an inflexible set of guidelines that might be inapplicable as forensic practice evolves. The use of these modifiers, and the recognition of the role of professional discretion and judgment, also reflects that forensic practitioners are likely to encounter facts and circumstances not anticipated by the *Guidelines* and they may have to act upon uncertain or incomplete evidence. The *Guidelines* may provide general or conceptual guidance in such circumstances. The *Guidelines* do not, however, exhaust the legal, professional, moral and ethical considerations that inform forensic practitioners, for no complex activity can be completely defined by legal rules, codes of conduct, and aspirational guidelines.

The *Guidelines* are not intended to serve as a basis for disciplinary action or civil or criminal liability. The standard of care is established by a competent authority not by the *Guidelines*. No ethical, licensure, or other administrative action or remedy, nor any other cause of action, should be taken *solely* on the basis of a forensic practitioner acting in a manner consistent or inconsistent with these *Guidelines*.

In cases in which a competent authority references the *Guidelines* when formulating standards, the authority should consider that the *Guidelines* attempt to identify a high level of quality in forensic practice. Competent practice is defined as the conduct of a reasonably prudent forensic practitioner engaged in similar activities in similar circumstances. Professional conduct evolves and may be viewed along a continuum of adequacy, and 3 "minimally competent" and "best possible" are usually different points along that continuum.

The *Guidelines* are designed to be national in scope and are intended to be consistent with state and federal law. In cases in which a conflict between legal and professional obligations occur, forensic practitioners make known their commitment to the EPPCC and the *Guidelines* and take steps to achieve an appropriate resolution consistent with the EPPCC and *Guidelines*.

The format of the *Guidelines* is different from most other practice guidelines developed under the auspices of APA. This reflects the history of the *Guidelines* as well as the fact that the Guidelines are considerably broader in scope than any other APA-developed guidelines. Indeed, these are the only APA-approved guidelines that address a complete specialty practice area. Despite this difference in format, the *Guidelines* function as all other APA guideline documents.

This document replaces the 1991 *Specialty Guidelines for Forensic Psychologists* which were approved by the American Psychology-Law Society, Division 41 of the American Psychological Association and the American Board of Forensic Psychology. The current revision has also been approved by the Council of Representatives of the American Psychological Association. Appendix I includes a discussion of the revision process, enactment, and current status of these *Guidelines*. Appendix II includes definitions and terminology as used for the purposes of these *Guidelines*.

1. RESPONSIBILITIES

1.01 Integrity

Forensic practitioners strive for accuracy, honesty, and truthfulness in the science, teaching, and practice of forensic psychology and they strive to resist partisan pressures to provide services in any ways that might tend to be misleading or inaccurate.

1.02 Impartiality and Fairness

When offering expert opinion to be relied upon by a decision maker, providing forensic therapeutic services, or teaching or conducting research, forensic practitioners strive for accuracy, impartiality, fairness, and independence (EPPCC Standard 2.01).

Forensic practitioners recognize the adversarial nature of the legal system and strive to treat all participants and weigh all data, opinions, and rival hypotheses impartially.

When conducting forensic examinations, forensic practitioners strive to be unbiased and impartial, and avoid partisan presentation of unrepresentative, incomplete, or inaccurate evidence that might mislead finders of fact. This guideline does not preclude forceful presentation of the data and reasoning upon which a conclusion or professional product is based.

When providing educational services, forensic practitioners seek to represent alternative perspectives, including data, studies, or evidence on both sides of the question, in an accurate, fair and professional manner, and strive to weigh and present all views, facts, or opinions impartially.

When conducting research, forensic practitioners seek to represent results in a fair and impartial manner. Forensic practitioners strive to utilize research designs and scientific methods that adequately and fairly test the questions at hand, and they attempt to resist partisan pressures to develop designs or report results in ways that might be misleading or unfairly bias the results of a test, study, or evaluation.

1.03 Avoiding Conflicts of Interest

Forensic practitioners refrain from taking on a professional role when personal, scientific, professional, legal, financial, or other interests or relationships could reasonably be expected to impair their impartiality, competence, or effectiveness, or expose others with whom a professional relationship exists to harm (EPPCC Standard 3.06).

Forensic practitioners are encouraged to identify, make known, and address real or apparent conflicts of interest in an attempt to maintain the public confidence and trust, discharge professional obligations, and maintain responsibility, impartiality, and accountability (EPPCC Standard 3.06). Whenever possible, such conflicts are revealed to all parties as soon as they become known to the psychologist. Forensic practitioners consider whether a prudent and competent forensic practitioner engaged in similar circumstances would determine that the ability to make a proper decision is likely to become impaired under the immediate circumstances.

When a conflict of interest is determined to be manageable, continuing services are provided and documented in a way to manage the conflict, maintain accountability, and preserve the trust of relevant others (also see Section 4.02 below).

2. COMPETENCE

2.01 Scope of Competence

When determining one's competence to provide services in a particular matter, forensic practitioners may consider a variety of factors including the relative complexity and specialized nature of the service, relevant training and experience, the preparation and study they are able to devote to the matter, and the opportunity for consultation with a professional of established competence in the subject matter in question. Even with regard to subjects in which they are expert, forensic practitioners may choose to consult with colleagues.

2.02 Gaining and Maintaining Competence

Competence can be acquired through various combinations of education, training, supervised experience, consultation, study, and professional experience. Forensic practitioners planning to provide services, teach, or conduct research involving populations, areas, techniques, or technologies that are new to them are encouraged to undertake relevant education, training, supervised experience, consultation, or study.

Forensic practitioners make ongoing efforts to develop and maintain their competencies

(EPPCC Section 2.03). To maintain the requisite knowledge and skill, forensic practitioners keep abreast of developments in the fields of psychology and the law.

2.03 Representing Competencies

Consistent with the EPPCC, forensic practitioners adequately and accurately inform all recipients of their services (e.g., attorneys, tribunals) about relevant aspects of the nature and extent of their experience, training, credentials, and qualifications, and how they were obtained (EPPCC Standard 5.01)

2.04 Knowledge of the Legal System and the Legal Rights of Individuals

Forensic practitioners recognize the importance of obtaining a fundamental and reasonable level of knowledge and understanding of the legal and professional standards, laws, rules, and precedents that govern their participation in legal proceedings and that guide the impact of their services on service recipients (EPPCC Standard 2.01).

Forensic practitioners aspire to manage their professional conduct in a manner that does not threaten or impair the rights of affected individuals. They may consult with, and refer others to, legal counsel on matters of law. Although they do not provide formal legal advice or opinions, forensic practitioners may provide information about the legal process to others based on their knowledge and experience. They strive to distinguish this from legal opinions, however, and encourage consultation with attorneys as appropriate.

2.05 Knowledge of the Scientific Foundation for Opinions and Testimony

Forensic practitioners seek to provide opinions and testimony that are sufficiently based upon adequate scientific foundation,

and reliable and valid principles and methods that have been applied appropriately to the facts of the case. 5

When providing opinions and testimony that are based on novel or emerging principles and methods, forensic practitioners seek to make known the status and limitations of these principles and methods.

2.06 Knowledge of the Scientific Foundation for Teaching and Research

Forensic practitioners engage in teaching and research activities in which they have adequate knowledge, experience, and education (EPPCC Standard 2.01), and they acknowledge relevant limitations and caveats inherent in procedures and conclusions (EPPCC Standard 5.01).

2.07 Considering the Impact of Personal Beliefs and Experience

Forensic practitioners recognize that their own cultures, attitudes, values, beliefs, opinions, or biases may affect their ability to practice in a competent and impartial manner. When such factors may diminish their ability to practice in a competent and impartial manner, forensic practitioners may take steps to correct or limit such effects, decline participation in the matter, or limit their participation in a manner that is consistent with professional obligations.

2.08 Appreciation of Individual and Group Differences

When scientific or professional knowledge in the discipline of psychology establishes that an understanding of factors associated with age, gender, gender identity, race, ethnicity, culture, national origin, religion, sexual orientation, disability, language, socioeconomic status, or other relevant individual and cultural differences affects implementation or use of their services or research, forensic practitioners consider the boundaries of their expertise, make an appropriate referral if indicated, or gain the necessary training, experience, consultation, or supervision (EPPCC Standard 2.01, American Psychological Association, 2003; American Psychological Association, 2004; American Psychological Association, 2011c; American Psychological Association, in press; American Psychological Association Task Force on Guidelines for Assessment and Treatment of Persons with Disabilities, 2011).

Forensic practitioners strive to understand how factors associated with age, gender, gender identity, race, ethnicity, culture, national origin, religion, sexual orientation, disability, language, socioeconomic status, or other relevant individual and cultural differences may affect and be related to the basis for people's contact and involvement with the legal system.

Forensic practitioners do not engage in unfair discrimination based on such factors or on any basis proscribed by law (EPPCC Standard 3.01). They strive to take steps to correct or limit the effects of such factors on their work, decline participation in the matter, or limit their participation in a manner that is consistent with professional obligations.

2.09 Appropriate Use of Services and Products

Forensic practitioners are encouraged to make reasonable efforts to guard against misuse of their services and exercise professional discretion in addressing such misuses.

3. DILIGENCE

3.01 Provision of Services

Forensic practitioners are encouraged to seek explicit agreements that define the scope of, time-frame of, and compensation for their services. In the event that a client breaches the contract or acts in a way that would require the practitioner to violate ethical, legal or professional obligations, the forensic practitioner may terminate the relationship.

Forensic practitioners strive to act with reasonable diligence and promptness in providing agreed-upon and reasonably anticipated services. Forensic practitioners are not bound, however, to provide services not reasonably anticipated when retained, nor to provide every possible aspect or variation of service. Instead, forensic practitioners may exercise professional discretion in determining the extent and means by which services are provided and agreements are fulfilled.

3.02 Responsiveness

Forensic practitioners seek to manage their workloads so that services can be provided thoroughly, competently, and promptly. They recognize that acting with reasonable promptness, however, does not require the forensic practitioner to acquiesce to service demands not reasonably anticipated at the time the service was requested, nor does it require the forensic practitioner to provide services if the client has not acted in a manner consistent with existing agreements, including payment of fees.

3.03 Communication

Forensic practitioners strive to keep their clients reasonably informed about the status of their services, comply with their clients' reasonable requests for information, and consult with their clients about any substantial limitation on their conduct or performance that may arise when they reasonably believe that their clients expect a service that is not consistent with their professional obligations. Forensic practitioners attempt to keep their clients reasonably informed regarding new facts, opinions, or other potential evidence that may be relevant and applicable.

3.04 Termination of Services

The forensic practitioner seeks to carry through to conclusion all matters undertaken for a client unless the forensic practitioner-client relationship is terminated. When a forensic practitioner's employment is limited to a specific matter, the relationship may terminate when the matter has been resolved, anticipated services have been completed, or the agreement has been violated.

4. RELATIONSHIPS

Whether a forensic practitioner-client relationship exists depends on the circumstances and is determined by a number of factors which may include the information exchanged between the potential client and the forensic practitioner prior to, or at the initiation of, any contact or service, the nature of the interaction, and the purpose of the interaction.

In their work, forensic practitioners recognize that relationships are established with those who retain their services (e.g., retaining parties, employers, insurers, the court) and those with whom they interact (e.g., examinees, collateral contacts, research participants, students). Forensic practitioners recognize that associated obligations and duties vary as a function of the nature of the relationship.

4.01 Responsibilities to Retaining Parties

Most responsibilities to the retaining party attach only after the retaining party has requested and the forensic practitioner has agreed to render professional services and an agreement regarding compensation has been reached. Forensic practitioners are aware that there are some responsibilities, such as privacy, confidentiality, and privilege that may attach when the forensic practitioner agrees to consider whether a forensic practitioner-retaining party relationship shall be established. Forensic practitioners, prior to entering into a contract, may direct the potential retaining party not to reveal any confidential or privileged information as a way of protecting the retaining party's interest in case a conflict exists as a result of pre-existing relationships.

At the initiation of any request for service, forensic practitioners seek to clarify the nature of the relationship and the services to be provided including the role of the forensic practitioner (e.g., trial consultant, forensic examiner, treatment provider, expert witness, research consultant); which person or entity is the client; the probable uses of the services provided or information obtained; and any limitations to privacy, confidentiality, or privilege.

4.02 Multiple Relationships

A multiple relationship occurs when a forensic practitioner is in a professional role with a person and, at the same time or at a subsequent time, is in a different role with the same person; is involved in a personal, fiscal, or other relationship with an adverse party; at the same time is in a relationship with a person closely associated with or related to the person with whom the forensic practitioner has the professional relationship; or offers or agrees to enter into another relationship in the future with the person or a person closely associated with or related to the person (EPPCC Standard 3.05).

Forensic practitioners strive to recognize the potential conflicts of interest and threats to objectivity inherent in multiple relationships. Forensic practitioners are encouraged to recognize that some personal and professional relationships may interfere with their ability to practice in a competent and impartial manner and they seek to minimize any detrimental effects by avoiding involvement in such matters whenever feasible or limiting their assistance in a manner that is consistent with professional obligations.

4.02.01 Therapeutic-
Forensic Role Conflicts

Providing forensic and therapeutic psychological services to the same individual or closely related individuals involves multiple relationships that may impair objectivity and/or cause exploitation or other harm. Therefore, when requested or ordered to provide either concurrent or sequential forensic and therapeutic services, forensic practitioners are encouraged to disclose the potential risk and make reasonable efforts to refer the request to another qualified provider. If referral is not possible, the forensic practitioner is encouraged to consider the risks and benefits to all parties and to the legal system or entity likely to be impacted, the possibility of separating each service widely in time, seeking judicial review and direction, and consulting with knowledgeable colleagues. When providing both forensic and therapeutic services, forensic practitioners seek to minimize the potential negative effects of this circumstance (EPPCC Standard 3.05).

4.02.02 Expert Testimony
by Practitioners Providing
Therapeutic Services

Providing expert testimony about a patient who is a participant in a legal matter does not necessarily involve the practice of forensic psychology even when that testimony is relevant to a psycholegal issue before the decision-maker. For example, providing testimony on matters such as a patient's reported history or other statements, mental status, diagnosis, progress, prognosis, and treatment would not ordinarily be considered forensic practice even when the testimony is related to a psycholegal issue before the decision-maker. In contrast, rendering opinions and providing testimony about a person on psycholegal issues (e.g., criminal responsibility, legal causation, proximate cause,

trial competence, testamentary capacity, the relative merits of parenting arrangements) would ordinarily be considered the practice of forensic psychology.

Consistent with their ethical obligations to base their opinions on information and techniques sufficient to substantiate their findings (EPPCC Standards 2.04, 9.01), forensic practitioners are encouraged to provide testimony only on those issues for which they have adequate foundation and only when a reasonable forensic practitioner engaged in similar circumstances would determine that the ability to make a proper decision is unlikely to be impaired. As with testimony regarding forensic examinees, the forensic practitioner strives to identify any substantive limitations that may affect the reliability and validity of the facts or opinions offered, and communicates these to the decision maker.

4.02.03 Provision of Forensic
Therapeutic Services

Although some therapeutic services can be considered forensic in nature, the fact that therapeutic services are ordered by the court does not necessarily make them forensic.

In determining whether a therapeutic service should be considered the practice of forensic psychology, psychologists are encouraged to consider the potential impact of the legal context on treatment, the potential for treatment to impact the psycholegal issues involved in the case, and whether another reasonable psychologist in a similar position would consider the service to be forensic and these *Guidelines* to be applicable.

Therapeutic services can have significant effects on current or future legal proceedings. Forensic practitioners are encouraged to consider these effects and minimize any unintended or negative effects on such proceedings or therapy when they provide therapeutic services in forensic contexts.

4.03 Provision of Emergency Mental Health Services to Forensic Examinees

When providing forensic examination services an emergency may arise that requires the practitioner to provide short term therapeutic services to the examinee in order to prevent imminent harm to the examinee or others. In such cases, the forensic practitioner is encouraged to limit disclosure of information and inform the retaining attorney, legal representative, or the court in an appropriate manner. Upon providing emergency treatment to examinees, forensic practitioners consider whether they can continue in a forensic role with that individual so that potential for harm to the recipient of services is avoided (EPPCC 3.04).

5. FEES

5.01 Determining Fees

When determining fees forensic practitioners may consider salient factors such as their experience providing the service, the time and labor required, the novelty and difficulty of the questions involved, the skill required to perform the service, the fee customarily charged for similar forensic services, the likelihood that the acceptance of the particular employment will preclude other employment, the time limitations imposed by the client or circumstances, the nature and length of the professional relationship with the client, the client's ability to pay for the service, and any legal requirements.

5.02 Fee Arrangements

Forensic practitioners are encouraged to make clear to the client the likely cost of services whenever it is feasible, and make appropriate provisions in those cases in which the costs of services is greater than anticipated or the client's ability to pay for services changes in some way.

Forensic practitioners seek to avoid undue influence that might result from financial compensation or other gains. Because of the threat to impartiality presented by the acceptance of contingent fees and associated legal prohibitions, forensic practitioners strive to avoid providing professional services on the basis of contingent fees. Letters of protection, financial guarantees, and other security for payment of fees in the future are not considered contingent fees unless payment is dependent on the outcome of the matter.

5.03 Pro Bono Services

Forensic psychologists recognize that some persons may have limited access to legal services as a function of financial disadvantage and strive to contribute a portion of their professional time for little or no compensation or personal advantage (EPPCC Principle E).

6. INFORMED CONSENT, NOTIFICATION AND ASSENT

Because substantial rights, liberties, and properties are often at risk in forensic matters, and because the methods and procedures of forensic practitioners are complex and may not be accurately anticipated by the recipients of forensic services, forensic practitioners strive to inform service recipients about the nature and parameters of the services to be provided (EPPCC Standards 3.04, 3.10).

6.01 Timing and Substance

Forensic practitioners strive to inform clients, examinees, and others who are the recipients of forensic services as soon as is feasible about thenature and extent of reasonably anticipated forensic services.

In determining what information to impart, forensic practitioners are encouraged to consider a variety of factors including the person's experience or training in psychological and legal matters of the type involved and whether the person is represented by counsel. When questions or uncertainties remain after they have made the effort to explain the necessary information, forensic practitioners may recommend that the person seek legal advice.

6.02 Communication with Those Seeking to Retain a Forensic Practitioner

As part of the initial process of being retained, or as soon thereafter as previously unknown information becomes available, forensic practitioners strive to disclose to the retaining party information that would reasonably be anticipated to affect a decision to retain or continue the services of the forensic practitioner.

This disclosure may include, but is not limited to, the fee structure for anticipated services; prior and current personal or professional activities, obligations and relationships that would reasonably lead to the fact or the appearance of a conflict of interest; the forensic practitioner's knowledge, skill, experience, and education relevant to the forensic services being considered, including any significant limitations; and the scientific bases and limitations of the methods and procedures which are expected to be employed.

6.03 Communication with Forensic Examinees

Forensic practitioners inform examinees about the nature and purpose of the examination (EPPCC Standard 9.03; American Educational Research Association, American Psychological Association, & National Council on Measurement in Education, 1999). Such information may include the purpose, nature, and anticipated use of the examination; who will have access to the information; associated limitations on privacy, confidentiality, and privilege including who is authorized to release or access the information contained in the forensic practitioner's records; the voluntary or involuntary nature of participation, including potential consequences of participation or non-participation, if known; and, if the cost of the service is the responsibility of the examinee, the anticipated cost.

6.03.01 Persons Not Ordered or Mandated to Undergo Examination

If the examinee is not ordered by the court to participate in a forensic examination, the forensic practitioner seeks his or her informed consent (EPPCC Standards 3.10, 9.03). If the examinee declines to proceed after being notified of the nature and purpose of the forensic examination, the forensic practitioner may consider postponing the examination, advising the examinee to contact his or her attorney, and notifying the retaining party about the examinee's unwillingness to proceed.

6.03.02 Persons Ordered or Mandated to Undergo Examination or Treatment

If the examinee is ordered by the court to participate, the forensic practitioner can conduct the examination over the objection, and without the consent, of the examinee (EPPCC Standards 3.10, 9.03). If the examinee declines to proceed after being notified of the nature and purpose of the forensic examination, the forensic practitioner may consider a variety of options including postponing the examination, advising the examinee to contact his or her attorney, and notifying the retaining party about the examinee's unwillingness to proceed.

When an individual is ordered to undergo treatment but the goals of treatment are determined by a legal authority rather than the individual receiving services, the forensic practitioner informs the service recipient of the nature and purpose of treatment, and any limitations on confidentiality and privilege (EPPCC Standards 3.10, 10.01).

6.03.03 Persons Lacking Capacity to Provide Informed Consent

Forensic practitioners appreciate that the very conditions that precipitate psychological examination of individuals involved in legal proceedings can impair their functioning in a variety of important ways, including their ability to understand and consent to the evaluation process.

For examinees adjudicated or presumed by law to lack the capacity to provide informed consent for the anticipated forensic service, the forensic practitioner nevertheless provides an appropriate explanation, seeks the examinee's assent, and obtain appropriate permission from a legally authorized person, as permitted or required by law (EPPCC Standards 3.10, 9.03).

For examinees whom the forensic practitioner has concluded lack capacity to provide informed consent to a proposed, on-court-ordered service, but who have not been adjudicated as lacking such capacity, the forensic practitioner strives to take reasonable steps to protect their rights and welfare (EPPCC Standard 3.10). In such cases, the forensic practitioner may consider suspending the proposed service or notifying the examinee's attorney or the retaining party.

6.03.04 Evaluation of Persons Not Represented by Counsel

Because of the significant rights that may be at issue in a legal proceeding, forensic practitioners carefully consider the appropriateness of conducting a forensic evaluation of an individual who is not represented by counsel. Forensic practitioners may consider conducting such evaluations or delaying the evaluation so as to provide the examinee with the opportunity to consult with counsel.

6.04 Communication with Collateral Sources of Information

Forensic practitioners disclose to potential collateral sources information that might reasonably be expected to inform their decisions about participating that may include, but may not be limited to, who has retained the forensic practitioner; the nature, purpose, and intended use of the examination or other procedure; the nature of and any limits on privacy, confidentiality, and privilege; and whether their participation is voluntary (EPPCC Standard 3.10).

6.05 Communication in Research Contexts

When engaging in research or scholarly activities conducted as a service to a client in a legal proceeding, forensic practitioners attempt to clarify any anticipated use of the research or scholarly product, disclose their role in the resulting research or scholarly products, and obtain whatever consent or agreement is required.

In advance of any scientific study, forensic practitioners seek to negotiate with the client the circumstances under and manner in which the results may be made known to others. Forensic practitioners strive to balance the potentially competing rights and interests of the retaining party with the inappropriateness of suppressing data, for example, by agreeing to report the data without identifying the jurisdiction in which the study took place. Forensic practitioners represent the results of research in an accurate manner (EPPCC Standard 5.01).

7. CONFLICTS IN PRACTICE

In forensic psychology practice conflicting responsibilities and demands may be encountered. When conflicts occur, forensic practitioners seek to make the conflict known to the relevant parties or agencies, and consider the rights and interests of the relevant parties or agencies in their attempts to resolve the conflict.

7.01 Conflicts with Legal Authority

When their responsibilities conflict with law, regulations, or other governing legal authority, forensic practitioners make known their commitment to the EPPCC, and take steps to resolve the conflict. In situations in which the EPPCC or *Guidelines* are in conflict with the law, attempts to resolve the conflict are made in accordance with the EPPCC (EPPCC Standard 1.02).

When the conflict cannot be resolved by such means, forensic practitioners may adhere to the requirements of the law, regulations, or other governing legal authority, but only to the extent required and not in any way that violates a person's human rights (EPPCC Standard 1.03).

Forensic practitioners are encouraged to consider the appropriateness of complying with court orders when such compliance creates potential conflicts with professional standards of practice.

7.02 Conflicts with Organizational Demands

When the demands of an organization with which they are affiliated or for whom they are working conflict with their professional responsibilities and obligations, forensic practitioners strive to clarify the nature of the conflict and, to the extent feasible, resolve the conflict in a way consistent with professional obligations and responsibilities (EPPCC Standard 1.03).

7.03 Resolving Ethical Issues with Fellow Professionals

When an apparent or potential ethical violation has caused, or is likely to cause, substantial harm, forensic practitioners are encouraged to take action appropriate to the situation and consider a number of

factors including the nature and the immediacy of the potential harm; applicable privacy, confidentiality, and privilege; how the rights of the relevant parties may be affected by a particular course of action; and any other legal or ethical obligations (EPPCC Standard 1.04). Steps to resolve perceived ethical conflicts may include, but are not be limited to, obtaining the consultation of knowledgeable colleagues, obtaining the advice of independent counsel, and conferring directly with the client.

When forensic practitioners believe there may have been an ethical violation by another professional, an attempt is made to resolve the issue by bringing it to the attention of that individual, if that attempt does not violate any rights or privileges that may be involved, and if an informal resolution appears appropriate (EPPCC Standard 1.04). If this does not result in a satisfactory resolution, the forensic practitioner may have to take further action appropriate to the situation, including making a report to third parties of the perceived ethical violation (EPPCC Standard 1.05). In most instances, in order to minimize unforeseen risks to the party's rights in the legal matter, forensic practitioners consider consulting with the client before attempting to resolve a perceived ethical violation with another professional.

8. PRIVACY, CONFIDENTIALITY, AND PRIVILEGE

Forensic practitioners recognize their ethical obligations to maintain the confidentiality of information relating to a client or retaining party, except insofar as disclosure is consented to by the client or retaining party, or required or permitted by law (EPPCC Standard 4.01).

8.01 Release of Information

Forensic practitioners are encouraged to recognize the importance of complying with properly noticed and served subpoenas or court orders directing release of information, or other legally proper consent from duly authorized persons, unless there is a legally valid reason to offer an objection. When in doubt about an appropriate response or course of action, forensic practitioners may seek assistance from the retaining client, retain and seek legal advice from their own attorney, or formally notify the drafter of the subpoena or order of their uncertainty.

8.02 *Access to Information*

If requested, forensic practitioners seek to provide the retaining party access to, and a meaningful explanation of, all information that is in their records for the matter at hand, consistent with the relevant law, applicable codes of ethics and professional standards, and institutional rules and regulations. Forensic examinees typically are not provided access to the forensic practitioner's records without the consent of the retaining party. Access to records by anyone other than the retaining party is governed by legal process, usually subpoena or court order, or by explicit consent of the retaining party. Forensic practitioners may charge a reasonable fee for the costs associated with the storage, reproduction, review, and provision of records.

8.03 *Acquiring Collateral and Third Party Information*

Forensic practitioners strive to access information or records from collateral sources with the consent of the relevant attorney or the relevant party, or when otherwise authorized by law or court order.

8.04 *Use of Case Materials in Teaching, Continuing Education, and Other Scholarly Activities*

Forensic practitioners using case materials for purposes of teaching, training, or research strive to present such information in a fair, balanced, and respectful manner. They attempt to protect the privacy of persons by disguising the confidential, personally identifiable information of all persons and entities who would reasonably claim a privacy interest; using only those aspects of the case available in the public domain; or obtaining consent from the relevant clients, parties, participants, and organizations to use the materials for such purposes (EPPCC Standard 4.07; also see Sections 11.06 and 11.07 of these guidelines).

9. METHODS AND PROCEDURES

9.01 *Use of Appropriate Methods*

Forensic practitioners strive to utilize appropriate methods and procedures in their work. When performing examinations, treatment, consultation, educational activities or scholarly investigations, forensic practitioners seek to maintain integrity by examining the issue or problem at hand from all reasonable perspectives and seek information that will differentially test plausible rival hypotheses.

9.02 *Use of Multiple Sources of Information*

Forensic practitioners ordinarily avoid relying solely on one source of data, and corroborate important data whenever feasible (American Educational Research Association, American Psychological Association, & National Council on Measurement in Education, in press). When relying upon data that have not been corroborated, forensic practitioners seek to make known the uncorroborated status of the data, any associated strengths and limitations, and the reasons for relying upon the data.

9.03 *Opinions Regarding Persons Not Examined*

Forensic practitioners recognize their obligations to only provide written or oral evidence about the psychological characteristics of particular individuals when they have sufficient information or data to form an adequate foundation for those opinions or to substantiate their findings (EPPCC Standard 9.01). Forensic practitioners seek to make reasonable efforts to obtain such information or data, and they document their efforts to obtain it. When it is not possible or feasible to examine individuals about whom they are offering an opinion, forensic practitioners strive to make clear the impact of such limitations on the reliability and validity of their professional products, opinions, or testimony.

When conducting a record review or providing consultation or supervision that does not warrant an individual examination, forensic practitioners seek to identify the sources of information on which they are basing their opinions and recommendations, including any substantial limitations to their opinions and recommendations.

10. ASSESSMENT

10.01 Focus on Legally Relevant Factors

Forensic examiners seek to assist the trier of fact to understand evidence or determine a fact in issue, and they provide information that is most relevant to the psycholegal issue. In reports and testimony forensic practitioners typically provide information about examinees' functional abilities, capacities, knowledge, and beliefs, and address their opinions and recommendations to the identified psycholegal issues (American Bar Association and American Psychological Assocation, 2008; Grisso, 1986, 2003; Heilbrun, Marczyk, DeMatteo, & Mack-Allen, 2007).

Forensic practitioners are encouraged to consider the problems that may arise by using a clinical diagnosis in some forensic contexts, and consider and qualify their opinions and testimony appropriately.

10.02 Selection and Use of Assessment Procedures

Forensic practitioners use assessment procedures in the manner and for the purposes that are appropriate in light of the research on or evidence of their usefulness and proper application (EPPCC Standard 9.02, American Educational Research Association, American Psychological Association, & National Council on Measurement in Education, in press9). This includes assessment techniques, interviews, tests, instruments, and other procedures and their administration, adaptation, scoring, and interpretation, including computerized scoring and interpretation systems.

Forensic practitioners use assessment instruments whose validity and reliability have been established for use with members of the population assessed. When such validity and reliability have not been established, forensic practitioners consider and describe the strengths and limitations of their findings. Forensic practitioners use assessment methods that are appropriate to an examinee's language preference and competence, unless the use of an alternative language is relevant to the assessment issues (EPPCC Standard 9.02).

Assessment in forensic contexts differs from assessment in therapeutic contexts in important ways that forensic practitioners strive to take into account when conducting forensic examinations. Forensic practitioners seek to consider the strengths and limitations of employing traditional assessment procedures in forensic examinations (American Educational Research Association, American Psychological Association, & National Council on Measurement in Education, in press). Given the stakes involved in forensic contexts, forensic practitioners strive to ensure the integrity and security of test materials and results (American Educational Research Association, American Psychological Association, & National Council on Measurement in Education, in press9).

When the validity of an assessment technique has not been established in the forensic context or setting in which it is being used, the forensic practitioner seeks to describe the strengths and limitations of any test results and explain the extrapolation of these data to the forensic context Because of the many differences between forensic and therapeutic contexts, forensic practitioners consider and seek to make known that some examination results may warrant substantially different interpretation when administered in forensic contexts (American Educational Research Association, American Psychological Association, & National Council on Measurement in Education, in press).

Forensic practitioners consider and seek to make known that forensic examination results can be affected by factors unique to, or differentially present in, forensic contexts including response style, voluntariness of participation, and situational stress associated with involvement in forensic or legal matters (American Educational Research Association, American Psychological Association, & National Council on Measurement in Education, in press).

10.03 Appreciation of Individual Differences

When interpreting assessment results forensic practitioners consider the purpose of the assessment as well as the various test factors, test-taking abilities, and other characteristics of the person being assessed, such as situational, personal, linguistic, and cultural differences that might affect their judgments or reduce the accuracy of their interpretations (EPPCC Standard 9.06). Forensic practitioners strive to identify any significant strengths and limitations of their procedures and interpretations.

Forensic practitioners are encouraged to consider how the assessment process may be impacted by any disability an examinee is experiencing, make accommodations as possible, and consider such when interpreting and communicating the results of the assessment (American Psychological Association Task Force on Guidelines for Assessment and treatment of Persons with Disabilities, 2011).

10.04 Consideration of Assessment Settings

In order to maximize the validity of assessment results, forensic practitioners strive to conduct evaluations in settings that provide adequate comfort, safety and privacy.

10.05 Provision of Assessment Feedback

Forensic practitioners take reasonable steps to explain assessment results to the examinee or a designated representative in language they can understand (EPPCC Standard 9.10). In those circumstances in which communication about assessment results is precluded, the forensic practitioner explains this to the examinee in advance (EPPCC Standard 9.10).

Forensic practitioners seek to provide information about professional work in a manner consistent with professional and legal standards for the disclosure of test data or results, interpretation of data, and the factual bases for conclusions.

10.06 Documentation and Compilation of Data Considered

Forensic practitioners are encouraged to recognize the importance of documenting all data they consider with enough detail and quality to allow for reasonable judicial scrutiny and adequate discovery by all parties. This documentation includes, but is not limited to, letters and consultations; notes, recordings, and transcriptions; assessment and test data, scoring reports and interpretations; and all other records in any form or medium that were created or exchanged in connection with a matter.

When contemplating third party observation or audio/video-recording of examinations forensic practitioners strive to consider any law that may control such matters, the need for transparency and documentation, and the potential impact of observation or recording on the validity of the examination and test security (American Psychological Association Committee on Psychological Tests and Assessment, 2007).

10.07 Provision of Documentation

Pursuant to proper subpoenas or court orders, or other legally proper consent from authorized persons, forensic practitioners seek to make available all documentation described in 10.05, all financial records related to the matter, and any other records including reports (and draft reports if they have been provided to a party, attorney, or other entity for review), that might reasonably be related to the opinions to be expressed.

10.08 Recordkeeping

Forensic practitioners establish and maintain a system of recordkeeping and professional communication (EPPCC Standard 6.01; American Psychological Association, 2007), and attend to relevant laws and rules. When indicated by the extent of the rights, liberties, and properties that may be at risk, the complexity of the case, the amount and legal significance of unique evidence in the care and control of the forensic practitioner, and the likelihood of future appeal, forensic practitioners strive to inform the retaining party of the limits of recordkeeping times. If requested to do so, forensic practitioners consider maintaining such records until notified that all appeals in the matter have been exhausted, or sending a copy of any unique components/aspects of the record in their care and control to the retaining party before destruction of the record.

11. PROFESSIONAL AND OTHER PUBLIC COMMUNICATIONS

11.01 Accuracy, Fairness, and Avoidance of Deception

Forensic practitioners make reasonable efforts to ensure that the products of their services, as well as their own public statements and professional reports and testimony, are communicated in ways that promote understanding and avoid deception (EPPCC Standard 5.01).

When in their role as expert to the court or other tribunals, the role of forensic practitioners is to facilitate understanding of the evidence or dispute.

Consistent with legal and ethical requirements, forensic practitioners do not distort or withhold relevant evidence or opinion in reports or testimony. When responding to discovery requests and providing sworn testimony, forensic practitioners strive to have readily available for inspection all data which they considered, regardless of whether the data supports their opinion, subject to and consistent with court order, relevant rules of evidence, test security issues, and professional standards (American Educational Research Association, American Psychological Association, & National Council on Measurement in Education, in press; American Psychological Association Committee on Legal Issues, 2006; Bank & Packer, 2007; Golding, 1990).

When providing reports and other sworn statements or testimony in any form, forensic practitioners strive to present their conclusions, evidence, opinions, or other professional products in a fair manner. Forensic practitioners do not, by either commission or omission, participate in misrepresentation of their evidence, nor do they participate in partisan attempts to avoid, deny or subvert the presentation of evidence contrary to their own position or opinion (EPPCC Standard 5.01). This does not preclude forensic practitioners from forcefully presenting the data and reasoning upon which a conclusion or professional product is based.

11.02 Differentiating Observations, Inferences, and Conclusions

In their communications, forensic practitioners strive to distinguish observations, inferences, and conclusions. Forensic practitioners are encouraged to explain the relationship between their expert opinions and the legal issues and facts of the case at hand.

11.03 Disclosing Sources of Information and Bases of Opinions

Forensic practitioners are encouraged to disclose all sources of information obtained in the course of their professional services, and to identify the source of each piece of information that was considered and relied upon in formulating a particular conclusion, opinion or other professional product.

11.04 Comprehensive and Accurate Presentation of Opinions in Reports and Testimony

Consistent with relevant law and rules of evidence, when providing professional reports and other sworn statements or testimony, forensic practitioners strive to offer a complete statement of all relevant opinions that they formed within the scope of their work on the case, the basis and reasoning underlying the opinions, the salient data or other information that was considered in forming the opinions, and an indication of any additional evidence that may be used in support of the opinions to be offered. The specific substance of forensic reports is determined by the type of psycholegal issue at hand as well as relevant laws or rules in the jurisdiction in which the work is completed.

Forensic practitioners are encouraged to limit discussion of background information that does not bear directly upon the legal purpose of the examination or consultation. Forensic practitioners avoid offering information that is irrelevant and that does not provide a substantial basis of support for their opinions, except when required by law (EPPCC Standard 4.04).

11.05 Commenting Upon Other Professionals and Participants in Legal Proceedings

When evaluating or commenting upon the work or qualifications of other professionals involved in legal proceedings, forensic practitioners seek to represent their disagreements in a professional and respectful tone, and base them on a fair examination of the data, theories, standards and opinions of the other expert or party.

When describing or commenting upon clients, examinees, or other participants in legal proceedings, forensic practitioners strive to do so in a fair and impartial manner. Forensic practitioners strive to report the representations, opinions, and statements of clients, examinees, or other participants in a fair and impartial manner.

11.06 Out of Court Statements

Ordinarily, forensic practitioners seek to avoid making detailed public (out-of-court) statements about legal proceedings in which they have been involved. However, sometimes public statements may serve important goals such as educating the public about the role of forensic practitioners in the legal system, the appropriate practice of forensic psychology, and psychological and legal issues that are relevant to the matter at hand. When making public statements, forensic practitioners refrain from releasing private, confidential, or privileged information, and attempt to protect persons from harm, misuse, or misrepresentation as a result of their statements (EPPCC Standard 4.05).

11.07 Commenting Upon
Legal Proceedings

Forensic practitioners strive to address particular legal proceedings in publications or communications only to the extent that the information relied upon is part of a public record, or when consent for that use has been properly obtained from any party holding any relevant privilege (also see Section 8.04).

When offering public statements about specific cases in which they have not been involved, forensic practitioners offer opinions for which there is sufficient information or data and make clear the limitations of their statements and opinions resulting from having had no direct knowledge of or involvement with the case (EPPCC Standard 9.01).

References

American Bar Association & American Psychological Association. (2008). *Assessment of older adults with diminished capacity: A handbook for psychologists.* Washington, DC: American Bar Association and American Psychological Association.

American Educational Research Association, American Psychological Association, & National Council on Measurement in Education (in press). *Standards for educational and psychological testing (third edition).* Washington, DC: American Educational Research Association.

American Psychological Association (in press). Guidelines for psychological practice with gay, lesbian, and bisexual clients. *American Psychologist.*

American Psychological Association (2003). Guidelines on multicultural education, training, research, practice, and organizational change for psychologists. *American Psychologist*, 58, 377–402.

American Psychological Association. (2004). Guidelines for psychological practice with older adults. *American Psychologist*, 59, 4, 236–260. Washington, DC: Author.

American Psychological Association (2007). Record keeping guidelines, *American Psychologist*, 62, 993–1004.

American Psychological Association (2010). *Ethical principles of psychologists and code of conduct:* Retrieved July 26, 2010, from http://www.apa.org/ethics/code/index.aspx

American Psychological Association (2010). Guidelines for child custody evaluations in legal proceedings. *American Psychologist*, 65, 863–867.

American Psychological Association (2011a). *Guidelines for psychological evaluations in child protection matters.* Washington, DC: Author.

American Psychological Association (2011b). *Guidelines for the practice of parenting coordination.* Washington, DC: Author.

American Psychological Assocation (2011c). *Guidelines for the evaluation of dementia and age related cognitive change.* Washington, DC: Author.

American Psychological Association Committee on Legal Issues (2006). Strategies for private practitioners coping with subpoenas or compelled testimony for client records or test data. *Professional Psychology: Research and practice, 37*, 215–222.

American Psychological Association Committee on Psychological Tests and Assessment (2007). *Statement on third party observers in psychological testing and assessment: A Framework for Decision Making.* Washington, DC: Author.

American Psychological Association Task Force on Guidelines for Assessment and treatment of Persons with Disabilities (2011). *Guidelines for assessment of and intervention with persons with disabilities.* Washington, DC: Author.

Bank, S., & Packer, R. (2007). Expert witness testimony: Law, ethics, and practice. In A.M. Goldstein (Ed.), *Forensic Psychology: Emerging topics and expanding roles* (pp. 421–445). Hoboken, NJ: J. Wiley & Sons.

Golding, S. L. (1990). Mental health professionals and the courts: The ethics of expertise. *International Journal of Law and Psychiatry*, 13, 261–307.

Grisso, T. (1986). *Evaluating competencies: forensic assessments and instruments*, New York: Plenum.

Grisso, T. (2003). *Evaluating competencies: forensic assessments and instruments (second edition)*, New York: Kluwer/Plenum.

Heilbrun, K., Marczyk, G., DeMatteo, D., & Mack-Allen, J. (2007). A principles-based approach to forensic mental health assessment: 18

Utility and update. In A.M. Goldstein (Ed.), *Forensic Psychology: Emerging topics and expanding roles* (pp. 45–72). Hoboken, NJ: J. Wiley & Sons.

Melton, G., Petrila, J., Poythress, N., & slobogin, 1987). *Psychological evaluations for the courts: A handbook for mental health professionals and lawyers.* New York: Guilford.

Melton, G., Petrila, J., Poythress, N., & Slobogin, C. (1997). *Psychological evaluations for the courts: A handbook for mental health professionals and lawyers (second edition).* New York: Guilford.

Melton, G., Petrila, J., Poythress, N., & Slobogin, C., Lyons, P., & Otto, R. K. (2007). *Psychological evaluations for the courts: A handbook for mental health professionals and lawyers (third edition).* New York: Guilford.

Monahan, J. (Ed.). (1980). *Who is the client? The ethics of psychological intervention in the criminal justice system* Washington, D. C.: American Psychological Association. [1]

Rogers, R. (Ed.)(1988). *Clinical assessment of malingering and deception.* New York: Guilford.

Rogers, R. (Ed.)(1997). *Clinical assessment of malingering and deception (second edition).* New York: Guilford.

Rogers, R. (Ed.)(2008). *Clinical assessment of malingering and deception (third edition).* New York: Guilford.

APPENDIX I:
BACKGROUND OF THE *GUIDELINES* AND THE REVISION PROCESS

A. History of the Guidelines

The previous version of the *Specialty Guidelines for Forensic Psychologists* (Committee on Ethical Guidelines for Forensic Psychologists, 1991) was approved by the American Psychology-Law Society, Division 41 of the American Psychological Association, and the American Academy of Forensic Psychology in 1991. The current revision, now called the *Specialty Guidelines for Forensic Psychology* (referred to as *Guidelines* throughout this document), replace the 1991 *Specialty Guidelines for Forensic Psychologists.*

B. Revision Process

This revision of the *Guidelines* was coordinated by the Committee for the Revision of the Specialty Guidelines for Forensic Psychology, which was established by the American Academy of Forensic Psychology and the American Psychology-Law Society (Division 41 of the American Psychological Association) in 2002 and operated through 2011. This Committee consisted of two representatives from each organization (Solomon Fulero, PhD, JD, Stephen Golding, PhD, ABPP, Lisa Piechowski, PhD, ABPP, Christina Studebaker, PhD) a Chairperson (Randy Otto, PhD, ABPP), and a liaison from APA Division 42 (Jeffrey Younggren, PhD, ABPP).

This document was revised in accordance with American Psychological Association Rule 30.08 and the APA policy document *Criteria for the development and evaluation of practice guidelines* (APA, 2001). The Committee posted announcements regarding the revision process to relevant electronic discussion lists and professional publications (i.e., Psylaw-L email listserve, American Academy of Forensic Psychology listserve, American Psychology-Law Society Newsletter). In addition, an electronic discussion list devoted solely to issues concerning revision of the *Guidelines* was operated between December 2002 and July 2007, followed by establishment of an e-mail address in February 2008 (sgfp@yahoo.com). Individuals were invited to provide input and commentary on the existing *Guidelines* and proposed revisions via these means. In addition, two public meetings were held throughout the revision process at biennial meetings of the American Psychology-Law Society.

Upon development of a draft that the Revisions Committee deemed suitable, the revised *Guidelines* were submitted for review to the Executive Committee of the American Psychology-Law Society and Division 41 of the American Psychological Association, and to the American Board of Forensic Psychology. Once the revised *Guidelines* were approved by these two organizations, they were submitted to the American Psychological Association for review, commentary, and acceptance, consistent with the American Psychological Association's Criteria for Practice Guideline Development and Evaluation (Committee on Professional Practice and Standards, 2001) and Rule 30–8. They were subsequently revised by the Revisions Committee and were adopted by the American Psychological Association Council of Representatives on August, 3, 2011.

C. Developers and Support

The *Specialty Guidelines for Forensic Psychology* were developed by the American Psychology-Law Society (Division 41 of the American Psychological Association) and the American Academy of Forensic Psychology.

D. Current Status

These *Guidelines* are scheduled to expire August 3, 2021. After this date, users are encouraged to contact the American Psychological Association Practice Directorate to confirm that this document remains in effect.

APPENDIX II: DEFINITIONS AND TERMINOLOGY

For the purposes of these *Guidelines*:

Appropriate, when used in relation to conduct by a forensic practitioner means that, according to the prevailing professional judgment of competent forensic practitioners, the conduct is apt and pertinent and is considered befitting, suitable and proper for a particular person, place, condition, or function. "Inappropriate" means that, according to the prevailing professional judgment of competent forensic practitioners, the conduct is not suitable, desirable, or properly timed for a particular person, occasion, or purpose; and may also denote improper conduct, improprieties, or conduct that is discrepant for the circumstances.

Agreement refers to the objective and mutual understanding between the forensic practitioner and the person or persons seeking the professional service and/or agreeing to participate in the service. See also Assent, Consent, and Informed Consent.

Assent refers to the agreement, approval, or permission, especially regarding verbal or nonverbal conduct, that is reasonably intended and interpreted as expressing willingness, even in the absence of unmistakable consent. Forensic practitioners attempt to secure assent when consent and informed consent can not be obtained or when, because of mental state, the examinee may not be able to consent.

Consent refers to agreement, approval, or permission as to some act or purpose.

Client refers to the attorney, law firm, court, agency, entity, party, or other person who has retained, and who has a contractual relationship with, the forensic practitioner to provide services.

Conflict of Interest refers to a situation or circumstance in which the forensic practitioner's objectivity, impartiality, or judgment may be jeopardized due to a relationship, financial, or any other interest that would reasonably be expected to substantially affect a forensic practitioner's professional judgment, impartiality, or decision-making.

Decisionmaker refers to the person or entity with the authority to make a judicial decision, agency determination, arbitration award, or other contractual determination after consideration of the facts and the law.

Examinee refers to a person who is the subject of a forensic examination for the purpose of informing a decision maker or attorney about the psychological functioning of that examinee.

Forensic Examiner refers to a psychologist who examines the psychological condition of a person whose psychological condition is in controversy or at issue.

Forensic Practice refers to the application of the scientific, technical, or specialized knowledge of psychology to the law and the use of that knowledge to assist in resolving legal, contractual, and administrative disputes.

Forensic Practitioner refers to a psychologist when engaged in forensic practice.

Forensic Psychology refers to all forensic practice by any psychologist working within any sub-discipline of psychology (e.g., clinical, developmental, social, cognitive).

Informed Consent denotes the knowledgeable, voluntary, and competent agreement by a person to a proposed course of conduct after the forensic practitioner has communicated adequate information and explanation about the material risks and benefits of, and reasonably available alternatives to, the proposed course of conduct.

Legal Representative refers to a person who has the legal authority to act on behalf of another.

Party refers to a person or entity named in litigation, or who is involved in, or is witness to, an activity or relationship that may be reasonably anticipated to result in litigation.

Reasonable or *Reasonably*, when used in relation to conduct by a forensic practitioner, denotes the conduct of a prudent and competent forensic practitioner who is engaged in similar activities in similar circumstances.

Record or ***Written Record*** refers to all notes, records, documents, memorializations, and recordings of considerations and communications, be they in any form or on any media, tangible, electronic, hand-written, or mechanical, that are contained in, or are specifically related to, the forensic matter in question or the forensic service provided.

Retaining Party refers to the attorney, law firm, court, agency, entity, party, or other person who has retained, and who has a contractual relationship with, the forensic practitioner to provide services.

Tribunal denotes a court or an arbitrator in an arbitration proceeding, or a legislative body, administrative agency, or other body acting in an adjudicative capacity. A legislative body, administrative agency or other body acts in an adjudicative capacity when a neutral official, after the presentation of legal argument or evidence by a party or parties, renders a judgment directly affecting a party's interests in a particular matter.

Trier of Fact refers to a court or an arbitrator in an arbitration proceeding, or a legislative body, administrative agency, or other body acting in an adjudicative capacity. A legislative body, administrative agency or other body acts in an adjudicative capacity when a neutral official, after the presentation of legal argument or evidence by a party or parties, renders a judgment directly affecting a party's interests in a particular matter.

Appendix B
DVCC-R

Your name: _____ Date _____

Please answer the following questions in the chart – about your relationship with your significant other (former partner) whose name is _____

#	Questions	Yes	No	If yes, Who? What? When? Where?	Corroboration: Name of person(s) who saw or heard this first hand or who was told about this by someone else.	Is this the first time you remembered/ reported this? If remembered/ reported before, when and where did you report this?
1.	Do you and your partner have a particular way that you resolve differences, and if so, please describe?					
2.	Do you and your partner argue, and if so, what happens when you and your partner argue? Describe what each of you does when you get angry.					
3.	Can you and/or your partner tell when the other is about to get angry?					
4.	Do you and your partner have a way that resolve fights and if so, how?					
5.	Are there "trigger events" that trigger fights or disagreements between you and your partner, and if so, what are they?					
6.	Do fights between the two of you ever "go wrong" and if so, what happens?					
7.	Do you or your partner control some things in your relationship? If so, who controls what – money, chores, children, social calendar, major decisions, etc.?					

(continued)

#	Questions	Yes	No	If yes, Who? What? When? Where?	Corroboration: Name of person(s) who saw or heard this first hand or who was told about this by someone else.	Is this the first time you remembered/ reported this? If remembered/ reported before, when and where did you report this?
8.	Does one of you in your relationship have more power and if so, who does and over what?					
9.	Have you felt controlled in this relationship? If yes, please describe.					
	Has your partner ever …					
10.	Called you a name or made fun of you?					
11.	Insulted you/put you down					
12.	Public humiliation					
13.	Yelled at you/Shouted					
14.	Teasing that includes insults					
15.	Constant criticisms					
16.	Made you think you were crazy					
17.	Harassed you because of your gender					
18.	Swearing					
19.	Taunting					
20.	Badgering					
21.	Telling a person's secrets					
22.	Extreme jealousy					
23.	Isolated you from your family and friends					
24.	Pouted when you spend time with friends					
25.	Told you that "family problems" should not be told to anyone outside of the immediate family					
26.	Ignored you?					
27.	Told you that you were a bad parent?					
28.	Refused to do housework or childcare?					

(continued)

#	Questions	Yes	No	If yes, Who? What? When? Where?	Corroboration: Name of person(s) who saw or heard this first hand or who was told about this by someone else.	Is this the first time you remembered/ reported this? If remembered/ reported before, when and where did you report this?
29.	Accused you of paying too much attention to someone or something else					
30.	Made you beg for forgiveness?					
31.	Demanded to be waited upon?					
32.	Intimidated you through his tone of voice?					
33.	Gave you angry looks or stares?					
34.	Put down your family or friends?					
35.	Put down your physical appearance?					
36.	Tried to change your physical appearance?					
37.	Not taken advantage of your strengths or accomplishments?					
38.	Told you that no one else would want you?					
39.	Accused you of cheating on the relationship?					
40.	Harassed you for information on past relationships?					
41.	Put you down or yelled at you in front of your children?					
42.	Bodily confined or held you against your will?					
43.	Prevented you from leaving a room or your home?					
44.	Prevented you from going to school or work?					
45.	Prevented you from seeing your family or friends?					
46.	Denied you the right to receive health care?					
47.	Prevented you from taking any medications?					
48.	Listened to your phone calls?					

(continued)

#	Questions	Yes	No	If yes, Who? What? When? Where?	Corroboration: Name of person(s) who saw or heard this first hand or who was told about this by someone else.	Is this the first time you remembered/ reported this? If remembered/ reported before, when and where did you report this?
49.	Disabled your telephone?					
50.	Opened your mail without your permission?					
51.	Had you followed?					
52.	Checked the mileage on your car?					
53.	Taken away your keys?					
54.	Phoned you repeatedly at work?					
55.	Got you fired from work?					
56.	Controlled your food intake?					
57.	Tried to control what you do					
58.	Controlled funds					
59.	Put you on a monetary allowance?					
60.	Made you ask or beg for money?					
61.	Made you explain how money was spent?					
62.	Does your partner have empathy for the effects of the violence on you? On the children?					
63.	Financially deprived the children in retaliation for partner's behavior					
64.	Used the Family Court system to drain funds					
65.	Got angry if you were late getting home?					
66.	Made you explain your whereabouts at all times?					
67.	Insisted on having the final say in all decisions?					
68.	Made you use drugs or alcohol against your will?					
69.	Damaged a car, home, or other prized possessions					
70.	Destroyed gifts, clothing, letters					

(continued)

#	Questions	Yes	No	If yes, Who? What? When? Where?	Corroboration: Name of person(s) who saw or heard this first hand or who was told about this by someone else.	Is this the first time you remembered/ reported this? If remembered/ reported before, when and where did you report this?
71.	Threatened to physically take your children away?					
72.	Threatened to make you lose custody of the children?					
73.	Threatened to hit you?					
74.	Threatened to throw objects at you?					
75.	Threatened to use a weapon against you?					
76.	Threatened to leave you in an unsafe location					
77.	Threatened to kill you?					
78.	Threatened to harm or kill your family and/or friends?					
79.	Threatened to harm or kill your children?					
80.	Threatened to harm or kill himself/herself?					
81.	Stalked you					
82.	Thrown or smashed objects in your presence?					
83.	Destroyed your personal property?					
84.	Hit walls or pounded his/her fist when angry at you?					
85.	Driven carelessly when you were in the car?					
86.	Abused family pets to hurt you?					
87.	Punished your children when he/she was angry with you?					
88.	Hurt or mutilated himself/ herself to scare you?					
89.	Tried to run you over with a vehicle?					
90.	Slapped you?					
91.	Pushed or shoved you?					

(continued)

#	Questions	Yes	No	If yes, Who? What? When? Where?	Corroboration: Name of person(s) who saw or heard this first hand or who was told about this by someone else.	Is this the first time you remembered/ reported this? If remembered/ reported before, when and where did you report this?
92.	Thrown you around (into walls, furniture, onto floor)?					
93.	Hit you with an open hand?					
94.	Hit you with a fist?					
95.	Hit you with an object?					
96.	Scratched you?					
97.	Pinched you?					
98.	Pulled your hair?					
99.	Grabbed you?					
100.	Tripped you?					
101.	Punched you?					
102.	Spit on you?					
103.	Bit you?					
104.	Kicked you?					
105.	Burned you?					
106.	Injured you by holding or squeezing you too tightly?					
107.	Choked or tried to strangle you?					
108.	Used a weapon against you (stabbed, shot, etc.)?					
109.	Hit you or run you over with a vehicle?					
110.	Attempted murder					
111.	Physically hurt you when you were pregnant?					
112.	Called you negative sexual names like "frigid" or "whore"?					
113.	Unwanted sexual touching					
114.	Made sexual advances that made you feel uncomfortable					
115.	Insisted, physically or verbally, that a person who said "no" have sex anyway					

(continued)

#	Questions	Yes	No	If yes, Who? What? When? Where?	Corroboration: Name of person(s) who saw or heard this first hand or who was told about this by someone else.	Is this the first time you remembered/ reported this? If remembered/ reported before, when and where did you report this?
116.	Used emotional blackmail to get one to have sex ("If you loved me, you would…")					
117.	Forced or pressured you to participate in sex with him or her against your					
118.	Pressured you to participate in a sexual activity that hurt you?					
119.	Pressured you to participate in a sexual activity that you feel ashamed of?					
120.	Forced you to have sex in the presence of others?					
121.	Used threatening objects or weapons during sex?					
122.	Prevented you from using birth control?					
123.	Lied about his/her use of birth control?					
124.	Withheld information about whether he/she had been exposed to a sexually transmitted disease or HIV?					
125.	Physically attacked the sexual parts of your body (breasts or genitalia)?					
126.	Pressured you to get pregnant against your will?					
127.	Have you ever received severe contusions from any physical assaults					
128.	Have you ever received bruises from any physical assaults					
129.	Have you ever received any cuts from any physical assaults?					
130.	Have you ever received any burns from any physical assaults					
131.	Have you ever received any broken bones from any physical assaults					

(continued)

#	Questions	Yes	No	If yes, Who? What? When? Where?	Corroboration: Name of person(s) who saw or heard this first hand or who was told about this by someone else.	Is this the first time you remembered/ reported this? If remembered/ reported before, when and where did you report this?
132.	Have you ever received any head or internal injuries from any physical assaults					
133.	Have you ever received wounds from a gun from any physical assaults					
134.	Have you ever received wounds from a knife from any physical assaults					
135.	Are there any weapons in the home?					
136.	Do you or your partner have access to any weapons?					
137.	Physically hurt you while he/ she was under the influence of alcohol or drugs?					
138.	Have either of you ever or do you now have a problem with any substance? Used? Misused? Abused? Been dependent upon any substance?					
139.	Have you or your partner been non-compliant with any court orders? Been arrested for anything? Not honored any restraining orders?					
140.	Have you or your partner had any psychiatric history (especially manic and psychotic features) for you and/or your partner?					
141.	Have either you or your partner been involved in any maltreatment of animals?					
142.	Have either you or your partner been involved in any fire setting?					
143.	Have you or your partner ever been violent in previous relationships? As an adult? As a teen? As a child? Been violent in the workplace? Been arrested for any kind of aggressive crime?					

(continued)

#	Questions	Yes	No	If yes, Who? What? When? Where?	Corroboration: Name of person(s) who saw or heard this first hand or who was told about this by someone else.	Is this the first time you remembered/ reported this? If remembered/ reported before, when and where did you report this?
144.	Have you or your partner ever threatened or attempted to commit suicide?					
145.	Have either you or your partner taken medication for mental health problems (e.g. depression)?					
146.	Have you or your partner been violent with/to children in the past?					
147.	Do you have a child that does not belong to your partner? If so, does s/he physically or emotionally abuse your child?					
148.	Have either you or your partner used pornography?					
149.	Have you or your partner been involved in "forced sex" either as the perpetrator or as the victim – at the hands of your partner and/or others?					
150.	Have you or your partner been involved in control of the other through the children?					
151.	Has your partner had a history of probation failures?					
152.	Has your partner had a criminal history?					
153.	Have you ever called the police because your partner assaulted you? Was s/he arrested or did s/he avoid arrest?					
154.	Have you ever left home because you were assaulted or emotionally abused by your partner?					
155.	Do you believe that your partner is capable of killing you? Capable of killing your children?					
156.	Does your partner threaten to harm your children?					

(continued)

#	Questions	Yes	No	If yes, Who? What? When? Where?	Corroboration: Name of person(s) who saw or heard this first hand or who was told about this by someone else.	Is this the first time you remembered/ reported this? If remembered/ reported before, when and where did you report this?
157.	Has your partner ever assaulted or abused you in the presence of your children? If so, did they directly witness it and/or were they in the home?					
	Victims Only, please continue to answer the questions below.					
158.	Please describe the conflict between the two of you as the relationship was coming to an end, at the time of separation, and since the separation.					
159.	Have you felt oppressed in this relationship? If yes, please describe.					
160.	Do you and your partner feel isolated from others? From friends? From family? If so, please describe.					
161.	Do you and/or your partner ever feel scared of the other and if so, when and about what?					
162.	Have you felt hopeless at times?					
163.	Have you felt helpless at times?					
164.	Did the abuse occur mainly around the time of the separation in the relationship? Is there a pattern of abuse that was prevalent before the separation? Or was the abuse prevalent at and about the time of the separation? Or has the abuse been prevalent only since the time of the separation or soon thereafter?					
165.	Was there a pattern or are the incidents solitary ones?					
166.	Do you believe that your partner has been chronically violent?					
167.	Was the abuse chronic, intermittent and/or reactionary?					

(continued)

#	Questions	Yes	No	If yes, Who? What? When? Where?	Corroboration: Name of person(s) who saw or heard this first hand or who was told about this by someone else.	Is this the first time you remembered/ reported this? If remembered/ reported before, when and where did you report this?
168.	Has the frequency increased? When/Over what period of time?					
169.	Has the severity increased? When/Over what period of time?					
170.	Has your partner been violent in any of the ways described in this questionnaire in previous relationships and if so, when, how, and with whom?					
171.	Has your partner had any kind of treatment for violence? If yes, please describe and indicate whether or not the treatment was successful.					
172.	What was the age of your partner the first time that you know that he was violent in any of the ways described in this questionnaire—whether that was in a relationship with you or someone else?					
173.	Does your partner blame you for the acts of abuse that you have described in this questionnaire and/or does your partner focus on you, rather than on himself or herself, in terms of who is responsible for the problems in your relationship?					
174.	Does your partner deny having done any or all of the things that you have described in this questionnaire? If yes, please describe that which is denied and that which your partner admits to having done.					
175.	Does your partner acknowledge the violence? And if so, please describe.					
176.	Does your partner have guilt and remorse for what s/he has done?					

(continued)

#	Questions	Yes	No	If yes, Who? What? When? Where?	Corroboration: Name of person(s) who saw or heard this first hand or who was told about this by someone else.	Is this the first time you remembered/ reported this? If remembered/ reported before, when and where did you report this?
177.	Does your partner seem to understand and appreciate the impact that the violent acts have had on you? On the child(ren)?					
178.	Does your partner have empathy for the effects of the violence on you? On the children?					
179.	Does your partner take responsibility for his/her behavior? And if so, how does he or she take responsibility? Please describe.					
180.	Has your partner followed through in the things that s/he has promised to change— in a proactive manner? Have the things that s/he has followedthrough with been concrete and noticed by you?					
181.	Is your partner aware of your child(ren)'s needs in a way that is appropriate to the age that your child is? Is your partner aware of how the abuse has served to maintain control in the relationship?					
In the next section, you are asked to describe YOUR OWN BEHAVIOR. Now please comment on **YOUR OWN BEHAVIOR**, not your former partner's behavior.						
This section is for the person filling it out to answer questions about their own behavior.						
	Have YOU ever...					
182.	Called your partner a name or made fun of you?					
183.	Insulted your partner/put him or her down					
184.	Humiliated your partner in public					
185.	Yelled/Shouted at him/her					
186.	Teased or insulted him/her?					
187.	Constantly criticized him/her?					

(continued)

#	Questions	Yes	No	If yes, Who? What? When? Where?	Corroboration: Name of person(s) who saw or heard this first hand or who was told about this by someone else.	Is this the first time you remembered/ reported this? If remembered/ reported before, when and where did you report this?
188.	Made him/her think s/he was crazy					
189.	Harassed him because of his/her gender					
190.	Sworn at him/her?					
191.	Taunted him/her?					
192.	Badgered him/her?					
193.	Told his/her secrets?					
194.	Had extreme jealousy about him/her?					
195.	Isolated him/her from his/her family and friends					
196.	Pouted when s/he spent time with friends					
197.	Made him/her think s/he was crazy					
198.	Harassed him because of his/her gender					
199.	Sworn at him/her?					
200.	Taunted him/her?					
201.	Badgered him/her?					
202.	Told his/her secrets?					
203.	Had extreme jealousy about him/her?					
204.	Isolated him/her from his/her family and friends					
205.	Had extreme jealousy about him/her?					
206.	Isolated him/her from his/her family and friends					
207.	Pouted when s/he spent time with friends					
208.	Told him/her that "family problems" should not be told to anyone outside of the immediate family					

(continued)

#	Questions	Yes	No	If yes, Who? What? When? Where?	Corroboration: Name of person(s) who saw or heard this first hand or who was told about this by someone else.	Is this the first time you remembered/ reported this? If remembered/ reported before, when and where did you report this?
209.	Ignored him/her?					
210.	Told him/her that s/he was a bad parent?					
211.	Refused to do housework or childcare?					
212.	Accused him/her of paying too much attention to someone or something else					
213.	Made him/her beg for forgiveness?					
214.	Demanded to be waited upon?					
215.	Intimidated him/her through your tone of voice?					
216.	Gave him/her angry looks or stares?					
217.	Put down his/her family or friends?					
218.	Put down his/her physical appearance?					
219.	Tried to change his/her physical appearance?					
220.	Not taken advantage of his/ her strengths or accomplishments?					
221.	Told him/her that no one else would want him/her?					
222.	Accused him/her of cheating on the relationship?					
223.	Harassed him/her for information on past relationships?					
224.	Put him/her down or yelled at him/her in front of the children?					
225.	Bodily confined or held him/ her against his/her will?					
226.	Prevented him/her from leaving a room or the home?					
227.	Prevented him/her from going to school or work?					

(continued)

#	Questions	Yes	No	If yes, Who? What? When? Where?	Corroboration: Name of person(s) who saw or heard this first hand or who was told about this by someone else.	Is this the first time you remembered/ reported this? If remembered/ reported before, when and where did you report this?
228.	Prevented him/her from seeing family or friends?					
229.	Denied him/her the right to receive health care?					
230.	Prevented him/her from taking any medications?					
231.	Listened to his/her phone calls?					
232.	Disabled his/her telephone?					
233.	Opened his/her mail without permission?					
234.	Had him/her followed?					
235.	Checked the mileage on his/her car?					
236.	Taken away his/her keys?.					
237.	Phoned him/her repeatedly at work?					
238.	Got him/her fired from work?					
239.	Controlled his/her food intake?					
240.	Tried to control what he or she does?					
241.	Controlled funds					
242.	Put him/her on a monetary allowance?					
243.	Made him/her ask or beg for money?					
244.	Made him/her explain how money was spent?					
245.	Gave an insufficient "allowance" to manage household					
246.	Financially deprived the children in retaliation for partner's behavior					
247.	Used the Family Court system to drain funds					
248.	Got angry if he or she was late getting home?					

(continued)

#	Questions	Yes	No	If yes, Who? What? When? Where?	Corroboration: Name of person(s) who saw or heard this first hand or who was told about this by someone else.	Is this the first time you remembered/ reported this? If remembered/ reported before, when and where did you report this?
249.	Made him/her explain his or her whereabouts at all times?					
250.	Insisted on having the final say in all decisions?					
251.	Made him/her use drugs or alcohol against his/her will?					
252.	Damaged a car, home, or other prized possessions					
253.	Destroyed gifts, clothing, letters					
254.	Threatened to physically take the children away?					
255.	Threatened to make him/her lose custody of the children?					
256.	Threatened to hit him/her?					
257.	Threatened to throw objects at him/her?					
258.	Threatened to use a weapon against him/her?					
259.	Threatened to leave him/her in an unsafe location?					
260.	Threatened to kill him/her?					
261.	Threatened to harm or kill his/ her family and/or friends?					
262.	Threatened to harm or kill the children?					
263.	Threatened to harm or kill yourself as a way to get back at him/her?					
264.	Stalked him/her?					
265.	Thrown or smashed objects in his/her presence?					
266.	Destroyed his/her personal property?					
267.	Hit walls or pounded your fist when angry at him/her?					
268.	Driven carelessly when s/he was in the car?					

(continued)

#	Questions	Yes	No	If yes, Who? What? When? Where?	Corroboration: Name of person(s) who saw or heard this first hand or who was told about this by someone else.	Is this the first time you remembered/ reported this? If remembered/ reported before, when and where did you report this?
269.	Abused family pets to hurt him/her?					
270.	Punished the children when you were angry with him/her?					
271.	Hurt or mutilated yourself to scare him/her?					
272.	Tried to run him/her over with a vehicle?					
273.	Slapped him/her?					
274.	Pushed or shoved him/her?					
275.	Thrown him/her around (into walls, furniture, onto floor)?					
276.	Hit him/her with an open hand?					
277.	Hit him/her with a fist?					
278.	Hit him/her with an object?					
279.	Scratched him/her?					
280.	Pinched him/her?					
281.	Pulled him/her hair?					
282.	Grabbed him/her?					
283.	Tripped him/her?					
284.	Punched him/her?					
285.	Spit on him/her?					
286.	Bit him/her?					
287.	Kicked him/her?					
288.	Burned him/her?					
289.	Injured him/her by holding or squeezing him/her too tightly?					
290.	Choked or tried to strangle him/her?					
291.	Used a weapon against him/her (stabbed, shot, etc.)?					
292.	Hit him/her or run him/her over with a vehicle?					
293.	Attempted murder					

#	Questions	Yes	No	If yes, Who? What? When? Where?	Corroboration: Name of person(s) who saw or heard this first hand or who was told about this by someone else.	Is this the first time you remembered/ reported this? If remembered/ reported before, when and where did you report this?
294.	Physically hurt him/her when she was pregnant?					
295.	Called him/her negative sexual names like "frigid" or "whore"?					
296.	Unwanted sexual touching					
297.	Made sexual advances that made him/her feel uncomfortable					
298.	Insisted, physically or verbally, that a person who said "no" have sex anyway					
299.	Used emotional blackmail to get him/her to have sex ("If you loved me, you would…")					
300.	Forced or pressured him/her to participate in sex with you against his/her will?					
301.	Pressured him/her to participate in a sexual activity that hurt him/her?					
302.	Pressured him/her to participate in a sexual activity that s/he felt ashamed of?					
303.	Forced him/her to have sex in the presence of others?					
304.	Used threatening objects or weapons during sex?					
305.	Prevented him/her from using birth control?					
306.	Lied about your use of birth control?					
307.	Withheld information about whether you have been exposed to a sexually transmitted disease or HIV?					
308.	Physically attacked the sexual parts of his/her body (breasts or genitalia)?					
309.	Pressured him/her to have a baby against his/her will?					

#	Questions	Yes	No	If yes, Who? What? When? Where?	Corroboration: Name of person(s) who saw or heard this first hand or who was told about this by someone else.	Is this the first time you remembered/ reported this? If remembered/ reported before, when and where did you report this?
310.	Has s/he ever received severe contusions from any physical assaults by you?					
311.	Has s/he ever received bruises from any physical assaults by you?					
312.	Have s/he ever received any cuts from any physical assaults by you?					
313.	Has s/he ever received any burns from any physical assaults by you?					
314.	Has s/he ever received any broken bones from any physical assaults by you?					
315.	Has s/he ever received any head or internal injuries from any physical assaults by you?					
316.	Have you physically assaulted him/her with a gun?					
317.	Have you physically assaulted him/her with a knife?					
318.	Are there any weapons in the home or do you/your partner have access to weapons?					
317.	Have you physically hurt him/her while either of you were under the influence of alcohol or drugs?					
318.	Have either of you ever or do you now have a problem with any substance? Used? Misused? Abused? Been dependent upon any substance?					
319.	Have you been non-compliant with any court orders? Been arrested for anything? Not honored any restraining orders?					
320.	Have had any psychiatric history (especially manic and psychotic features) for you and/or your partner?					

#	Questions	Yes	No	If yes, Who? What? When? Where?	Corroboration: Name of person(s) who saw or heard this first hand or who was told about this by someone else.	Is this the first time you remembered/ reported this? If remembered/ reported before, when and where did you report this?
321.	Have either you been involved in any maltreatment of animals?					
322.	Have either of you been involved in any fire setting?					
323.	Have you ever been violent in previous relationships? As an adult? As a teen? As a child? Been violent in the workplace? Been arrested for any kind of aggressive crime?					
324.	Have you ever threatened or attempted to commit suicide?					
325.	Have either of you taken medication for mental health problems (e.g. depression)?					
326.	Have you been violent with/to children in the past?					
327.	Does your partner have a child that is not your biological child? If so, have you physically/ emotionally abused this child?					
328.	Have either you used pornography?					
329.	Have you been involved in "forced sex" either as the perpetrator or as the victim – at the hands of your partner and/or others?					
330.	Have you used the children to control your partner?					
331.	Have you had a history of probation failures?					
332.	Has your partner had a criminal history?					

Corroboration. Please provide corroboration for each instance in which you answer in the affirmative.

Question #	Firsthand corroboration: Who saw or heard what you are reporting that happened? Or at the time of the event, who did you tell about what happened	Please provide contact information for each person who can corroborate any of the events you are speaking about (email address, phone #).	Specific questions to ask the collateral.

Note: Questions 1–157 are about the relationship between you and your former partner and things that you have experienced in that relationship as in what you believe your partner has done. IF you consider yourself to have been a victim of your partner, questions 158–181 are for you to answer. The next set of questions (#s 182–332) are about your own behavior towards your partner. Pages 29–30 are to be used to provide details about that which can be corroborated. This is there for the person to provide the names of those who can provide firsthand knowledge of those things that are reported. *It is important for you to provide the persons who can corroborate the information you have set forth in this document. This information can be provided in the far-right column. Should you need more space, please turn to the back pages of this document (pages 29–30) for space to provide information about what someone may have heard or saw or (were told about the incidents reported. Please provide their contact information or where that contact information may be acquired. Thank you.

Bibliography

AFCC Task Force on Court-Involved Therapy. (2009). Guidelines for court-involved therapy. *Family Court Review, 49*(3), 564–581.

Ahern, E. C., Lyon, T. D., & Quas, J. A. (2011). Young children's emerging ability to make false statements. *Developmental Psychology, 47*(1), 61–66. doi:10.1037/a0021272

American Academy of Matrimonial Lawyers. (2009). *What should we tell the children? A parents' guide for talking about separation and divorce.* Text by Joan B. Kelly, Ph.D. www.aaml.org.

American Academy of Matrimonial Lawyers. (2010). *What should we tell the children? A parents' guide for talking about separation and divorce.* Chicago, Illinois: AAML.

American Professional Society on the Abuse of Children. (2012). *Practice guidelines: Forensic interviewing in cases of suspected child abuse.* Published by the American Professional Society on the Abuse of Children and available for purchase. www.apsac.org.

American Psychological Association. (2012). Guidelines for the practice of parenting coordination. *American Psychologist, 67*, 63–71.

Association of Family and Conciliation Courts Task Force on Parenting Coordination. (2006). Guidelines for parenting coordination. *Family Court Review, 44*(1), 164–181. www.afccnet.org/resources/standards_practice.asp

Babb, B. A., & Pruett, M. K. (Eds.). (2020). Special issue: Parent-child contact problems: Concepts, controversies & conundrums. *Family Court Review, 58*, 2.

Bala, N., & Birnbaum, R. (2013). *Hearing the voice of children in the family justice process: The role of judicial interviews.* CBA Newsletter, April. www.cba.org/CBA/sections_family/newsletters2013/interviews.aspx

Bala, N., Birnbaum, R., & Bertrand, L. (2013). The role of the children's lawyers: Instructional advocate or best interests guardian – Comparing legal practice in Alberta & Ontario—Two provinces with different policies. *Family Court Review, 51*(4), 681–697.

Bala, N., Birnbaum, R., Cyr, F., & McColley, D. (2013). Children's voices in family court: Guidelines for judges meeting children. *Family Law Quarterly, 47*(3), 381–410.

Bala, N., Birnbaum, R., & Cyr, F. (in press). Judicial interviews of children in Canada's family courts: Growing acceptance but still controversial. In T. Gal & B. F. Duramy (Eds.), *Promoting the participation of children across the globe: From social exclusion to child-inclusive policies.* Oxford University Press.

Bala, N., Birnbaum, R., & Martinson, D. (2010). One judge for one family: Differentiated case management for families in continuing conflict. *Canadian Journal of Family Law, 26*(2), 395–450.

Bala, N., Lee, K., Lindsay, R. C. L., & Talwar, V. (2010). The competency of children to testify: Psychological research informing Canadian law reform. *International Journal of Children's Rights, 18*, 52–77.

Bala, N., Mitnick, M., Trocmé, N., & Houston, C. (2007). Sexual abuse allegations and parental separation: Smokescreen or fire? *Journal of Family Studies, 13*, 26–56.

Bala, N., Ramakrishna, B., Lindsay, R. C. L., & Lee, K. (2005). Judicial assessment of the credibility of child witnesses. *Alberta Law Review, 42*(4), 995–1017.

Belcher-Timme, S. H., Belcher-Timme, Z., & Gibblings, E. (2013). Exploring best practices in parenting coordination: A national survey of current practices and practitioners. *Family Court Review, 51*(4), 651–666.

Bijorklund, D. F. (2012). *Children's thinking: Cognitive development and individual differences* (5th ed.). Belmont, CA: Wadsworth Cengage Learning.

Birnbaum, R. (2009). *The voice of the child in separation/divorce mediation and other alternative dispute resolution processes: A literature review.* Family, Children and Youth Section Department of Justice Canada. https://www.justice.gc.ca/eng/rp-pr/fl-lf/divorce/vcsdm-pvem/index.html

Birnbaum, R., & Bala, N. (2009). The child's perspective on legal representation: Young adults report on their experiences with child lawyers. *Canadian Journal of Family Law, 25*(1), 11–71.

Birnbaum, R., & Bala, N. (2010). Towards a differentiation of "high conflict" families: An analysis of social science and Canadian case law. *Family Court Review, 48*(3), 403–416.

Birnbaum, R., & Bala, N. (2010). Judicial interviews with children in custody and access cases: Comparing experiences in Ontario and Ohio. *International Journal of Law, Policy and the Family, 24*(3), 300–337.

Birnbaum, R., & Bala, N. (2013, September). Judicial interviews with children: A voice but not a choice. *Family Law News: International Bar Association Family Law Newsletter, 6*(1), 49–52.

Birnbaum, R., & Bala, N. (2013, November). Interviewing children: The role of judges and mediators. *Family Mediation News*, California 5–8.

Birnbaum, R., & Bala, N. (2014). A survey of Canadian judges about their meetings with children: Becoming more common but still contentious. *Canadian Bar Review, 91*, 1–17.

Birnbaum, R., & Saini, M. (2012). A qualitative synthesis of children's participation in custody disputes. *Journal of Social Work Research Practice, 22*(4), 400–409.

Birnbaum, R., & Saini, M. (2012). A scoping review of qualitative studies on the voice of the child in child custody disputes. *Childhood, 20*(2), 260–282.

Birnbaum, R., Bala, N., & Bertrand, L. (2013). Judicial interviews with children: Attitudes and practices of Canadian lawyers for children. *New Zealand Law Review, 3*, 465–482.

Birnbaum, R., Bala, N., & Cyr, F. (2011). Children's experiences with family justice professionals and judges: A comparative analysis of Ontario and Ohio. *Ontario Bar Association*, Toronto, Feb 4, 2011.

Block, S. D., Shestowsky, D., Segovia, D. A., Goodman, G. S., Schaaf, J. M., & Alexander, K. W. (2012). "That never happened": Adults' discernment of children's true and false memory reports. *Law and Human Behavior, 36*(5), 365–374. doi:10.1037/h0093920

Boshier, P. (2006). Involving children in decision making: Lessons from New Zealand. *Australian Journal of Family Law, 20*(2), 145–153.

Boshier, P., & Caldwell, J. (2013). Judicial interviewing of children: The New Zealand Family Court. AFCC 50th Anniversary Conference – Riding the Wave of the Future: Global Voices, Expanding Choices. Workshop 77.

Bow, J., Gottlieb, M., & Gould-Saltman, D. (2011). Attorneys' belief and opinions about child custody evaluations. *Family Court Review, 49*(2), 301–312.

Brassard, M. S., Hart, S. N., Baker, A. A., & Chiel, Z. (2019). *The APSAC monograph on psychological maltreatment.* American Professional Society on the Abuse of Children. https://www.apsac.org.

Brubacher, S. P., Poole, D. A., Dickinson, J. J., La Rooy, D., Szojka, Z. A., & Powell, M. B. (2019). Effects of interviewer familiarity and supportiveness on children's recall across repeated interviews. *Law and Human Behavior, 43*(6), 507–516. http://dx.doi.org/10.1037/lhb0000346

Bruck, M., Ceci, S. J., & Hembrooke, H. (1998). Reliability and credibility of young children's reports: From research to policy and practice. *American Psychologist, 53*(2), 136–151.

Byrnes, B. (2011). Voices of children in the legal process. *Journal of Family Studies, 17*, 44.

Caldwell, J. (2011). Common law judges and judicial interviewing. *Child & Family Law Quarterly, 23*, 41.

Calloway, G. C., & Erard, R. E. (Eds.). (2009). Special issue on attachment and child custody. *Journal of Family Trauma, Child Custody and Child Development, 6* (1–2), 1–162.

Carter, D. (2011). *Parenting coordination: A practical guide for family law professionals.* New York: Springer Publishing.

Casey, B. J., Getz, S., & Galván, A. (2008). The adolescent brain. *Developmental Review, 28*, 62–77. doi:10.1016/j.dr.2007.08.003

Casey, B. J., Jones, R. M., & Hare, T. A. (2008). The adolescent brain. *Annals of the New York Academy of Sciences, 1124*, 111–126. https://doi.org/10.1196/annals.1440.010

Cashmore, J., & Parkinson, P. (2008). Children's and parents' perceptions on children's participation in decision making after parental separation and divorce. *Family Court Review, 46*, 91–104.

Ceci, S. J., & Bruck, M. (1993). The suggestibility of the child witness: A historical review and synthesis. *Psychological Bulletin*, 113, 403–439.

Ceci, S. J., & Bruck, M. (1995). *Jeopardy in the courtroom: A scientific analysis of children's testimony.* Washington, D.C.: American Psychological Association.

Ceci, S. J., & Bruck, M. (1998). The ontogeny and durability of true and false memories: A fuzzy trace account. *Journal of Experimental Child Psychology, 71*, 165–169.

Ceci, S. J., & Hembrooke, H. (1998). *Expert witnesses in child abuse cases.* Washington, D.C.: American Psychological Association.

Ceci, S. J., & Friedman, R. D. (2000). The suggestibility of children: Scientific research and legal implications. *Cornell Law Review, 86*, 33–106.

Chialdini, R. (2007). *Influence: The psychology of persuasion.* New York: Harper Collins.

Cicchetti, D., Rogosch, F., Maughan, A., Toth, S., & Bruce, J. (2003). False belief understanding in maltreated children. *Development and Psychopathology, 15*(4), 1067–1091. doi:10.1017/S0954579403000440

Clawar, S., & Rivlin, B. (1992). *Children held hostage: Dealing with programmed and brainwashed children.* Chicago: American Bar Association Family Law Section.

Cohen, A. O., Breiner, K., Steinberg, L., et al. (2016). When is an adolescent an adult? Assessing cognitive control in emotional and nonemotional contexts. *Psychological Science, 27*(4), 549–562. doi:10.1177/0956797615627625

Cooper, A., Wallin, A. R., Quas, J. A., & Lyon, T. D. (2010). Maltreated and nonmaltreated children's knowledge of the juvenile dependency court system. *Child Maltreatment, 15*(3), 255–260. doi:10.1177/1077559510364056

Cross, P. (Ed.). Hearing children: Should you interview a child – And, if so, how? *Journal of American Academy of Matrimonial Lawyers, 18*, 295–296.

Dale, M. (2014). Don't forget the children: Court protection from parent conflict is in the best interests of children. *Family Court Review, 52*(4), 648–654.

Darlington, Y. (2006). Experiences of custody evaluations: Perspectives of young adults who were the subject of family court proceedings as children. *Journal of Child Custody, 3*(1), 51–66.

Davies, J., & Wright, J. (2008). Children's voices: A review of the literature pertinent to looked after children's views of mental health services. *Child and Adolescent Mental Health, 13*(1), 26–31. doi:10.1111/j.1475-3588.2007.00458

Drozd. L., Saini, M., & Olesen, N. (Eds.). (2016). *Parenting plan evaluations: Applied research for the family court* (2nd ed.). New York: Oxford University Press.

Dunn, J., Davies, L. C., & O'Connor, T. G. (2001). Family lives and friendships: The perspectives of children in step-, single-parent, and non-step families. *Journal of Family Psychology, 15*, 272–287.

Ebling, R., Pruett, K., & Pruett, M. (2009). "Get over it": Perspectives on divorce from young children. *Family Court Review, 47*(4), 665–681.

Edelstein, R. S., Luten, T. L., Ekman, P., & Goodman, G. S. (2006). Detecting lies in children and adults. *Law and Human Behavior, 30*(1), 1–10. Retrieved from www.jstor.org/stable/4499456

Eisen, M. L., Quas, J. A., & Goodman, G. S. (2002). *Memory and suggestibility in the forensic interview.* Mahwah, NJ: Lawrence Erlbaum Associates.

Emery, R. (1999). *Marriage, divorce, and children's adjustment.* (2nd ed.). Thousand Oaks, CA: Sage.

Evans, A. D., Brunet, M. K., Talwar, V., Bala, N., Lindsay, R. C. L., & Lee, K. (2012). The effects of repetition on children's true and false reports. *Psychiatry, Psychology, and Law: An Interdisciplinary Journal of the Australian and New Zealand Association of Psychiatry, Psychology and Law, 19*(4). doi:10.1080/13218719.2011.615808

Fabricius, W. V. (2003). Listening to children of divorce: New findings that diverge from Wallerstein, Lewis, & Blakeslee (2000). *Family Relations, 52*, 385–396.

Fabricius, W. B., & Hall, J. A. (2000). Young adults' perspectives on divorce: Living arrangements. *Family and Conciliation Courts Review, 38*(4), 446–461.

Fernando, M. (2009). Conversations between judges and children. *Australian Journal of Family Law, 23*, 48.

Fidler, B. J. (2012). Parenting coordination: Lessons learned and key practice issues. *Canadian Family Law Quarterly, 31*(2), 237–273

Fidler, B. J., & Bala, N. (2010). Children resisting post separation contact with a parent: Concepts, controversies, and conundrums. *Family Court Review, 48*, 10–47.

Fidler, B. J., Bala, N., & Saini, M. A. (2012). *Children who resist post-separation parental contact: A differential approach for legal and mental health professionals. American Psychology-Law Book Series.* New York: Oxford University Press.

Fieldstone, L. B., & Coates, C. A. (2008). *Innovations in interventions with high conflict families.* Madison, WI: Association of Family and Conciliation Courts.

Fieldstone, L., Carter, D., King, T., & McHale, J. (2011). Training, skills and practices of parenting coordinators: Florida statewide study. *Family Court Review, 49*(4), 671–674.

Fieldstone, L., Mackenzie, C., Lee, B., Jason, K., & McHale, J. P. (2012). Perspectives on parenting coordination: Views of parenting coordinators, attorneys, and judiciary members. *Family Court Review, 50*(3), 441–454.

Galván, A. (2017). *The neuroscience of adolescence.* Cambridge fundamentals of neuroscience in psychology. Cambridge and New York: Cambridge University Press. doi:10.1017/9781316106143

Galván, A., Hare, T., Voss, H., Glover, G., & Casey, B. J. (2007). Risk-taking and the adolescent brain: Who is at risk? *Developmental Science, 10*(2), F8–F14. doi:10.1111/j.1467–7687.2006.00579.x. PMID: 17286837.

Gamache, S. (2004). The role of the child specialist. In N. J. Cameron (Ed.), *Collaborative practice: Deepening the dialogue* (pp. 213–221). Vancouver, B.C.: The Continuing Legal Education Society.

Garbarino, J., & Stott, F. (1990). *What children can tell us: Eliciting, interpreting & evaluating information from children.* San Francisco: Jossey-Bass.

Garber, B. D. (2010). *Developmental psychology for family law professionals: Theory, application and best interests of the child.* New York: Springer Publishing.

Garber, B. D. (2011). The voice of the child in high conflict divorce: Systemic, developmental and practice considerations. Paper presented at the Ontario Bar Association, Toronto, February 3–5, 2011.

Gardner, R. (1989). *Family evaluation in child custody mediation, arbitration, and litigation.* Creskill, NJ: Creative Therapeutics.

Garrity, C. B. & Baris, M. A. (1995). *Caught in the middle: Protecting the children of high-conflict divorce.* San Francisco, CA: Josey Bass.

Garwood, F. (1990). Children in conciliation: The experience of involving children in conciliation. *Family and Conciliation Courts Review, 28*(1), 43–51.

Gentry, D. G. (1997). Including children in divorce mediation and education: Potential benefits and cautions. *Families in Society, Journal of Contemporary Human Services, 78*(3). https://journals.sagepub.com/doi/abs/10.1606/1044-3894.779

Goldson, J. (2006). *Hello, I'm a voice, let me talk: Child-inclusive mediation in family separation.* Center for child and family policy research, Auckland University. www.familiescommission.govt.nz/download/innovativepractice-goldson.pdf.

Gollop, M., & Taylor, N. (2012). New Zealand children and young people's perspectives on relocation following parental separation. In M. Freeman (Ed.), *Law and childhood studies* (pp. 219–242). Oxford: Oxford University Press.

Gollop, M., Smith, A. B., & Taylor, N. J. (2000). Children's involvement in custody and access arrangements. *Child and Family Law Quarterly, 12*(4), 396–99.

Goodman, G. S., Quas, J. A., Bulkley, J., & Shapiro, C. (1999). Innovations for child witnesses: A national survey. *Psychology, Public Policy, and Law, 5*(2), 255–281. doi:10.1037/1076–8971.5.2.255

Goodman, G. S., Quas, J. A., & Ogle, C. (2010). Child maltreatment and memory. *Annual Review of Psychology, 61*, 325–354.

Gould, J. W. (2006). *Conducting scientifically crafted custody evaluations* (2nd ed.) Sarasota, FL: Professional Resource Exchange.

Gould, J. W., & Martindale, D. A. (2007). *The art and science of child custody evaluations.* New York: Guilford Press.

Graffam Walker, A. (2013). *Handbook on questioning children: A linguistic perspective* (3rd ed.). Washington, D.C.: ABA Center on Children and the Law.

Greenberg, L. R., & Sullivan, M. (2012). Parenting coordinator and therapist collaboration in high-conflict shared custody cases. *Journal of Child Custody, 9,* 85–107.

Greenberg, M. T., Cicchetti, D., & Cummings, E. M. (1990). *Attachment in the preschool years: Theory, research and intervention.* Chicago: University of Chicago Press.

Greenberg, S. A., & Shuman, D. W. (1997). Irreconcilable conflict between therapeutic and forensic roles. *Professional Psychology: Research and Practice, 28*(1), 50–57.

Grisso, T. (2013). *Forensic evaluation of juveniles* (2nd ed.). Sarasota, FL: Professional Resource Press.

Grisso, T. (2005). *Evaluating juveniles' adjudicative competence: A guide for clinical practice.* Sarasota, FL: Professional Resources Press.

Grisso, T., & Kavanaugh, A. (2016). Prospects for developmental evidence in juvenile sentencing based on *Miller v. Alabama. Psychology, Public Policy and Law, 22*(3), 235–249.

Grisso, T., & Quinlan, J. C. (2005). *Massachusetts youth screening instrument, version 2.* In T. Grisso, G. Vincent, & D. Seagrave (Eds.), (2005). *Mental health screening and assessment in juvenile justice* (pp. 99–111). New York: Guilford Press.

Grisso, T., & Romaine, C. L. R. (2013). Forensic evaluation of juveniles. In R. K. Otto & I. B. Weiner (Eds.), *Handbook of psychology, vol. 11: Forensic psychology* (2nd ed.). Hoboken, NJ: John Wiley & Sons.

Grisso, T., Steinberg, L., Woolard, J. et al. (2003). Juveniles' competence to stand trial: A comparison of adolescents' and adults' capacities as trial defendants. *Law Hum Behav, 27,* 333–363. https://doi.org/10.1023/A:1024065015717

Higuchi, S. A., & Lally, S. J. (Eds.). (2014). *Parenting coordination handbook.* Washington, D.C.: American Psychological Association.

Hobbs, S., Goodman, G. S., Oran, D., Block, S. D., Quas, J. A., Park, A., Widaman, K. F., & Baumrind, N. (in press). Child maltreatment victims' attitudes about appearing in dependency and criminal courts. *Children and Youth Services Review.*

Holtzworth-Munroe, A., Applegate, A., D'Onofrio, B., & Bates, J. (2010). Child informed mediation study CIMS: Incorporating the children's perspective into divorce mediation in an American pilot study. *Journal of Family Studies, 16,* 116–129.

Hritz, A. C., Royer, C. E., Helm, R. K., Burd, K. A., Ojeda, K., & Ceci, S. (2014). Children's suggestibility research: Things to know before interviewing a child. *Anuario de Psicología Jurídica, 25,* 3–12. doi:10/1016/j.api.2014.09.002

Hynan, D. J. (1998). Interviewing children in custody evaluations. *Family & Conciliation Courts Review, 36,* (4), 466–478.

Hynan, D. J. (2003). Parent–child observations in custody evaluations. *Family Court Review, 41,* 214–223.

International Institute for Child Rights and Development. (2007). Hear the child interviews. Kelowna Pilot Evaluation. iicrd@uvic.ca.

Jensen, F., & Ellis Nutt, A. (2014). *The teenage brain: A neuroscientist's survival guide to raising adolescents and young adults.* New York: HarperCollins Publishers.

Johnston, J. R. (1993). Children of divorce who refuse visitation. In C. Depner & J. Bray (Eds.), *Non-residential parenting* (ch. 6).Newbury Park, CA: Sage.

Johnston, J. R. (2003). Parental alignments and rejection: An empirical study of alienation in children of divorce. *Journal of the American Academy of Psychiatry and Law, 31,* 158–170.

Johnston, J. R. (2005). Children of divorce who reject a parent and refuse visitation: Recent research and social policy implications for the alienated child. *Family Law Quarterly, 38*(4), 757–775.

Johnston, J. R., & Roseby, V. (1997). *In the name of the child: A developmental approach to understanding and helping children of conflict and violent divorce.* New York: Free Press.

Johnston, J. R., Roseby, V., & Kuehnle, K. (2009). *In the name of the child: A development approach to understanding and helping children of conflicted and violent divorce* (2nd ed.). New York: Springer.

Karen, R. (1994). *Becoming attached: First relationships and how they shape our capacity to love.* Oxford and New York: Oxford University Press.

Karle, M., & Gathmann, S. (2016). The state of the art of child hearings in Germany. Results of a nationwide representative study in German courts. *Family Court Review*, *54*(2), 167–185.

Kelly, J. B. (2000). Children's adjustment in conflicted marriage and divorce: A decade review of research. *Journal of Child and Adolescent Psychiatry*, *39*, 8, 1–11.

Kelly, J. B. (2002). Psychological and legal interventions for parents and children in custody and access disputes: Current research and practice. *Virginia Journal of Social Policy and the Law*, *10*(1), 129–163.

Kelly, J. B. (2003). Parents with enduring child disputes: Multiple pathways to enduring disputes. *Journal of Family Studies*, *9*(1), 37–50.

Kelly, J. B. (2003). Parents with enduring child disputes: Focused interventions with parents in enduring disputes. *Journal of Family Studies*, *9*(1), 51–62.

Kelly, J. B. (2005). Developing beneficial parenting plan models for children following separation and divorce. *Journal of American Academy of Matrimonial Lawyers*, *19*, 237–254.

Kelly, J. B. (2007). Children's living arrangements following separation and divorce: Insights from empirical and clinical research. *Family Process*, *46*(1), 35–52.

Kelly, J. B. (2008). Preparing for the parenting coordination role: Training needs for mental health and legal professionals. *Journal of Child Custody*, *5*(1/2), 140–159.

Kelly, J. B. (2014). Including children in the parenting coordination process: A specialized role. In S. A. Higuchi & S. J. Lally (Eds.), *Parenting coordination handbook*. Washington, D.C.: American Psychological Association.

Kelly, J. B., & Emery, R. E. (2003). Children's adjustment to divorce: Risk and resiliency perspectives. *Family Relations*, *52*(4), 352–362.

Kelly, J. B., & Johnston, J. R. (2001). The alienated child: A reformulation of Parental Alienation Syndrome. *Family Court Review*, *39*(3), 249–266.

Kelly, J. B., & Kisthardt, M. K. (2009). Helping parents tell their children about separation and divorce: Social science frameworks and the lawyer's counseling responsibility. *Journal of American Academy of Matrimonial Lawyers*, *22*, 1401–1420.

Kelly, J., & Wallerstein, J. (1977). Brief Interventions with children in divorcing families. *American Journal of Orthopsychiatry*, *47*, 23–29.

Klemfuss, J. Z., Qua, J. A., & Lyon, T. D. (2014). Attorneys' questions and children's productivity in child sexual abuse criminal trials. *Applied Cognitive Psychology*, *28*, 780–788, doi:10.1002/acp.3048

Kuehnle, K. & Connell, M. (2009). *The evaluation of child sexual abuse allegations: A comprehensive guide to assessment and testimony*. Hoboken, NJ: John Wiley & Sons.

Kuehnle, K., & Drozd, L. (Eds.). (2012). *Parenting plan evaluations: Applied research for the family court*. New York: Oxford University Press.

Kuehnle, K., Greenberg, L. R., & Gottlieb, M. C. (2004). Incorporating the principles of scientifically based child interviews into family law cases. *Journal of Child Custody*, *1*(1), 97–114.

Kuehnle, K., Ludolph, P. S., & Brubacher, S. (2016). Assessing allegations of child sexual abuse in child custody litigation: Children's memory and behavior in the forensic evaluation. In L. Drozd, M. Saini, & N. Olesen (Eds.), *Parenting plan evaluations: Applied research for the family court* (2nd ed.). New York: Oxford University Press.

Lamb, M. E., La Rooy, D. J., Malloy, L. C., & Katz, C. (2011). *Children's testimony: A handbook of psychological research and forensic practice* (2nd ed.). Chichester: Wiley-Blackwell.

Lamb, M., Orbach, Y., Hershkowitz, I., Esplin, P. W., & Horowitz, D. (2007). A structured forensic interview protocol improves the quality and informativeness of investigative interviews with children: A review of research using the NICHD Investigative Interview Protocol. *Child Abuse & Neglect*, *31*, 1201–1231.

La Rooy, D., Katz, C., Malloy, L. C., & Lamb, M. E. (2010). Do we need to rethink guidance on repeated interviews? *Psychology, Public Policy, and Law*, *16*(4), 373–392. doi:10.1037/a0019909

Larson, K., & Grisso, T. (2016). Transfer and commitment of youth in the United States: Law, policy and forensic practice. In K. Heilbrun, D. DeMatteo and N. E. S. Goldstein (Eds.), *APA handbook of psychology and juvenile justice*, (pp. 445–466). Washington, D.C.: American Psychological Association.

Lawrence, J. A., Levin, D. B., Brady, K. L., Jhai, M., & Lyon, T. D. (2015). Ohio v. Clark: Brief of amicus curiae American Professional Society on the abuse of children in support of petitioner. *Psychology, Public Policy, and Law, 21*(4), 365–373. http://dx.doi.org/10.1037/law0000062

Lee, S. M., & Kaufman, R. L. (2009). Disorganized attachment in young children: Manifestations, etiology and implications for child custody. *Journal of Child Custody, 6*(1/2), 62–90.

Lee, S. M., Borelli, J. L., & West, J. L. (2011). Children's attachment relationships: Can attachment data be used in child custody evaluations? *Journal of Child Custody, 8*(3), 212–242.

Lippincott, J., & Deutsch, R. (2005). *7 Things your teenager won't tell you and how to talk about them anyway.* New York: Ballantine Books.

Lyon, T. D. (2005). *Ten step child investigative interviews.* (Adaptation of NICHD Investigative Interview Protocol). http://works.bepress.com/thomaslyon/5

Lyon, T. D., Carrick, N., & Quas, J. A. (2010). Young children's competency to take the oath: Effects of task, maltreatment, and age. *Law and Human Behavior, 34*(2), 141–149. doi:10.1007/s10979-009-9177-9

Lyon, T. D., Wandrey, L., Ahern, E., Licht, R., Sim, M., & Quas, J. A. (in press). Eliciting maltreated and non-maltreated children's transgression disclosures: Narrative practice, rapport building, and a putative confession. *Child Development.*

Mackenzie, M., Bosk, E., & Zeanah, C. (2017). Separating families at the border: Consequences for children's health and well-being. *The New England Journal of Medicine, 376.* doi:10.1056/NEJMp1703375

Malloy, L., Mugno, A., Rivard, J., Lyon, T. D., & Quas, J. (2016). Familial influences on recantation in substantiated child sexual abuse cases. *Child Maltreatment, 21*(256). https://ssrn.com/abstract=2773711

Martinson, D. (2010). *Hearing children's voices in alienation cases: The legal framework.* Prepared for the Association of Family and Conciliation Courts' 47th Annual Conference, *Traversing the Trail of Alienation,* Denver, Colorado, June 2–5, 2010. AFCCnet.org

Martinson, D., & Bell, N. (2014). *Legal professionalism and access to justice for children.* The Advocate (British Columbia Law Society). https://ethicsincanada.com/2014/02/20/d-martinson-and-n-bell-legal-professionalism-and-access-to-justice-lawyers-as-champions-for-children

McAuliff, B. D., Nicholson, E., Amarilio, D., & Ravanshenas, D. (2013). Supporting children in U. S. legal proceedings: Descriptive and attitudinal data from a national survey of victim/witness assistants. *Psychology, Public Policy, and Law, 19*(1), 98–113. doi:10.1037/a0027879

McColley, D. (November 2012). Top ten tips for judicial interview of children, AFCC Member Center – Ask The Experts.

McIntosh, J. (2000). Child inclusive divorce mediation: *Report on a qualitative research project. Mediation Quarterly, 18*(1), 55–69.

McIntosh, J., & Long, C. (2006). *Children beyond dispute: A prospective study of outcomes from child focused and child inclusive post-separation family dispute resolution. Final Report for Attorney General's Department, Canberra, Australia.* https://www.researchgate.net/publication/305355200_Children_beyond_dispute_a_prospective_study_of_outcomes_from_child_focused_and_child_inclusive_post-separation_family_dispute_resolution_Final_report

McIntosh, J. E., Wells, Y. D., & Long, C. M. (2007). Child-focused and child-inclusive family law dispute resolution: One year findings from a prospective study of outcomes. *Journal of Family Studies, 13*(1), 8–25.

McIntosh, J. E., Wells, Y. D., Smyth, B. M., & Long, C. M. (2008). Child-focused and child-inclusive divorce mediation: Comparative outcomes from a prospective study of post separation adjustment. *Family Court Review, 46*, 105–124.

McSweeney, L., & Leach, C. (2011). *Children's participation in family law decision-making: Considerations for striking the balance.* Paper presented to the Ontario Association of Family Mediators, May 27, 2011. https://www.oafm.on.ca

Melton, G. B. (1999). Parents and children: Legal reform to facilitate children's participation. *American Psychologist, 54*, 935–942.

Miller, W. R., & Rollnick, S. (2012). *Motivational interviewing: Helping people change* (3rd ed.). New York: Guilford Press.

Milojevich, H. M., Russell, M. A., & Quas, J. A. (2018). Unpacking the associations among maltreatment, disengagement coping, and behavioral functioning in high-risk youth. *Child Maltreatment, 23*(4), 355–364. doi:10.1177/1077559518778805

Mitnick, M. (Ed.). *Top ten tips for interviewing children.* AFCC e-news: Ask the Experts. www.afccnet.org.

Morag, T., Rivkin, D., & Sorek, Y. (2012). Child's participation in the family courts: Lessons from the Israeli pilot project, *International Journal Law, Policy and the Family, 26*(1), 1–30.

Morley, J. (2013). The impact of foreign law on child custody determinations. *Journal of Child Custody, 10*(3–4), 209–235.

Myers, J. E. B. (Ed.). (2011). *The APSAC handbook on child maltreatment* (3rd ed.). Los Angeles, CA: Sage Publications.

National Research Council. (2013). *Reforming juvenile justice: A developmental approach.* Washington, D.C.: The National Academies Press. https://doi.org/10.17226/14685.

Newell, S., Graham, A., & Fitzgerald, R. M. (2009). *Results of an international survey regarding children's participation in decision-making following parental separation.* Childwatch International Research Network's Children & the Law Thematic Study Group, Southern Cross University, Lismore, NSW, Australia. http://epubs.scu.edu.au/cgi/viewcontent.cgi-article=1350&context=educ_pubs

O'Donohue, W. T., & Fanetti, M. (Eds.). (2016). *Forensic interviews regarding child sexual abuse: A guide to evidence-based practice.* Cham, Switzerland: Springer Publishing. https://doi.org/10.1007/978-3-319-21097-1_8

Ornstein, P. A., Merritt, K. A., Baker-Ward, L., Furtado, E., Gordon, B. N., & Principe, G. (1998). Children's knowledge, expectation, and long-term retention. *Applied Cognitive Psychology, 12,* 387–405.

Paetsch, J. J., Bertrand, L. D., Walker, J., MacRae, L. D., & Bala, N. (2009). Consultation on the voice of the child at the 5th World Congress on Family Law and Children's Rights (National Judicial Institute and Canadian Research Institute for Law and the Family, for Department of Justice) Canada. https://prism.ucalgary.ca/bitstream/handle/1880/107463/Consultation%20on%20Voice%20of%20the%20Child%20-%20Dec%202009.pdf?sequence=1&isAllowed=y

Parkinson, P., & Cashmore, J. (2007). Judicial conversations with children in parenting disputes: The views of Australian judges. *International Journal of Law, Policy and the Family, 21*(2), 160–189.

Parkinson, P., & Cashmore, J. (2008). *The voice of a child in family law disputes.* Oxford: Oxford University Press.

Parkinson, P., Cashmore, J., & Single, J. (2005). Adolescents' views on the fairness of parenting and financial arrangements after separation. *Family Court Review, 43,* 429–444.

Parkinson, P., Cashmore, J., & Single, J. (2007). Parents' and children's views on talking to judges in parenting disputes in Australia. *International Journal of Law, Policy and the Family, 21,* 84–107.

Peterson, C. (1999). Children's memory for medical emergencies: Two years later. *Developmental Psychology, 35,* 1493–1506.

Peterson, C., Baker-Ward, L., Morris, G. and Flynn, S. (2014). Predicting which childhood memories persist: Contributions of memory characteristics. *Developmental Psychology, 50, 2,* 439–448. doi:10.1037/a0033221.

Pezdek, K., Morrow, A., Blandon-Gitlin, I., Goodman, G. S., Quas, J. A., Saywitz, K. J., & Brodie, L. (2004). Detecting deception in children: Event familiarity affects criterion-based content analysis ratings. *Journal of Applied Psychology, 89*(1), 119–126. doi:10.1037/0021–9010.89.1.119

Pipe, M.-E., Lamb, M., Orbach, Y., & Cederborg, A.-C. (2007). *Child sexual abuse: Disclosure, delay and denial.* New York: Routledge.

Poole, D. A. (2016). *Interviewing children: The science of conversation in forensic contexts.* Washington, D.C.: American Psychological Association.

Poole, D. A., & Lamb, M. E. (1998). *Investigative interviews of children: A guide for helping professionals.* Washington, D.C.: American Psychological Association.

Quas, J. A., & Goodman, G. S. (2011). Consequences of criminal court involvement for child victims. *Psychology, Public Policy, & Law, 18,* 392–414.

Quas, J. A., & Goodman, G. S. (2012). Consequences of criminal court involvement for child victims. *Psychology, Public Policy, and Law, 18*(3), 392–414. http://dx.doi.org/10.1037/a0026146

Quas, J. A., Davis, E. L., Goodman, G. S., & Myers, J. E. B. (2007). Repeated questions, deception, and children's true and false reports of body touch. *Child Maltreatment, 12*(1), 60–67. doi:10.1177/1077559506296141

Quas, J. A., Goodman, G. S., Ghetti, S., Alexander, K. W., Edelstein, R., Redlich, A. D., Cordon, I. M., & Jones, D. P. H. (2005). Childhood sexual assault victims: Long term outcomes after testifying in criminal court. *Monographs of the Society for Research in Child Development, 70*(2), vii, 1–128. doi:10.1111/j.1540–5834.2005.00336.x

Quas, J. A., Malloy, L. C., Melinder, A., Goodman, G. S., D'Mello, M., & Schaaf, J. (2007). Developmental differences in the effects of repeated interviews and interviewer bias on young children's event memory and false reports. *Developmental Psychology, 43*(4), 823–837. http://doi.org/10.1037/0012-1649.43.4.823

Quas, J. A., Thompson, W. C., & Clarke-Stewart, K. A. (2005). Do jurors "know" what isn't so about child witnesses?. *Law and Human Behavior, 29*(4), 425–456. www.jstor.org/stable/4499431

Quas, J. A., Wallin, A. R., Horwitz, B., Davis, E., & Lyon, T. (2009). Maltreated children's knowledge of and emotional reactions to dependency court involvement. *Behavioral and the Law, 27,* 97–117.

Reyna, V., & Rivers, S. (2008). Special issue: Current directions in risk and decision making. *Developmental Science, 28*(1), 1–152.

Rudolph, M. D., Miranda-Domínguez, O., Cohen, A. O., Breiner, K., Steinberg, L., Bonnie, R. J., Scott, E. S., Taylor-Thompson, K., Chein, J., Fettich, K. C., Richeson, J. A., Dellarco, D. V., Galván, A., Casey, B. J., & Fair, D. A. (2017). At risk of being risky: The relationship between "brain age" under emotional states and risk preference. *Developmental Cognitive Neuroscience, 24*(93). doi:10.1016/j.dcn.2017.01.010. Epub 2017 Feb 1. PMID: 28279917; PMCID: PMC584923.

Rush, E. B., Lyon, T. D., Ahern, E. C., & Quas, J. A. (2014). Disclosure suspicion bias and abuse disclosure: Comparisons between sexual and physical abuse. *Child Maltreatment, 19*(2), 113–118. doi:10.1177/1077559514538114

Saklofske, D., Reynolds, C. R., & Schwean, V. (2013). *The Oxford handbook of child psychological assessment.* New York: Oxford University Press.

Sanchez, E. A., & Kibler-Sanchez, S. (2004). Empowering children in mediation: An intervention model. *Family Court Review, 42*(3), 554–575.

Saposnek, D. T. (2004). Working with children in mediation. In J. Folberg, A. Milne, & P. Salem (Eds.), *Divorce and family mediation* (ch. 8). New York: Guilford Press.

Sattler, J. M. (1998). *Clinical and forensic interviewing of children and families.* San Diego, CA: Jerome Sattler.

Saywitz, K. J. (2002). Developmental underpinnings of children's testimony. In H. L. Westcott, G. M. Davies, & R. H.C Bull (Eds.), *Children's testimony.* New York: Wiley.

Saywitz, K. J. (2008). The art of interviewing young children in custody disputes. *Family Advocate, 30*(4), 26–29.

Saywitz, K. J., & Camparo, L. (1998). Interviewing child witnesses: A developmental perspective. *Child Abuse and Neglect, 22,* 825–843.

Saywitz, K. J., Camparo, L. B., & Ramanoff, A. (2010). Interviewing children in custody cases: Implications of research and policy for practice. *Behavioral Sciences and the Law, 28,* 542–562.

Schoffer, M. J. (2005). Bring children to the mediation table. *Family Court Review, 43*(2), 323–338.

Schuman, J. P., Bala, N., & Lee, K. (1999). Developmentally appropriate questions for child witnesses. *Queens Law Journal, 25,* 251–302.

Schutz, & Pruett, M. (2013). How to unearth important facts from your child client. Workshop #13, AFCC Kansas City, Missouri. AFCCnet.org

Semple, N. (2010). The silent child: A quantitative analysis of children's evidence in Canadian custody and access cases. *Canadian Family Law Quarterly, 29*(1), 1–24.

Siegel, D. (2012). *The developing mind* (2nd ed.). New York: Guilford Press.

Siegel, D. (2013). *Brainstorm: The power and purpose of the teenage brain.* New York: Penguin.

Smart, C. (2002). From children's shoes to children's voices. *Family Court Review, 40,* 307–319.

Smart, C., & Neale, B. (2000). "It's my life too" – Children's perspectives on post-divorce parenting. *Family Law* (30), 163–169.

Smith, A. B., & Gallop, M. M. (2001). What children think separating parents should know. *New Zealand Journal of Psychology, 30*, 23–31.

Smith, A. B., Taylor, N. J., & Tapp, P. (2003). Rethinking children's involvement in decision-making after parental separation. *Childhood, 10*(2), 210–216.

Solomon, J., & George, C. (1999). *Attachment disorganization*. New York: Guilford Press.

Sparta, S. N., & Koocher, G. P. (Eds.). (2006). *Forensic mental health assessment of children and adolescents*. New York: Oxford Press.

Sroufe, L. A., Egeland, B., Carlson, E. A., & Collins, W. A. (2005). *The development of the person: The Minnesota study of risk and adaptation from birth to adulthood*. New York: Guilford Press.

Stahl, P. R. (1994). *Conducting child custody evaluations*. Thousand Oaks, CA: Sage Publications.

Stahl, P. R. (2007). Don't forget about me: Implementing Article 12 of the United Nations Convention on the Rights of the Child. *Arizona J. & Int'l Comp., 50*, 803. http://arizonajournal. org/wp-content/uploads/2015/11/6.-Stahl-9x6-Text.pdf

Stahl, P. R. (2011). *Conducting child custody evaluations: From basic to complex issues*. New York: Sage Publications.

Steinberg, L. (2017). Adolescent brain science and juvenile justice policymaking. *Psychology, Public Policy, and Law, 23*(4), 410–420. http://dx.doi.org/10.1037/law0000128

Steinberg, L. (2014). *Age of opportunity: Lessons from the new science of adolescence*. Boston, MA: Houghton Mifflin Harcourt.

Stolzenberg, S. N., & Lyon, T. D. (2014). "Evidence summarized in attorneys' closing arguments predicts acquittals in criminal trials of child sexual abuse." *Child Maltreatment*. doi:1077559514539388

Strange, D., Sutherland, R., & Garry, M. (2006). Event plausibility does not determine children's false memories, *Memory, 14*(8), 937–951

Talwar, V., & Lee, K. (2008). Socio-cognitive correlates of children's lying behaviour: Conceptual understanding of lying, executive functioning, and false beliefs. *Child Development, 79*, 866–881.

Talwar, V., Gordon, H., & Lee, K. (2007). Lie -telling behavior in school-age children. *Developmental Psychology, 43*, 804–810.

Talwar, V., Lee, K., Bala, N., & Lindsay, R. C. L. (2002). Children's conceptual knowledge of lying and its relation to their actual behaviors: Implications for court competence examinations. *Law and Human Behavior, 26*, 395–415.

Talwar, V., Lee, K., Bala, N., & Lindsay, R. C. L. (2004). Children's lie-telling to conceal a parent's transgression: Legal implications. *Law & Human Behavior, 28*, 411–435.

Talwar, V., Lee, K., Bala, N., & Lindsay, R. C. L. (2006). Adults' judgments of children's coached reports. *Law and Human Behavior, 30*(5), 561–570. doi:10.1007/s10979–006–9038–8

Taylor, N. (2006). What do we know about involving children and young people in family law decision making? A research update. *Australian Journal of Family Law, 20*(2), 154–178.

Taylor, N. (2007). Discussions with children in the family court: The research evidence. Presentation at Family Court Update: Discussions with Children February 27–28, 2007, Wellington, New Zealand.

Taylor, N., Caldwell, J., & Boshier, P. (2013). Judicial interviews of children: Documenting practice within the New Zealand Family Court. Paper presented for Workshop 77, AFCC, May 29– June 1. AFCCnet.org

Trinder, L. (1997). Competing constructions of childhood: Children's rights and children's wishes in divorce. *Journal of Social Welfare and Family Law, 19*(3), 291–305.

Turoy-Smith, K. M., Brubacher, S. P., Earhart, B., & Powell, M. B. (2018). Eliciting children's recall regarding home life and relationships. *Journal of Child Custody*. doi:10.1080/15379418.2018.1530 629.

Walker, A. G. (1999). *Handbook on questioning children: A linguistic perspective* (2nd ed., pp. 1–14).Washington, D.C.: ABA Center for Children and Law.

Wallerstein, J., & Kelly, J. (1980). *Surviving the breakup: How children & parents cope with divorce*. New York: Basic Books.

Wandrey, L., Lyon, T. D., Quas, J. A., & Friedman, W. (2011). Maltreated children's ability to estimate temporal location and numerosity of placement changes and court visits. *Psychology, Public, Policy, and Law, 18*, 79–104.

Warshak, R. (1992). *The custody revolution: The father factor and the motherhood mystique*. New York: Poseidon Press.

Warshak, R. (2003). Payoffs and pitfalls of listening to children. *Family Relations, 52*(4), 373–384.

Westcott, H. L., Davies, G. M., & Bull, R. H. C. (2002). *Children's testimony: A handbook of psychological research and forensic practice*. Chichester: John Wiley & Sons.

Wier, K. (2011). High -conflict contact disputes: Evident of the extreme unreliability of some children's ascertainable wishes and feelings. *Family Court Review, 49*(4), 788–800.

Williams, S. S. (2006). *Through the eyes of young people: Meaningful child participation in BC family court processes*. www.iicrd.orgt/child participation.

Williams, S. S. (2010). Judges listening to children directly in separation and divorce proceedings: Individual, institutional and international guidelines. (Paper presented to the National Judicial Institute of Canada Family Law Program, Toronto, February 2010 [unpublished]. www.nji.inm.ca

Williams, S. S., & Helland, J. (2007). Hear the child interviews: Kelowna pilot evaluation: May 2007. IICRD. www.iicrd.orgt/childparticipation

Yasenik, L. A., & Graham, J. M. (2016). The continuum of including children in ADR processes: A child-centered continuum model. *Family Court Review, 54*(2), 186–202.

Zeanah, C. H. (2019). *Handbook of infant mental health* (4th ed.) New York: Guilford Press.

Index

Page numbers in *italics* refer to figures. Page numbers with 'n' refer to notes.

Abbott v. Abbott (2001) 262
acquiescence, defense of 262–263
adaptive functioning, measures of 301, 302–303
adjudication 15, 21, 22, 23, 38, 47
adjudicative competence 299, 303–304
adolescents: brain development 16–17, 24–25, 26, 28–29, 33–34, 307–308; developmental characteristics 307–308; gender non-conforming 253; guarded 187–188; identity of 192; psychopathology 308; and trauma 188, 190–191; *see also* juvenile courts; juvenile justice system
adoption 5, 145–147, 154, 240, 250; foster-adopt home 144–145; parental rights 128, 146, 153; by same-sex couples 242; *see also* surrogacy
Adoption Assistance and Child Welfare Act of 1980 130
adult courts, transfer of youth to 3, 12, 27, 29, 32–33, 46, 303
adverse childhood experiences (ACEs) 174, 314
advocates for children 311–315
advocates for the disabled 307
age: of child witness 98; raise the age legislation 4, 28–30, 31; -related changes in memory of children 58–60; sufficient age and maturity defense 257, 263, 264, 265, 269–271, 272
Ainsworth, Mary 152
Alabama Supreme Court 33
Alcala v. Hernandez (2015) 263
alcohol use 19, 192
alibi witness 99
alienation, and separation of families 230, 277–278, 281, 284
Alito, Samuel 264
almshouses 112
alternative dispute resolution (ADR) 267, 277
Alvarez, Anne 137, 148
amenability hearings 32–33
American Academy of Pediatrics 253
American Psychiatric Association 308
American Psychological Association (APA) 117, 316; Ethical Principles of Psychologists and Code of Conduct (EPPCC) 304, 317, 318, 327;

Psychological Bulletin 186; *see also* Specialty Guidelines for Forensic Psychology
Americans with Disabilities Act 183, 307
amygdala 16, 17, 63
Anderson, L. 96
Annie E. Casey Foundation 37
antisocial personality disorder 31
approach-oriented coping 72
Archer, R. P. 121
assent 297, 326
assessment of children 113–114; clinical *vs.* forensic assessment 116–118; criminal court 116; data collection 119–121; data organization 121–122; family court 115–116; juvenile court 114–115; multi-modal assessment 119; report writing 122; testimony 122–123
assisted conception 245, 246
assisted reproductive technologies (ART) 235, 244, 252
Association of Family and Conciliation Courts (AFCC) 226, 227
asylum seekers 116, 167–168
Atkins v. Virginia (2002) 25
attachment 152–153, 161; case study 154–157; Circle of Security 152, *153*, 161; and coercive control 227; definition of 152; disorganized 284; disruptions 157, 162, 171, 227, 228, 237; expert witness testimony 153, 156–157, 159–162; information about 120; and memory 73; and mothers 237; multiple attachment relationships 237; of out-of-home care children 142; parent–child 236–237; secure 161
attachment disorders 147
attention during encoding 64
attorney counsel for foster care children 132
attorney-questioning tactics 92
attorney representation for youth 13–14, 20, 21–22
Atwater, Ann 50–51
authoritarian parenting 172
autobiographical memory 55, 56, 61
automatic transfer laws 32
avoidant-oriented coping 72, 73

Baby, In re (2014) 249–251
Baiocco, Roberto 242
Baker-Ward, Lynne 61, 63, 64, 75, 188, 200
Bala, N. 216, 233
Baruch, R. 175
Batterers Intervention Program (BIP) 226
battering 227
Baxter v. Baxter (2005) 263
behavioral checklists 121
Behavior Assessment System for Children
    (BASC) 303
Berrick, Jill Doerr 127
best-interest advocacy model 312–313, *313*
best interest of the child (BIC) 166; and adop-
    tion 154, 155–156, 157; and CASA/GAL
    volunteers 312; family law 115, 118, 122;
    and Hague Convention cases 116, 257–258,
    272, 274; and immigrant children 164; and
    intimate partner violence 226; juveniles 13,
    15, 22, 43, 47–48; and parenting 238, 239; and
    reunification 132
birth control 237
Blackmun, Harry 38
Blackstone, William 300
Block, S. D. 196
body diagrams, use in interviews 71
Borelli, Jessica L. 120
Boswell, John 129
Bow, J. N. 224
Bowlby, John 73, 152, 157, 236–237
Boxer, P. 224
Brace, Charles Loring 112
brain development 14, 15–16, 27; adolescent
    16–17, 24–25, 26, 28–29, 33–34, 307–308; and
    coercive interrogation techniques 33–34; and
    diagnosis of personality disorders 31; effect
    of drugs, trauma, and mental health issues
    on 18; and legal policy 19; and minimum age
    of criminal responsibility 31; and raise the
    age legislation 28–29; and stress/trauma 175
brain stem 16
Breed v. Jones (1975) 23
Brennan, William J., Jr. 22
Brevard, K. C. 135
Breyer, Stephen 33
Brief Focused Assessment (BFA) 116
broken windows policing theory 13, 14
Bronfenbrenner, U. 167
Brown, D. A. 76, 205
Brown, E.-J. 76
Bruce v. Boardwine (2015) 246
Bruck, M. 74, 200
burden of proof 2–3, 131
Burgwyn-Bailes, E. 74–75

California: California Family Code section
    7612 241–242; California Welfare Code 300
    131; child custody evaluations, guidelines
    for performing 279; courts, child-friendly

approach in 133; intimate partner violence
    law 225; Safety Organization Practice 134;
    sperm donation statute 244–245, 246–247
Calloway, Ginger 5–6, 121, 282
Campaign for Youth Justice 29
Cannon, Cole 26
Caretaker's Perception of Youth's Adjudication
    299, 304
case law 10, 20, 27–28, 307
case materials, use by forensic practitioners 328
Cassidy, Jude 73, 152
Ceci, S. J. 200
Central America 165; authoritarian parenting
    in 172; gangs in 169, 172; health services in
    171; homicide rates in 169; inequity and ine-
    quality in 170; pre-immigration development/
    risks 170–173; reasons for migration from
    168–169; violence against vulnerable groups
    in 169; *see also* immigrant children
Central Park jogger case 12, 34
cerebellum 16
cerebral cortex 16
cerebrum 16
Chae, Y. 73, 89
child abuse cases 56, 119, 130, 233; *see also* child
    sexual abuse; intimate partner violence (IPV)
Child Abuse Prevention and Treatment Act
    (CAPTA) of 1974 95, 130, 131, 132
child advocacy 132, 134–135
child advocacy centers (CACs) 91, 92
Child Behavior Checklist (CBCL) 121, 283, 286
child-centered approach to child welfare 130
child custody 3, 277; cases, child sexual abuse
    allegations in 212–217; and gender identifi-
    cation 240–241; and gender non-conforming
    children 253; international disputes 257;
    rights, and Hague Convention cases 262
child custody evaluations (CCE) 117, 118, 212,
    259; case analysis 283–284; case background
    and referral 280–282; context of 278–280;
    data collection 119, 121; document review
    282; initial interview with parents 282; par-
    enting coordinator 292–293; plan of contact
    for parents 293; procedures employed by
    evaluator 282–283; treatment interventions
    292–293
child custody recommending counselor 252
childhood amnesia 59
childhood trauma *see* trauma
child protection. history of 129–130
Child Protective Services 127, 153, 166
child removal 131–132, 139, 140, 161
Children's Aid Society 112
child-responsive courts 133–134
child sexual abuse 6, 113, 172, 188–193, 196–197;
    and age of child witness 98; child custody
    case 212–217; context 199; criminal case
    202–206; dependency case 209–212; develop-
    ing and testing multiple hypotheses 201, 205,

211, 216; false allegations 196, 216; false negatives 197; false positives 196–197; interviewing practices 198–199; juvenile criminal cases 206–209; memory and suggestibility 199–200; rates of 196; soft psychosocial evidence 196; source monitoring 200–201, 204, 205; standards of proof 197–198; testimony of abused children 91–92

child welfare system 49, 127, 130, 131–132, 136

CHINS (Child in Need of Services) *see* undisciplined cases

Circle of Security 152, *153*, 161

civil cases 6; childhood sexual abuse 188–193; guarded adolescents 187–188; mental health expert witness 182, 183–184, 188; personal injury cases, history of 182–183; psychological testing 184–187, 190–191

Civil Rights Act 183

clear and compelling evidence 3, 119, 131, 197, 245, 263

Cleveland, K. 98

clinical assessment 116–118

closed-circuit television (CCTV) testimony 97, 98

coaching, and child sexual abuse cases 201

coercive control in intimate partner violence 227–228, 230–231

coercive interrogation techniques, elimination of 33–35

collateral sources of information 118, 265, 283, 284, 290, 326, 328

Columbine High School shooting 13

Commission on Juvenile Crime and Justice, North Carolina 47

communication of forensic practitioners 321; accuracy, fairness, and avoidance of deception 331–332; with collateral sources of information 326; commenting on other professionals/participants in legal proceedings 332; commenting upon legal proceedings 333; comprehensive/accurate presentation of opinions 332; differentiating observations, inferences, and conclusions 332; disclosing sources of information and bases of opinions 332; with examinees 325–326; out of court statements 332; in research contexts 326; with retaining party 325

competence of forensic practitioners: appreciation of individual/group differences 320–321; appropriate use of services/products 321; gaining and maintaining 319–320; and impact of personal beliefs/experience 320; knowledge of legal system and legal rights of individuals 320; knowledge of scientific foundation for opinions/testimony 320; knowledge of scientific foundation for teaching/research 320; representation of 320; scope of 319

competency, testimonial 92–94

competency restoration training 300, 306, 307

competency to proceed *see* competency to stand trial (CST)

competency to stand trial (CST) 303–304, 305–307

competent practice 318

confessions, juvenile 21, 27–28, 34–35

confidence of child witnesses 98, 99

confidentiality 20–21, 297, 327–328

conflict-driven intimate partner violence 228–229

conflicts of forensic practitioners 326–327; avoiding conflicts of interest 319; with legal authority 327; with organizational demands 327; resolving ethical issues with fellow professionals 327

Conflict Tactics Scale 283, 290

Connecticut, raise the age legislation in 29

consent, defense of 262–263, 268, 272

context specificity, and memory 60–61

conversation, effects on memory 65–67, 200, 204–205

Cooper, G. 152

co-parenting 278

coping behaviors, effects on memory 72–73

Corpening, Jay 36

corporal discipline 135

cortisol 18

Costa Rica 169

Cournos, Francine 127, 147

court-appointed special advocate (CASA): best-interest advocacy model 312–313, *313*; impact on lives of children 314–315; origin of 311–312; volunteers 314

court counselors 15, 38

creativity, and suggestibility 74

criminal court 9, 166; assessment of children 116, 119; child sexual abuse allegations in 202–209

Crooks, C. V. 233

cross-examination 92

Crouse, Ex parte (1839) 9

cruel and unusual punishment, ban on 23, 24, 25–26

culpability of juveniles 14, 19, 24, 25–26, 32, 33, 115

culture: cultural competence, and non-traditional families 251–252; differences, effect on interviews 208; and international family disputes 258; Latino 171, 172, 175; shifts, of family 237–241; and suggestibility 200; and views of sexuality 199

Cummings, C. 196

Dahl, L. 99

Daignault, I. 91

Daubert standard 158–159

death penalty for juveniles 23, 24, 25

decriminalization of normal teen behaviors 37

defensive violence 229–230
Deferred Action for Childhood Arrivals (DACA) 168
deinstitutionalization of status offenders (DSO) 11
delay interval 64, 70; complications in legal system 67; effects of conversation 65–67; effects of intervening experiences 64–65
De Mause, Lloyd 129
Denver Juvenile Court 10
Department of Social Services (DSS) 49, 114, 153, 154, 212
dependency advocacy programs 148
dependency court 2, 5, 131; child advocacy and representation 132; child removal 131–132; child-responsive courts 133–134; child sexual abuse allegations in 197, 209–212; duration of dependency hearings 133–134; programs for child participation 134–135; time frames for juvenile dependency process 131–132; training for judicial decision makers 134
depositions 187, 279
depression 87, 297, 299, 304, 306
desegregation of schools 50–51
De Silva v. Pitts (2007) 263
detention: alternatives to 35; hearing 131; pretrial 24
Developmental History Form 283, 286, 287, 299
developmentally normative sexual behavior in children 199
developmental psychopathology 308
Diagnostic and Statistical Manual of Mental Disorders, Fifth Edition (DSM-5) 31, 87, 88, 300, 308
Diagnostic Assessment of Post Traumatic Stress (DAPS) 299
Dickens, Charles 129
diligence of forensic practitioners: communication 321; provision of services 321; responsiveness 321; termination of services 322
Dilulio, John 12, 45, 47
direct file 12, 32
disorderly conduct 37
disorganized attachment 147, 285
dispositions 4, 15, 38, 47, 48, 119, 131
disproportionate minority contact (DMC) 11, 14
dissociation 87–88
dissociative identity disorder 192
divorce 6, 235, 277; and alienation 277–278, 281, 284; high conflict 277; parental alienation syndrome 277; *see also* child custody evaluations (CCE)
documentation, forensic assessment 330–331
document review in child custody evaluations 282
dolls, use in interviews 71, 198
domestic violence 2, 87, 171, 226, 280; *see also* intimate partner violence (IPV)

dopamine 17–18
double jeopardy 23, 44
drawings, use in interviews 71, 198
drawing task 137–138, *138, 139,* 140
Drozd, Leslie M. 274
drugs 18, 19, 190, 192
due process 10, 14, 20, 21, 44, 48
Duke University 50
Durham County Teen Court & Restitution Program 46
Dusky v. United States (1960) 300
Dykas, M. J. 73

E.C.L., In re (2009) 163n12
ecological model 167
Eddings v. Oklahoma (1982) 23
Edelman, Marian Wright 312
Eighth Amendment 23, 24, 25–26
Eisen, M. L. 89
Elischberger, H. B. 75
Elmi, M. 91
El Salvador 169
emotions: and adolescent brain development 16, 17; assessment of out-of-home care children 142–143; emotional damages 183; emotional dysregulation of children after separation 284–285; and memorability 59, 60, 62–64; negative 63, 86; support animals 96; and testifying on children 91
encoding context 62; knowledge and understanding 62; stress and emotions 62–64
environment, child-friendly 133
episodic memory 55, 198, 208
Erard, Robert E. 152
Erikson, Erik 24, 192
Esplin, P. W. 205
ethical issues of forensic practitioners 327
Ethical Principles of Psychologists and Code of Conduct (EPPCC) 304, 317, 318, 327
Evaluating Juvenile's Adjudicative Competence 303
event memory 58–60
experience of forensic practitioners, impact of 320
expert witness: *Daubert* standard 158–159; mental health 182, 183–184, 188, 193; qualifications 159–160, 163n12; selection of 158–159; testimony 153, 156–157; testimony, admission of 160–162; testimony by practitioners providing therapeutic services 323
exposure to intimate partner violence 232
expressed interest of the child 14, 48
externalizing behaviors of victimized children 86, 141
eyewitness testimony 88, 90, 98

Fair Housing Act 183
fairness 318–319, 331
false allegations of child sexual abuse 196, 216

false confessions 34–35

family court 3, 121, 224, 241, 277; assessment of children 115–116, 119; best interest of the child 115, 118, 122; child sexual abuse allegations in 197; *see also* child custody; non-traditional families, children in

family history 266, 272, 301, 304

family reunification programs 147

Faust, David 182

Fawcett, H. 99

Federal Bureau of Investigation (FBI) 12

Federal Rules of Evidence: Rule 601 93; Rule 702 158

fees of forensic practitioners 324

felony murder rule, prohibition of 33

Fifth Amendment 23, 27

fitness hearings *see* amenability hearings

Fivush, Robyn 58, 64

Floyd, George 1

Flynn, James 302

Flynn effect 302

Fong, Mei 130

Fontes, L. A. 208

forensic assessment 116–118; appreciation of individual differences 330; documentation and compilation of data 330–331; feedback 330; focus on legally relevant factors 329; procedures 329–330; provision of documentation 331; recordkeeping 331; settings 330

Forensic Evaluation Outline Form 299

forensic practitioners 317; *see also* Specialty Guidelines for Forensic Psychology

forensic psychology 316

forensic therapeutic services, provision of 323

Fortas, Abe 19–21, 35

foster-adopt home 144–145

foster care *see* out-of-home care

Foster Child's Bill of Rights 163n8

Fox, James 46

Fraser, Aaron 84

Freud, Anna 237

Freud, Sigmund 236

Freyd, J. J. 196

Friedrich v. Friedrich (1996) 262

frontal lobe 16, 17

functional magnetic resonance imaging (fMRI) 15

Gang Prevention, Intervention and Suppression Act 14

gangs 12–13, 14, 169, 172

Garb, H. N. 186

Gardner, Richard 277

Gartrell, Nanette 242

Gault, Gerald "Jerry" 21

Gault, In re (1967) 10, 20–21, 22, 26, 35, 44

Gelles, Richard 130

gender identity, and parenting 238–239, 251, 252–253

gender non-conforming children 253–255

genetics 241, 244, 249

gestational surrogacy 248–249

get tough era of juvenile justice 12, 13, 14, 24

Giannaris v. Giannaris (2007) 163n13

Gideon v. Wainwright (1963) 19

Ginsburg, Ruth Bader 261

Gitter v. Gitter (2005) 261

Goldfarb, D. 3, 66

Goodman, G. S. 66

Gordon, B. N. 64

Gould, J. W. 283

Graham, Terrence 25–26, 27

Graham v. Florida (2010) 25–26

Grano v. Martin (2020) 261

"grave risk of harm" exception 257, 260, 263–264

gray matter 16

Greenberg, Stuart A. 116

Greenhoot, A. F. 69, 74

grooming behaviors of sexual offenders 191, 213

Grotberg, E. 175

guardian ad litem (GAL) 13, 132; best-interest advocacy model 312–313, *313*; impact on lives of children 314–315; origin of 311–312; volunteers 314

Guatemala 168, 169

Gudjonsson, G. H. 74

Gudjonsson Suggestibility Scale 2 (GSS 2) 74

habitual residence 261–262

Hague Convention cases 116, 257–259; acclimatization of children 257, 261–262, 268; acquiescence 262–263; case illustrations 265–274; consent 262–263, 268, 272; custody proceedings 260–261; exercise of parental rights 262; "grave risk of harm" exception 257, 263–264; habitual residence 261–262; involvement of mental health professionals 264–265; jurisdictional issues 258; legal issues 259–264; objections and preferences of child 270, 271; parental influence 263, 266, 268, 271; settlement in new environment 264, 265–267; sufficient age and maturity defense 257, 263, 264, 265, 269–271, 272; voices of children 259, 275

Hahm, H. C. 86

Haim, Bonnie 84

Harlan, John Marshall 22

Hass, Giselle 6, 116, 206, 257

Hébert, M. 91

Heilbrun, K. 118, 121

helpless caregiving 228

Hershkowitz, I. 205

high conflict divorce 277

hippocampus 16, 63

historic child sexual abuse 90

HLA typing 244

Hoffman, K. 152

Honduras 169
House of Refuge 9
Hulette, A. C. 87
Hunt, James B. 47, 48
hyperarousal 143

identity: of adolescents 192; gender identity
238–239, 251, 252–253; of immigrant children
174; and out-of-home care 139–140
illegitimate children 237–238, 241
Illinois Juvenile Court Act of 1899 10
Imhoff, M. C. 75
immigrant children 164–165; case example
176–177; current socio-political state for 165;
ecological model 167; immigration journey
and resettlement 173–174; intersectional theory 167; in legal system 165–166; motivations
for and impact of migration 167–170; participation of 167; pre-immigration development/
risks 170–173; traumatic stress reactions of
174–175; venues and roles 166–167; vulnerability and resilience in 175–176
immigration courts 116, 166, 257
impartiality 318–319
incidental memory 56
Independent Living Skills Programs 148
Independent Medical Examination (IME) 188,
194n4
Individuals with Disabilities Education Act 49
infantile amnesia 59
information: access to 328; collateral sources
118, 265, 283, 284, 290, 326, 328; multiple
sources of 328; release of 328; seeking, and
recall performance 72–73; sources, disclosing
332; third party 328
informed consent 114, 280, 297, 325, 326
initial disclosure 68
integrity of forensic practitioners 318
intellectual disability (ID) 295, 296, 300, 301,
305–306
intelligence tests 185, 299, 302
internalizing behaviors of victimized children
86
internal working models (IWMs) 73
International Child Abduction Remedies Act
(ICARA) 259
interparental violence 85–86
interpreters 208
intersectional theory 167
intervening experiences, effects on memory
64–65
interview(s) 70–72, 113–114, 119; areas of assessment 120; child custody evaluations 282, 283,
286, 289, 290; contamination of 199; evaluation of psychological injuries 184; Hague
Convention cases 265; interviewer bias 71–72,
202, 203; interviewer support during retrieval
69–70; juvenile homicide cases 304–305; with
parents 120; practices, child sexual abuse

cases 198–199; protocols 75, 88, 113, 119, 198,
210; repeated, impact on memory 204; suggestive 60–61, 71–72, 204; techniques 203; use
of dolls and drawings in 71, 198; videotaped
119, 202
intimate partner violence (IPV) 86, 224; and
best interest of the child 226; case examples 230–232; and child abuse 233; coercive
control 227–228, 230–231; defensive or
reactive violence 229–230; driven by conflict 228–229; DVCC-R protocol 339–359;
exposure *vs.* victimization 232; involvement
of children in 230; and legal issues 225–226;
and mental health professionals 224–225; and
post-traumatic stress disorder 87; prevalence
of 224; and psychological issues 226–230;
separation-instigated violence 229; violence
stemming from mental illness 229, 232

Jackson, Kuntrell 26
Jaffe, P. G. 233
jail removal 11
Jardim, G. B. G. 86
Jason P. v. Danielle S. (2017) 245–246
J.D.B. v. North Carolina (2011) 27, 28, 34–35
Johnson, M. K. 200
Johnson v. Calvert (1993) 248
Johnston, J. R. 233
jurisdictional issues in Hague Convention cases
258
jurisdiction hearing 131
Jurney, Alicia 5, 120, 153
jury(ies): juror perceptions of child testimony
98–99; jury trials for child custody 3; juvenile-specific pattern jury instructions 35; teen
courts 47
Juvenile Adjudicative Competence Interview
(JACI) 208, 299, 303, 304–305
Juvenile Code, North Carolina 47–48, 49
Juvenile Court of Allegheny County 10
juvenile courts 43–44, 130; adjudication 15, 21,
22, 23, 38, 47; assessment of children 114–115;
bifurcated structure of 38–39; convening
power of judges 50; disposition stage 38; as
dumping ground 43, 48; language/vocabulary
of 15, 44; parental attendance in 48; reforms
31–38; rise of 10; social work nature of 44;
teen courts 46–47; undisciplined cases 44–45;
and youth of color 51
Juvenile Delinquency and Prevention Control
Act (1968) 11
Juvenile Detention Alternatives Initiative 37
juvenile homicide 6; and adolescent developmental characteristics 307–308; assessment findings 301–306; assessment process
298–300; behavioral and social/emotional
measures 303; behavioral observations 298;
case introduction/critical elements 295;
competency to stand trial 303–304, 305–307;

data collection 119, 298–300; framework for instant offense 296–297; intelligence and achievement measures 302–303; interviews 304–305; legal proceedings 306–307; relevant case background history 301–302
Juvenile Justice and Delinquency Prevention Act of 1974 (JJDP) 11, 12, 14
Juvenile Justice Reinvestment Act, North Carolina 36
juvenile justice system 3–4; alternatives to detention 35; attorney representation 13–14, 20; bifurcated juvenile court structure 38–39; and brain development 14, 15–19; broken windows policing theory 13; constitutional rights 10–11; court counselors 15; criminal cases, child sexual abuse allegations in 206–209; dependency cases, child sexual abuse allegations in 209–212; diversion from court system 36–38; early treatment of children 9; elimination of coercive interrogation techniques 33–35; elimination of transfer to adult courts without amenability hearing 32–33; federal legislation for protection of children 11; juvenile courts, rise of 10; juvenile-specific pattern jury instructions 35; minimum age of criminal responsibility, raising 31–32; prohibition of felony murder rule 33; punitive approach 46–48; racial and ethnic disparities 14, 50–51; raise the age legislation 28–30, 31; reforms needed in juvenile court 31–38; School Resource Officers 13; super predator 4, 12, 14, 24, 45–46; training schools 46, 47; twenty-first century juvenile law 14–15; and U.S. Constitution 19–28; youth gangs 12–13, 14
juvenile-specific pattern jury instructions 35

Kagan, Elena 27, 32
Kennedy, Anthony 31
Kent, Morris 20
Kent v. United States (1966) 10, 19–20, 30
Khalip v. Khalip (2011) 263
Kids' Court School (KCS) 94
"Kids for Cash" scandal 22
knowledge of events: impact on retrieval 68–69; and memorability 60, 61, 62
knowledge of forensic practitioners: legal system 320; scientific foundation for opinions and testimony 320; scientific foundation for teaching/research 320
Kohlberg, Lawrence 24
Kuehnle, K. 233

Lamb, M. E. 76, 204, 205, 208
language: abilities, and recall 75–76; abilities, and suggestibility 200; barriers, Hague Convention case interviews 265; child-friendly, in courts 133; differences, effect on interviews 208; of vocabulary 15, 44

Lauren P., In re (2004) 163n12
Lee, S. 72–73
Lee, S. Margaret 1, 6, 120, 297
legal knowledge of children 94
legal parentage, recognition of 238
legal rights of individuals 320
Lench, H. C. 70
Levy, Amy 6, 113, 120, 121, 282
Lewis, C. N. 76
life without the opportunity for parole (LWOP) 25–27
Lilienfeld, S. O. 186
limbic system 17
Lindsay, D. S. 200–201
Lindsey, Ben 10
live link testimony 97
Locklair, B. 118
Lozano v. Alvarez (2014) 264
Lyon, A. 66
Lyon, T. D. 56

McKeiver v. Pennsylvania (1971) 22–23, 38
magnet resonance imaging (MRI) 14, 16, 17
major depressive disorder (MDD) *see* depression
malingering 300
mandatory sentencing schemes 26–27
mandatory transfer schemes 27, 32
Marriage of Buzzanca, In re (1998) 248–249
Marriage of Moschetta, In re (1994) 249
Martin, R. P. 73
Martindale, D. A. 283
Marvin, R. 152
maximum age of juvenile court jurisdiction 50
mediation 37
Melnyk, L. 74, 200
Melton, G. B. 121, 297
memory of children 4–5, 76–77; age-related changes in 58–60; and approach to coping 72–73; and attachment 73; and child sexual abuse cases 199–200; and context specificity 60–61; delay interval 64–67; effect of trauma on 88–90; encoding context 62–64; impact of repeated interviews on 204; and language abilities 75–76; in legal proceedings 55–57; retrieval context 67–72; and suggestibility 74–75, 88; and temperament 73–74; *see also* testimony
memory system, basic operation of 57–58
Mendez v. State 55, 56
Mendoza, John F. 312
mental health: effect on brain development 18; IPV stemming from mental illness 229, 232; maternal 171; mentally handicapped adults, culpability of 25; provision of emergency mental health services to forensic examinees 324; services, privatization of 49; and testimony 91

mental health professionals (MHP) 114, 115,
119, 164–165; as expert witness 182, 183–184,
188, 193; and Hague Convention cases
264–265; and IPV cases 224–225; and same-
sex couples 242–243; as therapist 225
Mercer, Barbara 5, 114
Merritt, K. A. 63, 73
methods/procedures of forensic practitioners
328
#MeToo movement 191–192
Mexico 168
Meyers, Gregory J. 121
Michael H. v. Gerald D. (1989) 238
Michigan, best interest of the child list of 226
Mihura, Joni L. 121, 186
Miller, Evan 26, 32
Miller v. Alabama (2012) 25, 26, 27, 32–33, 115
Millon Clinical Multiaxial Inventory (MCMI)
121
minimum age of criminal responsibility, raising
31–32
Minnesota Multiphasic Personality Inventory-2
(MMPI-2) 185, 191; Adolescent-Restructured
Form (MMPIA-RF) 185; Adolescent Version
(MMPI-2-A) 121, 185; Restructured Form
(MMPI-2-RF) 185
Miranda Rights 27–28, 206, 207
Miranda Rights Comprehension Instrument
(MRCI) 207
Miranda v. Arizona (1966) 21, 27
Misdemeanor Diversion Program (MDP)
50
mock trial participation 94
Models for Change: Juvenile Diversion
Guidebook 37
Monasky v. Taglieri (2020) 261–262
Montgomery v Louisiana (2016) 115
Morey, Marcia 4, 36
Moses 129
mothers, and attachment 237
Mozes v. Mozes (2001) 261
multi-modal assessment 119, 283
multiple relationships of forensic practitioners
322–323
myelination 16, 17
Myers, John E. B. 129

Nagel, A. G. 308
narrative coherence 59, 75–76
narrative practice 76, 120, 198, 210
Nathanson, R. 95
National Advisory Commission on Criminal
Justice Standards and Goals 13
National Association of School Resource
Officers 13
National CASA/GAL Association for Children
311–312, 315
National Child Abuse and Neglect Data
Systems 196

National Collegiate Athletic Association
(NCAA) 43
National Council of Juvenile and Family Court
Judges (NCJFCJ) 312
National Gang Center 14
National Institute of Child Health and Human
Development (NICHD) 119, 120, 198, 210
National Juvenile Justice Network 38
National Youth Gang Center (NYGC) 12–13,
14
negative emotions: and internalizing behaviors
86; and memorability 63
negativity bias 63
neurotransmitters 17–18
neutrality in forensic evaluations 117
New Deal 130
New York Society for the Prevention of Cruelty
to Children 112
Nezworski, M. T. 186
Nicaragua 169
non-traditional families, children in 5, 235;
assisted reproductive technologies 235, 244,
252; cases 239–241; cultural competence
251–252; gender non-conforming children
253–255; historical views and social science
research 236–237; legal outgrowths from
cultural shifts 237–241; same-sex couples 235,
241, 242–243; sperm donation cases 244–248;
surrogacy cases 248–251; transgender parents
252–253
norepinephrine 17
norm obsolescence 302
North Carolina General Assembly 46, 49

oath, testimonial 92–94
Obama, Barack 165
O'Donohue, W. T. 196
Office of Children's Issues 259
Office of Juvenile Justice and Delinquency
Prevention (OJJDP) 11, 12, 14; juvenile
delinquency prevention efforts 36–37; Model
Programs Guide 37–38; Restorative Justice
Working Group 37
Olesen, Nancy 6
open-ended questions 59, 60, 63, 65, 77, 88, 187
opinions of forensic practitioners: comprehensive and accurate presentation of 332;
disclosing sources of information and bases
of 332; knowledge of scientific foundation for
320; regarding persons not examined 328–329
Orbach, Y. 205
organizational demands, conflicts with 327
Ornstein, P. A. 63, 64, 75, 188, 200
orphanages 112
out of court statements 332
out-of-home care 127–128; case study
140–147; child advocacy 132, 134–135;
child-responsive courts 133–134; and
danger 137–139, 143; long-term foster

placement and therapy 144–145; parental rights and adoption 145–147; population, current scope of 128–129; programs for child participation 134–135; psychological assessment 136–137, 141–144; racial and socioeconomic disproportionality 135–136; representation for children 132, 134; separation and identity 139–140; therapeutic assessment 142; time frames for juvenile dependency process 131–132; and trauma 136–139; and well-being of children 147–148

Padilla v. Troxell (2017) 262
parens patriae, doctrine of 9, 10, 15, 19, 20
parental alienation syndrome 277
parental rights: and adoption 128, 146, 153; in Hague Convention cases 262; and surrogacy 250, 251
parenting coordinator (PC) 292–293
parenting plan 293
Parenting Stress Index (PSI) 121, 283
Parenting Stress Index, 4th Edition (PSI-4) 286
parent(s): alienating behaviors of 277, 278, 281, 284; attendance in courts 48; behavioral checklists 121; foster 141–142, 145–147; influence, Hague Convention cases 263, 266, 268, 271; meaning of 238, 241; parent–child conversations, effects on memory 65–66; parent–child relationship 116, 120–121, 171, 236–237, 238; polyamorous families 242, 243, 244, 255n3; psychological assessment of 228; psychological parent 237; separation, emotional dysregulation of children after 284–285; transgender parents, children of 252–253; *see also* divorce; intimate partner violence (IPV); non-traditional families, children in
peer pressure 17
Penry v. Lynaugh (1989) 25
performance-based tests, psychological testing 185–187
permanency planning 132, 154, 156
personal beliefs of forensic practitioners, impact of 320
personal injury 182–183; *see also* civil cases
Personality Assessment Inventory (PAI) 185, 283, 290
Personality Assessment Inventory – Adolescent (PAI-A) 121, 185
personality disorders 31
Peterson, C. 59, 63
physician density in Central America 171
PINS (Person in Need of Services) *see* undisciplined cases
plasticity 18
play activities 138, 142, 143–144, 145
plea bargaining 45
polyamorous families 242, 243, 244, 255n3
Poole, D. A. 71

post-traumatic play 143
post-traumatic stress disorder (PTSD) 87, 147, 188, 215
poverty 18, 136, 171
Powell, B. 152
pre-immigration development/risks for immigrant children: early childhood 171–172; late childhood and adolescence 172–173; middle childhood 172; prenatal and infancy periods 170–171
preponderance of evidence 2, 3, 22, 119, 131, 197, 262
President's Commission of Law Enforcement and Justice (1967) 11
pre-trial anxiety 94–95
pre-trial detention of juveniles 24
pre-trial preparation 94–95
Price, H. 99
Principe, G. F. 64, 65
privacy 327–328
privatization of mental health services 49
pro bono services by forensic practitioners 324
procedural protections/safeguards 10, 12, 15, 20, 22, 27
procedural rights 23, 114
props, use in interviews 71
protective supervision 44–45
psychological assessment 215; of adolescents 190–191; child custody cases 283, 285, 289–290; evaluation of psychological injuries 184–187; Hague Convention cases 266–267, 268; of immigrant children 177; and intimate partner violence 228, 229, 231; juvenile homicide cases 298, 299–300; of out-of-home care children 136–137, 141–144
psychological injuries 183–187
psychological parent 237
psychopathology 86–88, 89, 192, 308
psychosis 299, 303, 306
psychosocial maturity 115
psychotherapy 166
"purpose of juvenile court" clauses 15

Quas, J. A. 66, 70, 91, 98

race: and adoption 145–146; disparities, in juvenile justice system 14, 50–51; and out-of-home dependency 128–129, 135–136; and undisciplined proceedings 45
raise the age effect 30
raise the age legislation 4, 28–30, 31
rapport building in child sexual abuse interviews 198
Rathore, Z. 175
reactive attachment disorder 147
reactive violence 229–230
realistic estrangement 278
"reasonable person" adult standard 28
rebuttable presumption 225–226

recantation 119, 210, 211–212
recidivism 29–30, 36, 216
records 298–299; access to 328; evaluation of psychological injuries 184; recordkeeping 331
recovery agents 258
Redmond v. Redmond (2013) 261
referral questions 118, 226, 277, 281, 297
reform schools 9, 10, 22
relationship, forensic practitioner-client 322; multiple relationships 322–323; provision of emergency mental health services to forensic examinees 324; responsibilities to retaining parties 322
report writing by evaluators 122, 283–284
research, forensic practitioners: contexts, communication in 326; knowledge of scientific foundation for 320
re-sentencing, juvenile 23, 115
resilience in immigrant children 175–176
resist/refuse dynamics 6, 230, 271, 278, 284, 292
responsibilities of forensic practitioners 318–319
responsiveness of forensic practitioners 321
restorative justice 37
restrictive gatekeeping 278
retention interval 56
retrieval context 67–68; impact of knowledge/ understanding 68–69; initial disclosure 68; interviews and interviewer bias 70–72; stress/ interviewer support 69–70
reunification: family reunification programs 147; of immigrant children 174; plan 128, 130, 131
reward system of brain 18
Reyes, Matias 12
right against self-incrimination 15, 21, 27
right to confrontation 96
right to counsel 19, 21–22, 26
right to remain silent by non-cooperation 23
right to trial by jury 22–23
risk-need-responsivity theory 115
Robb v. Robb (2004) 163n12
Robinson-Confer, Idelia 311
role confusion in adolescence 192
Roper v. Simmons (2005) 23, 24–25, 27, 31, 307–308
Rorschach Comprehensive System (CS) 185, 186
Rorschach inkblot test 121, 185, 283, 288, 290
Rorschach Performance Assessment System (R-PAS) 185–186, 191
Roseby, V. 233
Ross, M. 68–69

Safety House, The 134
Safety Organization Practice 134
same-sex couples 235, 241, 242–243
Saywitz, K. 95
scared straight programs 18, 35
Schall v. Martin (1984) 24

schizophrenia 118, 303
School-Justice Partnership (SJP) 36
School Resource Officers (SRO) 13
school-to-prison pipeline 4, 13, 36, 48
self-report psychological testing 184–185, 191, 283
semantic memory 55–56
sentencing: of juveniles 23, 24; mandatory sentencing schemes 26–27; re-sentencing, juvenile 23, 115
separation-instigated violence 229
serotonin 18
sexual abuse *see* child sexual abuse
Seymour, Brent 6
Shaver, Phillip 152
Shear, Leslie E. 274
Shuman, Daniel 116
Sieglein v. Schmidt (2016) 247
sight and sound separation 11
Simmons, Christopher 24
Simpson, O. J. 230
Singer, Jaqueline 6, 114, 282
Sixth Amendment 22
Smith, Colby 26
Smith v. Smith (2007) 253–254
Sneed v. Sneed (2018) 163n12
Social Security Act 130
Social Security Entitlement Act (1961) 131
socioeconomic status (SES) 135–136, 211
Sotomayor, Sonia 34–35
Soukup, David W. 311–312
source monitoring in child sexual abuse cases 200–201, 204, 205
Special Immigrant Juveniles Status (SIJS) 168
Specialty Guidelines for Forensic Psychologists 117, 316
Specialty Guidelines for Forensic Psychology 316–318; assessment 329–331; background and revision process 336; competence 319–321; conflicts in practice 326–327; definitions and terminology 337–338; diligence 321–322; fees 324; informed consent, notification, and assent 324–326; methods and procedures 328–329; privacy, confidentiality, and privilege 327–328; professional and public communications 331–332; relationships 322–324; responsibilities 318–319
specific learning disability (SLD) 301
sperm donation 244–248
Spousal Assault Risk Assessment Guide (SARA) 290
standard error of measurement (SEM) 302
Stanford v. Kentucky (1989) 25
Stansell, Mary 50, 296
status offenders 11
status offenses 44–45
statutory exclusion 32
Stevens, John Paul 24
Stolzenberg, S. N. 56

storytelling 137, 138, 139
stress 18, 72; effect on recall 60, 61, 62–64; at retrieval 69–70; and testimony 91, 92; toxic stress 171–172, 175; traumatic stress reactions of immigrant children 174–175
stress inoculation training 94
Stutman, S. 175
substance abuse 158, 229
sufficient age and maturity, defense of 257, 263, 264, 265, 269–271, 272
Sugarman, S. D. 182–183
suggestibility: and child sexual abuse cases 201, 204; definition of 200; and recall 74–75, 88; and repeated questioning 204
suggestive interviews 60–61, 71–72, 204
suicidal attempts: and depression 87; of immigrant children 177; of transgender youth 253; of victimized children 86–87
super predator 4, 12, 14, 24, 45–46
Supplemental Nutrition Assistance Program (SNAP) 136
support animals for child witnesses 96, 97
supportive interviews 67, 69–70, 76, 198
support persons for child witnesses 95–96, 97
surrogacy 248; gestational 248–249; traditional 248, 249–251
suspension from schools 49
synaptic pruning 16

teaching, forensic practitioners in 320, 328
teen courts 46–47
temperament, and recall performance 73–74
Temperament Assessment Battery for Children 73
tender years doctrine 236
termination of services by forensic practitioners 322
Teske, Steven 36, 37
testimony 5, 55, 84, 90–91, 100, 116; accommodations for child witnesses 92–98; adults' abilities to recall childhood trauma experiences 88–90; closed-circuit television/live link 97, 98; dependency cases 134; developmentally appropriate competence assessment and oath 92–94; and forensic evaluation 122–123; impact of testifying on children 91–92; juror perceptions of 98–99; knowledge of scientific foundation for 320; pre-trial preparation 94–95; support animals 96, 97; support persons 95–96, 97; temporal details of abuse 98–99; timing of 90; truncation of 96; victims *vs.* bystanders, child witness as 99; videotaped 96–97, 98; *see also* expert witness; memory of children
theory of mind 237
therapeutic assessment 142
therapeutic-forensic role conflicts 323
third party information, acquiring 328
Thoennes, N. 216

Thomas, Taylor E. 188, 200
Thompson v. Oklahoma (1988) 24, 25
Three Houses Tool 134
timelines, data organization 121–122
Title IV-(E) Act (1980) 131
Tjaden, P. G. 216
tort litigation 183
toxic stress 171–172, 175
traditional parenting style, and suggestibility 74–75
traditional surrogacy 248, 249–251
training schools 46, 47
Trajan 129
transfer hearings 32–33
transferred intent 33
transgender parents, children of 252–253
Transitional Age Youth Programs (TAYS) 148
trauma 5–6, 113, 314; and adolescence 188, 190–191; adults' abilities to recall childhood trauma experiences 89–90; and asylum seekers 116; and attachment disruptions 157, 162; childhood trauma rates in United States 85–86; and coercive control 228; effect on brain development 18; effect on memory 88–90; of immigrant children 173, 174–175; of out-of-home care children 136–139, 141–144; post-traumatic play 143; potential psychopathologies in victimized children 86–88; psychological impacts of victimization 86; of relocated children 270; responses, child sexual abuse 199
Trauma Symptom Inventory – 2 191
Trocmé, N. 216
Trump, Donald 165
T-visas 168

U.N. Convention on the Rights of the Child (UNCRC) 133, 177
understanding of events: impact on retrieval 68–69; and memorability 60, 62, 66
undisciplined cases 44–45
Uniform Parentage Act (UPA) 238, 246
United Nations Convention on the Rights of Children (UNCRC) 164, 259
U.N. Office on Drugs and Crime, (UNODC) 169
U.S. Constitution 15; Eighth Amendment 23, 24, 25–26; Fifth Amendment 23, 27; rights of children 10–11, 19–28; Sixth Amendment 22
U-visas 168

"Valid Court Order" exception, JJDP 11
validity scales, self-report psychological tests with 185
Van der Kolk, Bessel 137, 147
Vermont, raise the age legislation in 29
victim advocates 95
victimization: direct 85; indirect 85–86; psychological impacts of 86; *vs.* exposure, intimate partner violence 232

videotaped interviews 119, 202
videotaped testimony 96–97, 98
Violence Against Women Act (VAWA) immigration 168
Virginia, assisted conception statute of 245, 246
voluntary parent–child separations 236

Wald, Deborah 5
Walsh v. Walsh (2000) 264
weapon focus effect 64
Wechsler Abbreviated Scale of Intelligence (WASI) 283, 288
Wechsler Adult Intelligence Scale, Fourth Edition (WAIS-4) 299
Wechsler Intelligence Scale for Children – Fifth Edition (WISC-V) 269
Wechsler Intelligence Scale for Children – Fourth Edition (WISC-IV) 266, 268, 272
West, Jessica L. 120
Wheeler v. United States (1895) 93
white matter 16

Wide Range Achievement Test, Fourth Edition (WRAT-4) 299, 302
Williams, L. M. 196
Willis, B. 196
Wilson, Mary C. 4
Winship, In re (1970) 22
Winstanley, K. 99
Wood, J. M. 186
World Health Organization (WHO) 196

Yerkes-Dodson law 64
Youth Advocacy Program (YAP), West Coast Children's Clinic 148
youth gangs 12–13, 14
youth of color 14, 51

zero tolerance policies: and juvenile justice 13, 14; related to immigration 165; in schools 48–49, 304
Zimbardo, Philip 13
Ziskin, Jay 182